CLINICAL LABORATORY TESTS

VALUES AND IMPLICATIONS

SECOND EDITION

CLINICAL LABORATORY TESTS

VALUES AND IMPLICATIONS

SECOND EDITION

Springhouse Corporation
Springhouse, Pennsylvania

Staff

Senior Publisher
Minnie B. Rose, RN, BSN, MEd

Art Director
John Hubbard

Editors
Neal Fandek, David Moreau, Karyn C. Newell, Art Ofner

Copy Editors
Diane M. Armento, Kathryn A. Marino, Christina P. Ponczek, Pamela Wingrod

Designers
Stephanie Peters (associate art director), Kaaren Mitchel

Manufacturing
Deborah Meiris (director), T.A. Landis

Production Coordinator
Margaret A. Rastiello

The clinical procedures described and recommended in this publication are based on research and consultation with nursing, medical, and legal authorities. To the best of our knowledge, these procedures reflect currently accepted practice; nevertheless, they can't be considered absolute and universal recommendations. For individual application, all recommendations must be considered in light of the patient's clinical condition and, before administration of new or infrequently used drugs, in light of latest package-insert information. The contributors and the publisher disclaim responsibility for any adverse effects resulting directly or indirectly from the suggested procedures, from any undetected errors, or from the reader's misunderstanding of the text.

For those organizations that have been granted a photocopy license by CCC, a separate system of payment has been arranged. The fee code for users of the Transactional Reporting Service is 0874347963/95 $00.00 + .75.

Printed in the United States of America. For information, write Springhouse Corporation, 1111 Bethlehem Pike, P.O. Box 908, Springhouse, PA 19477-0908.

CLT2-010295

$\mathcal{R}$ A member of the Reed Elsevier plc group

Library of Congress Cataloging-in-Publication Data
Clinical laboratory tests: values and implications. — 2nd
    ed.
    p. cm.
    1. Diagnosis, Laboratory — Handbooks, manuals, etc.
2. Reference values (Medicine) — Handbooks, manuals,
etc. 3. Nursing — Handbooks, manuals, etc. I.
Springhouse Corporation.
[DNLM: 1. Diagnosis, Laboratory — handbooks. QY 39
    C6415 1995]
RB38.2.C56 1995
616.07'5 — dc20
DNLM/DLC   94-41011
ISBN 0-87434-796-3   CIP

Contents

Contributors

Catherine P.M. Hayward, MD, FRCP
Director of Regional Coagulation Laboratory
Chedoke-McMaster Hospitals, McMaster University Medical
 Center
Hamilton, Ontario, Canada

George M. Lawson, PhD, DABCC
Director, Drug Laboratory
Mayo Clinic
Rochester, MN

Paula J. Santrach, MD
Co-Director, Hospital Clinical Laboratories
Mayo Clinic
Rochester, MN

**Special thanks to the following, who served as
contributors for the first edition:**

Lolita M. Adrien, RN, MS, ET
Bonnie L. Anderson, MD
G. David Ball, PhD
Wendy L. Baker, RN, BSN, MS
Carol K. Barker, RN, MSN, MEd
Deborah M. Berkowitz, RN, MSN, FNP
Barbara Gross Braverman, RN, MSN, DS
Debra C. Broadwell, RN, PhD, ET
Frank Lowell Brown, CUT
Mary Buritt, PhD
Judith Byrne, BS, MT(ASCP)
Ricardo L. Camponovo, MD
Donald C. Cannon, MD, PhD
Raynell J. Clark, BA, MT
Deborah L. Dalrymple, RN, MSN
Gordon DeWald, PhD
William M. Dougherty, BS
Mahmoud A. ElSohly, PhD
John J. Fenton, PhD, DABcc, FNACB
Sr. Rebecca Fidler, MT(ASCP), PhD
Katherine L. Fulton, RN
Shirley Given, HTR(ASCP)
Thad C. Hagen, MD
Patrice M. Harman, RN
Annette L. Harmon, RN, MSN
Lenora R. Haston, RN, MSN
Kathy A. Hausman, RN, MS, CNRN
Tobie Virginia Hittle, RN, BSN, CCRN
Henry A. Homburger, MD
Richard Edward Honigman, MD

Jerry A. Katzmann, PhD
Alicia Beth Kavka, MD
Susan A. Kayes, BS, MT(ASCP)
Sr. Mary Brian Kelber, RN, DNS
Sherry L. Keramidas, PhD
Catherine E. Kirby, RN, BSN
George Klee, MD, PhD
William E. Kline, MS, MT(ASCP), SBB
Jeananne Krejci, RN, BA
Clarke Lambe, MD
Laurel Kareus Lambe, MS, RD
George Lawson, PhD
Dennis E. Leavelle, MD
Vanda A. Lennon, MD, PhD
Claire B. Mailhot, RN, MS
Elizabeth Anne Mallon, BS, MT(ASCP)
Harry G. McCoy, PharmD
Marylou K. McHugh, RN, EdD
Joan C. McManus, RN, MA
Malinda S. Mitchell, RN, MS
S. Breanndan Moore, MD, DCH, FCAP
Susan F. Morrow, RN
John O'Brien, PhD
Whyte G. Owen, PhD
Lynda Palmer, RN, BSN
Deborah S. Parziale, RN, MS
Dale Rabe, MLT(ASCP)
Frank C. Riggall, MD
Carolyn Robertson, RN, MSN
Suzanne G. Rotzell, RN, BSN
Janice Selekman, RN, MSN, DNSc
Ellen Shipes, RN, MN, MEd, ET
Thomas F. Smith, PhD
Mary C. Smolenski, MSN, RN,C, ARNP
Barbara L. Solomon, RN, DNSc, CCNS
Harvey Spector, MD
Howard F. Taswell, MD
Barry L. Tonkonow, MD
Ronald J. Wapner, MD
Beverly A. Zenk Wheat, RN, MA
Elaine Gilligan Whelan, RN, MSN, MA.

Clinical consultants

Gordon W. DeWald, PhD
Chairman, Division of Laboratory Genetics
Mayo Clinic
Rochester, MN

Catherine P.M. Hayward, BSc, MD, FRCP
Director of Regional Coagulation Laboratory
Chedoke-McMaster Hospitals, McMaster University Medical
 Center
Hamilton, Ontario, Canada

George M. Lawson, PhD, DABCC
Director, Drug Laboratory
Mayo Clinic
Rochester, MN

Douglas W. MacPherson, MD, MSC, FRCPC
Head, Parasitology Laboratory
St. Joseph's Hospital
Ontario, Canada

Mary Meihofer, MD, MS, MT (ASCP), SBB
Pathologist, Director Medical Technology Consortium
Mercy Hospital Systems
Scranton, PA

Gary M. Odera, PharmD, MPH
Professor and Chairman
University of Utah
Salt Lake City

John J. O'Shea, MD
Head, Leukocyte Cell Biology Section
National Cancer Institute
Frederick Cancer Research and Development Center
Frederick, MD

David L. Sawhill, MD
Director, Clinical Chemistry
Medical College of Pennsylvania

Paula J. Santrach, MD
Co-Director, Hospital Clinical Laboratories
Mayo Clinic
Rochester, MN

Chris Walker, MD
Laboratory Director
Chedoke-McMaster Hospitals
Hamilton, Ontario, Canada

Special thanks to the following, who served as consultants for the first edition:

Doris G. Bartuska, MD, FCAP
George J. Blake, RPh, MS
Marlene M. Ciranowicz, RN, MSN
Paul R. Finley, MD
John C. Hagarty, MD, FCAP
Dennis E. Leavelle, MD
Barbara McVan, RN
Linda Pacharzina Powers, MD
Harvey F. Watts, MD.

Foreword

Today's health care field finds itself in a paradoxical position. On the one hand, accelerated advances in basic sciences as well as in applied medical technology have resulted in the most sophisticated delivery of health care in history. Techniques for the diagnosis and treatment of infectious diseases, autoimmune disorders, malignant diseases, and a host of other pathological conditions are currently being applied not only to major body organs but even to the DNA nucleotides that comprise an individual gene. Some procedures that are now considered standard medical practice were not even conceived of 10 years ago.

On the other hand, the health care industry has never been more closely scrutinized because of escalating costs. At last estimate, the United States is devoting approximately 12% of its gross national product to health care. To a large extent, these two facets of health care are interdependent; development of more sophisticated technology will inevitably generate more expensive procedures. The challenge, as we look toward the next century, is to continue the assault on those refractory diseases which continue to extract a great toll on society, but do it in a manner that society can afford. To this end, it is incumbent on medical practitioners to select judiciously from among the plethora of diagnostic procedures currently available.

In the field of laboratory medicine, the growth of diagnostic tests has been especially rapid. Maintaining a knowledge base to select the appropriate test that will yield useful diagnostic information to supplement the clinical symptomology has become more demanding. *Clinical Laboratory Tests: Values and Implications, Second Edition* is a practical reference guide that serves to extend that knowledge base. It includes concise descriptions of more than 350 tests available in the clinical laboratory. The entries have been written by a diverse group of health care professionals who have expertise in a specific category of testing.

Each entry begins with a brief description of the test. *Purpose* lists the specific diagnostic indications for performing the test listed. *Patient preparation* includes specific instructions that must be given to the patient to ensure a valid result. *Procedure* describes the protocol for specimen collection, including the proper specimen container and any special handling requirements after the specimen has been collected. *Values* lists the normal test value or range of values, as well as those considered abnormal. *Implications of results* elaborates on the information provided under *Values* and summarizes the test results commonly observed in various pathophysiological states, thus providing pertinent interpretive information. *Post-test care* describes appropriate patient management resulting from the invasive process of specimen collection or subsequent testing that may be indicated by the original test result. *Interfering factors* lists the known factors that may interfere with the test and possibly yield specious results.

The book also includes additional features to further the reader's knowledge base. An introductory chapter describes proper techniques for collecting blood and urine samples. Informative tables and sidebars are scattered throughout the book to highlight key data. Two appendices offer quick-scan charts on critical laboratory values and a guide to common abbreviations. Selected references provide the reader with numerous suggestions for further research and review. Finally, a detailed index allows the reader to find any important topic quickly and easily.

Clinical Laboratory Tests: Values and Implications, Second Edition will thus serve as a valuable reference to assist in the appropriate selection and interpretation of laboratory tests at a time when the practice of efficient medicine is paramount. In addition, the practical information provided on patient preparation, sample collection, and potential interferences ensures that, if the procedures described herein are followed, valid diagnostic information will be obtained, thereby contributing to the quality of patient management, the ultimate concern of all health care professionals.

Collection techniques for blood and urine samples

Blood

The type of blood sample required for testing whole blood, plasma, or serum varies according to the test. Whole blood — containing all blood elements — is the sample of choice for most routine hematologic studies. For example, the complete blood count, erythrocyte sedimentation rate, reticulocyte and platelet counts, and the osmotic fragility test, all require a sample of whole blood.

Plasma is the liquid part of whole blood, which contains all the blood proteins; *serum,* the liquid that remains after whole blood clots. Plasma and serum samples, which contain most of the physiologically and clinically significant substances found in blood, are used for most biochemical, immunologic, and coagulation studies. They also provide useful electrolyte evaluation, enzyme analysis, glucose concentration, protein determination, and bilirubin level.

When collecting blood samples, be sure to use the proper techniques to avoid exposure to pathogens (see *Universal precautions,* page 2.)

Sample quantities and containers

Sample quantities needed for diagnostic studies depend on the laboratory, available equipment, and the type of test. Some laboratories, for example, use automated analyzer systems that require a serum sample of 100 µl or less; others use manual systems that require a larger sample. The desired sample quantity determines the collection procedure, and the type and size of the container. A single venipuncture with a conventional glass or disposable plastic syringe can provide 15 ml of blood — sufficient for many hematologic, immunologic, chemical, and coagulation tests, but hardly enough for a series of tests.

To avoid multiple venipunctures when tests require a large blood sample, use an evacuated tube system (Vacutainer, Corvac) with interchangeable glass tubes, optional draw capacities, and a selection of additives. Evacuated tubes are commercially prepared with or without additives (indicated by their color-coded stoppers) and with enough vacuum to draw a predetermined blood volume (2 to 20 ml per tube).

Microanalysis of minute amounts of capillary blood collected with micropipettes or glass capillary tubes allows numerous hematologic and routine laboratory studies on infants, children, and patients with severe burns or poor veins. Micropipettes are color-coded by sample capacity and hold 30 to 50 µl of whole blood; glass capillary tubes hold 80 to 130 µl of serum or plasma.

Equipment

The following equipment is commonly used for venipuncture: tourniquet, 70% alcohol or povidone-iodine solution, sterile syringes or evacuated tubes, sterile needle (20G or 21G for forearm; 25G for wrist, hand, or ankle, or for children), color-coded tubes containing appropri-

Universal precautions

In the late 1980s, the increased incidence of human immunodeficiency virus (HIV) infection led to the widespread use of "universal blood and body-fluid precautions," or simply "universal precautions." These precautions, which seek to protect medical personnel from exposure to HIV, hepatitis B, and other blood-borne diseases, are especially relevant for health care personnel who obtain or handle blood or other body-fluid specimens for laboratory testing. The Centers for Disease Control and Prevention and the Occupational Safety and Health Administration recommend following universal precautions during the routine care of all patients; this means treating *all* blood and body fluids as if they're infectious.

Use appropriate barrier precautions routinely to keep from exposing your skin or mucous membranes to patients' blood and body fluids. Use your judgment in deciding which types of barriers (gloves, gowns, masks, and protective eyewear) are needed for each clinical situation.

Recommended procedures

- Wear gloves when touching blood and body fluids, mucous membranes, or broken skin; when handling items or surfaces soiled with blood or related body fluids; and when performing vascular access procedures. Change your gloves between patients. Also, be sure to wear a gown and face and eye shields during procedures likely to generate droplets of blood or body fluids.

- Discard used surgical or examination gloves; don't wash or disinfect them for reuse. Washing with surfactants may enhance the penetration of liquids through undetected holes in the gloves. Disinfecting agents may cause deterioration. Use general-purpose utility gloves for cleaning instruments or other chores involving potential blood contact. You may decontaminate and reuse utility gloves, but discard gloves that are peeling, cracked, discolored, or torn, or that show any other evidence of deterioration.

- Wash any skin surfaces immediately and thoroughly if they're contaminated by blood or body fluids. Wash your hands immediately after removing your gloves.

- Take precautions to prevent injuries caused by needles and sharp instruments during procedures and when cleaning used instruments and disposing of used needles. To prevent needle-stick injuries, don't recap needles, bend or break them by hand, or remove them from disposable syringes. After use, place disposable syringes and needles and other sharp items in puncture-resistant containers for disposal. Keep containers nearby. Place large-bore, reusable needles in a puncture-resistant container for transport to the reprocessing area.

- You need not wear gloves when feeding patients and when wiping saliva from skin. However, consider minimizing the need for emergency mouth-to-mouth resuscitation by keeping mouthpieces, resuscitation bags, and other ventilation devices nearby.

- If you have exudative lesions or weeping dermatitis, don't give direct patient care or handle patient care equipment until the condition resolves.

- If you're pregnant, be especially familiar with precautions and follow them closely because of the risk of transferring infection to the fetus.

Guide to color-top collection tubes

Red

Red-top tubes contain no additives. Draw volume may be 2 to 20 ml. These tubes are used for tests performed on serum samples.

Lavender

Lavender-top tubes contain EDTA. Draw volume may be 2 to 10 ml. These tubes are used for tests performed on whole blood samples.

Green (heparinized)

Green-top tubes contain heparin (sodium, lithium, or ammonium). Draw volume may be 2 to 15 ml. These tubes are used for tests performed on plasma samples.

Blue

Blue-top tubes contain sodium citrate and citric acid. Draw volume may be 2.7 or 4.5 ml. These tubes are used for coagulation studies performed on plasma samples.

Black

Black-top tubes contain sodium oxalate. Draw volume may be 2.7 or 4.5 ml. These tubes are used for coagulation studies performed on plasma samples.

Yellow

Yellow-top tubes contain acid-citrate-dextrose (ACD) solution. Draw volume is 12 ml. These tubes are used for tests performed on whole blood samples.

Gray

Gray-top tubes contain a glycolytic inhibitor (such as sodium fluoride, powdered oxalate, or glycolytic/microbial inhibitor). Draw volume may be 3 to 10 ml. These tubes are used most often for glucose determinations in serum or plasma samples.

ate additives (see *Guide to color-top collection tubes,* above), labels for identification, 2″ × 2″ gauze pads, tape or adhesive bandage, iced specimen container, and labels for syringe and specimen bag to indicate patient's name and room number (if applicable), doctor's name, date, collection time, and details of oxygen therapy.

The following equipment is used to collect a specimen of capillary blood: sterile, disposable blood lancet; 2″ × 2″ gauze pads; 70% alcohol or povidone-iodine solution; glass slides; heparinized capillary tubes, or pipettes; appropriate solutions.

Venous sample

The nature of the test and the patient's age and condition determine the appropriate blood sample, collection site, and technique. Most tests require a sample of venous blood. Although a relatively simple procedure, venipuncture must be performed carefully to avoid hemolysis or hemoconcentration of the sample, to prevent hematoma formation, and to prevent damage to the patient's veins (see *Safeguards for venipuncture,* page 4).

Labeling. All specimen containers should be clearly marked with the patient's name and room number, physician's name, date, and collection time.

Safeguards for venipuncture

- Make sure the patient is adequately supported, in case syncope occurs.

- When using a syringe to draw a sample, avoid injecting air into a vein by checking that the plunger is fully depressed before injection.

- If possible, avoid drawing blood from an arm or leg used for I.V. infusion of blood, dextrose, or electrolyte solutions, because this dilutes the blood sample. If you must collect blood near an I.V. site, choose a location below it.

- For easier identification of veins in patients with tortuous or sclerosed veins, or with veins damaged by repeated venipuncture, antibiotic therapy, or chemotherapy, apply warm, wet compresses 15 minutes before attempting venipuncture.

- When you cannot find a vein quickly, release the tourniquet temporarily to avoid tissue necrosis and circulation problems.

- Be sure to insert the needle at the correct angle to reduce the risk of puncturing the opposite wall of the vein and causing a hematoma.

- Always release the tourniquet before withdrawing the needle, to prevent a hematoma. When drawing multiple samples, release the tourniquet within 1 minute after beginning to draw blood to prevent a hemoconcentrated sample.

Selecting a venipuncture site. The most common site of venipuncture is the antecubital fossa area; other sites include the wrist and dorsum of the hand or foot. When drawing the sample at bedside, instruct the patient to lie supine, with head slightly elevated and arms resting at his sides. When drawing blood from an ambulatory patient, have the patient sit in a chair, with his arm supported securely on an armrest or table.

Performing venipuncture

When using an evacuated tube, attach the needle to the holder before applying the tourniquet. Apply a soft rubber tourniquet above the puncture site to prevent venous blood return and to increase venous pressure: this makes the veins more prominent and increases the volume of blood at the puncture site. The tourniquet should be snug but not tight enough to constrict arteries. Using a tourniquet for a patient with large, distended, and highly visible veins increases the risk of hematoma. If the patient's veins appear distinct, you may not need to apply a tourniquet.

Instruct the patient to make a fist several times to further enlarge the veins. Select a vein by palpation and inspection. (If you can't feel a vein distinctly, *don't* attempt venipuncture.) Working in a circular motion from the center outward, clean the puncture site with alcohol or povidone-iodine solution, and dry it with a gauze pad. If you must touch the cleansed puncture site again to relocate the vein, palpate with an antiseptically clean finger, and wipe the area again with an alcohol swab.

Draw the skin tautly over the vein by pressing just below the puncture site with your thumb, to keep the vein from moving.

Hold the syringe or tube with the needle bevel up and the shaft parallel to the path of the vein at a 15-degree angle to the arm. Enter the vein with a single direct puncture of the skin and vein wall. If you use a syringe, venous blood will appear in the hub. Withdraw the blood slowly, gently pulling on the syringe to create steady suction until you obtain the desired amount. For an evacuated tube, when a drop of blood appears just inside the needle holder, grasp the needle holder

Promoting accuracy of laboratory tests

Problems in all aspects of laboratory testing can interfere with accurate determination of results. Here's a review of potential problem areas, with suggestions on ways to minimize errors that may alter test results.

Ordering the sample

An accurate laboratory test begins with an accurate requisition. All test requisitions must be filled out completely, including the patient's name, age, and sex; the ordering physician's name; the date and time of sample collection; and all other pertinent information. And, obviously, the correct test must be ordered for meaningful results. For example, a serum hexosaminidase test, a screening test for Tay-Sachs disease, will yield little diagnostically useful information from a pregnant patient; a leukocyte preparation is the proper test for such a patient. Accurate microbiological tests require that the culture site be specified. Failure to do so can lead to inaccurate or misleading results. If the laboratory assumes the wrong culture site, it may not investigate for the relevant microorganisms.

When filling out a laboratory slip, be sure to include all information requested on the form. If you have any questions, don't hesitate to call the laboratory or the physician who ordered the test.

Preparing the patient

Correct patient preparation also is crucial. Certain tests, such as carbohydrate metabolism tests (fasting plasma glucose, oral glucose tolerance, and so forth), require the patient to fast for a variable time before sample or specimen collection. Others call for special diets, activity restrictions, withholding of certain drugs, and other special preparation. The test entries in this volume specify such requirements. Following these recommendations precisely is necessary to ensure accurate test results.

Collecting the sample

One of the areas most critical to accurate testing is sample collection. Whether obtaining a urine specimen or blood sample, following the proper collection procedure is essential. Contamination of a clean-catch midstream urine specimen with organisms from the genitalia can invalidate test results, as can tissue contamination of blood samples from a faulty needlestick. When collecting a sample, make sure you understand exactly how to perform the required procedure, and take care to perform it properly.

Transporting and storing the sample

After obtaining a sample, arrange for its transport to the laboratory under proper conditions and within a certain time, or arrange for proper storage if analysis will be delayed. Failure to do so can result in deterioration or contamination of the specimen with subsequent invalidation of all test results.

securely and push down on the collection tube until the needle punctures the rubber stopper; blood flows into the tube automatically. When the tube is filled, remove it, and if drawing multiple samples, repeat the procedure with additional tubes.

To prevent stasis, release the tourniquet as soon as you establish adequate blood flow. If the flow is sluggish, you may want to leave the tourniquet in place longer. However, always remove the tourniquet before withdrawing the needle.

After drawing the desired sample and releasing the tourniquet, place a gauze pad over the puncture site, then withdraw the needle slowly and gently. Apply gentle pressure to the puncture site. Ask the alert and cooperative patient to hold the gauze in place for several minutes until the bleeding stops, to prevent hematoma. If the patient is not alert and cooperative, hold the pad in place, or apply a small adhesive bandage.

After collection with a syringe, remove the needle and carefully empty the sample into the appropriate test tube, without delay. To prevent foaming and possible hemolysis, *don't* eject the blood through the needle or force it out of the syringe.

Place the appropriate color-coded stoppers on the tubes. Gently invert a tube containing anticoagulant several times to mix the sample thoroughly. *Don't* shake the tube. Examine the sample for clots or clumps; if none appear, send the sample to the laboratory immediately. (For additional information on handling samples, see *Promoting accuracy of laboratory tests*, page 5.)

Before leaving, check the patient's condition. Instruct the patient who has lingering discomfort or undue bleeding to lie down and rest. Watch for anxiety and signs of shock, such as hypotension and tachycardia.

Make sure the specimen is sent to the laboratory immediately.

Arterial sample

Arterial blood is rarely required for routine studies. Because arterial puncture carries special risks, arterial samples are usually collected by a physician or a specially trained nurse.

Before drawing an arterial sample, administer a local anesthetic at the puncture site, if necessary.

To heparinize the syringe, first attach a 20G needle to the syringe; then break open the ampule of heparin and draw 1 ml into the syringe. While rotating the barrel, pull the plunger back past the 7-ml mark. Hold the syringe in an upright position, and slowly force the heparin toward the hub of the syringe, as you continue to rotate the barrel. Leave enough heparin — about 0.1 ml — to fill the syringe tip.

Heparinize the needle by removing the first needle and replacing it with a 23G needle. Continue holding the syringe upright, but slightly tilted. Then push the plunger all the way up to eject the remaining heparin.

Perform Allen's test to assess circulation in the radial artery (See *How to perform the Allen's test.)* Choose either the radial or brachial artery, whichever has the better circulation. *Don't* choose a site where

How to perform the Allen's test

Before drawing blood from a radial artery, perform the Allen's test. This test tells you whether or not the patient will receive enough blood through the ulnar artery to supply his hand if occlusion of the radial artery occurs.

First, have the patient rest his arm on the mattress or bedside stand, supporting his wrist with a rolled towel. Ask him to clench his fist. Then, using your index and middle fingers, exert pressure on both the radial and ulnar arteries. Hold this position for a few seconds.

Without removing your fingers from the patient's arteries, ask the patient to un-clench his fist and hold his hand in a relaxed position. The palm will be blanched, because you have impaired the normal blood flow with your fingers.

Now, release the pressure on the patient's ulnar artery. If the hand becomes flushed, indicating the rush of oxygenated blood to the hand, you can safely proceed with the ra-dial artery puncture. If it does not, repeat the test on the other arm. If neither arm pro-duces a positive result, use the brachial artery for arterial puncture.

the patient has had a vascular graft or has an atrioventricular fistula in place.

Next, using a circular motion, clean the selected puncture site with a swab soaked in povidone-iodine solution. Then wipe the site with a swab soaked in alcohol to remove the povidone-iodine solution, which is sticky and may hinder palpation. Palpate the artery with the forefinger and middle finger of one hand, while holding the syringe over the puncture site with the other hand.

With the needle bevel up, puncture the skin at a 45-degree angle for the radial artery, at a 60-degree angle for the brachial artery, and at a 90-degree angle for a femoral artery. Advance the needle, but don't pull the plunger back. When you've punctured the artery, blood will pulsate into the syringe. Allow it to fill 5 to 10 ml. If the syringe doesn't fill immediately, you may have pushed the needle through the artery. Pull the needle back slightly, but don't pull the plunger back. If the syringe still doesn't fill, withdraw the needle and start over with a fresh heparinized needle. Never make more than two attempts to draw blood from a single site.

After drawing the arterial sample, remove the needle and apply firm pressure to the puncture site with a gauze pad for at least 5 minutes, to prevent hematoma (a significant risk after arterial puncture). If the patient is receiving an anticoagulant or has a bleeding disorder, apply firm pressure to the puncture site for at least 15 minutes. *Don't* ask the patient to apply pressure to an arterial site. The patient may not apply the continuous, firm pressure that's needed.

Rotate the syringe to mix the heparin with the sample. If air bubbles appear, try to remove them by holding the syringe upright and tapping it lightly with your finger. If the bubbles don't disappear, hold the syringe upright and pierce a 2″ × 2″ gauze pad or alcohol swab with the needle (slowly forcing some of the blood out of the syringe eliminates the bubbles, and the gauze pad catches the ejected blood). After removing air bubbles, plunge the needle into a rubber stopper to seal it from the air, and transfer the sample to the iced specimen container.

Before drawing an arterial blood sample for blood gas studies, carefully check the patient's oxygen therapy. If ABG levels are being measured to monitor response to withdrawal of oxygen, but the patient continues to receive it, results will be misleading. For the same reason, don't draw an arterial sample immediately after suctioning or ventilating the patient. Wait at least 15 minutes to allow circulating blood levels to accurately reflect adjustment to such changes.

Note on the laboratory slip the patient's temperature, hemoglobin count, and the type and amount of oxygen therapy. Send the sample to the laboratory immediately.

After releasing pressure on the puncture site, tape a bandage firmly over it. (Don't tape the entire wrist, as this may restrict circulation.)

➤ *Clinical alert:* After arterial puncture, observe carefully for signs of circulatory impairment distal to the puncture site, such as numbness or tingling in the bandaged extremity.

Capillary sample

Collection of a capillary blood sample requires skin puncture of the fingertip or earlobe of adults, or puncture of the great toe or the heel of neonates.

To facilitate collection of a capillary sample, first dilate the vessels by applying warm, moist compresses to the area for about 10 minutes. Select the puncture site, wipe it with gauze and alcohol, and dry it thoroughly with another gauze pad so the blood will well up. Avoid cold, cyanotic, or swollen sites, to ensure an adequate blood sample.

To draw a sample from the fingertip, use a lancet smaller than 2 mm, and make the puncture perpendicular to the lines of the patient's fingerprints.

After drawing the sample, wipe away the first drop of blood to reduce the chance of sample dilution with tissue fluid. For the same reason, avoid squeezing the puncture site. After collecting the sample, briefly apply pressure to the puncture site to prevent painful extravasation of blood into the subcutaneous tissues. Ask the adult patient to hold a sterile gauze pad over the puncture site until bleeding has stopped. Then apply a small adhesive bandage.

Urine

The type of urine specimen required (random, second-voided, clean-catch midstream, first-morning, fasting, or timed) depends on the patient's condition and age and the purpose of the test. Random, second-voided, and clean-catch midstream specimens can be collected at any time; first-morning, fasting, or timed specimens require collection at specific times.

First-morning and *fasting* specimens must be collected when the patient awakes. Because the *first-morning* specimen is the most concentrated of the day, it's the specimen of choice for nitrate, protein, and urine sediment analysis. For this specimen, the patient voids and discards the urine just before going to bed, then collects the first voiding of the morning. For the *fasting* specimen, which is used for glucose testing, the patient collects a *first-morning* specimen after an overnight fast.

The *timed* specimen determines the urinary concentration of such substances as hormones, proteins, creatinine, and electrolytes over a specified period — usually over 2, 12, or 24 hours. The 24-hour collection, the most common timed specimen, provides a measure of average excretion for substances, such as hormones, eliminated in variable amounts during the day. Timed specimens also may be collected for administration of a challenge dose of a chemical, to measure physiologic efficiency — for example, ingestion of glucose to test for suspected diabetes mellitus or hypoglycemia. This type of specimen also is preferred for quantitative analysis of urobilinogen and amylase.

Equipment
Random, second-voided, first-morning, or fasting collection: clean, dry bedpan or urinal (for nonambulatory patients), specimen container, specimen labels, laboratory slip.

Clean-catch midstream collection: commercially prepared kit containing necessary equipment and directions for patient in several languages (English, Spanish, French) or antiseptic solution (green soap or povidone-iodine solution), water, cotton balls, sterile gloves, specimen labels, laboratory slip.

Timed collection (24-hour specimen): clean, dry gallon containers or commercial urine collection containers, preservative (as appropriate for the test), labels for collection container, display signs.

Pediatric urine collection: plastic disposable collection bags, specimen containers, laboratory slip, cotton swabs, soap and water, diapers.

Random and second-voided collections
For *random* collection, tell the ambulatory patient to void directly into a clean, dry specimen container. Tell the nonambulatory patient to void into a clean bedpan or urinal, to minimize bacterial or chemical contamination; then transfer about 30 ml of urine to the specimen container, and secure the cap.

For *second-voided* collection, instruct the patient to void and discard the urine. Then, offer at least one glass of water, to stimulate urine production. Collect the patient's urine 30 minutes later, using the random collection technique.

Label the container with the patient's name and room number (if applicable), physician's name, date, and collection time. Send the specimen and a completed request slip to the laboratory immediately. On the chart, record the time of the procedure and the time the specimen was sent to the laboratory.

First-morning and fasting collections
Unless the patient is an infant, is catheterized, or is unable to void, the following collection techniques are used for first-morning and fasting specimens.

For either specimen, instruct the patient to void and discard the urine before retiring for the night, then collect the first voiding of the next day in a clean, dry specimen container. (The patient who must void during the night should note the time on the specimen label — for example, "Urine specimen, 2:15 a.m. to 8:00 a.m.") For a fasting specimen, instruct the patient to restrict food and fluids after midnight the night before the test.

Label the container with the patient's name, room number (if applicable), physician's name, date, and collection time. Send the specimen and a completed request slip to the laboratory immediately. On the patient's chart, record the time of the procedure and the time the specimen was sent to the laboratory.

Clean-catch midstream collection

This aseptic technique for obtaining a *clean-catch midstream* urine specimen has become the acceptable procedure for collection random urine specimen. It's especially valuable for collecting urine specimens in women, because it provides a specimen that's virtually free of bacterial contamination.

Teach the correct procedure for obtaining a clean-catch midstream specimen (see *Patient-teaching aid* on page 11). After obtaining the specimen, send it to the laboratory immediately or refrigerate it to prevent bacterial growth. Record the time of the procedure and the time the specimen was sent to the laboratory.

Timed collection

All timed specimens (2-hour, 12-hour, and 24-hour) are collected virtually the same way. The following procedure is applicable for un-catheterized adults and continent children.

Explain the procedure and instruct the patient to collect all urine during the test period, to notify you after each voiding, and to avoid contaminating the specimen with toilet tissue or stool. Provide written instructions for home collection. Explain any necessary dietary, drug, or activity restrictions.

Obtain the proper preservative from the laboratory. Label a gallon jug or commercial urine collection container with the patient's name and room number (if applicable); physician's name; date and time the collection begins and ends; a warning "Do Not Discard"; and instructions to keep the container refrigerated. Prominently display signs indicating that a 24-hour urine collection is in progress: one at the head of the patient's bed, a second over the toilet bowl in the patient's bathroom, and a third over the utility room bedpan hopper.

Instruct the patient to void and discard the urine; then begin 24-hour collection with the next voiding. After placing the first voiding in the container, add the preservative. Add each voiding to the container immediately. If any urine is lost, restart the test, but consider that the test should end at a time when the laboratory is open to receive the specimen for processing. Just before the end of the collection period, instruct the patient to void, and add the urine to the gallon jug.

Send the labeled container to the laboratory immediately after the collection period. On the patient's chart, record the time urine collection ended and when the specimen was sent to the laboratory.

Patient-teaching aid

How to obtain a clean-catch midstream specimen

Procedure for males

1. Before attempting to collect this specimen, make sure your bladder is moderately full. This minimizes the risk of contamination by prostatic fluid.

2. Retract your foreskin, and clean the tip of your penis (urethral meatus and glans) with an antiseptic-moistened swab, wiping in a circular motion away from the urinary opening. Discard this swab, and use another swab to remove excess antiseptic.

3. Begin voiding into a toilet or urinal, and, without interrupting the flow, catch about 1 oz (30 ml) of urine in a sterile specimen container. (To prevent contamination of the specimen, don't touch the inner surface of the container or lid.)

4. Replace the lid of the specimen container. If you're not going to deliver the specimen to a laboratory immediately, refrigerate the specimen.

Procedure for females

1. If you're menstruating, your physician may want to postpone this test until after your menstrual period ends. However, if the test must be performed immediately, you can prevent contamination of the urine specimen with vaginal discharge or menstrual flow by inserting a tampon.

2. Kneel or squat over a bedpan or straddle the toilet bowl, to facilitate separating the folds of skin (labia) that cover the vagina and urinary opening.

3. Expose the urinary opening (urethral meatus) by separating the labia with your thumb and forefinger. Keep the labial folds separated during the collection.

4. Clean the area around the urinary opening with three antiseptic-moistened swabs: one for each side of the urethral meatus and the third for the meatus itself. Wipe with a front-to-back motion. Remove excess antiseptic with another swab.

5. Begin voiding into a bedpan or toilet bowl, and, without interrupting the flow, catch about 1 oz (30 ml) of urine in a sterile specimen container. (To prevent contamination of the specimen, don't touch the inner surface of the container or lid.)

6. Replace the lid of the specimen container. If you're not going to deliver the specimen to a laboratory immediately, refrigerate the specimen.

Special timed collections

Some tests require collection of the specimen at specified times — for example, the glucose tolerance test requires collection of urine 30 minutes, 1 hour, 2 hours, 3 hours, and, occasionally, 4 and 5 hours after a test meal. To ensure that the patient can void at the specified times, encourage the patient to drink some water at least every hour. For other tests (such as urea clearance) that require 2-hour collection periods, the patient should drink at least 2 oz (60 ml) of water 30 minutes before the test and one full glass each hour during the test.

Pediatric urine collection

Pediatric urine collection is used to obtain a random, second-voided, first-morning, fasting, or timed specimen from infants. Place the infant in the supine position, with hips externally rotated and abducted and knees flexed. Cleanse the perineal area with cotton swabs, soap, and water. Then, rinse the area with warm water; dry it thoroughly.

For *boys,* apply the collection device over the penis and scrotum, and press the flaps of the collection bag closely against the perineum to ensure a tight fit. For *girls,* tape the pediatric collection bag to the perineum, starting at the point between the anus and the vagina and working anteriorly. Cover the collection bag with a diaper to prevent the child from dislodging it. Elevate the head of the bed to facilitate drainage.

After collection is complete, remove the bag immediately to prevent skin excoriation. Transfer the urine to a clean, dry specimen container. Label the container with the patient's name and room number (if applicable), physician's name, date, and collection time. Send the specimen and the completed request slip to the laboratory immediately, and note the collection time on the patient's chart.

Catheter collection

Although catheter collection increases the risk of bacterial infection in the lower genitourinary tract, it may be necessary to obtain a random, second-voided, first-morning, fasting, or timed specimen in a patient who cannot void voluntarily.

To catheterize the patient, have ready the following equipment: Sterile catheterization set (sterile gloves, sterile catheter [for adults, #16 French; for children, #8 French]), sterile forceps, soap, water, towelette, sterile water-soluble lubricant, sterile cotton balls, antiseptic solution, sterile drapes, sterile specimen container, and labels for specimen container.

As appropriate, explain to the patient that you will collect a urine sample by inserting a small tube into the bladder through the urethra. Mention that this procedure may cause some transient discomfort.

Male catheterization: Wash the perineal area with soap and water. Place a sterile drape under the patient's buttocks and around the penis, making sure not to contaminate the drape. Put on sterile gloves. Moisten cotton balls with sterile cleaning solution. Arrange all sterile articles within easy reach on a sterile wrapper. Open the sterile specimen container, and lubricate the sterile catheter.

Grasp the shaft of the penis in one hand and elevate it about 90 degrees, hold it upright until the procedure is completed. Retract the foreskin and, with the forceps, grasp an antiseptic-moistened cotton ball. Cleanse the urethral meatus, wiping with a circular motion away from the urethral opening, toward the glans. Repeat the cleansing twice, each time with a fresh antiseptic-moistened cotton ball. Gently insert the lubricated catheter until urine flows. Allow a few milliliters to drain into the basin, then collect 10 to 60 ml in a sterile plastic container, depending on test requirements. After gently removing the catheter, clean and dry the periurethral area.

Send the specimen and the completed request slip to the laboratory within 10 minutes, or refrigerate the specimen. On the chart, record the procedure and the time the specimen is sent.

Female catheterization: After washing the perineal area with soap and water, place the patient in supine position with her knees flexed and feet on the bed. Place a sterile drape under the patient's buttocks and around the perineal area, making sure not to contaminate the drape. Put on sterile gloves, and moisten cotton balls with sterile cleaning solution. Lubricate the sterile catheter. Arrange all sterile articles within easy reach on a sterile wrapper, and open the sterile specimen container. Separate and keep the patient's labia majora open with one hand. With the other hand, take the forceps and grasp an antiseptic-moistened cotton ball. Make two vertical swipes of the cotton ball on the labia minora. (Use a new cotton ball for each swipe, cleaning from the urethral meatus toward the anus.)

Position the sterile tray with the lubricated catheter on the sterile field between the patient's legs. Then gently insert the catheter into the urethra until urine flows. Allow a few milliliters of urine to flow into a basin, then collect 10 to 60 ml in a sterile plastic container, depending on the test requirements. Gently remove the catheter; clean and dry the urethral area.

Send the specimen and completed request slip to the laboratory within 10 minutes, or refrigerate the specimen. On the patient's chart, record the procedure and the time the specimen was sent.

Collection from an indwelling catheter

You can minimize the risk of bacterial contamination by aspirating a urine specimen from an indwelling urinary catheter made of self-sealing rubber or from a collection tube with a special sampling port. (*Don't* aspirate from a Silastic, silicone, or plastic catheter.) This technique can provide random, second-voided, first-morning, fasting, or timed specimen.

Have ready the following equipment: Sterile syringe (10 to 20 ml), sterile needle (21G to 25G), alcohol sponge, sterile specimen container, specimen labels, laboratory slip.

About 30 minutes before collecting the specimen, clamp the collection tube. (*Note:* This procedure is contraindicated for patients who have just undergone genitourinary surgery.) If the collection tube has a sampling port, wipe the sampling port with an alcohol sponge, insert the needle at a 90-degree angle, and aspirate the urine into the syringe.

If the collection tube doesn't have a port and the catheter is made of rubber, you can obtain the specimen from the catheter. To do this, wipe the catheter with alcohol just above the connection of the collection tube to the catheter. Insert the needle at a 45-degree angle into the rubber catheter, and withdraw the urine specimen. Never insert the needle into the shaft of the catheter because this may puncture the lumen leading to the balloon.

Be sure to unclamp the tube after collecting the specimen. Failure to do so can cause bladder distention and may predispose the patient to a bladder infection. If you can't draw any urine, lift the tube slightly, but make sure urine doesn't return to the bladder. Aspirate the urine, and transfer the specimen to a sterile container for transport to the laboratory.

Legal implications

Testing for drugs of abuse, which usually occurs to confirm or detect suspected or known drug overdose or abuse, involves unique problems for specimen collection. For example, such tests — like those performed on specimens from homicide or rape victims — may require legal chain of custody protection for the test specimens. Legal chain of custody requires that each time a specimen changes hands, the person receiving it becomes the documented holder of the specimen and is responsible for its integrity. One particular source of difficulty in drug testing is that many persons being tested attempt to invalidate the screening tests performed on urine specimens. Such efforts may involve diluting the urine, adding a substance that would interfere with the test, or substituting another person's specimen. Possible dilution may be determined by checking the specimen for abnormal specific gravity, temperature (above or below body temperature), unusual color or appearance, abnormally high or low urine pH (normal urine pH is 4.5 to 8.0). To prevent substitution before collecting a specimen for a test with important legal implications, it may be necessary to verify the patient's identity through photographs.

An important consideration for all tests with legal implications is the requirement to maintain confidentiality. This is especially relevant during testing for human immunodeficiency virus (HIV) infection.

ABO blood typing

This test classifies blood according to the presence or absence of major antigens A and B on red cell surfaces and the presence of their reciprocal serum antibodies anti-A and anti-B. ABO blood typing, using both forward and reverse methods, is required before transfusion to prevent a lethal reaction.

In forward typing, the patient's red cells are tested with anti-A and anti-B sera. Cells that test negative are then tested with anti-A and anti-B antisera to detect weakly expressed subgroups of the A and B antigens. The presence or absence of agglutination determines the blood group. In reverse typing, the patient's serum is added to known group A and group B cells. Agglutination or hemolysis constitutes a positive reaction. Normally, antibodies are present in serum to counter any antigen not expressed on the red blood cells. Forward and reverse types should match; discrepancies must be resolved before transfusion.

Purpose
- To establish blood group according to the ABO system
- To check compatibility of donor and recipient blood before transfusion

Patient preparation
Explain that this test determines blood group, which is required for matching donor blood. Inform the patient that the test requires a blood sample. Check for recent administration of blood, dextran, or I.V. contrast media.

Procedure
Verify the patient's identity. Perform a venipuncture, and collect the sample in a *red-top* or *lavender-top* tube (for automated testing). Handle the sample gently. The specimen must be completely and properly labeled at the patient's bedside to prevent staff error or specimen misidentification. Send the sample with a properly completed request form to the laboratory immediately.

Precautions

Before the patient receives a transfusion, compare current and previous ABO typing and crossmatching to detect mistaken identification and to prevent transfusion reaction.

Findings and implications of results

In forward typing, if agglutination occurs when the patient's red cells are tested with anti-A serum, the A antigen is present and the blood is type A. If agglutination occurs when the patient's red cells are tested with anti-B serum, the B antigen is present and the blood is type B. If agglutination occurs with both anti-A and anti-B antisera, both A and B antigens are present and the blood is type AB. If agglutination does not occur with either anti-A or anti-B antisera, a third antibody, anti-A_1B, is used to detect weak subgroups of blood type A or B. A negative reaction confirms the absence of A and B antigens, making the blood type O.

In reverse typing, if agglutination or hemolysis occurs when B cells are tested with the patient's serum, anti-B is present and the blood is type A. If agglutination or hemolysis occurs when A cells are tested, anti-A is present and the blood is type B. If agglutination or hemolysis occurs when both A and B cells are mixed, anti-A and anti-B are present and the blood is type O. If agglutination or hemolysis does not occur with either A or B cells, neither anti-A nor anti-B is present and the blood is type AB. Unexpected agglutination of reverse typing cells indicates the presence of an atypical antibody in the serum which must be identified prior to transfusion. Unexpected absence of agglutination may be seen in hypogammaglobulinemia states.

Post-test care

If a hematoma develops at the venipuncture site, applying warm soaks eases discomfort.

Interfering factors

• Recent administration of dextran or I.V. contrast media causes cellular aggregation that resembles agglutination.
• Hemolysis caused by excessive agitation of the sample or poor venipuncture technique can result in a false-positive reaction in reverse typing.
• If a patient has previously received blood or been pregnant, atypical antibodies may develop, interfering with the reverse typing or compatibility testing. Provide the blood bank with the patient's history of prior transfusion or pregnancy when submitting specimens.

Acetaminophen, serum

This test uses high-performance liquid chromatography or an enzyme-multiplied immunoassay technique to measure serum acetaminophen levels. The test is essential for anticipating potential hepatotoxicity from an overdose; clinical effects of hepatotoxicity (jaundice, coagulation defects, encephalopathy, renal failure, and coma) don't appear until after liver damage occurs — generally 2 to 5 days after the ingestion of a toxic dose.

Absorbed rapidly from the GI tract, acetaminophen is metabolized by the liver and excreted in the urine. Acetaminophen overdose saturates the liver conjugation pathway, causing metabolism to hydroxamine-N-acetyl-P-aminophenol, a reactive toxic intermediate that injures liver cells and depletes hepatic glutathione, a substance that normally works to inactivate the toxic intermediate.

Concomitant ingestion of alcohol or barbiturates can significantly increase the amount of acetaminophen metabolized to the toxic intermediate, exaggerating the risk of hepatotoxicity.

Purpose
- To confirm acetaminophen toxicity suspected from history or onset of symptoms
- To monitor detoxification treatment with I.V. acetylcysteine
- To predict severity of acetaminophen poisoning

Patient preparation
Explain that this test determines blood levels of acetaminophen to prevent or check for toxicity. Inform the patient that the test requires multiple blood samples at timed intervals.

Check the patient's drug history, noting the time of acetaminophen ingestion and the dosage. Also check for use of alcohol and barbiturates.

Procedure
Perform the venipuncture and collect the sample in a 7-ml *red-top* tube. Send the sample to the laboratory immediately. Repeat the procedure 4, 8, and 12 hours after drug ingestion.

If the time of drug ingestion is unknown, collect two samples at least 4 hours apart so that the elimination half-life of the drug can be estimated.

Values
Generally, serum acetaminophen levels below 120 mcg/ml (800 µmol/L) 4 hours after ingestion rule out hepatotoxicity.

When ingestion time isn't known, elimination half-life helps determine possible toxicity. Normal elimination half-life is 2 to 4 hours.

Implications of results

Serum acetaminophen levels above 150 mcg/ml (1,000 µmol/L) 4 hours after ingestion indicate probable hepatotoxicity, as does an elimination half-life over 4 hours. An elimination half-life over 10 hours may indicate impending hepatic coma and death.

Liver function studies, such as serum bilirubin and alkaline phosphatase, may be necessary to assess liver damage.

Post-test care

- If acetaminophen levels indicate toxicity, begin treatment with I.V. acetylcysteine. Draw additional blood samples, as needed, to monitor the effectiveness of detoxification measures.
- If a hematoma develops at the venipuncture sites, applying warm soaks eases discomfort.

Interfering factor

Failure to observe the correct time intervals in serial testing of serum acetaminophen can interfere with accuracy of test results.

Acetylcholine receptor antibodies

The acetylcholine receptor (AChR) antibodies test is the most useful immunologic test for confirming acquired (autoimmune) myasthenia gravis (MG). This disorder of neuromuscular transmission can affect muscles innervated by cranial nerves, such as those of the face, lips, tongue, neck, and throat, as well as other muscle groups. In normal muscle contraction, acetylcholine (ACh) is released from the terminal end of the nerve and binds to AChR sites on the muscle motor end plate. In MG, however, antibodies block and destroy such sites, causing muscle weakness that can be either generalized or localized to the ocular muscles.

Two test methods — a binding assay and a blocking assay — can determine the relative concentration of AChR antibodies in serum. In the binding assay, purified AChRs are complexed with ^{125}I-labeled alpha-bungarotoxin (a molecule that binds specifically to AChRs and blocks them). A serum sample is added to this complex; after incubation, antihuman immunoglobulin is added. Antibodies bind to AChR –^{125}I-labeled alpha-bungarotoxin complexes that coprecipitate with the total human immunoglobulin. The amount of radioactivity is then measured to assay the available AChR sites.

When the AChR-binding assay is negative in a patient with MG symptoms, the AChR-blocking assay may be performed. Here, the patient's serum is incubated with purified AChRs before ^{125}I-labeled alpha-bungarotoxin is added to detect antibodies whose antigenic sites would otherwise be blocked. The blocking assay is specific for the autoimmune form of MG.

In tests for both binding and blocking AChR antibodies, a positive result is found in about 90% of patients with generalized MG and in about 80% of those with ocular MG. AChR-blocking antibodies are rarely found, except in patients with autoimmune MG; the antibodies are detectable in 52% of MG patients (in 30% of those with ocular MG). Determination of AChR antibodies by either method also helps monitor immunosuppressant therapy for MG, although antibody levels do not usually parallel the severity of the disease.

Purpose
• To confirm diagnosis of MG
• To monitor the effectiveness of immunosuppressant therapy for MG

Patient preparation
Explain that this test helps confirm MG or assesses the effectiveness of treatment. Inform the patient that the test requires a blood sample.

Check the patient's history for immunosuppressants that may affect test results. Note such use on the laboratory slip.

Procedure
Perform a venipuncture, and collect the sample in a 7-ml *red-top* tube. Keep the sample at room temperature and send it to the laboratory immediately.

Values
Results are reported as a percent loss of AChR. Normal human sera generally cause loss of less than 20% of AChR; sera from MG patients cause loss of more than 30%. Loss of 20% to 30% on repeat testing is considered an equivocal result.

Implications of results
Positive AChR antibodies in symptomatic adults confirm diagnosis of MG. Patients who have only ocular symptoms of MG tend to have lower anti-

body titers than those who have generalized symptoms.

Post-test care
- Because patients treated for autoimmune disease often are immunocompromised, check the venipuncture site for infection. Keep a clean, dry bandage over the site for at least 24 hours.
- If a hematoma develops at the venipuncture site, applying warm soaks eases discomfort.

Interfering factors
- Failure to maintain the sample at room temperature and to send it to the laboratory immediately may affect the accurate determination of test results.
- Thymectomy, thoracic duct drainage, immunosuppressant therapy, or plasmapheresis may cause reduced AChR-antibody levels.
- Patients with amyotrophic lateral sclerosis may show false-positive test results.
- Muscle relaxant drugs used during anesthesia can cause false-positive results in serum samples obtained perioperatively.

Acid mucopolysaccharides, urine

This quantitative test for mucopolysaccharidosis measures the urine level of acid mucopolysaccharides (AMPs), a group of polysaccharides or carbohydrates, in children with family histories of such disease. When an inborn error of metabolism causes enzymatic deficiencies, AMPs — especially dermatan sulfate and heparitin sulfate — accumulate in the tissues, producing a rare disorder called mucopolysaccharidosis. Its severest form, Hurler's syndrome (or gargoylism), results from deposition of these macromolecular complexes in several organs, particularly the heart and kidneys, and excretion of large amounts of mucopolysaccharides in the urine.

The measured AMP value is reported as mg glucuronic acid. This number, divided by the amount of creatinine in the same specimen (which reflects glomerular filtration rate), is a ratio that is used to overcome irregularities in the 24-hour urine collection. The values vary with age.

Purpose
To diagnose mucopolysaccharidosis

Patient preparation   Explain to the parents that this test helps determine the efficiency of carbohydrate metabolism. Inform them that they needn't restrict the child's food or fluids before the test, and that the test requires urine collection for 24 hours. If appropriate, instruct them on the proper method for collecting the specimen at home.

   If the child is receiving therapy with heparin and must continue it, note this on the laboratory slip.

Procedure   Obtain a 24-hour urine specimen. Add 20 ml of toluene as a preservative at the start of the collection. During the collection period, refrigerate the specimen or place it on ice and, if the patient's parents are collecting specimens at home, advise them to do the same. At the end of the 24-hour collection period, send the specimen to the laboratory immediately. Indicate the patient's age on the laboratory slip.

Values   Normal AMP values vary with age. They are reported as milligrams of glucuronic acid per day, or milligrams of glucuronic acid per grams of creatinine.

Age (years)	mg glucuronic acid/g creatinine	μmol glucuronic acid/mmol creatinine
2	8 to 30	5 to 20
4	7 to 27	4 to 19
6	6 to 24	4 to 18
8	4 to 22	3 to 15
10	2 to 18	2 to 12
12	0 to 15	0 to 10
14	0 to 12	0 to 8

Implications of results   Elevated AMP levels reliably indicate mucopolysaccharidosis. Supplementary quantitative analysis and detailed blood studies can identify the defective enzyme.

Post-test care   All adhesive from the urine collector should be removed from the child's perineum and the area washed gently with soap and water. Observe for irritation.

Interfering factors   • Failure to collect all urine during the test period, and improper specimen storage may interfere with accurate determination of test results.
   • Heparin elevates urine levels of AMPs.

Acid phosphatase

Acid phosphatase, a group of phosphatase enzymes most active at a pH of about 5.0, appears primarily in the prostate gland and semen and, to a lesser extent, in the liver, spleen, red blood cells, bone marrow, and platelets. Prostatic and erythrocytic enzymes are this group's two major isoenzymes; the prostatic isoenzyme is more specific for prostate cancer. The more widespread the tumor, the more likely it is to produce high serum acid phosphatase levels. The acid phosphatase assay is usually restricted to adult males to detect prostate cancer.

This test measures total acid phosphatase and the prostatic fraction by biochemical assay, or prostatic acid phosphatase by an immunochemical assay, such as radioimmunoassay.

Purpose	• To detect prostate cancer • To monitor response to therapy for prostate cancer; successful treatment decreases acid phosphatase levels
Patient preparation	Explain the purpose of the test and inform the patient that the test requires a blood sample.
Procedure	Perform a venipuncture, and collect the sample in a 7-ml *red-top* tube. Handle the collection tube gently to prevent hemolysis, and send the sample to the laboratory immediately. Acid phosphatase levels drop by 50% within 1 hour if the sample remains at room temperature without the addition of a preservative or if it's not packed in ice.
Precautions	Don't draw the sample within 48 hours of prostate manipulation (rectal exam).
Values	Serum values for total acid phosphatase range from 0 to 5 U/L. Normal range of immunoassay results is 2.5 to 3.7 ng/ml.
Implications of results	Generally, high prostatic acid phosphatase levels indicate a tumor that has spread beyond the prostatic capsule. If the tumor has metastasized to bone, high acid phosphatase levels are accompanied by high alkaline phosphatase levels, reflecting increased osteoblastic activity. Misleading results may occur if alkaline phosphatase levels are high because acid and alkaline

phosphatase enzymes are very similar and differ mainly in their optimum pH ranges. Total acid phosphatase levels (as measured by an enzymatic test) rise moderately in prostatic infarction, Paget's disease (some patients), Gaucher's disease, and occasionally, in other conditions, such as multiple myeloma.

Post-test care
- If a hematoma develops at the venipuncture site, applying warm soaks eases discomfort.
- The patient may resume medications discontinued before the test.

Interfering factors
- Prostate massage, catheterization, or rectal examination within 48 hours of the test may interfere with test results.
- Hemolysis of the sample, or improper sample storage may interfere with test results.

ACTH, plasma
Adrenocorticotropic hormone, corticotropin

This test measures the plasma levels of adrenocorticotropic hormone (ACTH) by radioimmunoassay. ACTH, a polypeptide hormone released by the basophilic cells of the anterior pituitary gland, stimulates the adrenal cortex to secrete cortisol and, to a lesser degree, androgens and aldosterone. ACTH also has some melanocyte-stimulating activity and increases the uptake of amino acids by muscle cells, promotes lipolysis by fat cells, stimulates pancreatic beta cells to secrete insulin, and may contribute to the release of growth hormone. ACTH levels vary diurnally, peaking between 6 a.m. and 8 a.m. and ebbing between 6 p.m. and 11 p.m.

Through a negative feedback mechanism, plasma cortisol levels control ACTH secretion — for example, high cortisol levels suppress ACTH secretion. Emotional and physical stress (pain, surgery, insulin-induced hypoglycemia) stimulate secretion and can override the effects of plasma cortisol levels.

The plasma ACTH test may be ordered for patients with signs of adrenal hypofunction (insufficiency) or hyperfunction (Cushing's syndrome). However, ACTH suppression or stimulation testing is usually necessary to confirm diagnosis. The instability of plasma ACTH greatly limits its diagnostic significance and reliability.

Purpose	• To facilitate differential diagnosis of primary and secondary adrenal hypofunction
	• To aid differential diagnosis of Cushing's syndrome

Patient preparation

Explain that this test helps evaluate hormonal secretion. Inform the patient that the test may require fasting and limiting carbohydrate intake for 2 days before the test, and limiting physical activity for 10 to 12 hours. Tell the patient that the test requires a blood sample.

Check the patient's history for the use of any drugs that may interfere with accurate test results, such as corticosteroids, and drugs that affect cortisol levels — estrogens, amphetamines, spironolactone, calcium gluconate, or alcohol. These drugs should be withheld for 48 hours or longer before the test. If these medications must be continued, note this on the laboratory slip.

Procedure

For a patient with suspected adrenal hypofunction, perform the venipuncture for a baseline level between 6 a.m. and 8 a.m. (peak secretion); for a patient with suspected Cushing's syndrome, perform the venipuncture between 6 p.m. and 11 p.m. (low secretion). Collect the sample in a *plastic* tube, since ACTH may adsorb to glass, or in a *green-top* (heparinized) tube. Because proteolytic enzymes in the plasma degrade ACTH, a temperature of 39.2° F (4° C) is necessary to retard enzyme activity. Immediate transfer of the sample, packed in ice, to the laboratory is essential for reliable test results. Because stress can itself cause increased secretion of ACTH, perform the venipuncture with as little trauma and in as tranquil an environment as possible. The collection technique may vary, depending on the laboratory.

Values

Reference values are not yet firmly established. Some clinics set peak values at less than 120 pg/ml (26 pmol/L), but these values may vary, depending on the laboratory.

Implications of results

A higher-than-normal plasma ACTH level in the presence of a low plasma cortisol level may indicate primary adrenal hypofunction (Addison's disease), in which the pituitary gland attempts to compensate for the unresponsiveness of the target organ by releasing excessive ACTH. The underlying cause of adrenocortical hypofunction may be idiopathic atrophy of the adrenal cortex, or partial destruction of the gland by granuloma, neoplasm, amyloidosis, or inflammatory necrosis.

A low-normal plasma ACTH level with a low cortisol level suggests secondary adrenal hypofunction resulting from pituitary or hypothalamic dysfunction. The primary determinant may be panhypopituitarism, absence of corticotropin-releasing hormone in the hypothalamus, or chronic blunting of ACTH levels by long-term corticosteroid therapy.

In suspected Cushing's syndrome, an elevated plasma ACTH level suggests Cushing's *disease*, in which pituitary dysfunction (caused by adenoma) causes continuous ACTH production which results in continuously elevated plasma cortisol levels without diurnal variations.

A low-normal ACTH level implies adrenal hyperfunction caused by an adrenocortical tumor or hyperplasia as the source of high cortisol levels; in such hyperfunction, ACTH levels are low-normal (or undetectable) because the high plasma cortisol levels suppress ACTH secretion through negative feedback.

Post-test care
- If a hematoma develops at the puncture site, applying warm soaks eases discomfort.
- The patient may resume diet and medications that were discontinued before the test.

Interfering factors
- Failure to observe restrictions of diet, medications, and physical activity; or trauma, pain, and emotional distress during venipuncture may interfere with accurate determination of the test results. ACTH levels are depressed by corticosteroids, including cortisone and its analogues, and by drugs that increase endogenous cortisol secretion (estrogens, calcium gluconate, amphetamines, spironolactone, and ethanol). Lithium carbonate decreases cortisol levels and may interfere with ACTH secretion. ACTH levels are also affected by the menstrual cycle and pregnancy.
- Radioactive scan performed within 1 week before the test may influence test results.

ACTH, rapid stimulation test
Cosyntropin test

The rapid adrenocorticotropic hormone (ACTH) test is gradually replacing the 8-hour ACTH stimulation test as the most effective diagnostic tool for evaluating adrenal hypofunction (insufficiency). Using cosyntropin, a synthetic analogue of the biologically active part of ACTH, the rapid ACTH test provides faster results and causes fewer allergic reactions than the 8-hour test, which uses natural ACTH from animal sources. This test requires prior determination of baseline plasma cortisol levels to evaluate the effect of cosyntropin administration on cortisol secretion. An unequivocally high morning cortisol level rules out adrenal hypofunction and makes further testing unnecessary.

Purpose
- To aid diagnosis of primary and secondary adrenal hypofunction
- To determine adrenal reserve function, especially in patients taking corticosteroids (corticosteroids may cause prolonged suppression of adrenal function, and sudden withdrawal may result in dangerous adrenal insufficiency)

Patient preparation
Explain that this test helps determine if the patient's condition is caused by a hormonal deficiency. Inform the patient that he may be required to fast for 10 to 12 hours before the test, and must be relaxed and resting quietly for 30 minutes before the test and that the test, which takes at least 1 hour to perform, requires three venipunctures and an injection.

This test may be given on an outpatient basis. If the patient receiving ACTH is also receiving concurrent corticosteroids, note this on the laboratory slip. Withdrawal of corticosteroids must be performed under medical supervision.

Procedure
Draw 5 ml of blood for a baseline value. Collect the sample in a 5-ml *green-top* (heparinized) tube. Label this sample "preinjection," and send it to the laboratory. Inject 250 mcg (0.25 mg) cosyntropin I.V. (preferably) or I.M. (I.V. administration affords more accurate determinations because ineffective absorption after I.M. administration may cause wide variations in response.)

Draw another 5 ml of blood 30 and 60 minutes following the cosyntropin injection. Collect the samples in 5-ml *green-top* (heparinized) tubes. Label the samples "30 minutes postinjection" and "60 minutes postinjection"; then send them to the laboratory. Indicate the actual collection times on the laboratory slip. These samples require no special precautions other than avoiding stasis.

Values   Normally, plasma cortisol levels rise 7 or more mcg/dl (200 nmol/L) above the baseline value to a peak of 18 mcg/dl (500 nmol/L) 60 minutes after the cosyntropin injection. Generally, a doubling of the baseline value indicates a normal response.

Implications of results   A normal result excludes primary adrenal hypofunction (insufficiency). In patients with primary adrenal hypofunction (Addison's disease), cortisol levels remain low. Thus, the rapid stimulation ACTH test provides an effective method of screening for adrenal hypofunction. However, if test results show subnormal increases in plasma cortisol levels, prolonged stimulation of the adrenal cortex may be required to differentiate between primary and secondary adrenal hypofunction.

Post-test care
- If a hematoma develops at the venipuncture sites, applying warm soaks eases discomfort.
- Observe the patient for signs of an allergic reaction to cosyntropin (rare), such as hives and itching, or tachycardia.
- The patient may resume diet and medications that were discontinued before the test.

Interfering factors
- Failure to observe restrictions of diet, medications, and physical activity may hinder accurate determination of test results. Drugs that increase plasma cortisol levels — including estrogens (which increase plasma cortisol-binding proteins) and amphetamines — may interfere with test results. Smoking and obesity may also increase plasma cortisol levels. Lithium carbonate decreases plasma cortisol levels.
- Radioactive scan performed within 1 week before the test may influence test results, because plasma cortisol levels are determined by radioimmunoassay.
- Hemolysis of the sample may interfere with accurate determination of test results.

Activated partial thromboplastin time

The activated partial thromboplastin time (APTT) test screens for intrinsic pathway factor deficiencies and also is an important test for monitoring heparin treatment. The test is performed by adding a contact activator and phospholipid emulsion, then calcium, to a plasma sample. The time elapsed, in seconds, from the addition of calcium to the formation of a fibrin clot is then reported. APTT is sensitive to factors II, V, VIII, IX, X, and XI and fibrinogen. However, because contact activators are used to initiate coagulation, the test also is sensitive to deficiencies of contact pathway factors (factor XII, prekallikrein, and high molecular weight kininogen), which do not cause bleeding. Depending on their phospholipid composition, some APTT reagents will also detect nonspecific coagulation inhibitors. (The partial thromboplastin time [PTT] test, which is similar but less sensitive and less frequently performed, relies on contact with the glass surface of a test tube to activate the sample.)

Purpose
- To detect congenital factor deficiencies (factors II, V, VIII, IX, X, and XI and fibrinogen) and acquired factor deficiencies (liver disease, disseminated intravascular coagulation)
- To monitor heparin therapy

Patient preparation
Explain to the patient that this test helps determine if his blood clots normally. Tell the patient that the test requires a blood sample. Tell the patient receiving heparin therapy that this test may be repeated to determine his heparin dosage requirements.

Procedure
Perform a venipuncture, and collect the sample in a 7-ml *blue-top* (citrated) tube. To prevent hemolysis, avoid excessive probing of venipuncture site and handle the sample gently. Fill the collection tube completely, invert it gently several times, and send it to the laboratory.

Values
Normally, a fibrin clot forms 25 to 36 seconds after addition of calcium reagent.

Implications of results
Prolonged times may indicate a deficiency of certain plasma clotting factors; the presence of heparin; or the presence of fibrin split products, fibrinol-

ysis, or circulating anticoagulants (antibodies to specific clotting factors and to phospholipid).

Post-test care If a hematoma develops at the venipuncture site, applying warm soaks eases discomfort.

Interfering factors

- Failure to use the proper anticoagulant, to fill the collection tube completely, or to mix the sample and the anticoagulant adequately may interfere with accurate test results.
- Collection of samples from heparinized lines may cause falsely prolonged results.
- Anemia and polycythemia can cause falsely short or prolonged results, because of improper dilution of test plasma with anticoagulant.
- Hemolysis caused by excessive agitation of the sample or by excessive probing at the venipuncture site may alter test results.
- Failure to send the sample to the laboratory immediately or to place it on ice may cause misleading test results.

Alanine aminotransferase (ALT), serum

Alanine transaminase, serum; glutamic-pyruvic transaminase (SGPT), serum

Alanine aminotransferase (ALT) is one of two enzymes that catalyzes a reversible amino group transfer reaction to urea via ammonia production in the Krebs-Henseleit cycle. Unlike aspartate aminotransferase, the other aminotransferase, ALT primarily appears in hepatocellular cytoplasm, with lesser amounts in the kidneys, heart, and skeletal muscles, and is a relatively specific indicator of acute hepatocellular damage. When such damage occurs, ALT is released from the cytoplasm into the bloodstream, often before jaundice appears, resulting in abnormally high serum levels that may not return to normal for days or weeks. This test measures serum ALT levels, using the spectrophotometric or the colorimetric method.

Purpose

- To help detect and evaluate treatment of acute hepatic disease — especially hepatitis and cirrhosis without jaundice

- To help distinguish between myocardial and hepatic tissue damage (used with aspartate aminotransferase [AST])
- To assess hepatotoxicity of some drugs

Patient preparation

Explain that this test, which requires a blood sample, helps assess liver function.

Procedure

Perform a venipuncture, and collect the sample in a 7-ml *red-top* tube. Handle the sample gently to prevent hemolysis. ALT activity is stable in serum for up to 3 days at room temperature.

Values

ALT levels by a commonly used method range from 10 to 32 U/L; in females, from 9 to 24 U/L. The normal range for infants is twice that of adults.

Implications of results

Very high ALT levels (up to 50 times normal) suggest viral or severe drug-induced hepatitis or other hepatic disease with extensive necrosis. (AST levels are also elevated but usually to a lesser degree.) Moderate-to-high levels may indicate infectious mononucleosis, chronic hepatitis, intrahepatic cholestasis or cholecystitis, early or improving acute viral hepatitis, or severe hepatic congestion caused by heart failure. Slight-to-moderate elevations of ALT (usually with higher increases in AST levels) may appear in any condition that produces acute hepatocellular injury — such as active cirrhosis and drug-induced or alcoholic hepatitis. Marginal elevations occasionally occur in acute myocardial infarction, reflecting secondary hepatic congestion or the release of small amounts of ALT from myocardial tissue.

Post-test care

- If a hematoma develops at the venipuncture site, applying warm soaks eases discomfort.
- Patient may resume medications that were withheld before the test.

Interfering factors

- Many medications produce hepatic injury by competitively interfering with cellular metabolism. Elevated ALT levels can follow use of barbiturates, griseofulvin, isoniazid, nitrofurantoin, methyldopa, phenothiazines, phenytoin, salicylates, tetracycline, chlorpromazine, para-aminosalicylic acid, and other drugs. High ALT levels may require discontinuation of therapy with such drugs.

- Ingestion of lead or exposure to carbon tetrachloride causes direct injury to hepatic cells and sharp elevations of ALT.
- Hemolysis caused by excessive agitation of the sample may interfere with accurate determination of ALT levels.

Aldosterone, serum

This test measures serum aldosterone levels by radioimmunoassay. Aldosterone, the principal mineralocorticoid secreted by the zona glomerulosa of the adrenal cortex, regulates ion transport across cell membranes in the renal tubules to promote reabsorption of sodium and chloride in exchange for potassium and hydrogen ions. Consequently, aldosterone helps to maintain blood pressure and blood volume and to regulate fluid and electrolyte balance.

Aldosterone secretion is controlled primarily by the renin-angiotensin system, by the circulating concentration of potassium and, to a lesser extent, by corticotropin. Thus, high serum potassium levels elicit secretion of aldosterone through a potent feedback system; similarly, hyponatremia, hypovolemia, and other disorders that provoke the release of renin stimulate aldosterone secretion.

This test identifies hyperaldosteronism and, when supported by plasma renin levels, distinguishes between the primary and secondary forms of this disorder. Thus, it's helpful in identifying adrenal adenoma and adrenal hyperplasia, which may cause primary hyperaldosteronism.

Evaluation of aldosterone secretion requires measurement of both blood and urine levels.

Purpose
To aid diagnosis of primary and secondary aldosteronism or hypoaldosteronism (salt-losing syndrome)

Patient preparation
Explain that this test, which requires a blood sample, helps determine if symptoms are caused by abnormal hormonal secretion.

Preparation is critical and varies according to the purpose of the test. For example, to test for excess secretion, the patient follows a high-salt diet for several days (usually 5) or follows a normal diet and receives a 4-hour normal saline infusion before aldosterone levels are measured. To test for hypoaldosteronism, the patient follows a low-salt diet and receives a diuretic (furosemide) before supine and upright levels of aldosterone and renin are measured.

All drugs that alter fluid, sodium, and potassium balance — especially diuretics, antihypertensives, steroids, cyclic progestational agents, and estrogens — should be withheld for at least 2 weeks or, preferably, for 30 days before the test. All renin inhibitors (such as propranolol) and calcium channel blockers should be withheld for 1 week before the test. If these medications must be continued, note this on the laboratory slip. Tell the patient to avoid licorice, which has an aldosterone-like effect, for at least 2 weeks before the test.

Procedure   Venipuncture should be performed with the patient standing, after the patient has been up and about for at least 4 hours. Collect the sample in a 7-ml *red-top* collection tube, and send it to the laboratory promptly.

Record on the laboratory slip that the patient was standing during the venipuncture. If the patient is a premenopausal female, specify the phase of her menstrual cycle because aldosterone levels may fluctuate during the menstrual cycle.

Values   Normally, serum aldosterone levels (in a standing, nonpregnant patient) range from 1 to 21 ng/dl (30 to 570 pmol/L). A normal supine (for at least 2 hours) serum aldosterone level for an adult male or female is 7.4 ± 4.2 ng/dl (200 ± 11 pmol/L); an upright (for 4 hours) level with unrestricted salt intake is 6 to 22 ng/dl (0.17 to 0.61 nmol/L) for an adult female, 5 to 30 ng/dl (0.14 to 0.83 nmol/L) for an adult male. Values vary greatly with method, and trends are significant.

Implications of results   Excessive aldosterone secretion may indicate a primary or secondary disease. Primary hyperaldosteronism (Conn's syndrome) may result from adrenocortical adenoma, bilateral adrenal hyperplasia or, less commonly, cancer. Elevated levels in secondary aldosteronism can result from external stimuli causing increased renin-angiotensin activity, for example, in salt depletion, potassium excess, treatment with corticotropin, renovascular hypertension, congestive heart failure, cirrhosis of the liver, nephrotic syndrome, idiopathic cyclic edema, or during the third trimester of pregnancy.

Depressed serum aldosterone levels may indicate primary hypoaldosteronism, salt-losing syndrome, toxemia of pregnancy, Addison's disease, renin deficiency, or hypokalemia.

Post-test care
- If a hematoma develops at the venipuncture site, applying warm soaks eases discomfort.
- The patient may resume diet and medications discontinued before the test.

Interfering factors
- Hemolysis caused by excessive agitation of the sample may interfere with accurate determination of test results.
- Failure to observe restrictions of diet, medications, or posture may interfere with accurate determination of test results.
- Some antihypertensive drugs — methyldopa, for example — promote sodium and water retention, and therefore may reduce aldosterone levels.
- Diuretics promote sodium excretion and may raise aldosterone levels.
- Some corticosteroids — fludrocortisone, for example — mimic mineralocorticoid activity and therefore may lower aldosterone levels.
- Excessive potassium intake increases aldosterone levels; deficient intake of potassium in the presence of aldosterone excess lowers aldosterone levels.
- Increased plasma concentration of potassium stimulates adrenal production of aldosterone.
- In conditions of severe physical stress (such as burns or hemorrhage), corticotropin may affect aldosterone production.
- Radioactive scan performed within 1 week before the test may influence test results.
- Ingestion of licorice or treatment with propranolol decreases aldosterone levels.
- Upright posture, acute stress, and late pregnancy may increase aldosterone levels. For example, upright posture in a salt-depleted state will raise aldosterone levels from two to five times the supine levels.

Aldosterone, urine

This test measures urine levels of aldosterone, the principal mineralocorticoid secreted by the zona glomerulosa of the adrenal cortex. Aldosterone promotes retention of sodium and excretion of potassium by the renal tubules, thereby helping to regulate blood pressure, and fluid and electrolyte balance. In turn, aldosterone secretion is controlled by the renin-angiotensin system. Potassium levels also influence aldosterone secretion: increased potassium concentration stimulates the adrenal cortex, triggering a substantial increase in aldosterone secretion to promote potassium excretion. This feedback mechanism is vital to maintaining fluid and electrolyte balance.

Urine aldosterone levels, measured by radioimmunoassay, are usually evaluated after measurement of serum electrolyte and renin levels.

Purpose
To aid diagnosis of primary and secondary aldosteronism

Patient preparation
Explain that this test evaluates hormonal balance. Instruct the patient to maintain a normal sodium diet (3 g/day) before the test; to avoid sodium-rich foods, and to avoid strenuous physical exercise and stressful situations during the collection period. Tell the patient the test requires collection of a 24-hour urine specimen, and teach the proper collection technique.

Check the patient's history for use of drugs that may affect aldosterone levels. As ordered, restrict these medications before the test.

Procedure
Collect a 24-hour specimen in a bottle containing a preservative to keep the specimen at a pH of 4.0 to 4.5. Refrigerate the specimen or place it on ice during the collection period. When the collection is completed, send the specimen to the laboratory immediately.

Values
Normally, urine aldosterone levels range from 2 to 16 mcg/day (5 to 45 nmol/day).

Implications of results
Elevated urine aldosterone levels suggest primary or secondary aldosteronism. The primary form usually arises from an aldosterone-secreting adenoma of the adrenal cortex but may also result from

adrenocortical hyperplasia. Secondary aldosteronism, the more common form, results from external stimulation of the adrenal cortex, such as that produced when the renin-angiotensin system is activated by hypertensive and edematous disorders (malignant hypertension, congestive heart failure, cirrhosis of the liver, nephrotic syndrome, and idiopathic cyclic edema).

Low urine aldosterone levels may result from Addison's disease, salt-losing syndrome, and toxemia of pregnancy. These levels normally rise during pregnancy but rapidly decline following parturition.

Post-test care The patient may resume medications and normal physical activity.

Interfering factors
- Antihypertensive drugs promote sodium and water retention, and may suppress urine aldosterone levels. Diuretics and most steroids promote sodium excretion and may raise aldosterone levels. Some corticosteroids, such as fludrocortisone, mimic mineralocorticoid activity and consequently may lower aldosterone levels.
- Failure to maintain a normal dietary intake of sodium can influence test results.
- Failure to collect *all* urine during the 24-hour specimen collection period or to store the urine specimen properly can interfere with accurate determination of test results.
- Strenuous physical exercise and emotional stress before the test stimulates adrenocortical secretions and thus increases aldosterone levels.
- Radioactive scan performed within 1 week before the test may interfere with the accurate determination of aldosterone levels using this radioimmunoassay method.

Alkaline phosphatase

This test measures serum levels of alkaline phosphatase, an enzyme that is most active at about pH 9.0. Alkaline phosphatase influences bone calcification and lipid and metabolite transport. Total serum levels reflect the combined activity of several alkaline phosphatase isoenzymes found in the liver, bones, kidneys, intestinal lining, and placenta. Bone and liver alkaline phosphatase are always present in adult serum, with liver alkaline phosphatase most prominent — except during the third trimester of pregnancy (when the placenta produces about half of all alkaline phosphatase). The intestinal variant of this enzyme can be a normal component (in less than 10% of normal patients; a genetically controlled characteristic found almost exclusively in the sera of blood groups B and O), or it can be an abnormal finding associated with hepatic disease.

The alkaline phosphatase test is particularly sensitive to mild biliary obstruction and is a primary indicator of space-occupying hepatic lesions; additional liver function studies are usually required to identify hepatobiliary disorders. Its most specific clinical application is in the diagnosis of metabolic bone disease.

Purpose
- To detect and identify skeletal diseases primarily characterized by marked osteoblastic activity
- To detect local hepatic lesions causing biliary obstruction, such as tumor or abscess
- To supplement information from other liver function studies and GI enzyme tests
- To assess response to vitamin D in the treatment of deficiency-induced rickets

Patient preparation
Explain that this test, which requires a blood sample, assesses liver or bone function. Instruct the patient to fast for 10 to 12 hours before the test because fat intake stimulates intestinal alkaline phosphatase secretion.

Procedure
Perform a venipuncture, and collect the sample in a 7-ml *red-top* tube. Handle the collection tube gently to prevent hemolysis, and send the sample to the laboratory immediately, because alkaline phosphatase activity increases at room temperature due to a rise in pH.

Values
The normal adult range of serum alkaline phosphatase is 30 to 110 U/L. Total alkaline phosphatase levels range from 30 to 120 U/L in adults, 40 to 300 U/L in children. Because alkaline phosphatase concentrations rise during active bone formation and growth, infants, children, and adolescents normally have levels that may be three times as high as those of adults. Pregnancy also causes a physiologic rise in alkaline phosphatase levels.

Implications of
results

Significant alkaline phosphatase elevations are most likely to indicate skeletal disease, or extrahepatic or intrahepatic biliary obstruction that causes cholestasis. Many acute hepatic diseases cause alkaline phosphatase elevations before any change occurs in serum bilirubin levels. Moderate rise in alkaline phosphatase levels may reflect acute biliary obstruction caused by hepatocellular inflammation in active cirrhosis, mononucleosis, and viral hepatitis. Moderate increases are also seen in osteomalacia and deficiency-induced rickets.

Sharp elevations of alkaline phosphatase levels may result from incomplete biliary obstruction by malignant or infectious infiltrations or fibrosis. Such markedly high levels are most common in Paget's disease and, occasionally, in biliary obstruction, extensive bone metastases, or hyperparathyroidism. Metastatic bone tumors resulting from pancreatic cancer raise alkaline phosphatase levels without a concomitant rise in AST levels.

Isoenzyme fractionation and additional enzyme tests — serum gamma glutamyl transferase, acid phosphatase, 5'-nucleotidase, and leucine aminopeptidase — are sometimes performed when the cause of alkaline phosphatase elevations (skeletal or hepatic disease) is in doubt (see *Alkaline phosphatase isoenzymes,* page 38, for more information). Rarely, low serum alkaline phosphatase levels are associated with hypophosphatasia, and protein or magnesium deficiency.

Post-test care

- If a hematoma develops at the venipuncture site, applying warm soaks eases discomfort.
- Patient may resume a normal diet.

Interfering
factors

- Recent ingestion of vitamin D may increase levels of alkaline phosphatase, because of the effect of vitamin D on osteoblastic activity.
- Recent infusion of albumin prepared from placental venous blood causes extreme increases in serum alkaline phosphatase levels.
- Drugs that influence liver function or cause cholestasis, such as barbiturates, chlorpropamide, oral contraceptives, isoniazid, methyldopa, phenothiazines, phenytoin, and rifampin, can mildly elevate alkaline phosphatase levels; halothane sensitivity may increase levels drastically. Clofibrate decreases alkaline phosphatase levels.

Alkaline phosphatase isoenzymes

Separation of alkaline phosphatase isoenzymes in the laboratory, using heat inactivation, electrophoresis, or chemical means, is sometimes used in place of serum gamma glutamyl transferase, leucine aminopeptidase, or 5′-nucleotidase to differentiate hepatic from skeletal diseases. Sixteen molecularly distinct isoenzyme fractions have been identified electrophoretically in human serum, stimulating continuing controversy about the origins, proportions, and methods of isoenzyme determination. Although the number and concentration of alkaline phosphatase isoenzymes in total serum levels vary with the laboratory separation methods used, the five isoenzymes of greatest clinical significance originate in the liver (includes kidney and bile fractions), bone (may also include bile fraction), intestine, and placenta.

On electrophoresis, the liver isoenzyme usually ranges from 24 to 158 U/L; the bone isoenzyme, from 24 to 146 U/L; and the intestinal fraction — which occurs almost exclusively in individuals with blood group B or O and is markedly elevated 8 hours after a fatty meal — from undetectable to 22 U/L. The placental isoenzyme first appears in the second trimester of pregnancy, accounts for roughly half of all alkaline phosphatase during the third trimester, and drops to normal levels the first month postpartum. Regan, another isoenzyme, resembles the placental isoenzyme and appears in a small percentage of patients with cancer; it may be used as a tumor marker.

- Healing long-bone fractures, age (infants, children, adolescents, and women over age 45), and pregnancy (third trimester) can produce physiologic elevations of alkaline phosphatase levels.
- Hemolysis caused by excessive agitation of the sample or a delay of more than 8 hours in sending the sample to the laboratory may interfere with accurate determination of alkaline phosphatase levels.

Alpha₁-antitrypsin

Alpha₁-antitrypsin is an alpha₁ globulin produced by the liver. It is the major inhibitor of the proteolytic enzymes trypsin and plasmin, which are released by macrophages in the alveoli and by bacteria in the lungs. Inherited deficiencies of alpha₁-antitrypsin are associated with unusually early development of emphysema and with increased incidence of neonatal hepatitis, usually progressing to cirrhosis. Such deficiencies are detectable by serum electrophoresis. Serum levels are estimated nephelometrically with the antihuman alpha₁-antitrypsin.

Purpose
- To detect alpha₁-antitrypsin deficiency in persons with family histories of associated diseases
- To identify alpha₁-antitrypsin deficiency as the cause of early onset emphysema in nonsmokers
- To aid diagnosis of suspected chronic inflammatory disorders
- To aid diagnosis of unexplained cirrhosis and jaundice in children and young adults

Patient preparation
Explain the purpose of the test. Inform the patient that the test requires a blood sample and fasting for 8 hours before the test. Oral contraceptives should be withheld for 24 hours before the test.

Procedure
Perform a venipuncture and collect a blood sample into a *red-top* tube. Handle the sample gently to prevent hemolysis and send it to the laboratory immediately.

Values
Normal values of alpha₁-antitrypsin are 126 to 226 mg/dl.

Implications of results
Deficiency of alpha₁-antitrypsin is associated with early onset emphysema and cirrhosis. Decreased levels of alpha₁-antitrypsin also occur in patients with nephrotic syndrome and malnutrition.

Elevated serum levels of alpha₁-antitrypsin are associated with chronic inflammatory disorders and also may occur during pregnancy, in patients with acute pulmonary infections, and in persons who are taking oral contraceptives, experiencing unusual stress, or exercising strenuously. Elevated levels also occur in rheumatoid arthritis, bacterial infections, vasculitis, and carcinomatosis.

Post-test care
- The patient may resume normal diet and any medications that were discontinued before the test.
- Patients with confirmed deficiencies of alpha₁-antitrypsin require appropriate medical follow-up and genetic counseling.

Interfering
factors

- Falsely elevated values may result from strenuous exercise, stress, or use of oral contraceptives.
- Failure to follow dietary restrictions before the test may influence test results.

Alpha-fetoprotein

Alpha-fetoprotein (AFP) is a glycoprotein produced by fetal tissue and tumors that differentiate from midline embryonic structures. During fetal development, AFP levels in serum and amniotic fluid rise; since this protein crosses the placenta, it also appears in maternal serum. In late stages of pregnancy, AFP concentrations in fetal and maternal serum and in amniotic fluid begin to diminish. During the first year of life, serum AFP levels continue to decline and characteristically persist at a low level thereafter.

High maternal serum AFP levels at 16 to 18 weeks' gestation may suggest fetal neural tube defects, such as spina bifida or anencephaly, but positive confirmation requires amniocentesis and ultrasonography. Other congenital anomalies may also be associated with high maternal serum AFP concentrations. Elevated AFP levels in those persons who aren't pregnant may occur in malignancy, such as hepatocellular carcinoma, or in such nonmalignant conditions as ataxia-telangiectasia; in these conditions, AFP assays are more useful for monitoring response to therapy than for establishing diagnosis.

AFP levels are best determined by enzyme immunoassay on plasma or serum. AFP is not measured alone, but in conjunction with hCG (see Human Chorionic Gonadotropin [hCG], Serum).

Purpose

- To monitor the effectiveness of therapy in malignant conditions, such as hepatomas, testicular and ovarian tumors, and in such nonmalignant conditions as ataxia-telangiectasia
- To screen neural tube defects

Patient
preparation

Explain that this test monitors response to therapy by measuring a special blood protein. Inform the patient that restriction of food, fluids, or medications before the test is not required, that this test requires a blood sample, and that further testing may be needed if levels of this protein are elevated.

Procedure
Perform a venipuncture, and collect the sample in a 7-ml *red-top* tube. Handle the sample gently to prevent hemolysis.

Values
In persons who aren't pregnant, serum AFP values normally are less than 15 ng/ml (µg/L). (See *Alpha-fetoprotein [AFP] values during pregnancy* for more information.)

Implications of results
Elevated maternal serum AFP levels may suggest neural tube defect or other tube anomalies after 14 weeks' gestation. AFP levels rise sharply in approximately 90% of fetuses with anencephaly and in 50% of those with spina bifida. However, definitive diagnosis requires ultrasonography and amniocentesis. High AFP levels may also indicate intrauterine death. Occasionally, such levels indicate other anomalies — for example, duodenal atresia, omphalocele, tetralogy of Fallot, and Turner's syndrome.

Elevated serum AFP levels in persons who aren't pregnant may indicate hepatocellular carcinoma (although low AFP levels don't rule it out) or germ cell tumor of gonadal, retroperitoneal, or mediastinal origin. Serum AFP levels rise in ataxia-telangiectasia and, occasionally, in cancer of the pancreas, the stomach, or the biliary system. Transient modest elevations sometimes occur in nonneoplastic

Alpha-fetoprotein (AFP) values during pregnancy

Gestational age (weeks)	AFP value (ng/ml)
15	33.9
16	37.1
17	40.5
18	45.5
19	55.4
20	68.0
21	68.6

hepatocellular disease, such as acute or chronic hepatitis and alcoholic cirrhosis.

In hepatocellular carcinoma, a gradual decrease in serum AFP levels indicates a favorable response to therapy. In germ cell tumors, serum AFP levels and serum human chorionic gonadotropin levels should be measured concurrently to assess the patient's response to therapy.

Post-test care If a hematoma develops at the venipuncture site, applying warm soaks eases discomfort.

Interfering factors
- Hemolysis caused by excessive agitation of the sample may alter serum AFP levels.
- Multiple pregnancy may cause false-positive test results.

Amebiasis antibody

Entamoeba histolytica antibody, serum

This test detects antibodies to *E. histolytica,* an intestinal parasite, which is the causative pathogen in amebiasis. Although stool examination that reveals cysts or trophozoites is the usual method of detecting amebiasis, a negative stool examination does not necessarily rule it out. Because extraintestinal infections — for example, liver abscess — commonly are not associated with organisms in the stool, this serologic test is often useful.

This test can be performed by indirect hemagglutination, latex agglutination, counterimmunoelectrophoresis, and enzyme-linked immunosorbent assay.

Purpose To aid diagnosis of amebiasis

Patient preparation Explain the purpose of the test and inform the patient that the test requires a blood sample.

Procedure Perform a venipuncture and obtain a 5-ml clotted blood sample.

Findings Normal test result is negative for antibodies to *E. histolytica.*

Implications of results A positive test result may indicate current or past infection, amebic liver abscess, or amebic dysentery. A positive hemagglutination titer of 1:128 or greater indicates active or recent infection; titer of 1:256 to 1:2,048 indicates current infection; titer of 1:32 to 1:64 is an ambiguous result that suggests repeat testing of an additional serum sample. A single positive serologic test result may not rule out infection, and the test may have to be repeated. Titers below 1:32 usually rule out invasive amebiasis, however.

Post-test care If a hematoma develops at the venipuncture site, applying warm soaks eases discomfort.

Interfering factors None

Amino acid screening, plasma

This qualitative test is an effective screen for inborn errors of amino acid metabolism. More than 50 aminoacidopathies are now recognized. They are associated with various genetic disorders that can cause mental retardation, reduced growth rates, and various unexplained symptoms.

Amino acids are the components of all proteins and polypeptides. Certain congenital enzymatic deficiencies interfere with normal metabolism of one or more amino acids and cause accumulation or deficiency of these amino acids. Excessive accumulation of amino acids typically produces overflow aminoacidurias. Congenital abnormalities of the amino acid transport system in the kidneys produce a second group of disorders called renal aminoacidurias.

Purpose To screen for inborn errors of amino acid metabolism

Patient preparation Explain to the parents that this test, which requires a blood sample, helps determine if their child can metabolize amino acids normally. The infant must fast for 4 hours before the test.

Procedure Perform a heelstick, and collect 0.1 ml of blood in a heparinized capillary tube.

Values Normal amino acid values are age dependent. (See *Amino acid normal values,* pages 44 and 45, and *Chromatographic identification of amino acid disorders,* pages 46 and 47.)

Amino acid normal values

Amino acid	Plasma amino acid Normal range (µmol/L)		Urine amino acid Normal range (µmol/L)	
	Children (3 to 16 years)	Adults (> 16 years)	Children (3 to 16 years)	Adults (> 16 years)
Alanine	200 to 450	230 to 510	65 to 190	160 to 690
Alpha-Aminoadipic Acid	Not measured		25 to 78	0 to 165
Alpha-Amino-N-Butyric Acid	8 to 37	15 to 41	7 to 25	0 to 28
Arginine	44 to 120	45 to 130	10 to 25	13 to 64
Asparagine	8 to 37	24 to 79	15 to 40	34 to 100
Aspartic acid	0 to 26	0 to 6	10 to 26	14 to 89
Beta-Alanine	0 to 49	0 to 29	0 to 42	0 to 93
Beta-Aminoiso-butyric Acid	Not measured		25 to 96	10 to 235
Carnosine	Not measured		34 to 220	16 to 125
Citrulline	16 to 32	16 to 55	0 to 13	0 to 11
Cystine	19 to 47	30 to 65	11 to 53	28 to 115
Glutamic acid	32 to 140	18 to 98	13 to 22	27 to 105
Glutamine	420 to 730	390 to 650	150 to 400	300 to 1,040
Glycine	110 to 240	170 to 330	195 to 855	750 to 2,400
Histidine	68 to 120	26 to 120	46 to 725	500 to 1,500
Hydroxyproline	0 to 5	Not measured	Not measured	
Isoleucine	37 to 140	42 to 100	3 to 15	4 to 23
Leucine	70 to 170	66 to 170	9 to 23	20 to 77
Lysine	120 to 290	150 to 220	19 to 140	32 to 290
Methionine	13 to 30	16 to 30	7 to 20	5 to 30

Amino acid normal values *(continued)*				
Amino acid	**Plasma amino acid** Normal range (µmol/L)		**Urine amino acid** Normal range (µmol/L)	
	Children (3 to 16 years)	**Adults (> 16 years)**	**Children (3 to 16 years)**	**Adults (> 16 years)**
1-Methylhistidine	Not measured		41 to 300	68 to 855
3-Methylhistidine	0 to 52	0 to 64	42 to 135	64 to 320
Ornithine	44 to 90	27 to 80	3 to 16	5 to 70
Phenylalanine	26 to 86	41 to 68	20 to 61	36 to 90
Phosphoserine	0 to 12	0 to 12	16 to 34	28 to 95
Phosphoetha-nolamine	0 to 12	0 to 55	24 to 66	17 to 95
Proline	130 to 290	110 to 360	Not measured	
Serine	93 to 150	56 to 140	93 to 210	200 to 695
Taurine	11 to 120	45 to 130	62 to 970	267 to 1,290
Threonine	67 to 150	92 to 240	25 to 100	80 to 320
Tyrosine	26 to 110	45 to 74	30 to 83	38 to 145
Valine	160 to 350	150 to 310	17 to 37	19 to 74

Implications of results The plasma urine amino acid patterns are abnormal in renal aminoacidurias and overflow aminoacidurias.

Total plasma amino acids are increased in aminoacidopathies, diabetes with ketosis, malabsorption, Reyes' syndrome, acute and chronic renal failure, and eclampsia; decreased in adrenal cortical hyperfunction, Huntington's chorea, phlebotomus fever, rheumatoid arthritis, Hartnup disease, fever, and malnutrition.

Post-test care
- If a hematoma develops at the heelstick site, applying warm soaks eases discomfort.
- The infant may resume a normal diet.

Interfering factor Failure to observe restrictions of diet may influence amino acid levels.

(Text continues on page 48.)

Chromatographic identification of amino acid disorders

In chromatography, amino acids migrate into multicolored bands in standard migratory patterns as listed below. When congenital enzyme deficiencies and subsequent metabolic disorders increase plasma and urine amino acid levels, these bands intensify.

Metabolic amino acid disorders

Band number	Amino acids	Phenylketonuria		Maple syrup urine disease		Cystinuria			
		Plasma	Urine	Plasma	Urine	Plasma	Urine		
1	Leucine, isoleucine			+	+				
2	Phenylalanine	+	+						
3	Valine, methionine			+	+				
4	Tryptophan, beta-aminoisobutyric acid								
5	Tyrosine								
6	Proline			+					
7	Alanine, ethanolamine								
8	Threonine, glutamic acid								
9	Homocitrulline, glycine, serine, hydroxyproline, aspartic acid, glutamine, citrulline			+					
10	Homocystine, asparagine								
11	Argininosuccinic acid, histidine, arginine, lysine, ornithine, cystathionine, cystine, cysteine, hydroxylysine						+		

Key: + Increased amino acids in the plasma or urine
Reproduced with permission from *The Bio-Science Handbook,* 14th ed. Van Nuys, Calif.: Bio-Science Enterprises, 1987.

Homocystinuria		Hartnup disease		Arginosuccinicaciduria		Histidinemia		Hyperprolinemia, type A		Citrullinuria	
Plasma	Urine	Plasma	Urine	Plasma	Urine	Plasma	Urine	Plasma	Urine	Plasma	Urine
			+								
			+								
			+								
			+								
			+								
								+	+		
			+				+			+	
							+			+	
	+		+		+			+	+	+	
			+		+	+			+		

Amino acid screening, urine

This test screens for aminoaciduria — elevated urine amino acid levels — a condition that may result from inborn errors of metabolism caused by the absence of specific enzymatic activities. (Normally, up to 200 mg of amino acids may be excreted in the urine in 24 hours [2 mmol/d]). Abnormal metabolism causes an excess of one or more amino acids to appear in plasma and, as the renal threshold is exceeded, in urine. Aminoacidurias may be classified as either primary (overflow) aminoacidopathies or as secondary (renal) aminoacidopathies. The latter type is associated with conditions marked by defective tubular reabsorption from congenital disorders. A defect such as cystinuria may cause one or more amino acids to appear in urine.

To screen newborns, children, and adults for congenital aminoacidurias, plasma or urine specimens may be used. The plasma test is the better indicator of overflow aminoacidurias; urine testing is used to confirm or monitor certain amino acid disorders and to screen for renal aminoacidurias.

Various laboratory techniques are available to screen for aminoacidurias, but chromatography is the preferred method. Positive findings on chromatography can be elaborated by fractionation, showing specific amino acid levels. Testing for specific amino acid levels is also necessary for infants or young children with acidosis, severe vomiting and diarrhea, and abnormal urine odor. Such testing is especially important in newborns, because early diagnosis of certain aminoacidurias may prevent mental retardation by allowing prompt treatment.

Purpose
- To screen for renal aminoacidurias
- To confirm plasma test findings when results of these tests suggest certain overflow aminoacidurias

Patient preparation
Explain to the patient or the parents that this test, which requires a urine specimen, helps detect amino acid disorders, and that additional tests may be necessary. The patient need not restrict food or fluids before the test.

Check the patient's history for drugs that may interfere with test results. If such drugs must be continued, note this on the laboratory slip. (If the patient is a breast-fed infant, record any drugs the mother is receiving.)

Procedure   If the patient is an infant, clean and dry the genital area, attach the collection device securely to prevent leakage, and observe for voiding. Transfer the collected urine — at least 20 ml — to a specimen container. If the patient is an adult or a child, collect a fresh random specimen. Send the specimen to the laboratory immediately.

Values   Normal values are age dependent. (See *Amino acid normal values,* pages 44 and 45.)

Implications of results   Total urine amino acids are increased in viral hepatitis, multiple myeloma, hyperparathyroidism, osteomalacia, galactosemia, cystinosis, Wilson's disease, and Hartnup disease.

   If thin-layer chromatography shows abnormal patterns, blood and 24-hour urine quantitative column chromatography are performed to identify specific amino acid abnormalities and to differentiate overflow and renal aminoacidurias (see *Chromatographic identification of amino acid disorders,* pages 46 and 47).

Post-test care   To prevent skin irritation, remove the collection device carefully from an infant.

Interfering factors
• Failure to send the urine specimen to the laboratory immediately may interfere with the accurate test results.
• Results are invalid in a newborn who has not ingested dietary protein in the 48 hours preceding the test.

Aminoglycoside antibiotics, serum

This quantitative immunoassay directly measures serum levels of aminoglycoside antibiotics to determine therapeutic concentrations and to detect toxic accumulations. Therapeutic levels are also measurable through assay of body fluids, but serum assay is more reliable.

   Aminoglycoside antibiotics that most often requires therapeutic monitoring are: amikacin, gentamicin, kanamycin, netilmicin, and tobramycin.

These drugs are used to treat infections from gram-negative bacilli and gram-positive cocci; resistant strains require high serum levels, with increased potential for ototoxicity, neurotoxicity, and nephrotoxicity. Although these antibiotics are normally excreted unmetabolized by the kidneys, toxic blood levels can damage the kidneys, allowing even higher blood levels to accumulate and produce ototoxicity.

Purpose
- To monitor therapeutic levels of aminoglycoside antibiotics
- To check for toxicity suspected from history or after onset of nephrotoxic symptoms (such as renal failure, proteinuria, oliguria, anuria, elevated serum creatinine and blood urea nitrogen, and low specific gravity and creatinine clearance) or ototoxic or neurotoxic symptoms

Patient preparation
Explain that this test measures blood concentration of antibiotics to help determine the most effective drug dosage. Inform the patient that the test requires a blood sample. Check the patient's recent medication history, noting drug, dosage, and route of administration.

Procedure
Perform a venipuncture, and collect a trough-level or peak-level sample in a 7-ml *red-top* tube. Record the date, time, and administration route of the last dose, and the sample collection time on the laboratory slip.

When monitoring therapeutic levels, observe the same time span between drug administration and sample collection in serial testing.

Send the sample to the laboratory immediately.

Findings
Peak-time, steady-state, and therapeutic and toxic serum levels vary, depending on the antibiotic being administered (see *Aminoglycoside antibiotic blood levels*).

Implications of results
Antibiotic blood levels allow dosage adjustment to maintain effective therapeutic levels and prevent excessive accumulation and toxicity.

Post-test care
If a hematoma develops at the venipuncture site, applying warm soaks eases discomfort.

Aminoglycoside antibiotic blood levels					
Drug	**Peak time**	**Steady state**	**Therapeutic level**	**Toxic peak**	**Toxic trough***
Amikacin	I.M.: 30 minutes to 1 hour I.V.: 15 to 30 minutes	1 to 2 days	8 to 16 mcg/ml	> 35 mcg/ml	> 8 mcg/ml
Gentamicin	I.M.: 30 minutes to 1 hour I.V.: 15 to 30 minutes	1 to 2 days	4 to 10 mcg/ml	> 12 mcg/ml	> 2 mcg/ml
Kanamycin	I.M.: 30 minutes to 1 hour	1 to 2 days	8 to 16 mcg/ml	> 35 mcg/ml	> 8 mcg/ml
Netilmicin	I.M.: 30 minutes to 1 hour I.V.: 15 to 30 minutes	1 to 2 days	0.5 to 10 mcg/ml	> 16 mcg/ml	> 4 mcg/ml
Tobramycin	I.M.: 30 minutes to 1 hour I.V.: 15 to 30 minutes	1 to 2 days	4 to 8 mcg/ml	> 12 mcg/ml	> 2 mcg/ml

*Trough toxic levels can be below therapeutic levels because of the nephrotoxic nature of aminoglycoside antibiotics.

Interfering factors   None

Amitriptyline and nortriptyline, serum

Amitriptyline and nortriptyline are tricyclic antidepressants (TCAs) used in the treatment of endogenous depression. These drugs inhibit the reuptake of the neurotransmitters norepinephrine and serotonin at the synaptic cleft, and their mechanism of action is thought to be related to the potentiation of synaptic transmission in the central nervous system. Because amitriptyline is metabolized to nortriptyline, administration of amitriptyline results in the presence of both drugs in serum. Reverse conversion does not occur, so patients taking nortriptyline will have only this drug present in serum.

Monitoring the serum levels of TCAs has proved useful because relief of depressive symptoms is a subjective evaluation and clinical studies have reported a superior response to these drugs in patients having serum levels within a defined therapeutic range. Evidence suggests a therapeutic window for these TCAs, particularly nortriptyline, in that patients with serum levels maintained either below or above the therapeutic range tend to show poor response as compared with patients maintained within the therapeutic range. Monitoring serum levels is also useful because overdose with TCAs is frequently associated with seizure activity and possible cardiac toxicity.

Amitriptyline and nortriptyline are most commonly measured in serum by enzyme immunoassay or high performance liquid chromatography.

Purpose
- To monitor drug dosage for optimal therapeutic efficacy
- To assess patient compliance
- To help assess the extent of toxicity in overdose situations

Patient preparation
On average, at least 7 days of treatment with amitriptyline or nortriptyline are required to achieve a steady-state serum level. Monitoring serum levels before the attainment of steady state is not recommended because the results cannot be interpreted. For the same reason, any change in the total daily dosage requires at least 7 days of therapy to establish a new steady state. For patients at steady state on a single daily dosage, samples should be collected between 10 and 14 hours after the last dose. For patients on a divided daily dosage, samples should be collected 4 to 6 hours after the last dose.

Describe the purpose of the test. Inform the patient that the test requires a blood sample, but does not require restriction of food before the test.

Procedure
Perform a venipuncture and collect the blood sample in a 7-ml *red-top* tube. Collection tubes containing a gel separator should not be used. Avoid hemolysis because these drugs are concentrated in erythrocytes and hemolyzed specimens may yield spuriously elevated results. Testing is performed on serum but heparinized plasma is also suitable.

Amitriptyline and nortriptyline are stable in serum for at least 5 days at room temperature and for extended periods when refrigerated at 39.2° F (4° C).

Values   For patients taking amitriptyline, the therapeutic range for the total of amitriptyline plus nortriptyline is 75 to 225 ng/ml (270 to 810 nmol/L).

For patients taking nortriptyline, the therapeutic range is 50 to 150 ng/ml (190 to 540 nmol/L).

A total tricyclic level greater than 450 ng/ml (1,700 nmol/L) is usually associated with toxicity; values greater than 1,000 ng/ml (3,700 nmol/L) are usually associated with serious toxicity.

Implications of results   Subtherapeutic serum levels are associated with an increased probability of therapeutic failure. Patients with steady-state levels in the therapeutic range who have not responded after 3 to 4 weeks of therapy may be candidates for a different antidepressant drug.

Post-test care   If a hematoma develops at the venipuncture site, applying warm soaks eases discomfort.

Interfering factors
- Collection of the sample before attainment of steady state interferes with accurate determination of test results.
- Hemolysis caused by excessive agitation of the sample may yield spuriously elevated results.

Ammonia, plasma

This test measures plasma levels of ammonia, a nonprotein nitrogen compound. Most ammonia is absorbed from the intestinal tract, where it is produced by bacterial action on urea and protein; a smaller amount is produced in the kidneys from hydrolysis of glutamine. Normally, the body converts ammonia to urea in the liver for excretion by the kidneys. In liver diseases, ammonia accumulates in the blood. Therefore, plasma ammonia levels may help indicate the severity of hepatocellular damage.

Purpose
- To help monitor the progression of severe hepatic disease and the effectiveness of therapy
- To recognize impending or established hepatic coma

Patient preparation	Explain that this test evaluates liver function. Inform the conscious patient that the test requires an overnight fast because protein intake may influence test results, and that the test requires a blood sample. Check the patient's medication history for use of antibiotics and other drugs that may influence ammonia levels.
Procedure	Perform a venipuncture, and collect the sample in a 10-ml *green-top* (heparinized) tube. Handle the sample gently to prevent hemolysis. Pack it in ice, and send it to the laboratory immediately. Because the test must be performed within 20 minutes, notify the laboratory before performing the venipuncture so that preliminary preparations can begin before you send the sample.
Values	Normally, plasma ammonia levels are less than 50 mcg/dl (35 µmol/L).
Implications of results	Elevated plasma ammonia levels are common in severe hepatic disease and hepatic coma caused by cirrhosis or acute hepatitis. Elevated ammonia levels occur also in Reye's syndrome, severe congestive heart failure, GI hemorrhage, erythroblastosis fetalis, pericarditis, and leukemia.
Post-test care	• Make sure bleeding has stopped before removing pressure from the venipuncture site because hepatic disease can prolong bleeding time. If a hematoma develops, applying warm soaks eases discomfort. • Watch for signs of impending or established hepatic coma if levels are high.
Interfering factors	• Acetazolamide, antibiotics, thiazides, ammonium salts, or furosemide raise ammonia levels, as can total parenteral nutrition or a portacaval shunt. Lactulose, neomycin, and kanamycin depress ammonia levels. • Hemolysis caused by excessive agitation of the sample may alter test results.

Amniotic fluid analysis

Amniocentesis is the transabdominal needle aspiration of 10 to 20 ml of amniotic fluid for laboratory analysis. Such analysis can detect several birth defects (especially Down's syndrome), identify increased risk of spina bifida, determine fetal maturity, detect hemolytic disease of the newborn, and, through karyotyping, detect gender and chromosomal abnormalities. This test can be performed only when the amniotic fluid level reaches 150 ml, usually after the 16th week of pregnancy.

Amniotic fluid reflects important metabolic changes in the fetus, the placenta, or the mother. It protects the fetus from external trauma, allows fetal movement, and provides an even body temperature and limited source of protein (10% to 15%) for the fetus. Although the origin of amniotic fluid is uncertain, it may arise as a water-permeable transudate from fetal skin, or as a dialysate from the maternal serum through the fetal membranes into the amniotic cavity. Its original composition is essentially the same as that of interstitial fluid. As the fetus matures, however, the amniotic fluid becomes progressively more diluted with hypotonic fetal urine.

One of the chief differences between amniotic fluid and maternal plasma during intrauterine development is the amniotic fluid's relatively high levels of uric acid, urea, and creatinine. The volume of amniotic fluid steadily rises from 50 ml at the end of the first trimester to an average of 1,000 ml near term; at 40 weeks' gestation, the volume decreases to 700 to 800 ml.

Amniocentesis is indicated during pregnancy associated with advanced maternal age (over 35); family history of genetic, chromosomal, or neural tube defects; increase in maternal serum alpha-fetoprotein; or previous miscarriage. Adverse effects from this test are rare; potential risks include spontaneous abortion, trauma to the fetus or placenta, bleeding, premature labor, infection, and Rh sensitization from fetal bleeding into the maternal circulation. However, because such complications are possible, amniocentesis is contraindicated as a general screening test. Abnormal test results or failure of the tissue cultures to grow may necessitate repetition of the test.

Purpose
- To detect fetal abnormalities, particularly chromosomal, and to determine risk of neural tube defects
- To detect hemolytic disease of the newborn
- To diagnose metabolic disorders, amino acid disorders, and mucopolysaccharidoses

- To determine fetal age and maturity, especially pulmonary maturity
- To assess fetal health by detecting the presence of meconium or blood, or measuring amniotic levels of estriol and fetal thyroid hormone
- To identify fetal sex when one or both parents are carriers of a sex-linked disorder

Patient preparation

Describe the procedure to the patient, and explain that this test detects fetal abnormalities. Assess her understanding of the test, and answer any questions she may have. Inform her that she needn't restrict food or fluids before the test. Tell her the test requires a specimen of amniotic fluid. Advise her that normal test results can't guarantee a normal fetus because some fetal disorders are undetectable.

Make sure the patient has signed a consent form. Explain that she'll feel a stinging sensation when the local anesthetic is injected. Reassure the patient before and during the test and reassure her that adverse effects are rare. Just before the test, ask her to void to minimize the risk of puncturing the bladder and aspirating urine instead of amniotic fluid.

Equipment

Sponge forceps, 70% alcohol or povidone-iodine solution, $2'' \times 2''$ gauze pads, local anesthetic (1% lidocaine), 25G sterile needle, 3-ml syringe, 20G sterile spinal needle with stylet, 10-ml syringe, amber or foil-covered sterile 10-ml test tube

Procedure

After determining fetal and placental position, usually through palpation and ultrasonic visualization, a pool of amniotic fluid is located. Following skin preparation with an antiseptic and alcohol, 1 ml of 1% lidocaine is injected with a 25G needle. A 20G sterile spinal needle with stylet is inserted into the amniotic cavity and the stylet is withdrawn. After a 10-ml syringe is attached to the needle, the fluid is aspirated and placed in an amber or foil-covered test tube. After the needle is withdrawn, an adhesive bandage is placed over the needle insertion site. The specimen is then sent to the laboratory.

Precautions

Instruct the patient to fold her hands behind her head during the test to prevent her from accidentally touching the sterile field and contaminating it.

Findings

Normal amniotic fluid is clear but may contain white flecks of vernix caseosa when the fetus is near term. For detailed analysis of the appearance and components of amniotic fluid, see *Analysis of amniotic fluid,* page 58.

Implications of results

Blood in amniotic fluid is usually of maternal origin and doesn't indicate abnormality. However, it does inhibit cell growth and changes the level of other amniotic fluid constituents.

Large amounts of *bilirubin,* a breakdown product of red blood cells, may indicate hemolytic disease of the newborn. Normally, the bilirubin level rises from the 14th to the 24th week of pregnancy, then declines as the fetus matures, essentially reaching zero at term. Testing for bilirubin usually isn't performed until the 26th week because that's the earliest time successful therapy for Rh sensitization can begin. Bilirubin level is determined by spectrophotometric measurement of the optic density of the amniotic fluid. The deviation of the scan at 450 mµ represents the bilirubin peak.

Meconium, a semisolid viscous material found in the fetal GI tract, consists of mucopolysaccharides, desquamated cells, vernix, hair, and cholesterol. Meconium passes into the amniotic fluid when hypoxia causes fetal distress and relaxation of the anal sphincter. Meconium is a normal finding in breech presentation. Meconium in the amniotic fluid produces a peak of 410 mµ on the spectrophotometric analysis. However, serial amniocentesis may show a clearing of meconium over a 2- to 3-week period. If meconium is present during labor, the newborn's nose and throat require thorough cleaning to prevent meconium aspiration.

Creatinine, a product of fetal urine, increases in the amniotic fluid as the fetal kidneys mature. Generally, the creatinine value exceeds 2 mg/100 ml (150 µmol/L) in a mature fetus.

Alpha-fetoprotein is a fetal alpha globulin produced first in the yolk sac and, later, in the parenchymal cells of the liver and GI tract. Fetal serum levels of alpha-fetoprotein are about 150 times more than amniotic fluid levels; maternal serum levels are far less than amniotic fluid levels. High amniotic fluid levels indicate neural tube defects, but the alpha-fetoprotein level may remain normal if the defect is small and closed. Elevated alpha-fetoprotein level may occur in multiple pregnancy; in disorders such as omphalocele, congenital nephrosis, eso-

Analysis of amniotic fluid

Test	Normal findings	Fetal implications of abnormal findings
Color	Clear, with white flecks of vernix caseosa in a mature fetus	Blood of maternal origin is usually harmless. "Port wine" fluid may indicate abruptio placentae. Fetal blood may indicate damage to the fetal, placental, or umbilical cord vessels.
Bilirubin	Absent at term	High levels indicate hemolytic disease of the newborn in isoimmunized pregnancy.
Meconium	Absent (except in breech presentation)	Presence indicates fetal hypotension or distress.
Creatinine	More than 2 mg/100 ml in a mature fetus	Decrease may indicate immature fetus (less than 37 weeks).
L/S ratio	More than 2 generally indicates fetal pulmonary maturity	Less than 2 indicates pulmonary immaturity and subsequent risk of respiratory distress syndrome.
Phosphatidylglycerol	Present	Absence indicates pulmonary immaturity.
Glucose	Less than 45 mg/100 ml	Excessive increase at or near term indicates hypertrophied fetal pancreas and subsequent neonatal hypoglycemia.
Alpha-fetoprotein	Variable, depending on gestational age and laboratory technique. Highest concentration (about 18.5 mcg/ml) occurs at 13 to 14 weeks)	Inappropriate increases indicate such neural tube defects as spina bifida or anencephaly, impending fetal death, congenital nephrosis, or contamination by fetal blood.
Bacteria	Absent	Presence indicates chorioamnionitis.
Chromosome	Normal karyotype	Abnormal karyotype may indicate fetal chromosome disorder.
Acetycholinesterase	Absent	Presence may indicate neural tube defects, exomphalos, or other serious malformations.

phageal or duodenal atresia, cystic fibrosis, exomphalos, Turner's syndrome, and fetal bladder neck obstruction with hydronephrosis; and in impending fetal death.

Estrone, estradiol, estriol, and *estriol conjugates* appear in amniotic fluid in varying amounts. Estriol, the most prevalent estrogen, increases from 26 ng/ml (100 nmol/L during the 16th to 20th weeks) to almost 1,000 ng/ml (3,700 nmol/L) at term. Severe erythroblastosis fetalis decreases the estriol level.

Blood in the amniotic fluid occurs in about 10% of amniocenteses and results from a traumatic tap. If the origin is maternal, the blood generally has not special significance; however, "port wine" fluid may be a sign of abruptio placentae, whereas blood of fetal origin may indicate damage to the fetal, placental, or umbilical cord vessels by the amniocentesis needle.

The Type II cells lining the fetal lung alveoli produce *lecithin* slowly in early pregnancy, and then markedly increase production around the 35th week.

The *sphingomyelin* level parallels that of lecithin until the 35th week, when it gradually decreases. Measuring the ratio of lecithin to sphingomyelin (L/S ratio) confirms fetal pulmonary maturity (L/S ratio greater than 2) or suggests a risk of respiratory distress (L/S ratio less than 2). However, fetal respiratory distress may develop in the fetus of a patient with diabetes, even though the L/S ratio is greater than 2, a level usually indicative of pulmonary maturity.

Phosphatidylglycerol levels are present with pulmonary maturity; *phosphatidylinositol* levels decrease. Measuring *glucose* levels in the fluid can aid in assessing glucose control in the patient with diabetes, but this isn't done routinely. A level greater than 45 mg/100 ml (2.5 mmol/L) indicates poor maternal and fetal control. *Insulin* levels normally increase slightly from the 27th to the 40th week but increase sharply (up to 27 times normal) in a patient with poorly controlled diabetes.

Elevated acetylcholinesterase levels may occur with neural tube defects, exomphalos, and other serious malformations.

When the mother carries an *X-linked disorder,* determination of fetal sex is important. If chromosome karyotyping identifies a male fetus, there's a

50% chance he'll be affected; a female fetus won't be affected but has a 50% chance of being a carrier.

Post-test care   Monitor fetal heart rate and maternal vital signs every 15 minutes for at least 30 minutes. If the patient feels faint or nauseated, or sweats profusely, position her on the left side to counteract uterine pressure on the vena cava. Before the patient is discharged, instruct her to watch for and immediately report abdominal pain or cramping, chills, fever, vaginal bleeding or leakage of serous vaginal fluid, fetal hyperactivity, or unusual fetal lethargy.

Interfering factors

- Failure to place the fluid specimen in an appropriate amber or foil-covered tube may result in abnormally low bilirubin levels.
- Blood or meconium in the fluid adversely affects the L/S ratio. Maternal blood in the fluid may lower creatinine levels. Fetal blood in the fluid specimen invalidates the alpha-fetoprotein results because even small amounts of fetal blood (50 µliter/10 ml [5 ml/L]) can double alpha-fetoprotein concentrations.
- Several disorders that are not associated with pregnancy (including infectious mononucleosis, cirrhosis, hepatic cancer, teratoma, endodermal sinus tumor, gastric carcinoma, pancreatic carcinoma, and subacute hereditary tyrosinemia) can cause increased alpha-fetoprotein levels.
- Collection of the specimen in a plastic disposable syringe can be toxic to amniotic fluid cells.

Amphetamines, urine

This quantitative analysis measures the urine levels of amphetamine, dextroamphetamine, methamphetamine, and phendimetrazine — sympathomimetic drugs that stimulate the medullary respiratory center, cerebral cortex, and reticular activating system. Serum concentrations of these drugs are usually too small to measure toxic levels. Laboratory methods for quantitative testing of urine amphetamines consist of enzyme-multiplied immunoassay technique or gas chromatography; for screening, thin-layer chromatography.

Purpose

- To monitor therapeutic levels of amphetamines
- To determine amphetamine toxicity suspected from history or after onset of symptoms

Urine amphetamine levels		
Drug	**Therapeutic**	**Toxic**
Amphetamine	2 to 3 mcg/ml	> 30 mcg/ml
Dextroamphetamine	1 to 1.5 mcg/ml	> 15 mcg/ml
Methamphetamine	3 to 5 mcg/ml	> 40 mcg/ml
Phendimetrazine	5 to 30 mcg/ml	> 50 mcg/ml

- To confirm the presence of amphetamines for medicolegal purposes

Patient preparation Explain that this test detects the presence or measures the levels of amphetamines in the body and that the test requires a urine specimen. If the test is being performed for medicolegal purposes, make sure the patient or responsible family member has signed a consent form. Check the patient's recent medication history.

Procedure Collect a random urine specimen. Seal the container to prevent air contamination, and send the specimen to the laboratory immediately or refrigerate it. For a medicolegal test, observe appropriate precautions.

Values Therapeutic and toxic levels vary depending on the amphetamine being measured (see *Urine amphetamine levels*).

Implications of results Quantitative analysis of serum amphetamine levels provides a basis for regulation of therapeutic dosage and for detoxification.

Presence of nonprescribed amphetamines has medicolegal implications.

Post-test care None

Interfering factor The rate at which amphetamines are excreted depends on urine Ph: acid urine increases the rate of excretion; alkaline urine decreases it.

Amylase, serum

Alpha-amylase (amylase), synthesized primarily in the pancreas and the salivary glands, is secreted into the GI tract. This enzyme helps digest starch and glycogen in the mouth, stomach, and intestine. In cases of suspected acute pancreatic disease, measurement of serum or urine amylase is the most important laboratory test.

More than 20 methods of measuring serum amylase exist, with different ranges of normal values. Unfortunately, values can't always be converted to a standard measurement. The method described here reports serum amylase in U/L.

Purpose
- To diagnose acute pancreatitis
- To distinguish between acute pancreatitis and other causes of abdominal pain that require immediate surgery
- To evaluate possible pancreatic injury caused by abdominal trauma or surgery

Patient preparation
Explain that this test, which requires a blood sample, helps assess pancreatic function. Inform the patient that he needn't fast before the test, but must abstain from alcohol. Withhold drugs that may elevate amylase levels, as appropriate. If these must be continued, note this on the laboratory slip.

Procedure
Perform a venipuncture, and collect the sample in a 7-ml *red-top* tube. Handle the sample gently to prevent hemolysis.

Precautions
If the patient has severe abdominal pain, draw the sample before diagnostic or therapeutic intervention. For accurate results, it's important to obtain an early sample.

Values
Serum levels range from 35 to 115 U/L.

Implications of results
Highest amylase levels occur 4 to 12 hours after onset of acute pancreatitis, then drop to normal in 48 to 72 hours. Determination of urine levels should follow normal serum amylase results, to rule out pancreatitis. Moderate serum elevations may accompany obstruction of the common bile duct, the pancreatic duct, or the ampulla of Vater; pancreatic injury from perforated peptic ulcer; pancreatic cancer; acute salivary gland disease; ectopic pregnan-

cy; peritonitis; and ovarian and lung cancers. Impaired renal function may raise serum levels.

Levels may be slightly elevated in a patient who is asymptomatic or who is responding unusually to therapy. An amylase fractionation test helps determine the source of the amylase and aids selection of additional tests.

Depressed levels can occur in chronic pancreatitis, pancreatic cancer, cirrhosis, hepatitis, and toxemia of pregnancy.

Post-test care
- If a hematoma develops at the venipuncture site, applying warm soaks eases discomfort.
- The patient may resume medications discontinued before the test.

Interfering factors
- The following conditions may produce false-positive test results:
  — ingestion of ethyl alcohol in large amounts; certain drugs, such as aminosalicylic acid, asparaginase, azathioprine, corticosteroids, cyproheptadine, narcotic analgesics, oral contraceptives, rifampin, sulfasalazine, or thiazide and loop diuretics
  — recent peripancreatic surgery, perforated ulcer or intestine, or abscess
  — spasm of the sphincter of Oddi or, rarely, macroamylasemia
  — coughing, sneezing, or talking near an open collection tube (saliva contains amylase).
- Hemolysis caused by excessive agitation of the sample may alter test results.

Amylase, urine

Amylase is a starch-splitting enzyme produced primarily in the pancreas and salivary glands, usually secreted into the alimentary tract, and absorbed into the blood; small amounts of amylase are also absorbed into the blood directly from these organs. Following glomerular filtration, amylase is excreted in the urine. In the presence of adequate renal function, serum and urine levels usually rise in tandem. However, within 2 or 3 days of onset of acute pancreatitis, serum amylase levels fall to normal, but elevated urine amylase persists for 7 to 10 days. Urine amylase may be elevated when serum amylase urine levels are normal, and the reverse is also true.

Purpose
- To diagnose acute pancreatitis when serum amylase levels are normal or borderline
- To aid diagnosis of chronic pancreatitis and salivary gland disorders

Patient preparation

Explain that this test evaluates the function of the pancreas and the salivary glands. Inform the patient that the test does not require restriction of food or fluids but requires urine collection for 2 or 24 hours. Encourage the patient to drink water during the test unless fluid intake is restricted; decreased urine output could reduce urine amylase levels. Evaluate urine output for 8 to 24 hours before and after the test.

Teach the patient how to collect a timed specimen. For example, instruct the patient not to contaminate the specimen with toilet tissue or stool, and be sure to collect all properly voided urine. Ensure that precise starting and ending times are recorded both on the specimen label and on the chart.

Withhold morphine, meperidine, codeine, pentazocine, bethanechol, thiazide diuretics, indomethacin, and alcohol, as appropriate, for 24 hours before the test. If these medications must be continued, note this on the laboratory slip.

If the female patient is menstruating, the test may have to be rescheduled.

Procedure

Collect a 2- or 24-hour specimen. Cover and refrigerate the specimen during the collection period. If the patient is catheterized, keep the collection bag on ice. Send the specimens to the laboratory immediately when the test is completed.

Values

Because urine amylase is reported in various units of measure, values differ among laboratories. For example, the Mayo Clinic reports urinary excretion of 10 to 80 amylase units/hour (0 to 17 U/hour) as normal.

Implications of results

Elevated amylase levels occur in acute pancreatitis; obstruction of the pancreatic duct, intestines, or salivary duct; carcinoma of the head of the pancreas; mumps; acute injury of the spleen; renal disease, with impaired absorption; perforated peptic or duodenal ulcers; and gallbladder disease.

Depressed levels occur in chronic pancreatitis, cachexia, alcoholism, liver cancer, cirrhosis, hepatitis, and hepatic abscess.

Post-test care　None

Interfering factors
- Heavy bacterial contamination of the specimen or blood in the urine may interfere with test results.
- Salivary amylase in the urine, caused by coughing or talking over the sample, may raise urine amylase levels.
- Failure to collect all urine during the test period and improper storage of the specimen may alter test results.
- Ingestion of morphine, meperidine, codeine, pentazocine, bethanechol, thiazide diuretics, indomethacin, or alcohol within 24 hours of the test may raise urine amylase levels. Fluorides may lower urine amylase levels.

Androstenedione

This test helps identify the causes of various disorders related to altered estrogen levels. Androstenedione, secreted by the adrenal cortex and the gonads, is converted to estrone (an estrogen of relatively low biologic activity) by adipose tissue and the liver. In premenopausal women, the amount of estrogen derived from androstenedione is relatively small compared with the amount of the more potent estrogen, estradiol, secreted by the ovaries. Usually, estrogen derived from androstenedione doesn't interfere with gonadotropin feedback during the menstrual cycle. But in such conditions as obesity, increased adrenal production of androstenedione or increased conversion of androstenedione to estrone may interfere with normal feedback, causing menstrual irregularities.

In children and postmenopausal women, estrone is a major source of estrogen. Increased androstenedione production or increased conversion to estrone may induce premature sexual development in children; and renewed ovarian stimulation, endometriosis, bleeding, and polycystic ovaries in postmenopausal women. In men, overproduction of androstenedione may cause feminizing signs, such as gynecomastia.

Purpose	To aid in determining the cause of gonadal dysfunction, menstrual or menopausal irregularities, and premature sexual development
Patient preparation	Explain that this test, which requires a blood sample, helps determine the cause of the patient's symptoms. If indicated, explain that the test should be done 1 week before or after her menstrual period and that it may have to be repeated. Withhold steroid and pituitary-based hormones. If these must be continued, note this on the laboratory slip.
Procedure	Perform a venipuncture, and collect a serum sample in a 10-ml *red-top* tube. (Collect a plasma sample in a *green-top* tube. If a plasma sample is taken, refrigerate it or place it on ice.) Record the patient's age, sex, and (if appropriate) phase of menstrual cycle on the laboratory slip, and send the specimen to the laboratory immediately. Handle the sample gently to prevent hemolysis.
Values	Premenopausal females: 0.6 to 3 ng/ml (2 to 10 nmol/L); postmenopausal females: 0.3 to 8 ng/ml (1 to 30 nmol/L); males: 0.9 to 1.7 ng/ml (3 to 6 nmol/L).
Implications of results	Elevated androstenedione levels are associated with Stein-Levanthal syndrome; Cushing's syndrome; ovarian, testicular, or adrenocortical tumors; ectopic corticotropin-producing tumors; late-onset congenital adrenal hyperplasia; and ovarian stromal hyperplasia. Elevated levels result in increased estrone levels, causing premature sexual development (children); menstrual irregularities (premenopausal women); bleeding, endometriosis, or polycystic ovaries (post-menopausal women); or feminizing signs, such as gynecomastia (men). Decreased levels occur in hypogonadism.
Post-test care	• If a hematoma develops at the venipuncture site, applying warm soaks eases discomfort. • The patient may resume medications discontinued before the test.
Interfering factors	• Hemolysis caused by excessive agitation of the sample may affect test results. • Ingestion of steroids or pituitary hormones may alter test results.

Angiotensin-converting enzyme

Angiotensin-converting enzyme (ACE) is found in high concentrations in lung capillaries and in lesser concentrations in blood vessels and kidney tissue. Its primary function is to help regulate arterial pressure by converting angiotensin I to angiotensin II, a powerful vasoconstrictor.

This test, which measures serum levels of ACE, is primarily used to diagnose sarcoidosis because of the high correlation between elevated serum ACE levels and this disease. Presumably, elevated serum levels reflect macrophage activity. This test also monitors response to treatment in sarcoidosis and helps confirm diagnosis of Gaucher's disease and Hansen's disease.

Purpose
- To aid diagnosis of sarcoidosis, especially pulmonary sarcoidosis
- To monitor response to therapy in sarcoidosis
- To help confirm Gaucher's disease or Hansen's disease

Patient preparation
Explain that this test helps diagnose sarcoidosis, Gaucher's disease, or Hansen's disease, or that it checks response to treatment for sarcoidosis. Inform the patient that the test requires fasting for 12 hours and a blood sample. If the patient is under age 20, the test may be postponed.

Procedure
Perform a venipuncture and collect the sample in a 7-ml *red-top* tube (a *green-top* tube may be required, depending on the laboratory method used). Note the patient's age on the laboratory slip. Avoid using a *lavender-top* tube or contaminating the sample with EDTA, because this can decrease ACE levels, altering test results.

Precautions
- Handle the collection tube gently to prevent hemolysis.
- Send the sample to the laboratory immediately, or freeze the sample and place it on dry ice until the test can be performed.

Values
In the colorimetric assay, normal values for serum ACE range from 18 to 67 U/L for patients over age 20. (Patients under age 20 have increased ACE lev-

els and their normal range is not established; therefore, they are not usually tested.)

Implications of results

Elevated serum ACE levels may indicate sarcoidosis, Gaucher's disease, or Hansen's disease, but results must be correlated with the patient's clinical condition. In some patients, elevated ACE levels may result from hyperthyroidism, diabetic retinopathy, and liver diseases.

Serum ACE levels decline as the patient responds to steroid or prednisone therapy for sarcoidosis.

Post-test care

If a hematoma develops at the venipuncture site, applying warm soaks eases discomfort.

Interfering factors

• Use of a *lavender-top* collection tube or other EDTA contamination can decrease ACE levels.
• Hemolysis caused by excessive agitation of the sample may interfere with accurate determination of ACE levels.
• Failure to fast before the test may cause significant lipemia of the sample, which may interfere with accurate test measurement.
• Failure to send the sample to the laboratory immediately or to freeze it and place it on dry ice may cause enzyme degradation and yield artificially low ACE levels.

Anion gap

The anion gap reflects serum anion-cation balance and helps distinguish types of metabolic acidosis. This test measures the difference between sodium (Na^+) and potassium (K^+) concentrations (the measured cations), and the sum of chloride (Cl^-) and bicarbonate (HCO_3^-) (the measured anions) for a quick calculation based on a simple physical principle: Because total concentrations of cations and anions are normally equal, thereby maintaining electrical neutrality in serum, the difference (gap) predominantly reflects the concentration of unmeasured anions. These are contributed by sulfates, phosphates, ketone bodies, lactic acid, and proteins.

An increased anion gap indicates an increase in one or more of these unmeasured anions, which may occur with acidoses characterized by excessive organic or inorganic acids, such as lactic acidosis or ketoacidosis.

A normal anion gap occurs in hyperchloremic acidoses, renal tubular acidosis, and severe bicarbonate-wasting conditions, such as biliary or pancreatic fistulas and poorly functioning ileal loops.

Purpose
- To distinguish types of metabolic acidosis
- To monitor renal function and I.V. total parenteral nutrition

Patient preparation
Explain the purpose of the test and inform the patient that the test requires a blood sample.

Check the patient's history for recent use of drugs (such as diuretics, corticosteroids, and antihypertensives) that may influence sodium, chloride, or bicarbonate blood levels. If these drugs must be continued, note this on the laboratory slip.

Procedure
Perform a venipuncture, and collect the sample in a 10- to 15-ml *red-top* tube. Handle the sample gently to prevent hemolysis.

Values
Normal values are 8 to 16 mEq/liter (mmol/L), using the formula $Na^+ - (Cl^- + HCO_3^-)$; normal values are 10 to 20 mEq/liter (mmol/L), using the formula $(Na^+ + K^+) - (Cl^- + HCO_3^-)$.

Implications of results
A normal anion gap doesn't rule out metabolic acidosis. When acidosis results from loss of bicarbonate in the urine or other body fluids, renal reabsorption of sodium promotes retention of chloride, and the anion gap remains unchanged. Thus, metabolic acidosis resulting from excessive chloride levels is known as a *normal anion gap acidosis*. Metabolic acidosis with a *normal anion gap* (8 to 14 mEq/liter) occurs with conditions characterized by loss of bicarbonate. The hypokalemic form of acidosis is caused by renal tubular acidosis, diarrhea, or ureteral diversions. The hyperkalemic form of acidosis is caused by acidifying agents (for example, NH_4Cl, HCl), renal diseases such as hydronephrosis, amyloidosis, nephritis, or sickle cell nephropathy.

When acidosis results from accumulation of metabolic acids — as occurs in lactic acidosis, for example — the anion gap increases (above 14 mEq/liter (mmol/L) with the increase in unmeasured anions. Metabolic acidosis caused by such accumulation is known as a *high anion gap acidosis*.

Metabolic acidosis with an *increased anion gap* (greater than 14 mEq/liter) occurs with conditions characterized by accumulation of organic acids, sulfates, or phosphates, such as renal failure; ketoacidosis caused by starvation, diabetes mellitus, or alcohol; lactic acidosis; or toxin ingestion, including salicylates, methanol, ethylene glycol (antifreeze), or paraldehyde.

Because the anion gap only determines the total anion-cation balance, it doesn't necessarily reflect abnormal values for individual electrolytes. Further investigation and diagnostic tests are usually necessary to determine the specific cause of metabolic acidosis.

A decreased anion gap (below 8 mEq/liter [μmol/L]) is rare. However, it may occur with hypermagnesemia and with paraproteinemic states, such as multiple myeloma and Waldenström's macroglobulinemia.

Post-test care
- If a hematoma develops at the venipuncture site, applying warm soaks eases discomfort.
- The patient may resume medications discontinued before the test.

Interfering factors
- Diuretics, lithium, chlorpropamide, and vasopressin suppress serum sodium, possibly decreasing the anion gap; corticosteroids and antihypertensives elevate serum sodium and may increase the anion gap.
- Salicylates, paraldehyde, methicillin, dimercaprol, ammonium chloride, acetazolamide, ethylene glycol, and methyl alcohol decrease serum bicarbonate, possibly increasing the anion gap; corticotropin, cortisone, mercurial or chlorthiazide diuretics, and excessive ingestion of alkalis or licorice elevate serum bicarbonate and may decrease the anion gap.
- Ammonium chloride, cholestyramine, boric acid, oxyphenbutazone, phenylbutazone, and excessive I.V. infusion of sodium chloride may elevate serum chloride and possibly decrease the anion gap.
- Thiazides, furosemide, ethacrynic acid, bicarbonates, or prolonged I.V. infusion of dextrose 5% in water can lower serum chloride and may increase the anion gap.
- Iodine absorption from wounds packed with povidone-iodine, or excessive use of magnesium-containing antacids (especially by patients with

renal failure) may cause a spuriously low anion gap.
- Hemolysis caused by excessive agitation of the sample may interfere with accurate determination of test results.

Antiarrhythmic drugs, serum

This quantitative test is performed to monitor antiarrhythmic therapy, because of a narrow margin of safety between therapeutic and toxic serum levels of antiarrhythmic drugs. Depending on the drug being measured and the laboratory performing the assay, the analytic method used can be high-performance liquid chromatography, gas-liquid chromatography, spectrofluorometry, or enzyme-multiplied immunoassay technique.

Purpose
- To monitor therapeutic levels of antiarrhythmic drugs
- To check for toxicity suspected from history or after onset of symptoms

Patient preparation
Explain that this test helps determine the most effective drug dosage. Inform the patient that the test requires a blood sample and that he needn't restrict food or fluids before the test. Check the patient's history for recent use of other drugs.

Procedure
Perform a venipuncture, collecting either a trough-level or peak-level sample, as appropriate, in the tube designated by the testing laboratory. Record the date and time of the last drug dose and the time of sample collection on the laboratory slip.

Observe the same time span between drug administration and sample collection for each test in the series.

If the patient is receiving quinidine, also note the use of acetazolamide, antacids, or sodium bicarbonate on the laboratory slip; if the patient is receiving lidocaine, note the use of barbiturates or phenytoin.

Handle the sample gently to prevent hemolysis, and send it to the laboratory immediately.

Values
Peak-time, steady-state, and therapeutic and toxic serum levels depend on the specific antiarrhythmic drug and on the route of administration (see *Antiarrhythmic blood levels,* page 72).

Antiarrhythmic blood levels

Drug	Peak time	Steady state	Therapeutic level	Toxic level
Disopyramide	P.O.: 2 hours	25 to 30 hours	2 to 4.5 mcg/ml	> 9 mcg/ml
Lidocaine	I.V.: immediate	5 to 10 hours	2 to 6 mcg/ml	> 7 mcg/ml
Procainamide	P.O.: 60 minutes			
	I.V.: 25 to 60 minutes	11 to 20 hours	4 to 8 mcg/ml	> 12 mcg/ml
N-acetylpro-cainamide	Not known	Not known	2 to 8 mcg/ml	> 30 mcg/ml
Propranolol	P.O.: 60 to 90 minutes	10 to 30 hours	40 to 85 ng/ml*	> 150 ng/ml†
	I.V.: 2 to 4 hours			
Quinidine	P.O.: 1 to 3 hours	20 to 35 hours	2.4 to 5 mcg/ml	> 6 mcg/ml
	I.V.: immediate			
	I.M.: 30 to 90 minutes			
Verapamil	P.O.: 1 to 2 hours	15 to 35 hours	0.08 to 0.3 mcg/ml	Not known
	I.V.: 5 minutes			

* If the patient's condition doesn't improve with serum level of 100 ng, treatment is unsuccessful.

† Toxic concentrations vary and require correlation with clinical status.

Implications of results Trough levels guide the adjustment of therapeutic dosage; peak levels can prevent or detect toxicity and monitor its treatment.

Post-test care If a hematoma develops at the venipuncture site, applying warm soaks eases discomfort.

Interfering factors • Hemolysis caused by excessive agitation of the sample can produce artifactual lowering of results for analysis by fluorometry or enzyme-multiplied immunoassay.

- Acetazolamide, antacids, and sodium bicarbonate elevate serum quinidine levels.
- Barbiturates and phenytoin suppress serum lidocaine and serum quinidine levels.

Antibody tests in diabetes mellitus

These tests detect various antibodies in the blood of patients with known or suspected diabetes mellitus. Antibody formation in diabetes mellitus can take three forms. The most common is formation of anti-insulin antibodies from exogenous insulin sources — beef, pork, or human insulin preparations. Detection of insulin antibodies confirms this process as the cause of insulin resistance and suggests the necessity for alternate therapy to control hyperglycemia.

Another type of antibody formed in diabetes mellitus, the anti-beta cell antibody, is directed against the insulin-producing cells of the pancreas. Research continues on the possible link between these antibodies, on diabetes mellitus with distinct HLA typing, and on using the tests for these antibodies as a predictor of diabetes. Still primarily a research tool, however, the test for anti-beta cell antibodies isn't commercially available at present.

A third type of antibody identified in diabetes, the anti-insulin receptor antibody, plays a role in the development of insulin resistance. Still largely experimental, measurement of these antibodies may help determine the cause of insulin resistance. Like the anti-beta cell antibody test, the test for anti-insulin receptor antibodies is also a research tool, not yet available for widespread clinical use.

Purpose
- To aid diagnosis of insulin resistance
- To assist in insulin management for control of hyperglycemia
- To aid diabetes research

Patient preparation
Explain to the patient that the test for anti–insulin antibodies evaluates diabetes and helps guide insulin therapy. If the patient is scheduled for the anti-beta cell antibody or anti-insulin receptor antibody test, explain that these tests help clinical researchers learn more about the nature of diabetes mellitus and its management. Tell the patient the test requires a blood sample.

Procedure	Perform a venipuncture, and collect the sample in a 7-ml *red-top* tube, or as directed by the testing laboratory.
Findings	Normally, no anti-insulin, anti-beta cell, or anti-insulin receptor antibodies are present in blood.
Implications of results	The presence of anti-insulin antibodies in a diabetic patient may indicate the need for an alternative type of insulin or for increased insulin dosage to achieve euglycemia. Both pork and beef insulin set up an antigen-antibody response by the human body. Pure pork insulin produces less anti-insulin antibodies than either beef-pork combinations or pure beef insulin. Human insulin was theoretically produced to eliminate antibody formation; however, such formation still occurs, although at lower levels than occur with pure pork insulin.

Positive anti-beta cell antibodies may indicate that the patient is at increased risk for diabetes mellitus, if it hasn't already developed. This finding may also indicate a greater risk for ketoacidosis, hypoglycemic reactions, and, possibly, long-term complications of diabetes.

The presence of anti-insulin receptor antibodies indicates a decreased ability of endogenous or exogenous insulin to exert an appropriate metabolic effect. In research studies, a positive test result usually confirms a diagnosis of insulin resistance of unknown etiology (as opposed to the more common diagnosis of insulin resistance caused by down-regulation of insulin receptors that occurs in obese Type II diabetic patients).

Post-test care	If a hematoma develops at the venipuncture site, applying warm soaks eases discomfort.
Interfering factors	None

Anticonvulsants, serum

This quantitative test uses an enzyme multiplied immunoassay technique to measure serum levels of anticonvulsants — notably carbamazepine, ethosuximide, phenobarbital, phenytoin, and primidone. It's useful in monitoring anticonvulsant therapy in children and mentally retarded persons (persons in whom toxicity is difficult to detect).

Anticonvulsant blood levels

Drug	Peak time	Steady state	Therapeutic level	Toxic level
Carbamazepine	2 to 6 hours	2 to 4 days	2 to 10 mcg/ml	> 12 mcg/ml*
Ethosuximide	1 to 2 hours	8 to 10 days	40 to 80 mcg/ml	> 100 mcg/ml
Phenobarbital	6 to 18 hours	14 to 21 days	20 to 40 mcg/ml	> 55 mcg/ml
Phenytoin	4 to 8 hours	5 to 11 days	10 to 20 mcg/ml	> 12 mcg/ml*

* Toxic concentrations vary; serum levels should be correlated with clinical symptoms.

Purpose
- To monitor therapeutic levels of anticonvulsants
- To confirm toxicity suspected from history or after onset of symptoms

Patient preparation
Explain that this test helps determine the most effective drug dosage. Inform the patient that the test requires a blood sample. Check the patient's recent medication history, noting dose, interval, and route of administration.

Procedure
Perform a venipuncture, and collect a trough-level sample in a 7-ml *red-top* tube. Record the date, time, and route of administration of the last drug dose, and the time of sample collection on the laboratory slip. Send the sample to the laboratory immediately. Observe the same time span between drug administration and sample collection in serial testing.

Values
Steady-state, peak-time, and therapeutic and toxic serum levels of anticonvulsants vary (see *Anticonvulsant blood levels*).

Implications of results
Anticonvulsant blood levels allow adjustment of dosage to maintain effective therapeutic levels and to prevent excessive accumulation and toxicity.

The slow rate of elimination of most anticonvulsants is an important consideration in treating drug toxicity.

Post-test care
If a hematoma develops at the venipuncture site, applying warm soaks eases discomfort.

Interfering factors

- Serum levels of carbamazepine are elevated by troleandomycin, erythromycin, and propoxyphene, and are lowered by phenytoin, phenobarbital, and primidone.
- Serum levels of phenobarbital are elevated by monoamine oxidase inhibitors and primidone, and are lowered by rifampin.
- Serum levels of phenytoin may be raised by oral anticoagulants, antihistamines, chloramphenicol, chlordiazepoxide, chlorpromazine hydrochloride, diazepam, diazoxide, disulfiram, ethosuximide, isoniazid, phenylbutazone, phenobarbital, propoxyphene, salicylates, sulfamethizole, and valproic acid; serum phenytoin levels may be suppressed by alcohol, phenobarbital, carbamazepine, folic acid, loxapine, and antacids.
- Serum levels of primidone are elevated by carbamazepine and phenytoin.

Antidepressants, plasma or serum

This quantitative toxicity test, which measures the plasma levels of antidepressant drugs, confirms overdose and monitors therapy. Major laboratory methods used to perform this test include gas chromatography, high-performance liquid chromatography, and, for screening, thin-layer chromatography.

Drugs currently used in the treatment of depression include tricyclic antidepressants (TCAs) — doxepin, amitriptyline, desipramine, imipramine, nortriptyline, and protriptyline — and the monoamine oxidase (MAO) inhibitors phenelzine and tranylcypromine. TCAs are preferred for treating depression because they are less toxic than MAO inhibitors. After oral administration, all antidepressants are distributed through the body, metabolized in the liver, and excreted in urine; TCAs are also eliminated in feces.

Purpose

- To check for antidepressant toxicity
- To monitor therapeutic levels of antidepressants
- To detect the presence of antidepressants for medicolegal purposes

Patient preparation

Explain that this test, which requires a blood sample, checks the level of antidepressants in the blood.

Tricyclic antidepressant blood levels

Drug	Therapeutic	Toxic
Amitriptyline (and metabo-lite, nortriptyline)	75 to 200 ng/ml	> 1,000 ng/ml
Desipramine	20 to 160 ng/ml	> 1,000 ng/ml
Doxepin (and metabolite, desmethyldoxepin)	90 to 250 ng/ml	> 1,000 ng/ml
Imipramine (and metabolite, desipramine)	200 ng/ml	> 1,000 ng/ml
Nortriptyline	75 to 150 ng/ml	> 300 ng/ml

If the test is being performed for medicolegal purposes, make sure the patient or responsible member of the family has signed a consent form. Check and record the patient's recent medication history, including dosage schedule and route of administration.

Procedure Perform a venipuncture, and collect the sample in a 7-ml *red-top* tube. For a monitoring test, draw the sample 2 hours before the next drug dose.

Send the sample to the laboratory immediately, or refrigerate it. For a medicolegal test, observe appropriate procedures.

Values Therapeutic and toxic antidepressant levels vary widely (see *Tricyclic antidepressant blood levels*) and do not correlate closely with clinical effects. Currently, no data are available on lethal levels of protriptyline, phenelzine, and tranylcypromine.

Implications of results Antidepressant blood levels allow regulation of therapeutic dosage and guide treatment of toxicity.

Post-test care If a hematoma develops at the venipuncture site, applying warm soaks eases discomfort.

Interfering factors Barbiturates lower blood TCA levels; methylphenidate raises them.

Antidiuretic hormone, serum
Vasopressin

Antidiuretic hormone (ADH) is a polypeptide produced by the hypothalamus and released from storage sites in the posterior pituitary gland on neural stimulation. The primary function of ADH is to promote water reabsorption, in response to *increased* osmolality (water deficiency with high concentration of sodium and other solutes). In response to *decreased* osmolality (water excess), reduced secretion of ADH allows increased excretion of water to maintain fluid balance. In an interlocking feedback mechanism with aldosterone, ADH helps regulate sodium, potassium, and fluid balance. It also stimulates vascular smooth-muscle contraction, causing an increase in arterial blood pressure.

This relatively rare test, a quantitative analysis of serum ADH level, may identify diabetes insipidus and other causes of severe homeostatic imbalance. It may be used as part of dehydration or hypertonic saline infusion testing, which determines the body's response to states of hyperosmolality.

Purpose To aid the differential diagnosis of pituitary diabetes insipidus, nephrogenic diabetes insipidus (congenital or familial), and syndrome of inappropriate antidiuretic hormone (SIADH)

Patient preparation Explain that this test measures hormonal secretion levels. Instruct the patient to fast and limit physical activity for 10 to 12 hours before the test. Tell him the test requires a blood sample and that he should relax and lie down for 30 minutes before the test.

Withhold conjugated estrogens, morphine, tranquilizers, hypnotics, oxytocin, anesthetics (such as ether), lithium carbonate, vincristine, carbamazepine, cyclophosphamide, and chlorothiazide; these drugs and others may cause SIADH. If these medications must be continued, note this on the laboratory slip.

Procedure Perform a venipuncture, and collect the sample in a *red-top,* plastic collection tube. Immediately send the sample to the laboratory, where serum must be separated from the clot within 10 minutes.

Note: The syringe and the collection tube *must* be plastic because the fragile ADH undergoes degradation when it comes in contact with glass.

Values   Normal ADH values range from 1 to 5 pg/ml (ng/L).

Implications of results   Absent or below-normal ADH levels indicate pituitary diabetes insipidus, resulting from a neurohypophyseal or hypothalamic tumor, viral infection, metastatic disease, sarcoidosis, tuberculosis, Hand-Schüller-Christian disease, syphilis, head trauma, or neurosurgical procedures.

Normal ADH levels, in the presence of typical clinical features of diabetes insipidus (such as polydipsia, polyuria, and hypotonic urine), may indicate the nephrogenic form of the disease, marked by renal tubular resistance to ADH. Levels may be elevated, however, if the pituitary attempts to compensate for renal resistance.

Elevated ADH levels may also indicate SIADH, possibly as a result of bronchogenic cancer, acute porphyria, hypothyroidism, Addison's disease, cirrhosis of the liver, infectious hepatitis, severe hemorrhage, or circulatory shock.

Post-test care   • If a hematoma develops at the venipuncture site, applying warm soaks eases discomfort.
• The patient may resume diet and medications discontinued before the test.

Interfering factors   • Failure to restrict diet, medications, or activity may hinder accurate determination of test results. Morphine, anesthetics, estrogens, oxytocin, chlorpropamide, vincristine, carbamazepine, cyclophosphamide, and chlorothiazide elevate ADH levels, as do stress, pain, and positive-pressure ventilation. Alcohol and negative-pressure ventilation inhibit ADH secretion.
• Radioactive scan performed within 1 week before the test may influence the results, because serum ADH level is determined by radioimmunoassay.

Antimicrosomal antibodies

Normally present in epithelial cytoplasm of thyroid follicles, free microsomes can act as antigens and stimulate the formation of antibodies against these follicular cells.

This test detects the presence of antibodies to thyroid microsomes, which are present in patients with primary hypothyroidism, thyroid tumors, and simple goiters, and in about 70% to 90% of patients with Hashimoto's thyroiditis (see Antithyroid Antibodies).

Purpose

To aid diagnosis of thyroid diseases, particularly Hashimoto's thyroiditis and juvenile lymphocytic thyroiditis

Patient preparation

Explain the purpose of the test and inform the patient that the test requires a blood sample.

Procedure

Perform a venipuncture and collect a blood sample of at least 2 ml.

Values

Normal titer of antimicrosomal antibodies is less than 1:100 and occurs in 5% to 10% of healthy persons.

Implications of results

Positive tests for antimicrosomal antibodies occur in 70% to 90% of patients with Hashimoto's thyroiditis and in 90% of patients with juvenile lymphocytic thyroiditis. Positive test results also occur in patients with myxedema, granulomatous thyroiditis, nontoxic nodular goiter, and in approximately 20% of patients with thyroid cancer.

Positive test results may also occur in patients with Sjögren's syndrome, systemic lupus erythematosus, rheumatoid arthritis, and autoimmune hemolytic anemia.

Post-test care

If a hematoma develops at the venipuncture site, applying warm soaks eases discomfort.

Interfering factors

None

Antimitochondrial antibodies

This test for antimitochondrial antibodies, which is usually performed with the test for anti–smooth-muscle antibodies, detects antibodies in serum by indirect immunofluorescence. Antimitochondrial antibodies react with mitochondria in the renal tubules, gastric mucosa, and other organs in which cells expend large amounts of energy. These autoantibodies are present in several hepatic diseases, although their etiologic role is unknown, and there is no evidence that they cause hepatic damage. Most commonly, they are associated with primary biliary cirrhosis and, sometimes, with chronic active hepatitis and drug-induced jaundice. Antimitochondrial antibodies are also associated with autoimmune diseases, such as systemic lupus erythematosus, rheumatoid arthritis, pernicious anemia, and idiopathic Addison's disease.

Purpose
- To aid diagnosis of primary biliary cirrhosis
- To distinguish between extrahepatic jaundice and biliary cirrhosis

Patient preparation
Explain that this test, which requires a blood sample, helps evaluate liver function. Check the patient's medication history for oxyphenisatin. Report use of this drug to the laboratory because it may produce antimitochondrial antibodies.

Procedure
Perform a venipuncture, and collect the sample in a 7-ml *red-top* tube.

Findings
Normally, serum is negative for antimitochondrial antibodies at a 1:5 dilution.

Implications of results
Although antimitochondrial antibodies appear in 79% to 94% of patients with primary biliary cirrhosis, this test alone doesn't confirm diagnosis. Further tests, such as serum alkaline phosphatase, serum bilirubin, alanine transaminase, aspartate aminotransferase or, possibly, liver biopsy or cholangiography, may also be necessary. The autoantibodies also appear in some patients with chronic active hepatitis, drug-induced jaundice, and cryptogenic cirrhosis. However, antimitochondrial antibodies rarely appear in patients with extrahepatic biliary obstruction, and a positive test helps rule out this condition.

Post-test care
Because patients with hepatic disease may bleed excessively, apply pressure to the venipuncture site until bleeding stops. If a hematoma develops at the venipuncture site, applying warm soaks eases discomfort.

Interfering factor
Confusion of antimitochondrial antibodies with heterophil antibodies, cardiolipin antibodies to syphilis, ribosomal antibodies, or microsomal hepatic or renal autoantibodies can cause inaccurate determination of test results.

Antinuclear antibodies (ANA)

In conditions such as systemic lupus erythematosus (SLE), scleroderma, and certain infections, the body's immune system may perceive portions of its own cell nuclei as foreign and may produce antinuclear antibodies (ANA). Specific ANA include antibodies to deoxyribonucleic acid (DNA), nucleoprotein, histones, nuclear ribonucleoprotein, and other nuclear constituents. Although ANA are harmless in themselves because they don't penetrate living cells, they sometimes form antigen-antibody complexes that cause tissue damage (as in SLE).

This test measures the relative concentration of ANA in a serum sample through indirect immunofluorescence. (Although there are other methods for measuring ANA — hemagglutination, counterimmunoelectrophoresis, radioimmunoassay, and enzyme immunoassay — indirect immunofluorescence is the method of choice.) Serial dilutions of serum are mixed with cell nuclei (usually taken from mouse liver or kidney). If the serum contains ANA, it forms antigen-antibody complexes with the cell nuclei. This preparation is then mixed with fluorescein-labeled antihuman serum and is examined under an ultraviolet microscope. If ANA are present, the nuclei fluoresce. About 99% of patients with SLE exhibit ANA; a large percentage of these persons do so at high titers.

Although this test is not specific for SLE, it is a useful screening tool. In elderly patients the incidence of false-positive results exceeds true positive results. A negative ANA result (titer less than 1:20) in an untreated patient essentially rules out active SLE. However, many investigators have reported patients with ANA-negative SLE. In these patients, nuclear antibodies do not react with the mouse substrate, but may react if another substrate is used. Generally, at least two substrates must be used before a specimen can be classified as negative; cryostat substrates generally yield a higher percentage of false-negative results. For example, the HEp-2 antigen produces a positive reaction in many ANA-negative patients. Therefore, the HEp-2 test is a follow-up to an ANA-negative test when SLE is suspected.

Purpose
- To screen for SLE
- To screen for SLE flare-ups in patients with established SLE

- To monitor the effectiveness of immunosuppressant therapy for SLE

Patient preparation

Explain that this test evaluates the immune system and that further testing is commonly required for accurate diagnosis. If appropriate, inform the patient that the test will be repeated to rule out false-positive results and to monitor response to therapy. Tell him that he needn't restrict food or fluids before the test and that the test requires a blood sample.

Check the patient's medication history for drugs that may affect test results, such as isoniazid, hydralazine, and procainamide. Note such drug use on the laboratory slip.

Procedure

Perform a venipuncture, and collect the sample in a 7-ml *red-top* tube.

Findings

The test for ANA is negative at a titer of 1:32 or less.

Implications of results

Although the test is a sensitive indicator of ANA, it is not specific for SLE. Low titers may occur in patients with viral diseases, chronic hepatic disease, collagen vascular disease and autoimmune diseases, and in some healthy adults; incidence increases with age. Consequently, the higher the titer, the more specific the test is for SLE (titer often exceeds 1:256).

The pattern of nuclear fluorescence helps identify the type of immune disease present. A peripheral pattern is almost exclusively associated with SLE because it indicates the presence of anti-DNA antibodies; anti-DNA antibodies are sometimes measured by radioimmunoassay if ANA titers are high or a peripheral pattern is observed. A homogeneous, or diffuse, pattern is also associated with SLE, as well as with related connective tissue disorders; a nucleolar pattern, with scleroderma; and a speckled, irregular pattern, with infectious mononucleosis and mixed connective tissue disorders (for example, SLE and scleroderma).

A single serum sample, especially one collected from a patient with collagen vascular disease, may contain antibodies to several parts of the cell's nucleus. In addition, as serum dilution increases, the fluorescent pattern may change because different antibodies are reactive at different titers.

Post-test care
- Observe the venipuncture site for signs of infection, especially in a patient being treated with immunosuppressants. Keep a clean, dry bandage over the site for at least 24 hours.
- If a hematoma develops at the venipuncture site, applying warm soaks eases discomfort.

Interfering factor

Certain drugs — most commonly isoniazid, hydralazine, and procainamide — can produce a syndrome resembling SLE; other such drugs include para-aminosalicylic acid, chlorpromazine, clofibrate, phenytoin, griseofulvin, ethosuximide, gold salts, methyldopa, oral contraceptives, penicillin, propylthiouracil, phenylbutazone, methysergide, streptomycin, sulfonamides, tetracyclines, quinidine, mephenytoin, primidone, reserpine, and trimethadione.

Antiparietal cell antibodies

Antibodies to gastric parietal cells occur in the serum of patients with pernicious anemia, atrophic gastritis, thyroid diseases, diabetes mellitus, and iron deficiency anemia. Such antibodies can be measured by the indirect immunofluorescence technique.

This test detects antiparietal cell antibodies in serum. A serum sample is applied to a slide containing tissue secretions of a combination substrate composed of mouse or rat kidney and stomach. Antiparietal cell antibodies in the serum bind to the gastric mucosa of the stomach tissue substrate, but not to the tubules in the kidney tissue. This distinguishes antiparietal cell antibodies from antimitochondrial antibodies, which bind to both tissue substrates.

Purpose

To aid diagnosis of pernicious anemia

Patient preparation

Explain that the purpose of this test is to help evaluate his condition. Tell the patient that he needn't restrict food or fluids before the test and explain that the test requires a blood sample.

Procedure

Perform a venipuncture, and collect the sample in a 5-ml *red-top* tube. Handle the specimen carefully to prevent hemolysis.

Findings
: Positive tests for antiparietal cell antibodies occur in 90% of patients with pernicious anemia; in 60% of those with atrophic gastritis; in 33% with gastric ulcers; in 33% with thyroid disease; and in 12% with diabetes.

 Fewer than 2% of normal persons test positive for antiparietal cell antibodies. However, this percentage increases with age, rising to 16% of persons over age 60.

Implication of results
: Antiparietal cell antibodies can be detected in 90% of patients with pernicious anemia; a positive test result helps distinguish autoimmune pernicious anemia from other megaloanemias.

Post-test care
: If a hematoma develops at the venipuncture site, applying ice eases discomfort.

Interfering factor
: Grossly hemolyzed or lipemic serum may produce increased background staining, interfering with accurate determination of test results.

Anti–smooth-muscle antibodies

By using indirect immunofluorescence, this test measures the relative concentration of anti–smooth-muscle antibodies in serum, and is usually performed with the test for antimitochondrial antibodies. The serum sample is exposed to a thin section of smooth muscle and incubated; then, a fluorescent-labeled antiglobulin is added. This antiglobulin binds only to antibodies that have formed a complex with smooth muscle and appears fluorescent when viewed through the microscope under ultraviolet light.

Anti–smooth-muscle antibodies appear in several hepatic diseases, especially chronic active hepatitis and, less often, primary biliary cirrhosis. Although anti–smooth-muscle antibodies are most commonly associated with hepatic diseases, their etiologic role is unknown, and no evidence that they cause hepatic damage exists.

Purpose
: To aid diagnosis of chronic active hepatitis and primary biliary cirrhosis

Patient preparation	Explain that this test helps evaluate liver function. Inform the patient that he needn't restrict food or fluids before the test and that this test requires a blood sample.
Procedure	Perform a venipuncture, and collect the sample in a 7-ml *red-top* tube.
Findings	Normal titer of anti–smooth-muscle antibodies is less than 1:20.
Implications of results	The test for anti–smooth-muscle antibodies is not very specific; these antibodies appear in about 66% of patients with chronic active hepatitis and in 30% to 40% of patients with primary biliary cirrhosis.
	Anti–smooth-muscle antibodies may also be present in patients with infectious mononucleosis, acute viral hepatitis, malignant tumor of the liver, and intrinsic asthma.
Post-test care	• Because patients with hepatic disease may bleed excessively, apply pressure to the venipuncture site until bleeding stops.
	• If a hematoma develops at the site, applying warm soaks eases discomfort.
Interfering factors	None

Antistreptolysin-O test
Streptococcal antibodies, serum

Because streptococcal infections are often overlooked, serologic testing is valuable in patients with glomerulonephritis and acute rheumatic fever to confirm antecedent infection by showing serologic response to streptococcal antigen. The antistreptolysin-O (ASO) test measures the relative serum concentrations of the antibody to streptolysin O, an oxygen-labile enzyme produced by group A beta-hemolytic streptococci.

In this test, a serum sample is diluted with a commercial preparation of streptolysin O and incubated. After the addition of rabbit or human red blood cells, the tube is reincubated and examined visually. If hemolysis fails to develop, ASO has formed a complex with the antigen, inactivated it, and prevented red blood cell destruction, indicat-

Test for anti-DNase B

The test for antideoxyribonuclease B (anti-DNase B), similar to the antistreptolysin-O (ASO) test, detects antibodies to DNase B, a potent antigen produced by all group A streptococci.

For adults, normal anti-DNase B titer is less than 85 Todd units/ml; for school-age children, less than 170 Todd units/ml; and for preschoolers, less than 60 Todd units/ml. Elevated anti-DNase B titers (greater than 120 Todd units/ml in adults and 240 Todd units/ml in children) appear in 80% of patients with acute rheumatic fever, in 75% of those with poststreptococcal glomerulonephritis (after streptococcal pharyngitis), and 60% of those with glomerulonephritis (after group A streptococcal pyoderma). This is a much higher percentage than those with ASO titer elevations (25%), making the test for anti-DNase B especially useful for detecting a reaction to group A streptococcal pyoderma.

ing recent beta-hemolytic streptococcal infection. The end point is read in Todd units, the reciprocal of the highest dilution (titer) that inhibits hemolysis. Excessively high ASO titers occur in post-streptococcal diseases, such as rheumatic fever or glomerulonephritis, and may occur in healthy carriers of beta-hemolytic streptococci.

Micro methods for detecting ASO, such as the ASO latex agglutination test, currently screen for beta-hemolytic streptococcal infection. When ASO titers are low, more sensitive tests may be performed for antibodies to hyaluronidase, streptokinase, deoxyribonuclease B, and nicotinamide, which are also produced in response to streptococcal infection. (See *Test for anti-DNase B,* above, and *Rapid tests for streptococcal pharyngitis,* page 88, for additional information.)

Purpose
- To confirm recent or current infection with beta-hemolytic streptococci
- To help diagnose rheumatic fever and post-streptococcal glomerulonephritis in the presence of clinical symptoms
- To distinguish between rheumatic fever and rheumatoid arthritis in a patient with joint pain

Patient preparation
Explain that this test detects an immunologic response to certain bacteria (streptococci). Inform

Rapid tests for streptococcal pharyngitis

These tests permit detection and identification of Group A streptococci directly from throat swabs in only 7 minutes. Through improved antibody-antigen technology, this test allows prompt diagnosis and treatment of streptococcal pharyngitis, but may yield false-positive reactions.

Other tests used to diagnose such infection depend on growing the organism in a culture, which can take from 24 to 48 hours.

This test will not identify the cause of pharyngitis as microorganisms other than Group A streptococci.

the patient he needn't restrict food or fluids before the test and that the test requires a blood sample.

If the test is to be repeated at regular intervals to identify active and inactive states of rheumatic fever or to confirm acute glomerulonephritis, tell the patient that measuring changes in antibody levels helps determine the effectiveness of therapy.

Check the patient's medication history for drugs that may suppress the streptococcal antibody response. If such drugs must be continued, note this on the laboratory slip.

Procedure
Perform a venipuncture, and collect the sample in a 7-ml *red-top* tube.

Values
Even healthy persons have a detectable ASO titer from previous minor streptococcal infections. For adults, normal ASO titer is less than 85 Todd units/ml; for school-age children, less than 170 Todd units/ml; and for preschoolers, less than 85 Todd units/ml.

Implications of results
High ASO titers usually occur only after prolonged or recurrent infections. Roughly 15% to 20% of patients with poststreptococcal disease don't have elevated ASO titers. Titers up to 250 Todd units may indicate inactive rheumatic fever. Higher titers of 500 to 5,000 Todd units suggest acute rheumatic fever or acute poststreptococcal glomerulonephritis.

Serial titers, determined at 10- to 14-day intervals, provide more reliable information than a single titer. A rise in titer 2 to 5 weeks after the acute infection, which peaks 4 to 6 weeks after the initial rise, confirms poststreptococcal disease.

Post-test care If a hematoma develops at the venipuncture site, applying warm soaks eases discomfort.

Interfering factors
- False-positive results are likely in patients with streptococcal skin infections.
- Antibiotic or corticosteroid therapy may suppress the streptococcal antibody response and may prevent accurate test results.
- Hemolysis caused by excessive agitation of the sample may interfere with accurate determination of test results.

Antithrombin level

Antithrombin (formerly antithrombin III) is an important coagulation regulator, a protein that inactivates factors IIa, IXa, Xa, and XIa. Deficiencies are associated with an increased risk of thrombosis. This test is generally used to identify individuals with inherited antithrombin deficiencies.

Tests for antithrombin levels measure antithrombin antigen (immunologic level) or function; functional assays measure the amount of antithrombin in plasma by inhibition of factor IIa or Xa. A chromogenic substrate (colorimetric reaction) is often used to measure any residual factor IIa or Xa activity. Many laboratories perform functional tests first and measure antigen levels only if the functional test shows a deficiency.

Using a fresh, citrated blood sample, this test measures the ability of antithrombin to inhibit thrombin's enzymatic cleavage of p-nitroaniline (p-NA) from a small polypeptide chain. Cleavage of colored p-NA is measured spectrophotometrically and compared with control samples.

Antithrombin can be assayed by several techniques, which can be divided into two groups: those that assay antithrombin activity (functional assay) and those that measure antithrombin molecules (immunologic assay) using antibody against antithrombin.

Purpose
- To detect inherited deficiencies of antithrombin in persons with predisposition to thrombosis
- To aid management of disseminated intravascular coagulation (DIC) or thrombotic disease

Patient
preparation

Explain that this test, which requires a blood sample, helps evaluate the coagulation system.

Procedure

Perform a venipuncture, and collect a blood sample. Some laboratories require a frozen specimen of citrated, platelet-poor plasma. Label the sample to include the patient's coagulation history and note any recent treatment with heparin.

Values

Normal functional values exceed 50% (0.50) of control and range from 77% to 122% (0.77 to 1.22). Immunologic values range from 65% to 110% (0.65 to 1.10) of control.

Implications of
results

Low antithrombin levels can result from heparin therapy or indicate inherited deficiencies, liver disease, malnutrition, DIC, sepsis, or nephrotic syndrome. If an inherited deficiency is suspected, results should be confirmed by both repeat testing and testing of the patient's family.

Interfering
factor

Recent thrombosis and heparin therapy may interfere with tests results, causing false-low levels; testing should be repeated after recovery from thrombosis.

Antithyroid antibodies

In autoimmune disorders such as Hashimoto's thyroiditis and Graves' disease (hyperthyroidism), thyroglobulin, the major colloidal storage compound, is released into the blood. Because thyroxine usually separates from thyroglobulin before its release into the blood, thyroglobulin doesn't normally enter the circulation. When it does, antithyroglobulin antibodies that attack this foreign substance are produced, and the ensuing autoimmune response damages the thyroid gland. The serum of a patient whose autoimmune system produces antithyroglobulin antibodies usually contains antimicrosomal antibodies, which react with the microsomes of the thyroid epithelial cells.

The tanned red cell hemagglutination test detects antithyroglobulin and antimicrosomal antibodies. In this assay, sheep red blood cells that have been pretreated with tannic acid and coated with thyroglobulin or with microsomal fragments are mixed with a serum sample. The mixture agglutinates in the presence of these specific antibodies,

Incidence of thyroid autoantibodies

Disorder	Antithyroglobulin	Antimicrosomal antibodies
Hashimoto's thyroiditis	50% to 86%	92% to 100%
Myxedema	50% to 64%	67% to 86%
Graves' disease	29% to 65%	71% to 86%
Adenomatous goiter	5% to 50%	27%
Thyroid cancer	20%	20%
Pernicious anemia	25%	10%

and serial dilutions can quantify the antibody concentration. Another laboratory technique, indirect immunofluorescence, can detect antimicrosomal antibodies.

Purpose
To detect circulating antithyroglobulin antibodies when clinical evidence indicates Hashimoto's thyroiditis, Graves' disease, or other thyroid diseases

Patient preparation
Explain that this test differentiates hypothyroidism from Hashimoto's thyroiditis. Advise the patient that he needn't restrict foods or fluids before the test and that the test requires a blood sample.

Procedure
Perform a venipuncture, and collect the sample in a 7-ml *red-top* tube.

Values
The normal titer is less than 1:100 for both antithyroglobulin and antimicrosomal antibodies. (Low levels of these antibodies are normal in up to 15% of the general population and in 20% or more of persons aged 70 or older.)

Implications of results
The presence of antithyroglobulin or antimicrosomal antibodies in serum can indicate subclinical autoimmune thyroid disease, Graves' disease, or idiopathic myxedema. High titers (which may be in the millions) strongly suggest Hashimoto's thyroiditis. The accompanying chart shows the approximate incidence of antithyroglobulin and antimicrosomal

antibodies in thyroid diseases and pernicious anemia. Such antibodies may also occur in some patients with other autoimmune disorders, such as systemic lupus erythematosus, rheumatoid arthritis, and autoimmune hemolytic anemia. (See *Incidence of thyroid autoantibodies,* page 91.)

Post-test care
If a hematoma develops at the venipuncture site, applying warm soaks eases discomfort.

Interfering factor
High titers of thyroid antibodies have been reported in patients with nonthyroid disorders (Addison's disease, myasthenia gravis, liver disease, and diabetes mellitus) and may interfere with accurate interpretation of results.

Arterial blood gas (ABG) analysis

Arterial blood gas (ABG) analysis evaluates gas exchange in the lungs by measuring the partial pressures of oxygen (PaO_2) and carbon dioxide ($PaCO_2$), and the pH of an arterial sample. PaO_2 indicates how much oxygen the lungs are delivering to the blood. $PaCO_2$ indicates how efficiently the lungs eliminate carbon dioxide. The pH indicates the acid-base level of the blood or the hydrogen ion (H^+) concentration. Acidity indicates H^+ excess; alkalinity, H^+ deficit. Oxygen content (O_2CT), oxygen saturation (O_2 Sat), and bicarbonate (HCO_3^-) values also aid diagnosis. A blood sample for ABG analysis may be drawn by percutaneous arterial puncture or from an arterial line.

Purpose
- To evaluate the efficiency of pulmonary gas exchange
- To assess the integrity of the ventilatory control system
- To determine the acid-base level of the blood
- To monitor respiratory therapy

Patient preparation
Explain that this test evaluates oxygen delivery to the blood and elimination of carbon dioxide. Inform the patient that the test requires a blood sample. Instruct the patient to breathe normally during the test, and warn that a brief cramping or throbbing pain may occur at the puncture site.

Procedure   Perform an arterial puncture and collect the blood in a heparinized syringe. Before sending the sample to the laboratory in ice water, include the following information on the laboratory slip:
• Indicate whether the patient was breathing room air or receiving oxygen therapy when the sample was drawn. If he was receiving oxygen therapy, give the flow rate.
• If the patient is receiving mechanical ventilation, note the FIO_2 and tidal volume.
• Record the patient's rectal temperature and respiratory rate.
• Record the patient's rectal temperature and respiratory rate.

Precautions   • If the patient has recently had an intermittent positive-pressure breathing treatment, wait at least 20 minutes before drawing arterial blood, because such treatment alters blood gas values.
• If the patient is receiving oxygen therapy, discontinue oxygen therapy for 15 to 20 minutes before drawing the sample to measure ABGs while he breathes room air.

Values   Normal ABG values fall within the following ranges:
PaO_2 : 75 to 100 mm Hg
$PaCO_2$: 35 to 45 mm Hg
pH: 7.35 to 7.42
O_2 CT: 15% to 23%
O_2 Sat: 94% to 100%
$HCO_3{}^-$: 22 to 26 mEq/liter.

Implications of results   Low PaO_2, O_2 CT, and O_2 Sat levels, combined with a high $PaCO_2$ value, may be the result of conditions that impair respiratory function, such as respiratory muscle weakness or paralysis (in Guillain-Barré syndrome or myasthenia gravis), respiratory center inhibition (from head injury, brain tumor, or drug abuse, for example), and airway obstruction (possibly from mucous plugs or a tumor). Similarly, low readings may result from bronchiole obstruction caused by asthma or emphysema, from an abnormal ventilation-perfusion ratio caused by partially blocked alveoli or pulmonary capillaries, or from alveoli that are damaged or filled with fluid because of disease, hemorrhage, or near-drowning.

When inspired air contains insufficient oxygen, PaO_2, O_2CT, and O_2 Sat also decrease, but $PaCO_2$ may be normal. Such findings are also seen in pneumothorax, impaired diffusion between alveoli and blood (caused by interstitial fibrosis, for example), or in an arteriovenous shunt that permits blood to bypass the lungs.

Low O_2CT — with normal PaO_2, O_2 Sat, and possibly, $PaCO_2$ values — may result from severe anemia, decreased blood volume, and reduced hemoglobin oxygen-carrying capacity.

In addition to clarifying blood oxygen disorders, ABGs can provide considerable information about acid-base disorders.

Post-test care
- After applying pressure to the puncture site for at least 5 minutes, tape a gauze pad firmly over it. (If the puncture site is on the arm, don't tape the entire circumference; this may restrict circulation.)
- Monitor vital signs, and observe for signs of circulatory impairment, such as swelling, discoloration, pain, numbness, or tingling in the bandaged arm or leg.
- Watch for bleeding from the puncture site.

Interfering factors
- Exposing the sample to air affects PaO_2 and $PaCO_2$ levels and interferes with accurate determination of results. Make sure the sample contains no air bubbles.
- Failure to heparinize the syringe prior to sample collection, to place the sample correctly in ice water, or to send the sample to the laboratory immediately adversely affects the test results.
- Excessive heparin solution in the sample can affect test results. Draw samples from arterial lines only after a sufficient amount of waste blood (containing residual heparin from the line) has been removed.
- Fever may cause false-high levels of PaO_2 and PaO_2; hypothermia, false-low levels.
- Venous blood in the sample may lower PaO_2 and elevate $PaCO_2$.
- Bicarbonate, ethacrynic acid, hydrocortisone, metolazone, prednisone, and thiazides may elevate $PaCO_2$ levels. Acetazolamide, methicillin, nitrofurantoin, and tetracycline may decrease $PaCO_2$ levels.

Arylsulfatase A, urine

Arylsulfatase A (ARS-A), a lysosomal enzyme that is found in every cell except the mature erythrocyte, is principally active in the liver, the pancreas, and the kidneys, where exogenous substances are detoxified into ester sulfates. When ARS-A is present in large amounts, it reverses this process by catalyzing the release of free phenylsulfates, such as benzidine and naphthyline, from ester sulfates. Elevated ARS-A levels are associated with cancers of the transitional bladder, colon, and rectum, granulocytic leukemia, lipid storage diseases, leukemia and mucolipidoses II and III. Decreased values are associated with metachromatic leukodystrophy. This test measures urine ARS-A levels by colorimetric or kinetic techniques.

Purpose To aid diagnosis of metachromatic leukodystrophy (an inherited lipid storage disease)

Patient preparation Explain that this test measures an enzyme that is present throughout the body. Tell the patient that the test requires 24-hour urine collection, and teach the correct procedure for collecting a timed specimen. Tell the patient not to contaminate the urine specimen with toilet tissue or stool.

If the female patient is menstruating, the test may have to be rescheduled because increased numbers of epithelial cells in the urine raise ARS-A levels.

Procedure Collect a 24-hour urine specimen. Keep the collection container refrigerated or on ice during the collection period, and send the specimen to the laboratory immediately at the end of the collection period. If the patient has an indwelling urinary catheter in place, keep the collection bag on ice for the duration of the test; the continuous urinary drainage apparatus should be changed before beginning the collection.

Values ARS-A values normally are greater than 1 U/L.

Implications of results Elevated ARS-A levels may result from cancer of the bladder, colon, or rectum, or from myeloid leukemia.

Depressed ARS-A levels can result from meta-chromatic leukodystrophy. In patients with this condition, urine studies show metachromatic granules in the urinary sediment.

Post-test care   None

Interfering
factors
- Failure to collect all urine during the test period may interfere with accurate test results.
- Contamination of the urine specimen by stool, mucus, or blood, or by the improper storage of the specimen may alter the test results.
- Surgery performed within 1 week before the test may raise ARS-A levels.

Aspartate aminotransferase (AST), serum
Aspartate transaminase, serum; glutamic-oxaloacetic transaminase (SGOT), serum

Aspartate aminotransferase (AST), is one of two enzymes that catalyze the transfer of the nitrogenous portion of an amino acid to an amino acid residue. AST is found in the cytoplasm and mitochondria of many cells, primarily in the liver, heart, skeletal muscles, kidneys, pancreas, and, to a lesser extent, in red blood cells. It is released into serum in proportion to cellular damage.

Although a high correlation exists between myocardial infarction (MI) and elevated AST, this test is sometimes considered superfluous for diagnosing MI because of its relatively low organ specificity; it doesn't enable differentiation between acute MI and the effects of hepatic congestion caused by heart failure.

Purpose
- To detect recent MI (together with creatine kinase and lactate dehydrogenase)
- To aid detection and differential diagnosis of acute hepatic disease
- To monitor patient progress and prognosis in cardiac and hepatic diseases

Patient
preparation
Explain to the patient that this test helps assess heart and liver function. Inform him that he needn't restrict food or fluids before the test. Tell him the test usually requires three venipunctures: one at admission and one each day for the next 2 days.

Procedure
Perform a venipuncture, and collect the sample in a 7-ml *red-top* tube. To avoid missing peak AST levels, draw serum samples at the same time each day. Handle the collection tube gently to prevent hemolysis, and send the sample to the laboratory immediately.

Values
AST levels by a commonly used method range from 8 to 20 U/L. Normal values for infants are as high as four times those of adults.

Implications of results
AST levels fluctuate in response to the extent of cellular necrosis and therefore may be transiently and minimally elevated early in the disease process, and extremely elevated during the most acute phase. Depending on when the initial sample was drawn, AST levels can rise — indicating increasing disease severity and tissue damage — or fall — indicating disease resolution and tissue repair. Thus, the relative change in AST values serves as a reliable monitoring mechanism.

Maximum elevations are associated with certain diseases and conditions. For example, very high elevations (more than 20 times normal) may indicate acute viral hepatitis, severe skeletal muscle trauma, extensive surgery, drug-induced hepatic injury, and severe passive liver congestion.

High levels (ranging from 10 to 20 times normal) may indicate severe MI, severe infectious mononucleosis, and alcoholic cirrhosis. High levels may also occur during the prodromal or resolving stages of conditions that cause maximal elevations.

Moderate-to-high levels (ranging from 5 to 10 times normal) may indicate Duchenne's muscular dystrophy, dermatomyositis, and chronic hepatitis. Moderate-to-high levels also occur during prodromal and resolving stages of diseases that cause high elevations.

Low-to-moderate levels (ranging from 2 to 5 times normal) may indicate hemolytic anemia, metastatic hepatic tumors, acute pancreatitis, pulmonary emboli, alcohol withdrawal syndrome, and fatty liver. AST levels rise slightly after the first few days of biliary duct obstruction. Also, low-to-moderate elevations occur at some time during any of the preceding conditions or diseases.

Post-test care
• If a hematoma develops at the venipuncture site, applying warm soaks eases discomfort.

- Patient may resume medications discontinued before the test.

Interfering factors
- Chlorpropamide, opiates, methyldopa, erythromycin, sulfonamides, pyridoxine, dicumarol, antitubercular agents, large doses of acetaminophen, salicylates, and vitamin A, and many other drugs known to affect the liver cause elevated AST levels. Strenuous exercise and muscle trauma caused by intramuscular injections also raise AST levels.
- Hemolysis caused by excessive agitation of the sample may hinder accurate determination of AST levels.
- Failure to draw the sample as scheduled, missing peak AST levels, may interfere with accurate determination of test results.

Aspergillus antibodies, serum

This immunodiffusion test is used to detect antibodies to the *Aspergillus* organism, including *A. flavus, A. fumigatus,* and *A. niger.* These organisms cause clinical conditions ranging from allergic bronchospasm to pulmonary aspergillosis to an invasive, usually fatal disease that occurs in immunosuppressed patients. *Aspergillus* infection is commonly associated with bronchopulmonary disease, endophthalmitis, and systemic disease affecting the kidneys, heart, brain, and bone.

Antibodies to an antigen derived from *A. fumigatus* and *A. niger* are detected by immunodiffusion, complement fixation, or counterimmunoelectrophoresis.

Purpose
To detect antibodies resulting from aspergillosis

Patient preparation
Explain the purpose of the test and inform the patient that the test requires a blood sample.

Procedure
Perform a venipuncture and obtain a blood sample of at least 2 ml.

Findings
The normal test result is negative for *Aspergillus* antibodies.

Implications of results
Serum that exhibits one to four strong precipitin lines with either antigen strongly suggests aspergil-

losis or other invasive diseases. Severely immunocompromised patients may not have detectable antibody levels and may develop an invasive fungal disease.

Post-test care If a hematoma develops at the venipuncture site, applying warm soaks eases discomfort.

Interfering factors In patients with inflammatory disease, C substance from aspergillus can react with C-reactive protein, causing false-positive results.

Atrial natriuretic factor, plasma
Atrial natriuretic hormone, atrionatriuretic peptides, atriopeptins

This radioimmunoassay test measures the plasma level of atrial natriuretic factor (ANF), a vasoactive and natriuretic hormone that is secreted from the heart when expansion of blood volume stretches the atrial tissue. ANF appears to be released in response to atrial stretching and is an extremely potent natriuretic agent, rapidly producing natriuresis and diuresis. ANF is vasoactive, producing vasodilation and increased glomerular filtration rate. Some researchers consider ANF part of the counter-regulation of the renin-angiotensin system. ANF is a potent vasodilator that overcomes the vasoconstriction produced by certain catecholamines and angiotensin II. ANF appears to block renin release by direct action on the kidney, and to act on the adrenal gland to block the secretion and, possibly, production of aldosterone.

This hormone appears to have a critical role in regulating extracellular fluid volume, blood pressure, and sodium metabolism. ANF promotes sodium excretion, inhibits the effect of the renin-angiotensin system on aldosterone secretion, and decreases atrial pressure by decreasing venous return, thereby reducing both blood pressure and blood volume.

Clinical investigators have found that patients with overt congestive heart failure (CHF) have highly elevated plasma levels of ANF. Patients with cardiovascular disease and elevated cardiac-filling pressure, but without CHF, also have markedly elevated ANF. Recent findings support ANF as a possible marker for early asymptomatic left ventricular dysfunction and increased cardiac volume.

Purpose
- To confirm CHF
- To identify asymptomatic cardiac volume overload

Patient preparation
Explain the purpose of the test and inform the patient that the test requires fasting and a blood sample. Check the patient's history for use of medications that can influence test results. Beta blocking agents, calcium antagonists, diuretics, vasodilators, and digitalis glycosides should be withdrawn for 24 hours before the blood sample is drawn.

Procedure
Perform a venipuncture and collect a blood sample into a prechilled potassium-EDTA tube. After chilled centrifugation, the EDTA plasma is promptly frozen and sent to the laboratory for analysis.

Values
Normal ANF levels range from 20 to 77 pg/ml.

Implications of results
Markedly elevated levels of ANF are found in patients with frank CHF and significantly elevated cardiac-filling pressure.

Post-test care
- If a hematoma develops at the venipuncture site, applying warm soaks eases discomfort.
- The patient may resume normal diet and medications restricted before the test.

Interfering factor
Cardiovascular medications, including beta blocking agents, calcium antagonists, diuretics, vasodilators and digitalis glycosides interfere with accurate measurement of ANF levels.

B

Barbiturates, serum

This quantitative analysis measures serum barbiturate levels. A prominent cause of drug-induced coma, barbiturates are classified by their length of action: long-acting (mephobarbital, phenobarbital); short- to intermediate-acting (amobarbital, pentobarbital, and secobarbital); and ultrashort-acting (thiamylal, hexobarbital, and thiopental).

The appropriate laboratory method for measuring serum barbiturate levels varies — for example, long-acting barbiturates require gas chromatography; short- to intermediate-acting barbiturates require the enzyme-multiplied immunoassay technique. Although the serum level usually correlates with the patient's clinical condition, many factors can influence it (including route of administration, the degree of central nervous system [CNS] excitability, the patient's barbiturate tolerance, and the additive effects of such compounds as alcohol, opiates, and tranquilizers).

Purpose
- To check for barbiturate toxicity suspected from the patient's history or after the onset of toxic symptoms, such as headache, confusion, ataxia, respiratory and CNS depression, flaccid muscles, hypothermia to hyperthermia, hypotension, low urinary output, areflexia, or shock syndrome
- To monitor therapeutic barbiturate levels
- To confirm the presence of barbiturates for medicolegal purposes

Patient preparation
Explain that this test determines the concentration of barbiturates in the body. Tell the patient that the test requires a blood sample. If the test is being performed for medicolegal purposes, make sure the patient or responsible family member has signed a consent form. Obtain a recent drug history, including doses, times, and administration routes.

Procedure
Perform a venipuncture, and collect the sample in a 7-ml *red-top* tube.

Handle the sample gently to prevent hemolysis, and send the sample to the laboratory immediately or refrigerate it.

Barbiturate blood levels and possible effects

Drug	Therapeutic	Moderately toxic	Toxic
Phenobarbital	10 to 40 mcg/ml	> 55 mcg/ml	> 70 mcg/ml
Amobarbital	≤ 15 mcg/ml	> 30 mcg/ml	> 50 mcg/ml
Pentobarbital	4 mcg/ml	> 15 mcg/ml	> 20 mcg/ml*
Secobarbital	5 mcg/ml	> 15 mcg/ml	> 20 mcg/ml
Primidone	5 to 12 mcg/ml	†	†

* In some patients, toxicity may not occur until levels are as high as 30 to 40 mcg/ml.

† Because phenobarbital is a metabolite of primidone, patients receiving long-term therapy with primidone may have plasma phenobarbital levels two or three times that of primidone.

For a medicolegal test, observe appropriate precautions.

Values   Generally, short-acting barbiturates (amobarbital, pentobarbital, secobarbital) produce both therapeutic and toxic effects at lower serum concentrations than long-acting barbiturates (phenobarbital). (See *Barbiturate blood levels and possible effects*.) These values are not absolute, but severe toxicity usually follows ingestion of approximately 10 times the usual hypnotic dose.

Implications of results   Individual tolerance influences the clinical effects of barbiturates and should be considered in regulating therapeutic dosage. Prolonged use of barbiturates often induces tolerance and physical dependence, which are closely related. Abrupt withdrawal after chronic intoxication causes withdrawal syndromes that are consistently dose-related; the higher the intoxicating dose, the more severe the withdrawal syndrome. While tolerance to the sedative and intoxicating effects of barbiturates may be considerable, the lethal dose is not much greater in persons addicted to drugs than in other persons. Thus, acute toxicity may develop abruptly in barbiturate addicts. Physical dependence also occurs with long-term use and is a concern for discontinuation of the drug.

The anesthesia induced by ultrashort-acting barbiturates begins rapidly (onset at less than 1 minute) and disappears rapidly. Toxicity after I.V. use varies according to the patient's susceptibility to respiratory depression and apnea. I.V. use requires precautions to maintain pulmonary ventilation.

Paradoxically, children, elderly persons, and patients with severe pain may respond to administration of barbiturates with excitement, restlessness, hyperactivity, or delirium.

Post-test care If a hematoma develops at the venipuncture site, applying warm soaks eases discomfort.

Interfering factors

- Hemolysis caused by excessive agitation of the sample causes false-high levels in a sample analyzed by the enzyme-multiplied immunoassay technique.
- Salicylates and sulfonamides interfere with the test.
- Monoamine oxidase inhibitors, disulfiram, and alcohol ingestion can raise barbiturate blood levels; rifampin may lower them.
- Long-term therapy with primidone may elevate phenobarbital blood levels.
- Concurrent use of barbiturates and other CNS depressants causes additive sedative effects that can exceed the safe level.

Bence-Jones proteins, urine

Bence-Jones proteins are monoclonal light-chains of immunoglobulins that appear in the urine of 50% to 80% of patients with multiple myeloma and in most patients with Waldenström's macroglobulinemia.

In most cases, these proteins — thought to be synthesized by malignant plasma cells in the bone marrow — are rapidly cleared from the plasma and don't usually appear in serum. When these proteins exceed renal tubular capacity to reabsorb them, they overflow and are excreted in the urine (overflow proteinuria). Eventually, the effort to reabsorb excess amounts of protein causes the renal tubular cells to degenerate. Consequently, protein precipitates and inclusions occur in the renal tubular cells. If renal failure results from such precipitation or from hypercalcemia, increased uric acid, or infiltration by abnormal plasma cells, more Bence-Jones proteins and other proteins then appear in the urine because the dysfunctional nephrons no longer control protein excretion.

Urine screening tests, such as thermal coagulation and Bradshaw's test, are unreliable indicators of Bence-Jones proteins. Immunofixation or electrophoresis are the methods of choice for definitive identification of monoclonal light chains. Both urine and serum studies are used for patients suspected of having multiple myeloma.

Purpose
: To confirm the presence of multiple myeloma in patients with characteristic clinical signs such as bone pain (especially in the back and thorax) and persistent anemia and fatigue

Patient preparation
: Explain that this test can detect abnormal protein in the urine. Tell the patient the test requires an early-morning urine specimen, and teach the correct procedure for collecting a clean-catch specimen. Instruct the patient not to contaminate the urine specimen with toilet tissue or stool.

Procedure
: Collect an early-morning urine specimen of at least 50 ml. Send the specimen to the laboratory immediately. If transport is delayed, refrigerate the specimen.

Findings
: Normal urine should contain no Bence-Jones proteins.

Implications of results
: The presence of Bence-Jones proteins in urine suggests multiple myeloma or Waldenström's macroglobulinemia. Excessively low levels, in the absence of other symptoms, may result from benign monoclonal gammopathy. However, clinical evidence figures prominently in diagnosis of multiple myeloma.

Post-test care
: None

Interfering factors
: • False-positive results may occur in connective tissue disease, renal insufficiency, or certain malignant diseases.
• Contamination of the specimen with menstrual blood, prostatic secretions, or semen may cause false-positive results.
• Failure to send the specimen to the laboratory immediately or to keep the specimen refri-

gerated may cause a false-positive result, because heat-coagulable protein denatures or decomposes at room temperature.

Beta-glucosidase, fibroblasts or leukocytes

Beta-glucosidase, a lysosomal enzyme that influences the hydrolysis of glucocerebroside, is normally present in many body tissues, including the fibroblasts and leukocytes. In Gaucher's disease (a lysosomal storage disease transmitted by autosomal recessive inheritance), a deficiency of beta-glucosidase causes increased storage of glucosylceramide. Gaucher's disease occurs as one of three clinical types: adult-chronic; infantile-acute neuropathic; and juvenile-subacute neuropathic. It is usually associated with splenomegaly and hepatomegaly; central nervous system symptoms are limited to the infantile type. Characteristic Gaucher's cells are large histiocytes derived from endothelial cells and found in the spleen, liver, bone marrow, lymph nodes, and lungs.

Beta-glucosidase can be measured in both fibroblasts and leukocytes by fluorometric testing.

Purpose To detect Gaucher's disease

Patient preparation Explain the purpose of the test. Inform the patient that the test will require a blood sample for testing of leukocytes, or a skin biopsy for testing of fibroblasts.

Procedure For testing of leukocytes, perform a venipuncture and draw a 7-ml sample into a *yellow-top* tube. Send the refrigerated (but not frozen) specimen to the laboratory promptly. This analysis should be performed within 48 hours of drawing the blood specimen.

For testing of fibroblasts, a 4-mm punch skin biopsy is obtained, prepared with an appropriate fixative, and sent to the laboratory for cell culture and analysis.

Values Normal beta-glucosidase in leukocytes is 0.08 to 0.35 U/10 10 cells; in fibroblasts, 3.80 to 8.70 U/g of cellular protein.

Implications of results
Decreased levels of beta-glucosidase are associated with Gaucher's disease.

Post-test care
The biopsy site is closed and a sterile dressing is applied.

Interfering factors
None

B-hydroxybutyrate, serum

B-hydroxybutyrate is one of three ketone bodies whose relative proportion (78%) in the blood is greater than acetoacetate (20%) or acetone (2%). A small amount of acetoacetate and B-hydroxybutyrate is formed during the normal hepatic metabolism of free fatty acids and is then metabolized in the peripheral tissues. In some conditions, increased acetoacetate production may exceed the metabolic capacity of the peripheral tissues. As acetoacetate accumulates in the blood, a small portion is converted to acetone by spontaneous decarboxylation. The remaining and greater portion of acetoacetate is converted to B-hydroxybutyrate. The accumulation of all three ketone bodies is called ketosis.

Purpose
• To aid diagnosis of carbohydrate deprivation resulting from starvation or frequent vomiting (anorexia or bulimia)
• To aid diagnosis of diabetes mellitus
• To aid diagnosis of type I glycogen storage disease (Von Gierke's disease)

Patient preparation
Explain the purpose of this test and inform the patient that this test requires a blood sample. Either a fasting or nonfasting specimen is acceptable for analysis. Values will increase with increased fasting time.

Procedure
Perform a venipuncture and collect 5 ml of whole blood. Draw the sample into a 5-ml *red-top* tube. Allow the specimen to clot. Centrifuge and remove the serum. If an acetone level is requested, perform this analysis first. Serum B-hydroxybutyrate is stable for at least 1 week at 35.6° to 46.4° F (2° to 8° C). Plasma is also an acceptable specimen for analysis.

Values

The normal value for serum or plasma B-hydroxy-butyrate levels is less than 0.4 mmol/L.

➤ *Clinical alert:* Values greater than 2.0 mmol/L indicate a critical limit that mandates immediate notification of the patient's physician.

Implications of results

The determination of ketone bodies in the blood, rather than in the urine, is extremely helpful in the diagnosis of any unexplained increase in the anion gap. Although once used to monitor insulin therapy in treating diabetic ketoacidosis, B-hydroxybutyrate levels are now seen as contributing to overtreatment. Monitoring the patient's blood sugar remains the optimum method of monitoring therapy.

Post-test care

If hematoma develops at the venipuncture site, applying warm soaks eases discomfort.

Interfering factors

- Hemolysis, jaundice, or lipemia have little or no effect on results. Heparin does not interfere with the reaction.
- The presence of both lactic dehydrogenase, at high concentrations, and lactic acid, at concentrations greater than 10 mmol/L, may elevate the B-hydroxybutyrate value by at least 0.2 mmol/L.
- Sodium fluoride, at concentrations greater than 2.5 nmol/L, appears to decrease the B-hydroxybutyrate value by at least 0.1 mmol/L.

Bilirubin, serum

This test measures serum levels of bilirubin. Bilirubin is the major product of hemoglobin catabolism. After being formed in the reticuloendothelial cells, bilirubin is bound to albumin and is transported to the liver, where it is conjugated with glucuronic acid to form bilirubin glucuronide and bilirubin diglucuronide — compounds that are then excreted in bile.

Effective conjugation and excretion of bilirubin depends on a properly functioning hepatobiliary system and a normal red blood cell (RBC) turnover rate. Therefore, measurement of unconjugated (indirect or prehepatic) bilirubin, and conjugated (direct or posthepatic) bilirubin can help evaluate hepatobiliary and erythropoietic functions. Serum bilirubin measurements are especially significant in neonates because elevated unconjugated bilirubin can accumulate in the brain (kernicterus) and cause irreparable tissue damage.

Elevated indirect serum bilirubin levels often indicate hepatic damage in which the parenchymal cells can no longer conjugate bilirubin with glucuronide. Consequently, indirect bilirubin reenters the bloodstream. High levels of indirect bilirubin are also likely in severe hemolytic anemia, when excessive indirect bilirubin overwhelms the liver's conjugating mechanism. If hemolysis continues, both direct and indirect bilirubin levels may rise.

Purpose
- To evaluate liver function
- To aid differential diagnosis of jaundice and to monitor the progression of this disorder
- To aid diagnosis of biliary obstruction and hemolytic anemia
- To determine whether a neonate requires an exchange transfusion or phototherapy because of dangerously high levels of unconjugated bilirubin

Patient preparation
Explain that this test evaluates liver function and the condition of RBCs. If the patient is a neonate, explain the importance of this test to his parents. Advise the adult patient to fast for at least 4 hours before the test. (Fasting is not necessary for a neonate.) Tell the patient that the test requires a blood sample; inform the parents that a small amount of blood will be drawn from the neonate's heel.

Check the patient's medication history for use of drugs that are known to interfere with serum bilirubin levels. Such drugs may be withheld for 24 hours before the test.

Procedure
If the patient is an adult, perform a venipuncture, and collect the sample in a 10- to 15-ml *red-top* tube.

If the patient is a neonate, perform a heelstick, and fill the microcapillary tube with blood to the designated level.

Protect the sample from any source of light because bilirubin breaks down when exposed to light. Handle the sample gently to prevent hemolysis, and send it to the laboratory immediately.

Values
Normally in an adult, indirect serum bilirubin measures 1.1 mg/dl (18 μmol/L) or less; direct serum bilirubin, less than 0.5 mg/dl (8 μmol/L). Total se-

rum bilirubin in neonates ranges from 1 to 12 mg/dl (17 to 205 µmol/L).

Implications of results

Elevated serum levels of indirect bilirubin indicate hemolysis (for example, in glucose-6-phosphate dehydrogenase deficiency, autoimmunity, or transfusion reaction); hemolytic or pernicious anemia or hemorrhage; hepatocellular dysfunction (possibly resulting from viral hepatitis or congenital enzyme deficiencies, such as Gilbert's disease and Crigler-Najjar syndrome); or neonatal hepatic immaturity.

Elevated levels of direct conjugated bilirubin usually indicate biliary obstruction, in which direct bilirubin, blocked from its normal pathway from the liver into the biliary tree, overflows into the bloodstream. Biliary obstruction may be intrahepatic (viral hepatitis, cirrhosis, chlorpromazine reaction), extrahepatic (gallstones, gallbladder or pancreatic cancer), or result from bile duct disease. If biliary obstruction continues, both direct and indirect bilirubin may be eventually elevated because of hepatic damage. In severe chronic hepatic damage, direct bilirubin concentrations may return to normal or near-normal levels, but elevated indirect bilirubin levels persist.

In neonates, total bilirubin levels that reach or exceed 20 mg/dl (340 µmol/L) indicate the need for exchange transfusion.

Post-test care

- If a hematoma develops at the venipuncture or heelstick site, applying warm soaks eases discomfort.
- The patient may resume diet and medications withheld before the test.

Interfering factors

- Treatment with allopurinol, antibiotics, antineoplastic agents, barbiturates, caffeine, steroids, sulfonamides, sulfonylureas, propylthiouracil, theophylline, indomethacin, and any hepatotoxic drug may elevate bilirubin levels.
- Exposure of the patient or of the sample to direct sunlight or ultraviolet light may depress bilirubin levels.
- Hemolysis caused by excessive agitation of the sample may alter test results.

Bilirubin, urine

This screening test, based on a color reaction with a specific reagent, detects abnormally high urine concentrations of direct (conjugated) bilirubin. The reticuloendothelial system produces bilirubin from hemoglobin breakdown. The pigment bilirubin then binds to albumin, a plasma protein, and is transported to the liver as indirect (unconjugated) bilirubin. In the liver, most indirect bilirubin is combined with glucuronic acid to form bilirubin glucuronide and bilirubin diglucuronide, which are water-soluble compounds almost totally excreted into the bile (together known as direct bilirubin).

In the intestine, bacterial action converts direct bilirubin to urobilinogen. Normally, only a small amount of direct bilirubin passes from the liver to plasma, where it is mostly bound to albumin. The kidneys filter the unbound portion, which may appear in trace amounts in the urine. Fat-soluble indirect bilirubin can't be filtered by the glomeruli and is never present in urine. Bilirubin in the urine indicates liver disease due to cholestasis, either within the liver or in the bile duct or caused by rare inherited disorders of bilirubin metabolism.

When combined with urobilinogen measurements, this test helps identify disorders that can cause jaundice. The analysis can be performed at bedside, using a bilirubin reagent strip, or in the laboratory.

Purpose

To help identify the cause of jaundice

Patient preparation

Explain that this test helps determine the cause of jaundice. Inform the patient that the test requires a random urine specimen and whether the specimen will be tested at the bedside or in the laboratory.

Procedure

Collect a random urine specimen in the container provided. For bedside analysis, use one of the following procedures:

Dipstrip: Dip the reagent strip into the specimen and remove it immediately. After 20 seconds, compare the strip color with the color standards. Record the test results on the patient's chart.

Ictotest: This test is easier to read and more sensitive than the dipstrip method. Place five drops of urine on the asbestos-cellulose test mat. If bilirubin is present, it will be absorbed into the mat. Next, put a reagent tablet on the wet area of the mat, and

Values of bilirubin and urobilinogen in jaundice

Causes of jaundice	Serum		Urine		Feces
	Indirect bilirubin	Direct bilirubin	Bilirubin	Urobi-linogen	Urobi-linogen
Unconjugated hyperbilirubinemia					
Hemolytic disorders (hemolytic anemia, erythroblastosis fetalis)	▲	●	○	▲	▲
Gilbert's disease (constitutional hepatic dysfunction)	▲	●	○	▽●	▽●
Crigler-Najjar syndrome (congenital hyperbilirubinemia)	▲▲	●	○	▽●	▽●
Conjugated hyperbilirubinemia					
Extrahepatic obstruction (calculi, tumor, scar tissue in common bile duct or hepatic excretory duct)	●	▲	▲	○▽	○▽
Hepatocellular disorders (viral, toxic, or alcoholic hepatitis; cirrhosis; parenchymal injury) *or intrahepatic obstruction* (drug-induced cholestasis; some familial defects, such as Dubin-Johnson syndrome and Rotor's syndrome; viral hepatitis; primary biliary cirrhosis)	▲	▲	▲	▽●▲	▽●

Key

○	absent	○▽	absent or reduced
▽	reduced	▽●	reduced or normal
●	normal	▽●▲	variable
▲	increased	▲▲	markedly increased

place two drops of water on the tablet. If bilirubin is present, a blue-to-purple coloration will develop on the mat. Pink or red indicates the absence of bilirubin — a negative test.

Use only a freshly voided specimen. Bilirubin decomposes on exposure to light.

If the specimen is to be analyzed in the laboratory, send it to the laboratory immediately. Record the time of collection on the patient's chart. If the specimen is tested at bedside, make sure 20 seconds elapse before interpreting the color change on the dipstrip. Be sure lighting is adequate to make an accurate color determination.

➤ *Clinical alert:* Regard any sample as a potential source of hepatitis, and always affix the correct biohazard label to the specimen.

Findings
Normally, bilirubin is not found in urine in a routine screening test.

Implications of results
High concentrations of direct (conjugated) bilirubin in urine may be evident from the specimen's appearance (dark, with a yellow foam). To identify the cause of jaundice, however, the presence or absence of direct bilirubin in urine must be correlated with serum test results, and with urine and fecal urobilinogen levels (see *Values of bilirubin and urobilinogen in jaundice,* page 111).

Post-test care
None

Interfering factors
• Dipstrip testing is affected by large amounts of ascorbic acid and nitrite, which may lower bilirubin levels and cause false-negative test results.
• Phenazopyridine and phenothiazine derivatives, such as chlorpromazine and acetophenazine maleate, can cause false-positive results.
• Exposure of the specimen to light can cause bilirubin degradation and lower bilirubin levels.

Bleeding time

This test measures the duration of bleeding after a standardized skin incision. Bleeding time depends on the elasticity of the blood vessel wall and on the number and functional capacity of platelets. This test is usually performed on patients with personal or family histories of bleeding disorders; it is of no value in preoperative screening unless a hemostatic defect is suspected. Bleeding time may be measured by one of four methods: template, modified template, Ivy, or Duke. The template methods are the most frequently used and the most accurate, because they standardize the incision size, making test results more reproducible.

Purpose   To investigate congenital and acquired platelet function disorders

Patient preparation   Explain that this test measures the time required to form a clot and stop bleeding. Tell the patient he needn't restrict food or fluids before the test, and that the test will require two small, hairline incisions. Warn him that these incisions may scar when healed.

Check the patient's history for recent ingestion of drugs that prolong bleeding time. If the patient has taken such drugs, check with the laboratory for special instructions. If the test is being used to identify a suspected bleeding disorder, it should be postponed and the drugs discontinued.

Equipment   Blood pressure cuff, disposable lancet, template with 9-mm slits (template method) or 5-mm slits (modified template method), spring-loaded blade (modified template method), 70% alcohol or povidone-iodine solution, filter paper, small pressure bandage, stopwatch

Procedure   *Template and modified template methods:* Wrap the pressure cuff around the upper arm and inflate the cuff to 40 mm Hg. Select an area on the forearm that is free of superficial veins, and clean it with antiseptic. Allow the skin to dry *completely* before making the incision. Apply the appropriate template lengthwise to the forearm. For the template method, use the lancet to make two incisions, 1 mm deep and 9 mm long. For the modified template method, use the spring-loaded blade to make two incisions, 1 mm deep and 5 mm long. Start the stopwatch. Taking care not to touch the cuts, gently blot the drops of blood with filter paper every 30 seconds, until the bleeding stops in both cuts. Average the bleeding time of the two cuts, and record the result.

Ivy method: After applying the pressure cuff and preparing the test site, make three small punctures with a disposable lancet. Start the stopwatch immediately. Taking care not to touch the punctures, blot each site with filter paper every 30 seconds until the bleeding stops. Average the bleeding time of the three punctures, and record the result.

(*Duke method*, which involves earlobe puncture, is rarely used.)

Precautions — If the bleeding doesn't diminish after 15 minutes, discontinue the test by applying compression to the incision site.

Findings — The normal range of bleeding time is from 2 to 8 minutes in the template method; from 2 to 10 minutes in the modified template method; and from 1 to 7 minutes in the Ivy method.

Implications of results — Bleeding time is sensitive to defects of platelet number and function. Severe coagulation factor deficiencies that limit wound thrombin generation can also cause prolonged bleeding time.

Post-test care
- In a patient with a bleeding tendency (hemophilia, for example), maintain a pressure bandage over the incision for 24 to 48 hours to prevent further bleeding. Keep the edges of the cuts aligned to minimize scarring. Otherwise, a piece of gauze held in place by an adhesive bandage is sufficient. Check the test area frequently.
- Patient may resume medications discontinued before the test.

Interfering factor — Nonsteroidal anti-inflammatory drugs, such as aspirin and aspirin compounds, are the most common causes of prolonged bleeding times.

Blood culture

A blood culture is performed by inoculating a culture medium with a blood sample and incubating it for isolation and identification of the pathogens in fungemia or bacteremia (fungal or bacterial invasion of the bloodstream) and septicemia (systemic spread of such infection). Blood culture can identify about 90% of pathogens within 24 hours.

Bacteria from local tissue infection usually invade the bloodstream through the lymphatic system by way of the thoracic duct (occasionally, directly through infusion lines, thrombophlebitis, or bacterial endocarditis from prosthetic heart valve replacements). Bacteremia may be transient, intermittent, or continuous. Timing of the specimens for blood cultures is somewhat debatable. Usually, it reflects the suspected type of bacteremia (intermittent or continuous) and the need to begin drug therapy.

Purpose
- To confirm bacteremia or fungemia
- To identify the causative organism

Patient preparation
Explain that this procedure may identify the organism causing infection. Inform the patient how many blood samples the test will require.

Equipment
Tourniquet; small adhesive bandages; alcohol sponges; povidone-iodine sponges; 10- to 20-ml syringe for an adult; 6-ml syringe for a child, three or four sterile needles; two blood culture bottles, one vented (aerobic) and one unvented (anaerobic); or a lysis-centrifugation tube.

Procedure
After cleaning the venipuncture site with an alcohol sponge, clean it again with an iodine sponge, starting at the site and working outward in a circular motion. Wait at least 1 minute for the skin to dry, and remove the residual iodine with an alcohol sponge. (Or you can remove the iodine after venipuncture.)

Perform a venipuncture; draw 10 to 20 ml of blood for an adult, and one syringe of 2 to 6 ml for a child. Clean the diaphragm tops of the culture bottles with alcohol or iodine, and change the needle on the syringe. If you're using broth, add blood to each bottle until you obtain a 1:5 or 1:10 dilution. For example, add 10 ml of blood to a 100-ml bottle. (Size of the bottle may vary depending on individual hospital protocol.) Draw the blood directly into a special collection or processing tube if you're using the lysis-centrifugation technique. Indicate the tentative diagnosis on the laboratory slip, and note any current or recent antibiotic therapy. Send samples to the laboratory immediately after collection.

Findings
Normally, blood cultures should be sterile.

Implications of results
Positive blood cultures do not necessarily confirm pathologic septicemia because many organisms may temporarily invade the bloodstream during the early stages of infection. Mild, transient bacteremia may occur during the course of many infectious dis-

eases or may complicate other disorders. Persistent, continuous, or recurrent bacteremia reliably confirms the presence of serious infection.

Isolation of most organisms takes about 24 hours; however, negative cultures are held for 1 week or more before being reported as negative. For example, cultures for suspected *Brucella* are generally held for 4 weeks before they are reported as negative.

Common blood pathogens include *Neisseria meningitidis, Streptococcus pneumoniae, Haemophilus influenzae,* other *Streptococcus* species, *Staphylococcus aureus, Pseudomonas aeruginosa,* Bacteroidaceae, *Brucella,* and Enterobacteriaceae. Although 2% to 3% of blood samples cultured are contaminated by skin bacteria, such as *Staphylococcus epidermidis,* diphtheroids, and *Propionibacterium,* these organisms may be clinically significant when isolated from multiple cultures.

Post-test care
If a hematoma develops at the venipuncture site, applying warm soaks eases discomfort.

Interfering factors
• Improper collection technique may contaminate the sample.
• Previous or current antimicrobial therapy may result in negative cultures or delayed growth.
• Removal of culture bottle caps at the bedside may prevent anaerobic growth; use of incorrect bottle and media may prevent aerobic growth.

Blood urea nitrogen (BUN)

This test measures the nitrogen fraction of urea, the chief end product of protein metabolism. Formed in the liver from ammonia and excreted by the kidneys, urea constitutes 40% to 50% of the blood's nonprotein nitrogen. The blood urea nitrogen (BUN) level reflects protein intake and renal excretory capacity, but is a less reliable indicator of uremia than the serum creatinine level.

Purpose
• To evaluate renal function and aid diagnosis of renal disease
• To aid assessment of hydration

Patient preparation
Tell the patient this test evaluates kidney function. Inform him he needn't restrict food or fluids before

the test and that it requires a blood sample. Check the history for drugs that influence BUN levels.

Procedure   Perform a venipuncture, and collect the sample in a 10- to 15-ml *red-top* tube. Handle the sample gently to prevent hemolysis.

Values   BUN values normally range from 8 to 20 mg/dl (3.0 to 7.1 mmol/L).

Implications of results   Elevated BUN levels occur in renal disease, reduced renal blood flow (caused by dehydration, for example), urinary tract obstruction, in increased protein catabolism (as in burns), in intestinal bleeding, and in steroid therapy.

Depressed BUN levels occur in severe hepatic damage, malnutrition, and overhydration.

Post-test care   If a hematoma develops at the venipuncture site, applying warm soaks eases discomfort.

Interfering factors
- Nephrotoxic drugs, such as aminoglycosides, amphotericin B, and methicillin can elevate BUN levels.
- Chloramphenicol can depress BUN levels.
- Hemolysis caused by excessive agitation of the sample may affect test results.

Bone biopsy

Bone biopsy is the removal of a piece or core of bone for histologic examination. It's performed either by using a special drill needle with a local anesthetic, or by surgical excision with the patient receiving general anesthesia. Bone biopsy is indicated in patients with bone pain and tenderness when bone scan, computed tomography (CT) scan, X-ray, or arteriography reveals a mass or deformity. Excision provides a larger specimen than drill biopsy, and permits immediate surgical treatment if quick histologic analysis of the specimen reveals malignant disease. In the presence of tumors, bones bow slightly, thicken, and sometimes fracture — the result of increased osteoblastic or osteoclastic activity, or both.

Possible complications of bone biopsy include bone fracture, damage to surrounding tissue, and infection (osteomyelitis).

Purpose   To distinguish between benign and malignant bone
           tumors

Patient   Describe the procedure and answer the patient's
preparation questions. Explain that this test permits microscop-
           ic examination of a bone specimen. If the patient is
           to have a drill biopsy, inform him he needn't restrict
           food or fluids. If the patient is to have an open biop-
           sy, instruct him to fast overnight before the test.
               Tell the patient that a local anesthetic will be ad-
           ministered but some discomfort and pressure will
           occur when the biopsy needle enters the bone. Ex-
           plain that a special bone drill forces the needle into
           the bone. Stress the importance of cooperation dur-
           ing the biopsy.
               Make sure the patient or a responsible family
           member has signed a consent form. Check the pa-
           tient's history for hypersensitivity to the local anes-
           thetic.

Procedure *Drill biopsy:* The patient is properly positioned, and
           the biopsy site is shaved and meticulously pre-
           pared. After the local anesthetic is injected, a small
           incision (usually about 3 mm) is made and the biop-
           sy needle with pointed trocar is pushed into the
           bone, using firm, even pressure. Once the needle is
           engaged in the bone, it is rotated about 180 de-
           grees, while continuous pressure is applied. When
           the bone core is obtained, the trocar is withdrawn
           by reversing the drilling motion, and the specimen
           is placed in a properly labeled bottle containing 10%
           formaldehyde solution. Pressure is then applied to
           the site with a sterile gauze pad. When bleeding
           stops, remove the gauze and apply a topical antisep-
           tic (povidone-iodine ointment) and an adhesive
           bandage or other sterile covering, to close the
           wound and prevent infection.
               Open biopsy: The patient is anesthetized, and the
           biopsy site is prepared by shaving the area, clean-
           ing it with surgical soap and then disinfecting it with
           an iodine wash and alcohol. The surgeon makes an
           incision, removes a piece of bone, and sends it to
           the histology laboratory immediately for analysis.
           Further surgery can then be performed, depend-
           ing on bone specimen findings.

Precautions • Bone biopsy should be performed cautiously in
             patients with coagulopathy.

• Send the specimen to the laboratory immediately.

Findings

Normal bone tissue consists of fibers of collagen, osteocytes, and osteoblasts.

Normal bone is of two histologic types: compact and cancellous. Compact bone has dense, concentric layers of mineral deposits, or lamellae. Cancellous bone has widely spaced lamellae, with osteocytes and red and yellow marrow lying between them.

Implications of results

Histologic examination of a bone specimen can reveal benign or malignant tumors. Benign tumors, generally well-circumscribed and nonmetastasizing, include osteoid osteoma, osteoblastoma, osteochondroma, unicameral bone cyst, benign giant-cell tumor, and fibroma. Malignant tumors, which spread irregularly and rapidly, most commonly include both multiple myeloma and osteosarcoma, although the most lethal is Ewing's sarcoma. Most malignant tumors spread to the bone through the blood and lymph systems from the breast, lungs, prostate or thyroid gland, or kidneys.

Post-test care

• Monitor vital signs and the dressing at the biopsy site for excessive drainage.
• If the patient experiences pain at the biopsy site, administer an analgesic, as appropriate.
• For several days after the biopsy, monitor for indications of bone infection: fever, headache, pain on movement, and tissue redness or abscess at or near the biopsy site.
• The patient may resume his usual diet.

Interfering factor

Failure to obtain a representative bone specimen, to use the proper fixative, or to send the specimen to the laboratory immediately may interfere with accurate determination of test results.

Bone marrow aspiration and biopsy

Bone marrow, the soft tissue contained in the medullary canals of long bone and in the interstices of cancellous bone, may be removed by aspiration or needle biopsy under local anesthetic. In an aspiration biopsy, a fluid specimen in which pustula of marrow are suspended is removed from the bone marrow. In a needle biopsy, a core of marrow — cells, not fluid — is removed. These methods are often used concurrently to obtain the best possible marrow specimens. Because bone marrow is the major site of hematopoiesis, the histologic and hematologic examinations of its contents provide reliable diagnostic information about blood disorders. Marrow removed from the bone may be red or yellow. Red marrow, which comprises about 50% of an adult's marrow, actively produces red blood cells; yellow marrow contains fat cells and connective tissue, and is inactive. Because yellow marrow can become active in response to the body's needs, an adult has a large hematopoietic capacity. An infant's marrow is primarily red and, consequently, reflects a small hematopoietic capacity.

Bleeding and infection may result from bone marrow biopsy at any site, but the most serious complications occur at the sternum. Such complications are rare but include puncture of the heart and major vessels — causing severe hemorrhage — and puncture of the mediastinum — causing mediastinitis or pneumomediastinum.

Purpose
- To diagnose thrombocytopenia; leukemias; granulomas; and aplastic, hypoplastic, and pernicious anemias
- To diagnose primary and metastatic tumors
- To determine the cause of infection
- To aid staging of disease, such as Hodgkin's disease
- To evaluate the effectiveness of chemotherapy and help monitor myelosuppression

Patient preparation
Describe the procedure and answer the patient's questions. Explain that the test permits microscopic examination of a bone marrow specimen. Inform the patient that he needn't restrict food or fluids before the test.

Inform the patient that more than one bone marrow specimen may be required, and that a blood sample will be collected before biopsy, for laboratory testing.

Make sure the patient or a responsible family member has signed a consent form. Check the patient's history for hypersensitivity to the local anesthetic. Tell the patient which bone — sternum, anterior or posterior iliac crest, vertebral spinous process, rib, or tibia — will be the biopsy site. Explain that a local anesthetic will be administered, but warn the patient to expect some pressure on insertion of the biopsy needle and a brief, pulling pain on removal of the marrow. The patient may benefit from administration of a mild sedative 1 hour before the test.

Procedure   After positioning, instruct the patient to remain as still as possible. Offer emotional support during the biopsy by talking quietly to the patient, describing what is being done, and answering any questions.

Aspiration biopsy: After the skin over the biopsy site is prepared and the area is draped, the local anesthetic is injected. With a twisting motion, the marrow aspiration needle is inserted through the skin, the subcutaneous tissue, and the cortex of the bone. The stylet is removed from the needle, and a 10- to 20-ml syringe is attached. The examiner aspirates 0.2 to 0.5 ml of marrow, then withdraws the needle. Apply pressure to the site for 5 minutes while the marrow slides are being prepared. (If the patient has thrombocytopenia, apply pressure to the site for 10 to 15 minutes.) The biopsy site is cleaned again, and a sterile adhesive bandage is applied.

If an adequate marrow specimen has not been obtained on the first attempt, the needle may be repositioned within the marrow cavity, or may be removed and reinserted in another site within the anesthetized area. If the second attempt fails, a needle biopsy may be necessary.

Needle biopsy: After preparing the biopsy site and draping the area, the examiner marks the skin at the site with an indelible pencil or marking pen. A local anesthetic is then injected intradermally, subcutaneously, and at the surface of the bone. Then the biopsy needle is inserted into the periosteum, and the needle guard is set, as indicated. The needle is advanced with a steady boring motion until the outer needle passes through the cortex of the bone. The inner needle with trephine tip is inserted into the outer needle, and the stylet is removed. By alternately rotating the inner needle clockwise and counterclockwise, the examiner directs the needle into the marrow cavity and then removes a tissue plug. The needle assembly is withdrawn, and the marrow is expelled into a labeled bottle containing Zenker's acetic acid solution. After the biopsy site is cleaned, a sterile adhesive bandage or a pressure

Bone marrow: Cell types and normal values

Cell types	Normal mean values		
	Adults	Children	Infants
Normoblasts, total	25.6%	23.1%	8.0%
Pronormoblasts	0.2% to 1.3%	0.5%	0.1%
Basophilic	0.5% to 2.4%	1.7%	0.3%
Polychromatic	17.9% to 29.2%	18.2%	6.9%
Orthochromatic	0.4% to 4.6%	2.7%	0.5%
Neutrophils, total	56.5%	57.1%	32.4%
Myeloblasts	0.2% to 1.5%	1.2%	0.6%
Promyelocytes	2.1% to 4.1%	1.4%	0.8%
Myelocytes	8.2% to 15.7%	18.3%	2.5%
Metamyelocytes	9.6% to 24.6%	23.3%	11.3%
Bands	9.5% to 15.3%	0	14.1%
Segmented	6.0% to 12.0%	12.9%	3.6%
Eosinophils	3.1%	3.6%	2.6%
Basophils	0.01%	0.06%	0.1%
Lymphocytes	16.2%	16.0%	49.0%
Plasma cells	1.3%	0.4%	0.02%
Megakaryocytes	0.1%	0.1%	0.05%
Myeloid: Erythroid ratio	2:3	2:9	4:4

dressing is applied. The tissue specimen or slides are sent to the laboratory immediately.

Precautions   Bone marrow biopsy is contraindicated in patients with severe bleeding disorders.

Findings   Yellow marrow contains fat cells and connective tissue; red marrow contains hematopoietic cells, fat cells, and connective tissue. (See *Bone marrow: Cell types and normal values*.)

In addition, special stains that detect hematologic disorders produce these normal findings: the iron stain, which measures hemosiderin (storage iron), has a +2 level; the Sudan Black B (SBB) stain, which shows granulocytes, is negative; and the periodic acid-Schiff (PAS) stain, which detects glycogen reactions, is negative.

Implications of results

Histologic examination of a bone marrow specimen can help detect myelofibrosis, granulomas, lymphoma, or cancer. Hematologic analysis, including the differential count and myeloid-erythroid ratio, can implicate a wide range of disorders. Elevated normoblast values are associated with polycythemia vera; depressed values with vitamin B_{12} or folic acid deficiency and hypoplastic or aplastic anemia. Elevated neutrophils are associated with acute myeloblastic or chronic myeloid leukemia; depressed values with lymphoblastic, lymphatic, or monocytic leukemia, and aplastic anemia. Elevated eosinophils are associated with bone marrow carcinoma, lymphadenoma, myeloid leukemia, eosinophilic leukemia, and pernicious anemia (in relapse). Elevated lymphocytes are associated with chronic lymphocytic leukemia, other lymphatic leukemias, lymphoma, mononucleosis, aplastic anemia, and macroglobulinemia. Elevated plasma cells are associated with myeloma, collagen disease, infection, antigen sensitivity, and malignant disease. Elevated megakaryocytes are associated with old age, chronic myeloid leukemia, polycythemia vera, megakaryocytic myelosis, infection, idiopathic thrombocytopenic purpura, and thrombocytopenia; depressed values, with pernicious anemia. Elevated myeloid-erythroid ratio is associated with myeloid leukemia, infection, leukemoid reactions, and depressed hematopoiesis; depressed ratio with agranulocytosis, hematopoiesis after hemorrhage or hemolysis, iron deficiency anemia, and polycythemia vera.

In an iron stain, decreased hemosiderin levels may indicate a true iron deficiency. Increased levels may accompany other types of anemias or blood disorders. A positive SBB stain can differentiate acute granulocytic leukemia from acute lymphocytic leukemia (which is SBB negative) or may indicate granulation in myeloblasts. A positive PAS stain may indicate acute or chronic lymphocytic leukemia, amyloidosis, thalassemia, lymphomas, infectious mononucleosis, iron-deficiency anemia, or sideroblastic anemia.

Post-test care
- Monitor for bleeding and inflammation.
- Observe the patient for signs of hemorrhage and infection, such as rapid pulse rate, low blood pressure, and fever.

Interfering factor

Failure to obtain a representative specimen, to use a fixative (for histologic analysis), or to send the specimen to the laboratory immediately may alter test results.

Breast biopsy

Although X-rays, mammography, and thermography aid diagnosis of breast masses, only histologic examination of breast tissue obtained by biopsy can confirm or rule out cancer. Needle biopsy or fine-needle biopsy can provide a core of tissue or a fluid aspirate, but needle biopsy should be restricted to fluid-filled cysts and advanced malignant lesions. Both methods have limited diagnostic value because of the small and perhaps unrepresentative specimens they provide. Open biopsy provides a complete tissue specimen, which can be sectioned to allow more accurate evaluation. All three techniques require only a local anesthetic and can often be performed on outpatients; however, open biopsy may require a general anesthetic if the patient is fearful or uncooperative.

Breast biopsy is indicated in patients with palpable masses, suspicious areas in mammography, or persistently encrusted, inflamed, or eczematoid breast lesions or bloody discharge from the nipples. Breast tissue analysis often includes an estrogen and progesterone receptor assay to help select therapy if the mass proves malignant. This assay measures quick-frozen tumor tissue to determine binding capacity of its estrogen and progesterone receptors.

Purpose

To differentiate between benign and malignant breast tumors

Patient preparation

Obtain a complete medical history, including when the patient first noticed the lesion, the presence or absence of pain, a change in the lesion's size, association with the patient's menstrual cycle, nipple discharge, and nipple or skin changes, such as the characteristic "orange-peel" skin that may indicate an underlying inflammatory carcinoma.

Describe the procedure to the patient, and explain that this test permits microscopic examination of a breast tissue specimen. Offer her emotional support, and assure her that breast masses don't always indicate cancer. It may help to mention that

80% of breast lumps aren't malignant. If the patient is to receive a local anesthetic, tell her she needn't restrict food, fluids, or medication before the test. If she is to receive a general anesthetic, advise her to fast from midnight the night before the test. Tell her that pretest blood studies, urinalysis, and a chest X-ray may be required.

Make sure the patient or an appropriate family member has signed a consent form. Check the patient's history for hypersensitivity to anesthetics.

Procedure *Needle biopsy:* Instruct the patient to undress to the waist. After guiding her to a sitting or recumbent position, with her hands at her sides, tell her to remain still. The biopsy site is prepared, a local anesthetic is administered, and the syringe (luer-lock syringe for aspiration, Vim-Silverman needle for tissue specimen) is introduced into the lesion. Fluid aspirated from the breast is expelled into a properly labeled, heparinized tube; the tissue specimen is placed in a labeled specimen bottle containing normal saline solution or formaldehyde. (With fine-needle aspiration, a slide is made for cytology and viewed immediately under a microscope.) Pressure is exerted on the biopsy site and, after bleeding stops, an adhesive bandage is applied. (Since breast fluid aspiration is not considered diagnostically accurate, some clinicians aspirate fluid only from cysts. If such fluid is clear yellow and the mass disappears, the aspiration procedure is both diagnostic and therapeutic, and the aspirate is discarded. If aspiration yields no fluid, or if the lesion recurs two or three times, an open biopsy is then considered appropriate.)

Open biopsy: After the patient receives a general or local anesthetic, an incision is made in the breast, to expose the mass. The examiner may then *incise* a portion of tissue or *excise* the entire mass. If the mass is smaller than ¾″ (2 cm) and appears benign, it is usually excised; if it is larger or appears malignant, a specimen is usually incised before the mass is excised. (Incisional biopsy generally provides an adequate specimen for histologic analysis.) The specimen is placed in a properly labeled specimen bottle containing 10% formaldehyde solution. Tissue that appears malignant is sent for frozen section and receptor assays. (Receptor assay specimens must not be placed in formaldehyde.) The wound is sutured, and an adhesive bandage is applied. Send the specimen to the laboratory immediately.

Precautions   Open breast biopsy is contraindicated in patients with conditions that preclude surgery

Findings   Normally, breast tissue consists of cellular and non-cellular connective tissue, fat lobules, and various lactiferous ducts. It's pink, more fatty than fibrous, and shows no abnormal development of cells or tissue elements.

Implications of results   Abnormal breast tissue may exhibit a wide range of malignant or benign pathology. Breast tumors are common in women and account for 27% of female cancers; such tumors are rare in men (0.2% of male cancers). Benign tumors include fibrocystic disease, adenofibroma, intraductal papilloma, mammary fat necrosis, and plasma cell mastitis (mammary duct ectasia). Malignant tumors include adenocarcinoma, cystosarcoma, intraductal carcinoma, infiltrating carcinoma, inflammatory carcinoma, medullary or circumscribed carcinoma, colloid carcinoma, lobular carcinoma, sarcoma, and Paget's disease.

Special testing by receptor assays that shows a binding capacity of greater than or equal to 3 fmol/mg of protein indicates an estrogen- or progesterone- positive tumor. Over half of all estrogen-positive, protesterone-negative tumors respond to ablative endocrine therapy, such as oopherectomy, adrenalectomy, or hypophysectomy, or anti-estrogen medication. Tumors that are estrogen- *and* progesterone-positive are even more likely to respond to therapy.

Post-test care
- If the patient has received a local anesthetic during needle or open biopsy, monitor vital signs, and provide medication for pain, as appropriate. Watch for and report bleeding, tenderness, or redness at the biopsy site.
- If the patient has received a general anesthetic, check vital signs every 30 minutes for the first 4 hours, every hour for the next 4 hours, and then every 4 hours. Administer an analgesic. Watch for bleeding, tenderness, or redness at the biopsy site.
- Provide emotional support for the patient who is awaiting diagnosis. If the biopsy confirms cancer, the patient will require follow-up tests, including radiographic tests, blood studies, bone scans,

and urinalysis, to determine appropriate treatment.

Interfering factor
Failure to obtain an adequate tissue specimen or to place the specimen in the proper solution container may interfere with test results.

Bronchodilators, serum

Through high-performance liquid chromatography and immunoassay, this highly accurate test monitors serum levels of bronchodilators (aminophylline and theophylline) and detects toxicity. Because the margin of safety between therapeutic and toxic levels is narrow, this analysis is usually performed on patients beginning therapy with these drugs.

Bronchodilators — especially theophylline and aminophylline — relax smooth muscle, particularly in the bronchi; consequently, these drugs are useful for treating asthma and bronchospasm. Theophylline can also effectively treat neonatal and Cheyne-Stokes respiration apnea, probably because it directly stimulates the medullary respiratory center. Bronchodilators are absorbed in the GI tract, metabolized in the liver, and excreted by the kidneys.

Purpose
• To monitor therapeutic levels of bronchodilators
• To check for toxicity suspected from the medication history or after onset of symptoms

Patient preparation
Explain that this test helps determine the most effective drug dosage. Tell the patient that the test requires a blood sample.

Check the patient's history for recent ingestion of dietary xanthines, caffeine, and drugs that may affect test results.

Procedure
Perform a venipuncture, and obtain a trough-level sample by drawing blood just before a scheduled drug dose; obtain a peak-level sample by drawing blood 2 hours after the last dose. Collect the sample in a 7-ml *red-top* tube.

Record on the laboratory slip the specific bronchodilator administered, the time and amount of the last dose the patient has received, and the time of sample collection. Observe the same time span between drug administration and sample collection for serial testing.

Send the sample to the laboratory immediately.

Values

Serum concentrations of theophylline depend on the patient's age and metabolism. Generally, normal values range as follows:

Peak time: 2 to 3 hours, if administered P.O.; 15 minutes, if administered I.V.

Steady state: 15 to 40 hours in adults; 5 to 40 hours in children

Therapeutic level: 10 to 20 mcg/ml (55 to 110 µmol/L)

Toxic level: usually over 20 mcg/ml (110 µmol/L).

However, smaller serum concentrations have been associated with toxicity and greater serum concentrations aren't toxic for all patients. In some patients, doses of 20 mcg/ml are required to relieve bronchospasm. Sinus toxicity may occur at low serum concentrations in elderly patients or after chronic exposures. In general, elderly patients are at higher risk of severe toxicity at lower levels than younger patients.

Implications of results

Peak and trough serum concentrations guide adjustment of therapeutic dosage, especially in children and patients with cardiac, hepatic, pulmonary, or renal dysfunction.

Simultaneous dietary intake of xanthine derivatives (coffee, tea, or chocolate) can account for 2 mcg/ml (11 µmol/L) of serum concentration.

Simultaneous administration of more than one bronchodilator, by more than one route or with ephedrine or other sympathomimetics, increases the hazard of serious toxicity. Gastric symptoms result from irritation, not direct toxicity.

Post-test care

If a hematoma develops at the venipuncture site, applying warm soaks eases discomfort.

Interfering factors

- Caffeine and other xanthines may falsely elevate serum bronchodilator concentrations.
- Cimetidine, troleandomycin, erythromycin, and lincomycin raise serum bronchodilator levels by inhibiting these drugs' hepatic clearance; barbiturates lower them.

C

Calcitonin, plasma
Thyrocalcitonin

This radioimmunoassay measures plasma levels of calcitonin, a polypeptide hormone secreted by interstitial or parafollicular cells of the thyroid gland (C cells) in response to rising serum calcium levels. Calcitonin is known to inhibit bone resorption by osteoclasts, and to increase calcium excretion by the kidneys, thereby acting as an antagonist to parathyroid hormone and lowers serum calcium levels. The usual clinical indication for this test is suspected medullary carcinoma of the thyroid, which causes hypersecretion of calcitonin (without associated hypocalcemia). Equivocal results require provocative testing with I.V. pentagastrin and calcium to rule out disease.

Purpose
To aid diagnosis of thyroid medullary carcinoma in patients known to have a familial predisposition

Patient preparation
Explain that this test helps evaluate thyroid function. Instruct the patient to fast overnight, because eating may interfere with calcium homeostasis and, subsequently, calcitonin levels. Tell the patient that this test requires a blood sample and may require repeat testing after an injection of calcium or pentagastrin.

Procedure
Draw venous blood into a 10-ml *green-top* (heparinized) tube. Handle the sample gently to prevent hemolysis, and send it to the laboratory immediately.

For provocative testing, calcium is infused over 4 hours (2.4 mg/kg). Samples are taken just before the infusion and at 3 and 4 hours postinfusion.

Another test involves I.V. infusion of pentagastrin 0.5 mcg/kg over 5 to 10 seconds. A blood sample is drawn just before the I.V. infusion, and at 90 seconds, 5 minutes, and 10 minutes postinfusion.

A third method, which has been found more effective in some patients, is the combined infusion of calcium and pentagastrin. In this test, 2 mg/kg calcium gluconate is infused I.V. over 1 minute, and followed immediately by an infusion of pentagastrin, 0.5 mg/kg over 5 seconds. Calcitonin is measured just before infusion and again at 2 minutes, 5 minutes, and 10 minutes after the infusion.

Values

Serum calcitonin levels (basal) normally are less than or equal to 19 pg/ml (ng/L) in males; in females, less than or equal to 14 pg/ml (ng/L).

Values after provocative testing with 4-hour calcium infusion are less than or equal to 190 pg/ml (ng/L) in males; in females, less than or equal to 130 pg/ml (ng/L).

Values after provocative testing with pentagastrin infusion are less than or equal to 110 pg/ml (ng/L) in males; in females, less than or equal to 30 pg/ml (ng/L).

Detection limit of assay is 30 pg/ml (ng/L).

Implications of results

Elevated serum calcitonin levels are associated with medullary thyroid cancer, C-cell hyperplasia, chronic renal failure, pernicious anemia, and Zollinger-Ellison syndrome. Occasionally, increased calcitonin levels may be caused by ectopic calcitonin production by oat cell carcinoma of the lung or by breast carcinoma.

Post-test care

If a hematoma develops at the venipuncture site, applying warm soaks eases discomfort.

Interfering factors

- Failure to fast overnight before the test may interfere with accurate determination of test results.
- Hemolysis caused by excessive agitation of the sample may interfere with accurate determination of test results.

Calcium and phosphates, urine

This test measures the urine levels of calcium and phosphates, elements essential for the formation and resorption of bone. Urine calcium and phosphate levels generally parallel serum levels.

Normally absorbed in the upper intestine and excreted in feces and urine, calcium and phosphates help maintain tissue and fluid pH, electrolyte balance in cells and extracellular fluids, and permeability of cell membranes. Calcium promotes enzymatic processes, aids blood coagulation, and lowers neuromuscular irritability; phosphates aid carbohydrate metabolism. Factors that affect the calcium level and, indirectly, the phosphate level include parathyroid hormone level, calcitonin, and plasma proteins.

Purpose
- To evaluate calcium and phosphate metabolism and excretion
- To monitor treatment of calcium or phosphate deficiency
- To assess bone resorption

Patient preparation
Explain that this test measures the amount of calcium and phosphates in the urine. Encourage the patient to be as active as possible before the test. Tell the patient the test requires 24-hour urine specimen collection. If the patient is to collect the specimen, teach the proper technique. Tell the patient not to contaminate the specimen with toilet tissue or stool.

Use the Albright-Reifenstein diet (which contains about 130 mg of calcium/day) for 3 days before the test, or provide a copy of the diet for the patient to follow at home. Note recent use of thiazide diuretics, sodium phosphate, or glucocorticoids on the laboratory slip.

Procedure
Collect a 24-hour urine specimen using either a plastic container or acid-washed bottle. Label the container with the patient's name, the date, and the time the collection started.

Values
Normal values depend on dietary intake. The normal amount of calcium excreted may range from 100 to 250 mg/24 hours (2.5 to 6.2 mmol/day); normal phosphorus, from 900 to 1,300 mg/24 hours (29 to 42 mmol/day).

Implications of results
Urine calcium and urine phosphate levels vary (see *Disorders that affect urine calcium and urine phosphate levels,* page 132).

Post-test care
Observe a patient with low urine calcium levels for tetany.

Interfering factors
- Failure to collect all urine during test period may alter test results.

Disorder	Calcium level	Phosphate level
Hyperparathyroidism	Elevated	Elevated
Vitamin D intoxication	Elevated	Suppressed
Metastatic bone cancer	Elevated	Normal
Sarcoidosis	Elevated	Suppressed
Renal tubular acidosis	Elevated	Elevated
Multiple myeloma	Elevated or normal	Elevated or normal
Paget's disease	Elevated	Normal
Milk-alkali syndrome	Suppressed or normal	Suppressed or normal
Vitamin D deficiency	Suppressed	Elevated
Hypoparathyroidism	Suppressed	Suppressed
Pseudohypoparathyroidism	Suppressed	Suppressed
Acute nephrosis	Suppressed	Suppressed or normal
Chronic nephrosis	Suppressed	Suppressed
Acute nephritis	Suppressed	Suppressed
Renal insufficiency	Suppressed	Suppressed
Osteomalacia	Suppressed	Suppressed
Steatorrhea	Suppressed	Suppressed

Disorders that affect urine calcium and urine phosphate levels

- Thiazide diuretics decrease excretion of calcium. Prolonged inactivity and ingestion of corticosteroids, sodium phosphate, and calcitonin increase excretion. Vitamin D increases phosphate absorption and excretion.
- Parathyroid hormone increases urinary excretion of phosphates and decreases urinary excretion of calcium.

Calcium, serum

This test measures serum levels of calcium, a predominantly extracellular cation that helps regulate and promote neuromuscular and enzyme activity, skeletal development, and blood coagulation. The body absorbs calcium from the GI tract, provided sufficient vitamin D is present, and excretes it in the urine and feces. Over 98% of the body's calcium is found in the bones and teeth. However, calcium can shift in and out of these structures. For example, when calcium concentrations in the blood fall below normal, calcium ions can move out of the bones and teeth to help restore blood levels.

Parathyroid hormone, vitamin D, and to a lesser extent, calcitonin and adrenal steroids control calcium blood levels. Calcium and phosphorus are closely related, usually reacting together to form insoluble calcium phosphate. To prevent formation of a precipitate in the blood, calcium levels vary inversely with phosphorus; as serum calcium levels rise, phosphorus levels should decrease through renal excretion. Because the body excretes calcium daily, regular ingestion of calcium in food (at least 1 g/day) is necessary for normal calcium balance.

Purpose To aid diagnosis of neuromuscular, skeletal, and endocrine disorders; arrhythmias; blood-clotting deficiencies; and acid-base imbalance

Patient preparation Explain that this test determines the blood calcium level. Inform the patient that restriction of food or fluids is not required and that the test requires a blood sample.

Procedure Perform a venipuncture, and collect the sample in a 10- to 15-ml *red-top* tube.

Values Normally, serum calcium levels range from 8.9 to 10.1 mg/dl (atomic absorption; 2.25 to 2.75 mmol/L). In children, serum calcium levels are higher than in adults. Calcium levels can rise as high as 12 mg/dl (3.0 mmol/L) during phases of rapid bone growth.

Implications of results Abnormally high serum calcium levels (hypercalcemia) may occur in hyperparathyroidism and parathyroid tumors (caused by oversecretion of parathyroid hormone), Paget's disease of the bone, multiple myeloma, metastatic cancer, multiple fractures, or prolonged immobilization. Elevated serum calcium levels may also result from inadequate excretion of calcium, as in adrenal insufficiency and renal disease; from excessive calcium ingestion; or from overuse of antacids such as calcium carbonate.

Low calcium levels (hypocalcemia) may result from hypoparathyroidism, total parathyroidectomy, chronic liver disease, or malabsorption. Decreased serum levels of calcium may follow calcium loss in Cushing's syndrome, renal failure, acute pancreatitis, and peritonitis.

➤ *Clinical alert:* Observe the patient with hypercalcemia for deep bone pain, flank pain caused by renal calculi, and muscle hypotonicity. Hypercalcemic crisis begins with nausea, vomiting, and dehydration, leading to stupor and coma, and can end in cardiac arrest.

In a patient with hypocalcemia, be alert for circumoral and peripheral numbness and tingling, muscle twitching, Chvostek's sign (facial muscle spasm), tetany, muscle cramping, Trousseau's sign (carpopedal spasm), seizures, and arrhythmias.

Post-test care
If a hematoma develops at the venipuncture site, applying warm soaks eases discomfort.

Interfering factors
• Excessive ingestion of vitamin D or its derivatives (dihydrotachysterol, calcitriol), and the use of androgens, calciferol-activated calcium salts, progestins-estrogens, and thiazides can elevate serum calcium levels.
• Chronic use of laxatives, massive transfusions of citrated blood, and administration of acetazolamide, corticosteroids, and plicamycin can suppress calcium levels.
• Prolonged use of a tourniquet and fist clenching during sample collection may falsely increase serum calcium levels.

Cancer antigen 125, serum

Cancer antigen 125 (CA 125), an antigen detected by a monoclonal antibody, is used as a tumor marker in ovarian cancer. It is normally found in structures that develop from body cavity epithelium or ducts, such as the endocervix, endometrium, and fallopian tubes as well as the pericardium, peritoneum, and pleura. CA 125 levels may be elevated months to years before a patient presents with the clinical disease. Although this test is the most easily and commonly used screening test, it is unreliable when used alone because it is neither highly specific nor sensitive enough to detect early stage ovarian cancer and cannot distinguish benign from malignant tumors. Both benign and malignant conditions may increase serum CA 125 levels, creating false-positive results.

Purpose
- To monitor the progression or recurrence of ovarian cancer
- To detect advanced extrauterine endometrial cancer

Patient preparation
Explain the purpose of this test, and inform the patient that the test requires a blood sample.

Procedure
Perform a venipuncture, and collect the sample in a 7-ml *red-top* tube. Handle the sample gently and send it to the laboratory immediately; if this is not feasible, refrigerate the specimen. The Mayo Clinic requires that the frozen specimen be sent to the laboratory in a plastic vial on dry ice.

Values
Normal serum values are less than 35 U/ml (less than 35 kU/L).

Implications of results
CA 125 levels are elevated in 50% of patients with stage I ovarian cancer and in 90% of patients with stages III and IV ovarian cancer. Elevated levels also are present in patients with cancers of the breast, colon, fallopian tube, lung, pancreas, and uterus; hepatic cirrhosis; peritonitis; and, possibly, in benign conditions (such as endometriosis), liver disease, pregnancy, and uterine fibrosis. CA 125 levels greater than 65 U/ml are associated with pelvic malignant disease.

Absence of elevated CA 125 levels does not prove that a patient is tumor-free, but escalating levels indicate a poor prognosis.

Post-test care
If a hematoma develops at the venipuncture site, applying warm soaks eases discomfort.

Interfering factor
Hemolysis caused by excessive agitation of the specimen tube can affect test results.

Carbamazepine, serum

Carbamazepine is an anticonvulsant drug used to manage patients with generalized tonic-clonic seizures, partial complex seizures, or mixed seizures; it is used alone or in conjunction with other anticonvulsants. Carbamazepine is also the drug of choice for treating pain associated with trigeminal neuralgia. Oral bioavailability usually exceeds 80%, and the drug is cleared primarily by hepatic metabolism with an initial elimination half-life of 25 to 65 hours, which may decrease during chronic treatment to 8 to 20 hours because of autoinduction of hepatic enzymes. One of the major metabolites, carbamazepine-10, 11-epoxide retains the therapeutic properties and toxicity of the parent drug. Early signs and symptoms of toxicity include fever, sore throat, mouth ulcers, or easy bruising or bleeding.

Purpose	• To determine appropriate drug dosage
	• To assess patient compliance, particularly in patients who show a poor therapeutic response
	• To assess suspected toxicity

Patient preparation Explain the purpose of this test and inform the patient that the test requires a blood sample.

Procedure Perform a venipuncture and collect a minimum of 0.5 ml of blood in a *red-top* tube. For consistency, trough concentrations are usually monitored and should be collected one hour prior to the next dose. A fasting specimen is not required.

Values Normal carbamazepine therapeutic range is 2 to 10 µg/ml (8.5 to 42 µmol/L)

Implications of results Concentrations greater than or equal to 12 µg/ml (50.8 µmol/L) are toxic. Because of individual variation, some patients may exhibit toxic symptoms at a concentration within the therapeutic range. In patients taking concomitant medications that induce hepatic enzyme activity, toxicity can result from an elevated concentration of carbamazepine's active metabolite, carbamazepine-10, 11-epoxide, which has its own therapeutic range of 0.4 to 4.0 µg/ml.

Post-test care If a hematoma develops at the venipuncture site, applying warm soaks eases discomfort.

Interfering
factors

- Coadministration of phenobarbital, phenytoin, or primidone may significantly reduce serum carbamazepine concentrations.
- Coadministration of cimetidime, erythromycin, propoxyphene, isoniazid, fluoxetine, or calcium channel blockers may elevate serum carbamazepine concentrations and induce toxic symptoms.
- Collecting a blood sample before a steady-state serum concentration of carbamazepine is achieved, which typically takes 2 to 3 weeks after the initiation of therapy, may result in underestimated values.

Carbon dioxide content, total

Carbon dioxide (CO_2) is present in small amounts in the air, and in the body as an end product of food metabolism. When the pressure of CO_2 in the red blood cells exceeds 40 mm Hg, CO_2 spills out of the cells and dissolves in plasma. There it may combine with water (H_2O) to form carbonic acid (H_2CO_3), which, in turn, can dissociate into hydrogen (H^+) and bicarbonate ions (HCO_3^-).

This test measures the total concentration of all such forms of CO_2 in serum, plasma, or whole blood samples. Because about 90% of CO_2 in serum is in the form of bicarbonate, this test closely assesses bicarbonate levels. Total CO_2 content reflects the adequacy of gas exchange in the lungs and the efficiency of the carbonic acid – bicarbonate buffer system, which maintains acid-base balance and normal pH. Consequently, this test is commonly ordered for patients with respiratory insufficiency and is usually included in any assessment of electrolyte balance. For maximum clinical significance, test results must be considered with both pH and arterial blood gas values.

Purpose

To help evaluate acid-base balance

Patient
preparation

Explain that this test measures the amount of CO_2 in the blood. Inform the patient that restriction of food or fluids is not required and that this test requires a blood sample. Check the patient's history for medications that may influence CO_2 blood levels.

Procedure Perform a venipuncture. Because the CO_2 content is usually measured along with electrolytes, a 10- to 15-ml *red-top* tube may be used. When this test is performed alone, a *green-top* (heparinized) tube is appropriate. Completely fill the tube, to prevent diffusion of CO_2 into the vacuum.

Values Normally, total CO_2 levels range from 22 to 30 mEq/liter (mmol/L).

Implications of results High CO_2 levels may occur in metabolic alkalosis (caused by excessive ingestion or retention of base bicarbonate), respiratory acidosis (from hypoventilation, for example, as in emphysema or pneumonia), primary aldosteronism, and Cushing's syndrome. CO_2 levels may also rise above normal after excessive loss of acids, as in severe vomiting and continuous gastric drainage.

Decreased CO_2 levels are common in metabolic acidosis (as in diabetic acidosis, or renal tubular acidosis resulting from renal failure). Decreased total CO_2 levels in metabolic acidosis also result from loss of bicarbonate (as in severe diarrhea or intestinal drainage). Levels may fall below normal in respiratory alkalosis (from hyperventilation, for example, after trauma).

Post-test care If a hematoma develops at the venipuncture site, applying warm soaks eases discomfort.

Interfering factors
- CO_2 levels rise with administration of excessive adrenocorticotropic hormone, cortisone, or thiazide diuretics, or with excessive ingestion of alkalis or licorice.
- CO_2 levels decrease with administration of salicylates, paraldehyde, methicillin, dimercaprol, ammonium chloride, acetazolamide, and the accidental ingestion of ethylene glycol or methyl alcohol.

Carcinoembryonic antigen, serum or plasma

Carcinoembryonic antigen (CEA), a glycoprotein secreted onto the glycocalyx surface of cells lining the GI tract, appears during the first or second trimester of fetal life. Normally, production of CEA ends before birth but may begin again later if a neoplasm develops. Because CEA levels are raised by biliary obstruction, alcoholic hepatitis, chronic heavy smoking, and other conditions, as well as by benign or malignant neoplasms, this test can't be used as a general indicator of cancer. A grossly elevated value, however, justifies further cancer diagnostic efforts, especially in a nonsmoking or nondrinking patient. It is also useful for staging, assessing the adequacy of surgical resection, and monitoring colorectal cancer therapy because serum CEA levels, measured by enzyme immunoassay, usually return to normal within 6 weeks if cancer treatment is successful.

Purpose
- To monitor the effectiveness of cancer therapy
- To aid preoperative staging of colorectal and other cancers and to test for recurrence

Patient preparation
Explain to the patient that this test detects and measures a special protein that's not normally present in adults and that the test will be repeated to monitor the effectiveness of therapy.

Advise the patient that restriction of food, fluids, or medications is not required before the test and that the test requires a blood sample.

Procedure
Perform a venipuncture, and collect the sample in a 7-ml *red-top* tube. Handle the sample gently to prevent hemolysis, and send it to the laboratory immediately to ensure reliable test results. If there is a delay in sending, refrigerate the sample.

Values
Normal serum CEA values are less than 5 ng/ml (μg/L) in healthy nonsmokers.

Implications of results
If serum CEA levels exceed normal before surgical resection, chemotherapy, or radiation therapy, their return to normal within 6 weeks suggests successful treatment. Persistent elevation of CEA levels, however, suggests residual or recurrent tumor.

High CEA levels are characteristic in various malignant conditions, particularly endodermally derived neoplasms of the GI organs and the lungs, and in certain nonmalignant conditions, such as benign hepatic disease, hepatic cirrhosis, alcoholic pancreatitis, and inflammatory bowel disease.

Elevated CEA concentrations may also be associated with nonendodermal carcinoma; for example, breast and ovarian cancers typically elevate CEA levels.

Post-test care If a hematoma develops at the venipuncture site, applying warm soaks eases discomfort.

Interfering factors
- Chronic cigarette smoking may elevate serum CEA levels, causing inaccurate interpretation of test results.
- Hemolysis caused by excessive agitation of the sample may elevate serum CEA levels, thereby altering test results.

Cardiolipin antibodies

This test measures serum concentrations of immunoglobulin G or M (IgG or IgM) class antibodies to the phospholipid cardiolipin. These antibodies are found in the serum of some systemic lupus erythematosus (SLE) patients whose serum also contains a coagulation inhibitor (lupus anticoagulant). They are also found in some patients who do not fulfill all the diagnostic criteria for SLE but who experience recurrent episodes of spontaneous thrombosis, fetal loss, or thrombocytopenia.

Serum concentrations of anticardiolipin antibodies are measured using enzyme-linked immunosorbent assay.

Purpose To aid diagnosis of anticardiolipin antibody syndrome in patients with or without SLE who experience recurrent episodes of spontaneous thrombosis, thrombocytopenia, or fetal loss

Patient preparation Explain the purpose of this test. Tell the patient that the test requires a blood sample and that food or fluids need not be restricted before the test.

Procedure Perform a venipuncture, and collect the sample in a 5-ml *red-top* tube. Handle the sample gently to prevent hemolysis, and send the sample to the laboratory immediately.

Findings Anticardiolipin antibody results are reported as dilution titers obtained by making 1:2 serial dilutions of serum. The highest dilution is reported. A 1:4 titer is a borderline result. A lower titer (1:2) is negative; a higher titer (1:8, 1:16), positive.

Implications of results

A positive test result associated with recurrent spontaneous thrombosis, thrombocytopenia, or repeated fetal loss suggests anticardiolipin antibody syndrome. Treatment may involve anticoagulant or platelet-inhibitor therapy.

Post-test care

If a hematoma develops at the venipuncture site, applying warm soaks eases discomfort.

Interfering factors

None

Catecholamines, plasma

This test, a quantitative (total or fractionated) analysis of plasma catecholamines, has significant clinical importance in patients with hypertension and signs of adrenal medullary tumor, and in patients with neural tumors that affect endocrine function. Elevated plasma catecholamine levels necessitate supportive confirmation by urinalysis that shows catecholamine degradation products such as vanillylmandelic acid (VMA) and metanephrine. Measurement of VMA, metanephrine, epinephrine, and norepinephrine using 24-hour urine samples is more common and is more sensitive for detecting pheochromocytoma (see Catecholamines, Urine).

Major catecholamines include the hormones epinephrine, norepinephrine, and dopamine, which are produced almost exclusively in the brain, sympathetic nerve endings, and adrenal medulla. When secreted into the bloodstream, adrenal medullary catecholamines prepare the body for the fight-or-flight reaction to stress: they increase heart rate and contractility; constrict peripheral and visceral blood vessels, and redistribute circulating blood toward the skeletal and coronary muscles; mobilize carbohydrate and lipid reserves; and sharpen mental alertness. These effects are similar to those produced by direct stimulation of the sympathetic nervous system, although greatly intensified and prolonged.

Because many factors influence catecholamine secretion, diurnal variations are common; for example, plasma levels may fluctuate in response to temperature, stress, postural change, diet, smoking, and many drugs.

Purpose
- To rule out adrenal medullary or extra-adrenal pheochromocytoma in patients with hypertension
- To help identify neuroblastoma, ganglio-neuroblastoma, and ganglioneuroma
- To distinguish between adrenal medullary tumors and other catecholamine-producing tumors, through fractional analysis. Urinalysis for catecholamine degradation products is recommended to support diagnosis. Analysis of a 24-hour urine collection for VMA, metanephrine, epinephrine and norepinephrine is more sensitive for pheochromocytoma and is more commonly used for this purpose
- To aid diagnosis of autonomic nervous system dysfunction, such as idiopathic orthostatic hypotension

Patient preparation

Explain that this test helps determine if hypertension or other symptoms are related to improper hormonal secretion. Because the action of catecholamines is so transitory, advise the patient to strictly follow pretest instructions for a reliable test result. Instruct the patient to observe these restrictions before the test: to refrain from using self-prescribed medications (especially cold or hay fever remedies that may contain sympathomimetics) for 2 weeks; to exclude amine-rich foods and beverages (such as bananas, avocados, cheese, coffee, tea, cocoa, beer, and Chianti) for 48 hours; to abstain from smoking for 24 hours (nicotine may alter test results); and to fast for 10 to 12 hours before the test.

Tell the patient that this test requires two blood samples. If the patient is hospitalized, withhold medications that affect catecholamine levels, such as amphetamines, phenothiazines (chlorpromazine), sympathomimetics, and tricyclic antidepressants (TCAs), as appropriate.

An indwelling venous catheter (heparin lock) may be inserted 24 hours before the test. This may be necessary, because the stress of the venipuncture itself may significantly raise catecholamine levels. The patient should be warm, relaxed, and recumbent for 45 to 60 minutes before the test. Low temperatures stimulate catecholamine secretion.

Procedure

Perform a venipuncture between 6 a.m. and 8 a.m. Collect the sample in a 10-ml chilled *lavender-top* tube containing EDTA, which can be obtained from the laboratory on request. Then have the patient stand for 10 minutes, and draw a second sample into another tube, exactly like the first. If a heparin lock is used, it may be necessary to discard the first 1 or 2 ml of blood. Check with the laboratory for the preferred procedure.

Precautions   After collecting each sample, roll the tube slowly between your palms to distribute the EDTA without agitating the blood. Then, pack the tube in crushed ice to minimize deactivation of catecholamines, and send it to the laboratory immediately. Indicate on the laboratory slip whether the patient was supine or standing, and the time the sample was drawn.

Values   In fractional analysis, catecholamine levels range as follows —
Supine: epinephrine, undetectable to 110 pg/ml (0 to 600 pmol/L); norepinephrine, 70 to 750 pg/ml (0.4 to 4.4 nmol/L); dopamine, undetectable to 30 pg/ml (0 to 150 pmol/L)
Standing: epinephrine, undetectable to 140 pg/ml (0 to 900 pmol/L); norepinephrine, 200 to 1,700 pg/ml (1.2 to 10 nmol/L); dopamine, undetectable to 30 pg/ml (0 to 150 pmol/L).

Implications of results   High catecholamine levels may indicate pheochromocytoma, neuroblastoma, ganglioneuroblastoma, or ganglioneuroma. Similar elevations are possible in thyroid disorders, hypoglycemia, or cardiac disease but do not directly confirm these disorders. Electroconvulsive therapy and shock resulting from hemorrhage, endotoxins, or anaphylaxis also may cause catecholamine levels to rise.

In the patient with normal or low baseline catecholamine levels, failure to show increased catecholamine levels in the sample taken after standing suggests autonomic nervous system dysfunction. Standing plasma values are less useful for pheochromocytoma and are not usually done.

Fractional analysis helps identify the specific abnormality that is producing elevated catecholamine levels. For example, adrenal medullary tumors secrete epinephrine; ganglioneuromas, ganglioblastomas, and neuroblastomas secrete norepinephrine.

Post-test care   • If a hematoma develops at the venipuncture site, applying warm soaks eases discomfort.

- The patient may resume diet and medications discontinued before the test.

<table>
<tr><td>Interfering
factors</td><td>

- Failure to observe pretest restrictions may interfere with accurate determination of test results.
- Epinephrine, levodopa, amphetamines, phenothiazines (chlorpromazine), sympathomimetics, decongestants, and tricyclic antidepressants raise plasma catecholamine levels. Reserpine lowers plasma catecholamine levels.
- Radioactive scan performed within 1 week before the test may influence results because plasma catecholamine levels are determined by radioimmunoassay.
</td></tr>
</table>

Catecholamines, urine

This test uses spectrophotofluorometry to measure urine levels of the major catecholamines — epinephrine, norepinephrine, and dopamine. Epinephrine is secreted by the adrenal medulla; dopamine, by the central nervous system; and norepinephrine, by both. Catecholamines can be secreted by certain tumors, most commonly by pheochromocytomas, which usually cause intermittent or persistent hypertension.

The preferred specimen for this test is a 24-hour urine specimen, because catecholamine secretion fluctuates diurnally and in response to pain, heat, cold, emotional stress, physical exercise, hypoglycemia, injury, hemorrhage, asphyxia, and drugs. However, a random specimen may be useful for evaluating catecholamine levels after a hypertensive episode.

For a complete diagnostic workup of catecholamine secretion, urine levels of catecholamine metabolites are measured concurrently. These metabolites — metanephrine, normetanephrine, homovanillic acid (HVA), and vanillylmandelic acid (VMA) normally appear in the urine in greater quantities than the catecholamines.

<table>
<tr><td>Purpose</td><td>

- To aid diagnosis of pheochromocytoma in a patient with unexplained hypertension
- To aid diagnosis of neuroblastoma, ganglio-neuroma, and dysautonomia
</td></tr>
<tr><td>Patient
preparation</td><td>Explain that this test evaluates adrenal function. Inform the patient that restriction of food or fluids is</td></tr>
</table>

not required before the test, but stressful situations and excessive physical activity should be avoided during the collection period. Tell the patient that either a 24-hour or a random urine specimen is required, and explain the approximate collection procedure.

Check the patient's drug history for medications (such as those listed below) that may affect catecholamine levels. Restrict such medications before the test, as appropriate.

Procedure

Collect a 24-hour urine specimen in a bottle containing a preservative to keep the specimen acidified to a pH of 3.0 or less. (If a random specimen is ordered, collect it immediately after a hypertensive episode.)

Refrigerate a 24-hour specimen or place it on ice during the collection period. At the end of the collection period, send the specimen to the laboratory immediately.

Values

Normally, urine catecholamine values range from undetectable to 135 mcg/day (0 to 730 nmol/day), or from undetectable to 18 mcg/dl (0 to 1,000 nmol/day) in a random specimen.

Implications of results

In a patient with undiagnosed hypertension, elevated urine catecholamine levels following a hypertensive episode usually indicate a pheochromocytoma. With the exception of HVA — a metabolite of dopamine — catecholamine metabolites may also be elevated. Abnormally high HVA levels rule out pheochromocytoma, because this tumor mainly secretes epinephrine, whose primary metabolite is VMA, not HVA. If tests indicate a pheochromocytoma, the patient may also be tested for multiple endocrine neoplasia.

Elevated catecholamine levels, without marked hypertension, may be caused by a neuroblastoma or a ganglioneuroma, although HVA levels reflect these conditions more accurately. Neuroblastomas and ganglioneuromas are primarily composed of immature cells and secrete large quantities of dopamine and HVA. Myasthenia gravis and progressive muscular dystrophy commonly cause urine catecholamine levels to rise above normal, but this test cannot diagnose these disorders.

Consistently low-normal catecholamine levels may indicate dysautonomia, marked by orthostatic hypotension.

Post-test care The patient may resume activity restricted during the test and may resume medications withheld before the test.

Interfering factors

- Caffeine, insulin, nitroglycerin, aminophylline, ethanol, sympathomimetics, methyldopa, tricyclic antidepressants, chloral hydrate, quinidine, quinine, tetracycline, B-complex vitamins, isoproterenol, levodopa, and monoamine oxidase inhibitors may raise urine catecholamine levels.
- Clonidine, guanethidine, reserpine, and iodine-containing contrast media may suppress the levels of urine catecholamine.
- Phenothiazines, erythromycin, and methenamine compounds may raise or suppress levels.
- Failure to comply with drug restrictions, to collect all urine during the test period, or to store the specimen properly may interfere with test results.
- Excessive physical exercise or emotional stress raises catecholamine levels.

Cerebrospinal fluid analysis

Cerebrospinal fluid (CSF), a clear fluid that circulates in the subarachnoid space, has many vital functions. It protects the brain and spinal cord from injury and transports products of neurosecretion, cellular biosynthesis, and cellular metabolism through the central nervous system. For qualitative analysis, CSF is most commonly obtained by lumbar puncture (usually between the third and fourth lumbar vertebrae [L3 and L4]) and, occasionally, by cisternal or ventricular puncture. A sample of CSF for laboratory analysis is frequently obtained during other neurologic tests, including myelography and pneumoencephalography.

Purpose

- To measure CSF pressure as an aid in detecting obstruction of CSF circulation
- To aid diagnosis of viral or bacterial meningitis, and subarachnoid or intracranial hemorrhage, tumors, and brain abscesses
- To aid diagnosis of neurosyphilis and chronic central nervous system infections

Patient preparation Describe the procedure and explain that this test analyzes the fluid within the spinal cord. Inform the patient that restriction of food or fluids is not required. Advise the patient that a headache is the most common side effect of a lumbar puncture. Emphasize that cooperation during the test minimizes such an effect. Make sure that the patient or a responsible family member has signed a consent form.

Equipment Lumbar puncture tray, sterile gloves, local anesthetic (usually 1% lidocaine), povidone-iodine, small adhesive bandage

Procedure Position the patient on his side at the edge of the bed, with knees drawn up to abdomen and chin to the chest. Provide pillows to support the spine on a horizontal plane. With the patient in this position, full flexion of the spine and easy access to the lumbar subarachnoid space are possible. Help the patient maintain this position by placing one arm around his knees and the other arm around his neck. If a sitting position is preferred, have the patient sit up and bend his chest and head toward his knees. Help the patient maintain this position throughout the procedure.

After the skin is prepared for injection, the area is draped. Warn the patient to expect a transient burning sensation when the local anesthetic is injected and, when the spinal needle is inserted, some local, transient pain as the needle transverses the dura mater. Ask the patient to report any pain or sensations that differ from or continue after this expected discomfort, as these may indicate irritation or puncture of a nerve root, requiring repositioning of the needle. Instruct the patient to remain still and breathe normally; movement and hyperventilation can alter pressure readings or cause injury.

The anesthetic is injected, and the spinal needle is inserted in the midline, between the spinous processes of the vertebrae (usually between L3 and L4). When the stylet is removed from the needle, CSF will drip from it if the needle is properly positioned. A stopcock and manometer are attached to the needle to measure initial (or opening) CSF pressure. After the specimen is collected, label the containers in the order in which they were filled, along with any specific instructions for the laboratory. A final pressure reading is taken, and the needle is removed. Clean the puncture site with a local antiseptic, such as povidone-iodine solution, and apply a small adhesive bandage.

Record the collection time on the test request form. Send it and all labeled specimens to the laboratory immediately.

Precautions Infection at the puncture site contraindicates removal of CSF; in a patient with increased intracranial pressure, CSF should be removed with extreme caution because the rapid reduction in pressure that follows withdrawal of fluid can cause cerebellar tonsillar herniation and medullary compression.

➤ *Clinical alert:* During the procedure, observe closely for signs of adverse reactions, such as elevated pulse rate, pallor, or clammy skin.

Findings Normally, the physician records CSF pressure and checks the appearance of the specimen. Three tubes are collected routinely and are sent to the laboratory for analysis of protein, sugar, and cells, as well as for serologic testing, such as the Venereal Disease Research Laboratory test for neurosyphilis. A separate specimen is also sent to the laboratory for culture and sensitivity testing. A Gram stain may be ordered as a supplementary test. (See *CSF findings,* pages 149 and 150, for a summary of normal and abnormal findings in CSF analysis.)

Post-test care
- Usually the patient must lie flat for 8 hours after lumbar puncture. Some physicians, however, allow a 30-degree elevation of the head of the bed. Warn the patient that he must not raise his head to prevent a headache.
- Encourage fluid intake.
- Check the puncture site for redness, swelling, and drainage every hour for the first 4 hours, then every 4 hours for the next 20 hours.
- If CSF pressure is elevated, assess neurologic status every 15 minutes for 4 hours. If the patient is stable, assess every hour for 2 hours, then every 4 hours or according to pretest schedule.

➤ *Clinical alert:* Watch for complications of lumbar puncture, such as reaction to the anesthetic, meningitis, bleeding into the spinal canal, and cerebellar tonsillar herniation and medullary compression. Signs of meningitis include fever, neck rigidity, and irritability; signs of herniation include

CSF findings

Test	Normal	Abnormal	Implications
Pressure	50 to 180 mm H_2O	Increased	Increased intracranial pressure from hemorrhage, tumor, or edema caused by trauma
		Decreased	Spinal subarachnoid obstruction above puncture site
Appearance	Clear, colorless	Cloudy	Infection (elevated white blood cell [WBC] count and protein, or many microorganisms)
		Bloody	Subarachnoid, intracerebral, or intraventricular hemorrhage; spinal cord obstruction; traumatic tap (usually noted only in initial specimen)
		Brown, orange, or yellow (xantho-chromic)	Elevated protein, red blood cell (RBC) breakdown (blood present for at least 3 days)
Protein	15 to 45 mg/dl	Marked increase	Tumors, trauma, hemorrhage, diabetes mellitus, polyneuritis, blood in cerebrospinal fluid (CSF)
		Marked decrease	Rapid CSF production
Gamma globulin	3% to 12% of total protein	Increased	Demyelinating disease (such as multiple sclerosis), neurosyphilis, Guillain-Barré syndrome
Glucose	45 to 85 mg/dl	Increased	Systemic hyperglycemia
		Decreased	Systemic hypoglycemia, bacterial or fungal infection, meningitis, mumps, postsubarachnoid hemorrhage
Cell count	0 to 5 WBCs	Increased	Active disease: meningitis, acute infection, onset of chronic illness, tumor, abscess, infarction, demyelinating disease (such as multiple sclerosis)
	No RBCs	RBCs	Hemorrhage or traumatic tap

(continued)

CSF findings *(continued)*			
Test	**Normal**	**Abnormal**	**Implications**
VDRL and other serologic tests	Nonreactive	Positive	Neurosyphilis
Gram stain	No organisms	Gram-positive or gram-negative organisms	Bacterial meningitis

decreased level of consciousness, changes in pupil size and equality, altered vital signs (including widened pulse pressure, decreased pulse rate, and irregular respirations), or respiratory failure.

Interfering factors
- The patient's position and activity can alter CSF pressure. Crying, coughing, or straining may increase pressure.
- Delay between collection time and laboratory testing can invalidate results, especially cell counts.

Cerebrospinal fluid, immunofixation

This test, which uses electrophoresis to analyze cerebrospinal fluid (CSF) and serum samples for immunoglobulins, helps confirm diagnosis of multiple sclerosis (MS). Increased total protein content of CSF, primarily caused by increased CSF immunoglobulin synthesis, is characteristic of MS and certain other degenerative neurologic disorders. The CSF immunoglobulins in MS electrophorese as discrete populations, known as oligoclonal bands, rather than as the broad, homogeneous polyclonal bands characteristic of normal, polyclonal immunoglobulin. These discrete immunoglobulins presumably come from restricted clones of immune cells in the CSF of MS patients. Although establishing the presence of oligoclonal bands in CSF through electrophoresis may give sufficient diagnostic information in most cases (see also Multiple Sclerosis [MS] Screening Panel), immunofixation provides confirmation by ruling out rare bands that aren't composed of immunoglobulin.

In this test, a sample of CSF is concentrated to approximately 200 mg/dl (2 g/L) of the immunoglobulin G (IgG) concentration, then analyzed through an agarose gel electrophoresis technique. Specific antibodies to IgG, IgM, IgA, and other immunoglobulins are added to the electrophoresed proteins; these react to form insoluble precipitates in the agarose. After unreacted protein (nonimmunoglobulin) is removed by washing, the precipitates are visualized by staining with amido black. In the final evaluation, the oligoclonal band pattern of the CSF sample is compared to the stained immunofixation pattern, and the immunoglobulin and light chain classes of the oligoclonal bands are recorded. As a cross-check, a serum sample is also analyzed for oligoclonal bands. (The bands aren't clinically significant if the same bands occur in both CSF and serum.)

Purpose

To help confirm diagnosis of MS

Patient preparation

Explain the purpose of this test. Advise the patient that the test requires both blood and CSF samples but does not require restriction of food or fluids. Describe the procedure and warn that it may cause some stinging from injection of the anesthetic and local pain from insertion of the spinal needle during lumbar puncture for CSF sampling. Advise the patient that he may experience headache during the procedure; emphasize that cooperation during the procedure will minimize this and other possible discomfort.

Before the test, make sure that the patient or a responsible family member has signed a consent form. The patient may need a mild sedative to ease anxiety and promote relaxation before lumbar puncture.

Procedure

Perform a venipuncture, and collect a blood sample in a 7-ml *red-top* tube. Then, within 2 hours of blood sampling, perform a lumbar puncture, and collect at least 3 ml of CSF in a sterile tube that contains no additives. Label the samples properly and send them to the laboratory immediately after collection. If the test can't be performed on the day of collection, the samples should be refrigerated, but not frozen.

Precautions | During the lumbar puncture, observe the patient for any signs of adverse reactions, such as elevated pulse rate, pallor, or cool, clammy skin.

Findings | Normally, CSF contains no oligoclonal bands or only one band of any immunoglobulin class and light chain.

Implications of results | Positive test results (two or more oligoclonal bands found in CSF but not in the concomitant serum sample) support a diagnosis of MS *only* in conjunction with characteristic clinical findings. This test may also be positive in a variety of central nervous system disorders, including cryptococcal meningitis, idiopathic polyneuritis, neurosyphilis, chronic rubella panencephalitis, and subacute sclerosing panencephalitis.

Post-test care |
• If a hematoma develops at the venipuncture site, apply ice.
• The patient should remain supine for at least 8 hours after lumbar puncture, and should be encouraged to increase fluid intake.
• For the patient's comfort, the head of the patient's bed may be raised 20 degrees.
• Monitor vital signs and neurologic status frequently, and check the lumbar puncture site for redness, swelling, and drainage.

Interfering factors |
• Freezing and thawing of specimens can cause false-negative results.
• Delay between collection time and laboratory testing can invalidate results.

Ceruloplasmin, serum

This test measures serum levels of ceruloplasmin, an alpha$_2$-globulin that binds about 95% of serum copper (virtually no copper exists in a free state), usually in the liver. Because ceruloplasmin catalyzes oxidation of ferrous compounds to ferric ions, it is thought to regulate iron uptake by transferrin, making iron available to reticulocytes for heme synthesis. The usual clinical indications for this assay are Menkes' (kinky hair) syndrome, suspected copper deficiency from total parenteral nutrition, and suspected Wilson's disease.

Purpose	To aid diagnosis of Wilson's disease, Menkes' syndrome, and copper deficiency
Patient preparation	Explain that this test helps determine the copper content of blood and that the test requires a blood sample. Check the patient's history for medications that may influence ceruloplasmin levels.
Procedure	Perform a venipuncture, and collect the sample in a 7-ml *red-top* tube. Send the sample to the laboratory immediately.
Values	Serum ceruloplasmin levels normally range from 23 to 43 mg/dl (230 to 430 mg/L).
Implications of results	Low ceruloplasmin levels usually indicate Wilson's disease; this is confirmed by Kayser-Fleischer rings (copper deposits in the corneas that form green-gold rings) and liver biopsy results that show more than 250 mcg of copper/g (4.0 µmol/g) of dry weight. Low ceruloplasmin levels may also occur in Menkes' syndrome, nephrotic syndrome, and hypocupremia caused by total parenteral nutrition. Elevated levels may indicate certain hepatic diseases and infections.
Post-test care	If a hematoma develops at the venipuncture site, applying warm soaks eases discomfort.
Interfering factor	Estrogen, methadone, and phenytoin may elevate serum ceruloplasmin levels.

Cervical punch biopsy

Cervical punch biopsy is the excision by sharp forceps of a tissue specimen from the cervix for histologic examination. Generally, multiple biopsies are done to obtain specimens from all areas with abnormal tissue, or from the squamocolumnar junction and other sites around the cervical circumference. This procedure is indicated in patients with suspicious cervical lesions and should be performed when the cervix is least vascular (usually 1 week after menses). Biopsy sites are selected by direct visualization of the cervix with a colposcope — the most accurate method — or by Schiller's test, which stains normal squamous epithelium a dark mahogany but fails to color abnormal tissue.

Purpose
• To evaluate suspicious cervical lesions
• To diagnose cervical cancer

Patient preparation
Describe this procedure, and explain that it provides a cervical tissue specimen for microscopic study. Tell the patient that she may experience mild discomfort during and after the biopsy. Advise the outpatient to have someone accompany her home after the biopsy.

Make sure that the patient or a responsible family member has signed a consent form. Just before the biopsy, ask the patient to void.

Procedure
Place the patient in the lithotomy position. Tell her to relax as the unlubricated speculum is inserted.

Direct visualization: The colposcope is inserted through the speculum, the biopsy site is located, and the cervix is cleaned with a cotton-tipped applicator soaked in 3% acetic acid solution. The biopsy forceps are then inserted through the speculum or the colposcope, and tissue is removed from any lesion or from selected sites, starting from the posterior lip to avoid obscuring other sites with blood. Each specimen is immediately put in 10% formaldehyde solution in a labeled bottle. To control bleeding after biopsy, the cervix is swabbed with 5% silver nitrate solution (cautery or sutures may be used instead). If bleeding persists, the examiner may insert a tampon.

Schiller's test: An applicator stick saturated with iodine solution is inserted through the speculum. This stains the cervix to identify lesions for biopsy.

Label the specimens appropriately and send them to the laboratory immediately. Record the biopsy sites on the laboratory slip.

Findings
Normal cervical tissue is composed of columnar and squamous epithelial cells, loose connective tissue, and smooth-muscle fibers, with no dysplasia or abnormal cell growth.

Implications of results
Histologic examination of a cervical tissue specimen identifies abnormal cells and differentiates the tissue as intraepithelial neoplasia or invasive cancer. If the cause of an abnormal Papanicolaou test isn't demonstrated by cervical biopsy, or if the specimen shows advanced dysplasia or carcinoma in situ, a cone biopsy is performed in the operating room, under general anesthetic. Cone biopsy gar-

ners a larger tissue specimen and allows a more accurate evaluation of dysplasia.

Post-test care

- Instruct the patient to avoid strenuous exercise for 8 to 24 hours after the biopsy. Encourage the outpatient to rest briefly before leaving the office.
- If a tampon was inserted after the biopsy, tell the patient to leave it in place for 8 to 24 hours, as directed. Inform her that some bleeding may occur, but tell her to promptly report heavy bleeding (heavier than menstrual) to her physician. Warn the patient to avoid using tampons, which can irritate the cervix and provoke bleeding, according to her physician's directions.
- Tell the patient to avoid douching and intercourse for 2 weeks, or as directed.
- Inform the patient that a foul-smelling, gray-green vaginal discharge is normal for several days after biopsy and may persist for 3 weeks.

Interfering factor

Failure to obtain representative specimens or to place them in the preservative immediately may alter results.

Chlamydia antibodies, serum

Chlamydia are small, obligate intracellular bacteria that develop within inclusion bodies in the cytoplasm of host cells. These organisms divide by binary fission, contain both deoxyribonucleic acid and ribonucleic acid, possess enzymatic activities, contain cell-wall material, and are susceptible to several antibiotics. Although similar to viruses in their parasitism of eucaryotic cells, *Chlamydia* utilize their own ribosomes and enzymes for the synthesis of proteins and nucleic acids. The genus *Chlamydia* includes three species: *C. trachomatis, C. psittaci,* and *C. pneumoniae. C. trachomatis,* which consists of 15 serotypes, is the most common microbial cause of urethritis and cervicitis (serotypes D to K) and may lead to other complications in adults such as pelvic inflammatory disease and the sexually transmitted lymphogranuloma venereum (serotypes L1, L2, L3); in infants, the organism causes conjunctivitis and pneumonia (serotypes A, B, Ba, C). *C. psittaci* is transmitted from birds to humans resulting in lower respiratory tract infections (psittacosis). A newly recognized organism,

C. pneumoniae has been associated with acute respiratory tract infections of children and adults.

The single-antigen indirect immunofluorescence test (*C. trachomatis* L2-infected cell cultures as substrate) detects antibodies to the lipopolysaccharide group antigen of *Chlamydia*; this test assays antibodies developed after infection with *C. trachomatis, C. psittaci,* and *C. pneumoniae.*

The microimmunofluorescence test detects and differentiates chlamydial antibodies directed to each of the 15 serotypes of *C. trachomatis*. This test is extremely difficult to perform and is available only in research laboratories. Other testing techniques, such as direct fluorescent antibody staining, are available, however.

Purpose To detect chlamydial infection in patients with genital or respiratory tract disease

Patient preparation Explain the purpose of this test and inform the patient that the test requires a blood sample. Restriction of food, fluids, or medication is not required before the test. Also explain that a second test, or a test for the specific causative agent, may be required.

Procedure Perform a venipuncture to collect 5 ml of sterile blood in a *red-top* tube. Allow the blood to clot for at least 1 hour at room temperature. Handle the sample gently to prevent hemolysis. Transfer the serum to a sterile tube or vial and send it to the laboratory promptly. If transmittal of the serum must be delayed, it may be stored for 1 to 2 days at 39.2° F (4° C), or longer at –4° F (–20° C) to avoid microbial contamination.

Values Serum specimens from patients who have never been infected with *Chlamydia* will have no detectable antibodies to the organism (titer greater than 1:5). Sera from patients with uncomplicated oculogenital infections usually show low levels of antibody to *Chlamydia* in serum (1:5 to 1:160); sera from patients with manifestations of systemic chlamydial infection (such as pelvic inflammatory disease, infant pneumonia, lymphogranuloma venereum) usually show titers of greater than 1:640 in serum specimens.

Implications of results	Chlamydial infection can be ruled out in acute and convalescent patients whose serum specimens have no detectable antibody to the organism. High levels of the antibody (greater than 1:640) suggest, but do not prove, recent infection with *Chlamydia*. To confirm such infection, specimens for culture or antigen detection could be submitted for additional testing to specifically determine infection with *C. trachomatis, C. psittaci,* or *C. pneumoniae*.
Post-test care	If a hematoma develops at the venipuncture site, applying warm soaks eases discomfort.
Interfering factors	None

Chlamydia trachomatis, culture

C. trachomatis is the most common cause of sexually transmitted disease in the United States. The organism is an obligate intracellular parasite that must be cultivated in the laboratory by infection of susceptible cells. In this procedure, the elementary bodies of *C. trachomatis* attach to specific receptor sites on McCoy cells and are engulfed by the cytoplasm of the cells where the organisms divide within inclusion bodies. After 48 hours' incubation, *Chlamydia*-infected cells can be detected by fluorescein isothiocyanate-conjugated monoclonal antibodies (FITC-MoAb). Optimal conditions for recovery of *C. trachomatis* include: infection of McCoy cells in shell vials, centrifugation at 700×G, incubation for 48 hours, and staining with FITC-MoAb rather than iodine. Recovery of *C. trachomatis* is considered the laboratory method of choice, although rapid noncultural (antigen detection) procedures are available for processing specimens from most clinical sites. Strains of *C. psittaci* and *C. pneumoniae* are not detected in these cell cultures without specific technical manipulations and reagents for detecting these species.

Purpose	To confirm infections caused by *C. trachomatis*
Patient preparation	Explain the purpose of the test and the procedure for collecting the specimen for culture. If the specimen will be collected from a male's genital tract,

instruct the patient not to urinate for 3 to 4 hours before the specimen is taken.

Procedure   Obtain a specimen of the epithelial cells from the infected site. Acceptable sites in adults are the eye, urethra, endocervix, or rectum. Epithelial cells are collected from the urethra rather than from the purulent exudate that may be present. A specimen is obtained by inserting a cotton-tipped applicator into the urethra for a distance of ¾″ to 2″ (2 to 5 cm). (A new urine test for detecting *Chlamydia* in males has recently been approved by the Food and Drug Administration. This test, available from Abbott Laboratories, offers an easier and less painful method for identifying males with *Chlamydia* infections.) To collect a specimen from the endocervix, a microbiological transport swab or cytobrush is used. The specimen is then extracted into sucrose phosphate (2SP) transport medium. Specimens collected from the throat, eye, nasopharynx, and aspirates from infants should be extracted into 2SP transport medium. The specimens are sent to the laboratory at 39.2° F (4° C).

If the anticipated time between collection of the specimen and inoculation into cell culture is more than 24 hours, freeze the 2SP transport medium and send it to the laboratory with dry ice.

Note: All specimens from patients suspected of being sexually abused should be processed for *C. trachomatis* by culture rather than antigen detection methods.

Findings   The detection of infected inclusion bodies by FITC-MoAb specific to *C. trachomatis* confirms infection with this organism.

Implications of results   Detection of *C. trachomatis* in cell culture indicates active infection with the organism.

Post-test care   Patients with sexually transmitted disease should receive counseling regarding treatment of their partners.

Interfering factor   If the patient has taken antibiotics within a few days before collection of the specimen, *C. trachomatis* may not be recovered.

Chloride, serum

This test, a quantitative analysis, measures serum levels of chloride, the major extracellular fluid anion. Interacting with sodium, chloride helps maintain the osmotic pressure of blood and therefore helps regulate blood volume and arterial pressure. Chloride levels also affect acid-base balance. Serum concentrations of this electrolyte are regulated by aldosterone secondarily to regulation of sodium. Chloride is absorbed from the intestines and is excreted primarily by the kidneys.

Purpose
To detect acid-base imbalance (acidosis and alkalosis) and to aid evaluation of fluid status and extracellular cation-anion balance

Patient preparation
Explain to the patient that this test evaluates the chloride content of blood and that the test requires a blood sample. Check the patient's medication history for recent therapy with drugs that may influence chloride levels.

Procedure
Perform a venipuncture, and collect the sample in a 10- to 15-ml *red-top* tube. Handle the sample gently to prevent hemolysis.

Values
Normally, serum chloride levels range from 97 to 107 mEq/liter (mmol/L).

Implications of results
Chloride levels relate inversely to those of bicarbonate and thus reflect acid-base balance. Excessive loss of gastric juices or of other secretions containing chloride may cause hypochloremic metabolic alkalosis; excessive chloride retention or ingestion may lead to hyperchloremic metabolic acidosis.

Elevated serum chloride levels (hyperchloremia) may result from severe dehydration, complete renal shutdown, and head injury (producing neurogenic hyperventilation).

Low chloride levels (hypochloremia) are usually associated with overhydration, and low sodium and potassium levels. Possible underlying causes include prolonged vomiting, gastric suctioning, intestinal fistula, chronic renal failure, primary aldosteronism, and Addison's disease. Congestive heart failure or edema resulting in excess extracellular fluid can cause dilutional hypochloremia.

➤ *Clinical alert:* Observe a patient with hypochlor-emia for hypertonicity of muscles, tetany, and depressed respirations. In a patient with hyperchloremia, be alert for signs of developing stupor, rapid deep breathing, and weakness that may lead to coma.

Post-test care
If a hematoma develops at the venipuncture site, applying warm soaks eases discomfort.

Interfering factors
- Elevated serum chloride levels may result from administration of ammonium chloride, cholestyramine, boric acid, oxyphenbutazone, phenylbutazone, or excessive I.V. infusion of sodium chloride solution.
- Serum chloride levels are decreased by thiazides, furosemide, ethacrynic acid, bicarbonates, or prolonged I.V. infusion of dextrose 5% in water.
- Hemolysis caused by excessive agitation of the sample may interfere with accurate determination of test results.

Cholesterol, total

This test, the quantitative analysis of serum cholesterol, measures the circulating levels of cholesterol and cholesterol esters; it reflects the level of the two forms in which this compound appears in the body. Total cholesterol is the only cholesterol routinely measured.

Cholesterol, a structural component in cell membranes and plasma lipoproteins, is both absorbed from the diet and synthesized in the liver and other body tissues. It contributes to the formation of adrenocorticosteroids, bile salts, androgens, and estrogens.

A diet high in saturated fat raises cholesterol levels by stimulating absorption of lipids, including cholesterol, from the intestine; a diet low in saturated fat lowers them. Elevated total serum cholesterol levels are associated with an increased risk of atherosclerotic cardiovascular disease, particularly coronary artery disease (CAD).

Purpose
- To assess the risk of CAD
- To evaluate fat metabolism
- To aid diagnosis of nephrotic syndrome, pancreatitis, and hepatic disease

Patient preparation	Explain that this test determines the body's fat metabolism. If the patient is hospitalized, impose overnight fast and abstention from alcohol for 24 hours before the test. Tell the patient the test will require a blood sample. As appropriate, withhold medications that influence cholesterol levels.
Procedure	Perform a venipuncture, and collect the sample in a 7-ml *red-top* tube. Send the sample to the laboratory immediately, because cholesterol isn't stable at room temperature.
Values	Total cholesterol concentrations vary with age and sex, and commonly range from 150 to 200 mg/dl (3.87 to 5.17 mmol/L).
Implications of results	The desirable blood cholesterol level is below 200 mg/dl. Cholesterol levels of 200 to 240 mg/dl are considered borderline or at high risk for CAD, depending on other concurrent risk factors. Cholesterol levels that exceed 250 mg/dl indicate high risk of cardiovascular disease and require treatment.

Elevated serum cholesterol (hypercholesterolemia) may occur in hepatitis, lipid disorders, bile duct blockage, nephrotic syndrome, obstructive jaundice, pancreatitis, and hypothyroidism. Hypercholesterolemia caused by high dietary intake requires modification of eating habits and, possibly, medication to retard absorption of cholesterol.

Low serum cholesterol (hypocholesterolemia) is commonly associated with malnutrition, cellular necrosis of the liver, and hyperthyroidism. Abnormal cholesterol levels frequently necessitate further testing to pinpoint the disorder, depending on the type of abnormality and the presence of overt signs. Abnormal levels associated with cardiovascular diseases, for example, may necessitate lipoprotein phenotyping.

Post-test care	• If a hematoma develops at the venipuncture site, applying warm soaks eases discomfort. • The patient may resume diet and medications discontinued before the test.
Interfering factors	• Cholesterol levels are lowered by cholestyramine, clofibrate, colestipol, colchicine, dextrothyroxine, estrogen, dilantin, glucagon, heparin, kanamycin, haloperidol, neomycin, niacin,

nitrates, para-aminosalicylic acid, and chlortetracycline. Levels are raised by adrenocorticotropic hormone, corticosteroids, androgens, bile salts, epinephrine, chlorpromazine, trifluoperazine, oral contraceptives, salicylates, thiouracils, and trimethadione. Androgens may have a variable effect on cholesterol levels.

- Failure to follow dietary restrictions may interfere with test results.

Cholinesterase

The cholinesterase test measures the amounts of two similar enzymes that hydrolyze acetylcholine: pseudocholinesterase (serum cholinesterase or acylcholine acylhydrolase) and acetylcholinesterase (true cholinesterase). Acetylcholinesterase — present in nerve tissue and red blood cells — inactivates acetylcholine at nerve junctions and is essential for normal transmission of impulses across nerve endings to muscle fibers. Pseudocholinesterase — which is produced primarily in the liver — appears in the serum. It is active against acetylcholine and other choline esters. Both cholinesterases are inhibited by organophosphates. Declining cholinesterase levels in serum provide a sensitive marker of exposure to organophosphate insecticides.

Measuring cholinesterase is also important for evaluating a patient's potential risk of prolonged apnea during succinylcholine administration, which develops not from the drug itself, but because the patient lacks adequate pseudocholinesterase, which normally inactivates the muscle relaxant. Atypical pseudocholinesterases, which cause such reactions to muscle relaxants, can be detected by their resistance to inhibition by dibucaine or by the fluoride ion. Normal pseudocholinesterase shows about 78% inhibition by dibucaine; atypical homozygotes show about 15% inhibition by dibucaine. This percentage of inhibition is called the *dibucaine number*. Similar measurement of inhibition of pseudocholinesterase of the fluoride ion is expressed as the *fluoride number*.

Cholinesterase levels also decline in patients with hepatocellular diseases, but are not used to detect these conditions.

Purpose
- To evaluate the patient's potential response to succinylcholine (which is hydrolyzed by cholinesterase) before surgery or electroconvulsive therapy
- To identify atypical forms of pseudocholinesterase and thereby detect patients who may experience prolonged respiratory depression after receiving succinylcholine
- To assess suspected exposure to organophosphate insecticides
- To assess liver function and aid diagnosis of liver disease (a rare purpose)

Patient preparation

Explain that this test assesses muscle function or the extent of exposure to poisoning. Inform the patient that the test requires a blood sample but does not require fasting before the test.

Withhold substances that affect serum cholinesterase levels, as appropriate. If such substances must be continued, note this on the laboratory slip.

Procedure

Perform a venipuncture, and collect the sample in a 7-ml *red-top* tube. Handle the collection tube gently to prevent hemolysis. If the sample can't be sent to the laboratory within 6 hours after being drawn, refrigerate it.

Values

Total serum pseudocholinesterase levels range from 8 to 18 U/ml (determined by kinetic colorimetric technique).

Implications of results

Severely depressed pseudocholinesterase levels suggest a congenital deficiency or organophosphate insecticide poisoning. In acute poisoning, cholinesterase activity is less than 50% of normal. Levels near zero necessitate emergency treatment.

Pseudocholinesterase levels are usually normal in early extrahepatic obstruction, and are variably decreased in hepatocellular damage, such as hepatitis or cirrhosis (especially cirrhosis with ascites and jaundice). Levels also decline in acute infections, chronic malnutrition, anemia, myocardial infarction, obstructive jaundice, and metastasis.

Post-test care
- If a hematoma develops at the venipuncture site, applying warm soaks eases discomfort.
- The patient may resume medications that were discontinued before the test.

Interfering
factors

- Hemolysis caused by excessive agitation of the sample may interfere with accurate determination of test results.
- Pregnancy or recent surgery may interfere with accurate test results.
- Serum cholinesterase levels can be falsely depressed by cyclophosphamide, echothiophate iodide, monoamine oxidase inhibitors, succinylcholine, neostigmine, quinine, quinidine, chloroquine, caffeine, codeine, theophylline, epinephrine, ether, barbiturates, atropine, morphine, codeine, phenothiazines, vitamin K, and folic acid.

Chorionic villus sampling

Chorionic villus sampling is used to detect fetal abnormalities resulting from genetic disorders. This test, which can be performed as early as the 8th week of pregnancy, can detect chromosomal defects. It does not, however, detect neural tube defects, which require amniocentesis.

Chorionic villi are fingerlike projections that cover the developing embryo and attach it to the uterine lining before development of the placenta. Chorionic villus samples are best obtained between the eighth and tenth weeks of pregnancy. These tissue cells are cultured, and the resulting cells are examined microscopically for chromosome abnormalities.

Purpose

- To screen for fetal abnormalities such as Down's syndrome
- To establish fetal sex when the mother is a known carrier of a sex-linked genetic disorder

Patient
preparation

Describe the procedure and explain the purpose of the test. Inform the patient that she will be prepared for the procedure as for a gynecological examination; that a small catheter will be inserted through the cervix to a site between the wall of the uterus and the developing embryo; and that a small tissue sample will be removed by gentle suction. Answer the patient's questions about the procedure and ensure that the patient has signed a consent form.

Just before the procedure, the patient's vital signs should be taken and compared to baseline, and the patient should void.

Procedure   With the patient in lithotomy position, the examiner inserts a suction catheter via the speculum through the cervical os to the biopsy site. Suction is applied to the catheter to remove about 30 mg of tissue from the villi. The sample is withdrawn, placed in a Petri dish with an appropriate culture medium. The sample is labeled and sent to the laboratory immediately.

Precautions   Chorionic villus sampling is contraindicated in patients with a history of incompetent cervix.

Findings   Normally, no chromosomal abnormalities are detected.

Implications of results   Chromosomal abnormalities of structure or number identify genetic disorders, except neural tube defects.

Post-test care
- Clean the patient's perineum and take her vital signs. Encourage her to remain supine and rest for a few minutes after the procedure.
- Advise the patient to promptly report cramping or bleeding.
- Explain the test results and their implications. If necessary, recommend appropriate genetic or other counseling and follow-up care.

Interfering factors
- Chemotherapy may cause abnormal results, such as chromosome breaks.
- Contamination of tissue with bacteria, fungus, or a virus may inhibit growth of the culture.
- Inclusion of maternal cells may cause false results.

Chromium, serum

This analysis by atomic absorption spectroscopy measures serum levels of chromium, a trace element found in most body tissues. Chromium aids the transport of amino acids to the liver and heart cells, and appears to enhance the effects of insulin in glucose utilization. In fact, when combined in a complex with nicotinic acid, trivalent chromium (the biologically active form) is known as the glucose tolerance factor because of its special role in glucose metabolism. The primary natural sources of chromium are meats, brewer's yeast, and whole-grain cereals. Chromium toxicity can result from industrial overexposure to the metal, which is used in the tanning, electroplating, and steelmaking industries.

Purpose
- To detect chromium toxicity or exposure
- To monitor patients receiving total parenteral nutrition (TPN) containing chromium
- To assess insulin resistance in nonseptic patients during TPN
- To evaluate acquired glucose intolerance in patients receiving enteral or parenteral feedings

Patient preparation
Explain that this test helps detect excessive levels of chromium. Inform the patient that restriction of food or fluids is not required and that the test requires a blood sample. Check the patient's history for diagnostic tests performed during the previous 3 months in which radioactive hexavalent chromium was used (such as in red blood cell survival studies).

Procedure
Perform a venipuncture, and collect the sample in a metal-free collection tube. Laboratories provide special kits for this test on request. Handle the sample gently to prevent hemolysis, and send it to the laboratory immediately.

Values
Normally, serum chromium values range from 0.05 to 0.15 ng/ml (1 to 3 nmol/L). Some laboratories report higher normal values to compensate for poor handling and collection technique.

Implications of results
High chromium levels are normal at birth but steadily decrease with age. Significant elevations indicate chromium toxicity, which usually causes dermatitis and liver and kidney impairment.

Low chromium levels may diminish protein synthesis because of decreased utilization of amino acids, but little evidence exists to verify clinical chromium deficiency.

Post-test care
If a hematoma develops at the venipuncture site, applying warm soaks eases discomfort.

Interfering factors
- Recently performed diagnostic tests in which radioactive hexavalent chromium was used may interfere with accurate determination of test results.

- Failure to use a metal-free collection tube may interfere with accurate determination of test results.

Chromosome analysis

Chromosomes — threadlike bodies in the cellular nucleus — each contain thousands of genes with biochemical programs for cell function that are stored in deoxyribonucleic acid (DNA), the basic genetic material. Chromosome analysis can be essential for detecting certain genetic disorders, for identifying abnormalities of chromosomal structure or number, and for aiding sex determinations in patients with ambiguous genitalia.

Additional cytogenic tests frequently used for prenatal diagnosis of chromosome abnormalities include blood sampling, amniotic fluid analysis (see Amniotic Fluid Analysis), chorionic villus sampling (see Chorionic Villus Sampling), and percutaneous umbilical chord sampling.

Purpose
- To identify chromosomal abnormalities of number or structure as the underlying cause of malformation, maldevelopment, or disease
- To determine the cause of multiple miscarriages
- To detect carriers of chromosome abnormalities
- To aid in sex determination
- To aid diagnosis of neoplastic disorders

Patient preparation
Explain the purpose of this test and inform the patient (or the patient's parents) about collection of the necessary specimen.

Procedure
Collect a blood sample (in a 5- to 10-ml *green-top* [heparinized] tube), a tissue specimen, 1 ml of bone marrow, or at least 20 ml of amniotic fluid. (For additional information, see Bone Marrow Aspiration and Biopsy as well as Amniotic Fluid Analysis.)

Precautions
- Keep all specimens sterile, especially those requiring a tissue culture.
- To facilitate interpretation of test results, send the specimen to the laboratory immediately, with a brief patient history and indication for the test. If transport must be delayed, refrigerate the specimen but *never* freeze it.
- Before a skin biopsy, clean the site with antibacterial soap. Avoid povidone-iodine solution,

which is toxic to cells and will prevent cell growth in a tissue culture.

Findings   The normal cell contains 46 chromosomes: 22 pairs of autosomes and 1 pair of sex chromosomes (two Xs in normal females, and X and Y in normal males). To evaluate chromosomes for anomalies of number or structure, a karyotype is prepared, arranging chromosomes by homologous pairs according to size and structure — the largest placed first, and the smallest last. The 23 pairs of homologous chromosomes are arranged in seven groups (A through G). Individual chromosomes are distinguished by length, location of the primary constriction or centromere, arm ratios, secondary constrictions, presence of satellites, and staining patterns.

Implications of   See *Chromosome analysis findings,* pages 169 and
results   170, for common implications of test results.

Chromosome abnormalities may be numerical or structural. Numerical deviation from the norm of 46 chromosomes is called aneuploidy. Less than 46 chromosomes is called hypodiploidy; more than 46, hyperdiploidy. Special designations exist for whole multiples of the haploid number 23: diploidy for the normal somatic number of 46, triploidy for 69, tetraploidy for 92, and so forth. When the deviation occurs within a single pair of chromosomes, the suffix *somy* is used, as in trisomy for the presence of three chromosomes instead of the usual pair, or monosomy for the presence of only one chromosome.

Aneuploidy most commonly follows failure of the chromosomal pair to separate (nondisjunction) during anaphase, the mitotic stage that follows metaphase. It may also result from anaphase lag, in which one of the normally separated chromosomes fails to move to a pole and is left out of the daughter cells. Errors in mitotic division after the formation of the zygote will produce more than one cell line (mosaicism).

Structural chromosome abnormalities result from chromosome breakage. Intrachromosomal rearrangement occurs within a single chromosome in various forms —
Deletion: loss of an end (terminal) or middle (interstitial) portion of a chromosome
Inversion: end-to-end reversal of a chromosome segment, which may be pericentric inversion (in-

Chromosome analysis findings

Specimen and indications	Results	Implications
Blood To evaluate abnormal appearance or development suggesting chromosomal irregularity	Normal or abnormal chromosome number (aneuploidy) or arrangement; if normal, suggests problem is not cytogenic	Identifies specific chromosome abnormality
To evaluate couple with history of miscarriages, or to identify balanced translocation carriers having unbalanced offspring	Normal chromosomes	Miscarriage unrelated to partial chromosomal abnormality
	Parental balanced translocation or inversion carrier	Increased risk of repeated abortion or unbalanced offspring indicates need for amniocentesis, chorionic villi sampling, or percutaneous umbilical cord sampling in future pregnancies
To detect chromosomal rearrangements in rare genetic diseases or chromosome breakage caused by toxic agents, both predisposing patient to malignant neoplasms	Chromosomal rearrangements, gaps, and breaks	Occurs in Bloom's syndrome, Fanconi's syndrome, or telangiectasia; patient predisposed to malignant neoplasms
Blood or bone marrow To identify Philadelphia chromosome and confirm chronic myelogenous leukemia	Reciprocal translocation, usually between chromosomes 9 and 22 (long arm)	Aids diagnosis of chronic myelogenous leukemia
	Aneuploidy (usually caused by abnormalities in chromosomes 8 and 12)	Occurs in 158 different conditions, including acute myelogenous leukemia
	Trisomy 12	Occurs in 158 different conditions, including chronic lymphocytic leukemia
Skin To evaluate abnormal appearance or development suggesting chromosomal irregularity	All chromosomal abnormalities possible	Same as chromosomal abnormality in blood; rarely, patient with mosaicism has normal blood but abnormal skin chromosomes
Amniotic fluid To evaluate developing fetus with possible chromosomal abnormality	All chromosomal abnormalities possible	Same as chromosomal abnormality in blood or fetus

(continued)

Chromosome analysis findings *(continued)*		
Specimen and indications	**Results**	**Implications**
Placental tissue To evaluate products of conception after a miscarriage to determine if abnormality is fetal or placental in origin	All chromosomal abnormalities possible	Over 50% of spontaneously aborted tissue is chromosomally abnormal
Tumor tissue Clinical research	Many chromosomal abnormalities possible	Solid tumors are often associated with numeric and structural abnormalities; more than 20, such as synovial and Ewing's sarcomas, are tumor-specific

cluding the centromere) or paracentric inversion (occurring in only one arm of the chromosome)
Ring chromosome formation: breakage of both ends of a chromosome and reunion of the ends
Isochromosome formation: abnormal splitting of the centromere in a transverse rather than a longitudinal plane.

Interchromosomal rearrangements (of more than one chromosome, usually two) also occur. The most common rearrangement is translocation, or exchange, of genetic material between two chromosomes. Translocations may be balanced, in which the cell neither loses nor gains genetic material; unbalanced, in which a piece of genetic material is gained or lost from each cell; or reciprocal, in which two chromosomes exchange material.

Post-test care
- Provide appropriate post-test care, depending on the procedure used to collect the specimen.
- Explain the test results and their implications to the patient or to the parents.
- Recommend appropriate genetic or other counseling and follow-up care, such as an infant stimulation program for Down's syndrome.

Interfering factors
- Chemotherapy may cause abnormal results, such as chromosome breaks.
- Contamination of tissue with bacteria, fungus, or a virus may inhibit growth of the culture.

- Inclusion of maternal cells in a specimen may cause false results.

Coagulation factor assays
Assays for factors II, V, VII, and X

When prothrombin time (PT) and activated partial thromboplastin time (APTT) are abnormal (prolonged), factor assays help determine which factor is deficient. If PT is abnormal but APTT is normal, factor VII may be deficient. If both tests yield abnormal results, factors V and X and fibrinogen deficiencies should be excluded. (See *Factor nomenclature,* page 172, for additional information.)

In this test, samples of the patient's plasma deficient in a single factor are added to plasma. The activity of each factor in the patient's plasma is compared with normal plasma activity plotted on a predetermined standard curve for each factor. Observing which deficient plasma corrects the coagulation deficiency allows identification of specific factor deficiencies (see *Hereditary coagulation defects,* page 173).

Purpose
- To identify a specific factor deficiency in persons with prolonged PT or APTT
- To study patients with congenital or acquired coagulation defects

Patient preparation
Explain that this test assesses the function of the blood coagulation system. Inform the patient that restriction of food or fluids is not required, and that the test requires a blood sample.

Procedure
Perform a venipuncture, and collect the sample in a 7-ml *blue-top* tube. Completely fill the collection tube, and invert it gently several times to mix the sample and the anticoagulant adequately. Handle the sample gently to prevent hemolysis, and send it to the laboratory immediately, or place it on ice.

Precautions
If the patient has a suspected coagulation defect, avoid excessive probing during a venipuncture; don't leave the tourniquet on too long (it will cause bruising); and, after collecting the sample, apply pressure to the puncture site for 5 minutes, or until the bleeding stops.

Factor nomenclature	
Factor I	Fibrinogen
Factor II	Prothrombin
Factor III	Tissue thromboplastin
Factor IV	Calcium ions
Factor V	Accelerator proglobulin (AcG), proaccelerin, labile factor
Factor VII	Proconvertin, autoprothrombin I, serum prothrombin conversion accelerator (SPCA)
Factor VIII	Antihemophilic factor (AHF), antihemophilic globulin (AHG)
Factor IX	Christmas factor, plasma thromboplastin component (PTC), autoprothrombin II
Factor X	Stuart-Prower factor, Stuart factor, autoprothromin III
Factor XI	Plasma thromboplastin antecedent (PTA)
Factor XII	Hageman factor
Factor XIII	Fibrin-stabilizing factor (FSF)

Values Most factor levels range from 50% to 150%. Neonates have lower levels of vitamin K-dependent factors (II, VII, IX, and X).

Implications of results Deficiency of factor II, factor VII, or factor X may indicate hepatic disease, vitamin K deficiency, or warfarin therapy. Factor V deficiency suggests severe hepatic disease, disseminated intravascular coagulation, or fibrinolysis. Inherited deficiencies are rare and, if suspected, family studies should be performed.

Post-test care If a hematoma develops at the venipuncture site, applying warm soaks eases discomfort.

Interfering factors
- Hemolysis caused by excessive agitation of the sample may interfere with accurate determination of test results.
- Failure to mix the sample and anticoagulant adequately, or to send the sample to the laboratory

Hereditary coagulation defects	
Deficient factor	**Coagulation disorder**
Extrinsic pathway	
II	Hypoprothrombinemia
V	Parahemophilia
VII	Factor VII deficiency
X	Stuart factor deficiency
Intrinsic pathway	
VII	Hemophilia A (classic hemophilia), von Willebrand's disease (vascular hemophilia)
IX	Hemophilia B (Christmas disease)
XI	Plasma thromboplastin antecedent deficiency (PTA deficiency)

immediately or to place it on ice may alter test results.

- Oral anticoagulants reduce the levels of clotting factors II, VII, and X.

Coagulation factor assay, intrinsic

Assays for factors VIII, IX, XI, and XII

When prothrombin time (PT) is normal but activated partial thromboplastin time (APTT) is abnormal, specific factor assays help identify a deficiency in the intrinsic coagulation system — factor VIII, factor IX, factor XI, or factor XII (see *Factor nomenclature,* page 172, for additional information).

In this test, samples of the patient's plasma are added to deficient plasmas, each lacking a single factor. The activity of each factor in the patient's plasma is compared with normal plasma activity plotted on a predetermined standard curve for each factor. Observing which factor corrects the coagulation deficiency can identify disorders of factors VIII, IX, and XI. Additionally, contact factor deficiencies that do not cause bleeding (factor XII, prekallikrien, and high molecular weight kininogen) can be identified using plasmas deficient in these factors. (See *Hereditary coagulation defects,* page 173, for additional information.)

Purpose
- To identify a specific factor deficiency
- To study patients with congenital or acquired co-agulation defects

Patient preparation
Explain that this test assesses the function of the blood coagulation system. Inform the patient that restriction of food or fluids is not required and that the test requires a blood sample. Withhold oral anticoagulants before the test, as ordered. If such medications must be continued, note this on the laboratory slip.

Procedure
Perform a venipuncture, and collect the sample in a 7-ml *blue-top* (citrated) tube. Completely fill the collection tube, and invert it gently several times to mix the sample and the anticoagulant adequately. Handle the sample gently to prevent hemolysis, and send it to the laboratory immediately, or place it on ice.

Precautions
If a coagulation defect is suspected, avoid excessive probing during a venipuncture, don't leave the tourniquet on too long (it will cause bruising), and apply pressure to the puncture site for 5 minutes, or until the bleeding stops.

Values
Most factor levels range from 50% to 150%.

Implications of results
Factor VIII deficiency may indicate hemophilia A, von Willebrand's disease, or a factor VIII inhibitor. An acquired deficiency of factor VIII may result from disseminated intravascular coagulation or fibrinolysis. Factor VIII antigen and ristocetin cofactor tests distinguish between hemophilia A (and its carrier state) and von Willebrand's disease.

Factor IX deficiency may suggest hemophilia B, or it may be acquired as a result of hepatic disease, a factor IX inhibitor, vitamin K deficiency, or coumarin therapy. (Factors VIII and IX inhibitors occur after transfusions in patients deficient in either factor, and are antibodies specific to each factor; acquired inhibitors are rare.)

Factor XI deficiencies may be inherited and appear transiently in neonates. Factor XII deficiencies may be inherited or acquired (as in nephrosis) and, like factor XI deficiencies, may appear transiently in neonates. Unlike factor XI deficiency, inherited deficiencies of factor XII are not associated with bleeding.

Post-test care
- If a hematoma develops at the venipuncture site, applying warm soaks eases discomfort.
- A patient with a bleeding disorder may require a pressure bandage to stop bleeding at the venipuncture site.
- The patient may resume medications discontinued before the test.

Interfering factors
- Hemolysis caused by excessive agitation of the sample may interfere with accurate determination of test results.
- Failure to mix the sample and the anticoagulant adequately, or to send the sample to the laboratory immediately or to place it on ice may alter test results.
- Oral anticoagulants decrease factor IX levels; pregnancy elevates factor VIII.

Cocaine confirmation, urine

Because cocaine and its major metabolite, benzoylecgonine, are excreted in urine, screening tests to detect cocaine use commonly employ enzyme immunoassay or radioimmunoassay to detect benzoylecgonine in urine. Used correctly, these techniques offer a high degree of reliability; however, a positive result should be considered only presumptive. For definitive confirmation of the presence of cocaine or benzoylecgonine, a screen-positive urine sample should be reanalyzed by a second method. Gas chromatography-mass spectrometry (GCMS) has become the accepted standard for confirmatory testing. This method is both specific and highly sensitive: it provides qualitative confirmation of the presence of cocaine or benzoylecgonine in urine; it also yields a quantitative measure of their urinary concentration, which is critical to the interpretation of test results. Urine levels of benzoylecgonine or cocaine equal to or exceeding 150 ng/ml (500 nmol/L) by GCMS are considered positive in most laboratories. Although high-performance laboratories can detect lower levels, the 150 ng/ml threshold has been established to prevent the reporting of false positive results that might result from the normal variables associated with any analytical process. Because cocaine is rapidly converted to benzoylecgonine, it is commonly undetectable in a urine sample that is positive for benzoylecgonine. Such results are considered definitive evidence for cocaine use. Some laboratories confirm only benzoylecgonine by GCMS because a cocaine-positive, benzoylecgonine-negative specimen is unlikely.

Some investigators are studying the possible use of urinary cocaine-benzoylecgonine ratios to establish approximate time of last ingestion, but have offered no recommendations.

Purpose

To prove recent use of cocaine by providing definitive evidence for the presence of cocaine or its major metabolite, benzoylecgonine, in urine

Patient preparation

Explain the purpose of this test and inform the patient that the test requires a random urine specimen. Explain the procedure for collecting the specimen.

Procedure

The test requires a random urine specimen; collect a minimum volume of 25 ml.

Precautions

If the results might be challenged in a court of law, the specimen should be collected under chain-of-custody conditions. Special containers, security seals, chain-of-custody forms, and instructions for their use should be obtained from the testing laboratory. Urine collection must be carefully controlled because drug users may attempt to submit a bogus specimen. If direct visual observation is not part of the collection procedure, the facility for collection must minimize the possibility of dilution with water or addition of other adulterants such as bleach, vinegar, or table salt. A laboratory associated with the collection facility may be able to determine some combination of urine temperature, pH, specific gravity, or creatinine to aid detection of a diluted or adulterated specimen.

Values

Benzoylecgonine 150 ng/ml (500 nmol/L) or cocaine 150 ng/ml (500 nmol/L) constitutes a positive result for most laboratories. Benzoylecgonine less than 150 ng/ml (500 nmol/L) and cocaine less than 150 ng/ml (500 nmol/L) constitute a negative result for most laboratories.

Implications of results	A confirmed positive result establishes recent cocaine use. There is no established relationship between the quantity of cocaine or benzoylecgonine in urine and extent of intoxication, if any, at the time of collection. After moderate use, urine usually tests positive for 2 to 3 days after use; after heavy use, the detection time may be extended, allowing positive test results for up to a week after use.
Post-test care	None
Interfering factors	None

Cold agglutinins

Cold agglutinins are antibodies (usually of the immunoglobulin [Ig] type) that cause red blood cells (RBCs) to aggregate at low temperatures, and may occur in small amounts in healthy persons. Transient elevations of these antibodies develop during certain infectious diseases, notably primary atypical pneumonia. This test reliably detects such pneumonia within 1 to 2 weeks after onset. However, only half of patients with *Mycoplasma pneumoniae* show any appreciable rise in cold agglutinins; therefore, the test is not considered a useful diagnostic instrument.

Although cold agglutinins are inert at inner body temperatures, some become active in exposed areas of skin at 82.4° to 89.6° F (28° to 32° C), producing pallor and acrocyanosis (Raynaud's phenomenon), and numbness of hands and feet. Intense agglutination of a whole blood sample occurs on cooling to temperatures between 32° and 68° F (0° and 20° C), peaking at 39.2° F (4° C), and is reversible by rewarming to 98.6° F (37° C). However, after rewarming, complement remains on the cell and may produce hemolysis. Consequently, patients with high cold agglutinin titers, such as those with primary atypical pneumonia, may develop acute transient hemolytic anemia after repeated exposure to cold; patients with persistently high titers may develop chronic hemolytic anemia.

Purpose	• To help confirm primary atypical pneumonia, such as *M. pneumoniae*
	• To provide additional diagnostic evidence for cold agglutinin disease associated with many vi-

ral, bacterial, or parasitic infections, lymphoreticular malignant disease, or autoimimmune diseases

Patient preparation   Explain that this test detects antibodies in the blood that attack RBCs after exposure to low temperatures, and that the test may be repeated to monitor response to therapy. Tell the patient that restriction of food or fluids is not required and that the test requires a blood sample. If the patient is receiving antibiotics, note this on the laboratory slip because such medications may interfere with the development of cold agglutinins.

Procedure   Perform a venipuncture, and collect the sample in a 7-ml *red-top* tube that has been prewarmed to 98.6° F (37° C). Handle the sample gently to prevent hemolysis, and send it to the laboratory immediately. Don't refrigerate the sample; cold agglutinins will coat the RBCs, leaving none in the serum for testing.

Values   Normal titers are less than 1:16 but may be higher in elderly persons.

Implications of results   High titers may occur as primary phenomena, or secondary to infections or lymphoreticular malignant disease. They may be present in infectious mononucleosis, cytomegalovirus infection, hemolytic anemia, multiple myeloma, scleroderma, malaria, cirrhosis, congenital syphilis, peripheral vascular disease, pulmonary embolism, trypanosomiasis, tonsillitis, staphylococcemia, scarlatina, influenza, and, occasionally, in pregnancy. Chronically elevated titers are most commonly associated with pneumonia and lymphoreticular malignant disease; an acute transient elevation commonly accompanies many viral infections.

In primary atypical pneumonia, cold agglutinins appear in serum in one-half to two-thirds of all patients during the 1st week of acute infection, even before antimycoplasmal antibodies can be detected by complement fixation or metabolic inhibition tests. Thus, titers usually become positive at 7 days, peak above 1:32 in 4 weeks, and commonly disappear rapidly after 6 weeks. When sequential titers verify this pattern and clinical evidence of pneumonia exists, diagnosis is confirmed.

Extremely high titers (1:1,000 to 1:1,000,000) can occur with idiopathic cold agglutinin disease that precedes development of lymphoma. Patients with titers this high are susceptible to intravascular agglutination, which causes significant clinical problems.

Post-test care
- If cold agglutinin disease is suspected, keep the patient warm. If the patient is exposed to low temperatures, agglutination may occur within peripheral vessels, possibly leading to frostbite, anemia, Raynaud's phenomenon or, rarely, focal gangrene.
- Watch for signs of vascular abnormalities, such as mottled skin, purpura, jaundice, or pallor; pain or swelling of extremities; and cramping of fingers and toes. Hemoglobinuria may result from severe intravascular hemolysis on exposure to severe cold.
- If a hematoma develops at the venipuncture site, applying warm soaks eases discomfort.

Interfering factors
- Hemolysis caused by excessive agitation of the sample can falsely depress titers, as can refrigeration of the sample before serum is separated from RBCs.
- Antibiotics can interfere with the development of cold agglutinins.

Complement assays

Complement is a collective term for a system of at least 20 serum proteins designed to destroy foreign cells and to help remove foreign materials. Complement components are numerically designated as C1 through C9, with C1 having three subcomponents (C1q, C1r, and C1s), alternative pathways (factor B, factor D), and regulatory proteins (factor H, factor I). It comprises 3% to 4% of total serum globulins and plays a key role in antibody-mediated immune reactions. Complement can function as a defense by promoting removal of infectious agents, or as a threat by triggering destructive reactions in host tissues. Therefore, complement deficiency can increase susceptibility to infection and can predispose to other diseases, such as autoimmune diseases. Complement assays are thus indicated in patients with known or suspected immunomediated disease or repeatedly abnormal response to infection.

Normally, complement is present in serum in an inactive state until "fixed," or activated, in the classic pathway by binding to an antibody-coated surface. In the classic pathway, a specific antibody identifies and coats an antigen that enters the body. C1 then recognizes and binds with this specific antibody, activating the complement cascade — a series of enzymatic reactions involving all complement components — producing a coordinated inflammatory response, and usually resulting in cell lysis or some other damaging outcome.

In the alternate pathway, substances such as polysaccharides, bacterial endotoxins, and aggregated immunoglobulins react with properdin and factors B, D, H, and I, producing an enzyme that activates C3. In turn, C3 activates the remainder of the complement cascade.

In both pathways, specific inhibitors regulate the sequential activation of complement components. The C1 esterase inhibitor, the most commonly studied inhibitor, regulates the classic pathway. The C3b inhibitor is a fragment of C3b, a breakdown product that does not actually inhibit or regulate C3b.

Although various laboratory methods are used to evaluate and measure total complement and its components, hemolytic assay, laser nephelometry, and radial immunodiffusion are the most common. Hemolytic assay evaluates the lytic capacity of complement and is expressed as hemolytic units per millimeter, which is the dilution of serum needed to lyse 50% of the erythrocytes in the assay. In the hemolytic assay, sheep RBCs are mixed with a specific antiserum that lacks complement. Antibody-antigen complexes form, but because complement is absent, lysis can't occur. After the patient's serum sample is serially diluted, equal volumes of these sensitized sheep RBCs are added to each dilution. Complement activity, reported in CH_{50} units, is the dilution capable of lysing 50% of available RBCs.

Laser nephelometry measures C1 esterase inhibitor, C3, C4, properdin, and factor B; immunodiffusion measures C3, C4, C5, properdin, factor B, and C1 inhibitor. In laser nephelometry, the serum sample is mixed with monospecific antiserum for C1 esterase inhibitor. They react to form a precipitate that scatters light from a laser beam directed through it. The amount of light scattered reflects the amount of C1 esterase inhibitor in the serum.

In radial immunodiffusion, an agar slide is impregnated with monospecific antibody for the factor to be studied. Known standards of complement and the patient's serum are placed in appropriate wells punched in the agar. Within 24 hours, a precipitation ring forms around this well where antigen and antibody react; its diameter is proportional to the concentration of complement component.

Although complement assays provide valuable information about the patient's immune system, the results must be considered in light of serum immunoglobulin and autoantibody tests for definitive diagnosis of immunomediated disease or abnormal response to infection.

Purpose
- To measure complement levels in patients with systemic lupus erythematosus (SLE) suspected of incipient flare-up, and major organ (such as kidney) disease
- To monitor effectiveness of immunosuppressive SLE therapy
- To diagnose hereditary angioedema

Patient preparation
Explain that this test measures a group of proteins that fight infection. Inform the patient that restriction of food or fluids is not required and that the test requires a blood sample. If the patient is scheduled for C1q assay, check the patient's history for recent heparin therapy. Report such therapy to the laboratory because it may affect test results.

Procedure
Perform a venipuncture, and collect the sample in a 7-ml *red-top* tube. Handle the sample gently to prevent hemolysis, and send it to the laboratory immediately because complement is heat labile and deteriorates rapidly.

Values
Normal values for complement may vary, depending upon the laboratory and precisely how it performs the assay. Typically, however, normal values for complement range as follows —
Total complement: 41 to 90 hemolytic units
C1 esterase inhibitor: 16 to 33 mg/dl (160 to 330 mg/L)
C3: in males, 88 to 252 mg/dl (880 to 2500 mg/L); in females, 88 to 206 mg/dl (880 to 2100 mg/L)

C4: in males, 12 to 72 mg/dl (120 to 720 mg/L); in females, 13 to 75 mg/dl (130 to 750 mg/L).

Implications of results

Complement abnormalities may be genetic or acquired; acquired abnormalities are most common. Depressed total complement levels (which are clinically more significant than elevations) may result from excessive formation of antigen-antibody complexes, insufficient synthesis of complement, inhibitor formation, or increased complement catabolism, and are characteristic in conditions such as SLE, acute poststreptococcal glomerulonephritis, and acute serum sickness. Low levels may also occur in some patients with advanced cirrhosis of the liver, multiple myeloma, hypogammaglobulinemia, and rapidly rejecting allografts.

Elevated total complement may occur in obstructive jaundice, thyroiditis, acute rheumatic fever, rheumatoid arthritis, acute myocardial infarction, ulcerative colitis, and diabetes.

C1 esterase-inhibitor deficiency is characteristic in hereditary angioedema, the most common genetic abnormality associated with complement; C3 deficiency is characteristic in recurrent pyogenic infection; and congenital C4 deficiency may be a risk factor for developing SLE.

Post-test care

- Because many patients with complement defects have a compromised immune system, the venipuncture site should be kept clean and dry.
- If a hematoma develops at the venipuncture site, applying warm soaks eases discomfort.

Interfering factors

- Hemolysis of the sample or failure to send the sample to the laboratory immediately may interfere with accurate determination of test results.
- Recent heparin therapy can affect test results.

Complete blood count

Blood cell profile, blood count, CBC

A complete blood count (CBC) usually includes hemoglobin (Hb), hematocrit (HCT), red blood cell (RBC) count, red blood cell indices, platelet count, white blood cell (WBC) count, and differential white cell count tests. The CBC, a basic diagnostic procedure for all patients, is one of the most commonly prescribed clinical laboratory tests. The CBC may reveal considerable data about the patient, including diagnosis, prognosis, treatment response, and recovery.

Purpose
- To assess anemia, leukemia, polycythemia, and hemolytic disease of infants
- To evaluate reaction to inflammation, infection, dehydration, hydration, and chemotherapy management

Patient preparation
Tell the patient that these blood tests will help to determine if hematologic diseases are present and if treatments for dehydration and infection are effective. Explain that a CBC can be used to ascertain if chemotherapy is being managed appropriately. Inform the patient that food and fluids do not need to be restricted.

Procedure
Perform a venipuncture, and collect a blood sample in a 7-ml *lavender-top* tube. Fill the collection tube completely, and invert it gently several times to adequately mix the sample with the anticoagulant.

Values
Check the values for individual tests, presented alphabetically elsewhere in this book. Critical values include: HCT of less than 18% or more than 58%, Hb of less than 6 g/dl or more than 18 g/dl, platelet count of less than 20,000/mm^3 or more than 1,000,000/mm^3, and WBC of less than 2,500/mm^3 or more than 30,000/mm^3.

Implications of results
The presence of the following values may merit further investigation: hemoglobin less than 10 g/dl or more than 18 g/dl, mean corpuscular volume less than 80 μm^3 or more than 100 μm^3, mean corpuscular hemoglobin concentration more than 37%, and WBC less than 2,000/mm^3 or more than 20,000/mm^3.

Post-test care
If a hematoma occurs, applying warm soaks eases discomfort.

Interfering factor
Check individual tests.

Connective tissue disease test panel

These three test series aid the differential diagnosis of a variety of immune-mediated connective tissue diseases, including systemic lupus erythematosus (SLE), rheumatoid arthritis, Sjögren's syndrome, mixed connective tissue disease, and psoriatic arthritis.

Purpose   To aid differential diagnosis of immune-mediated connective tissue disease and help monitor disease activity

Patient preparation   Explain that this test panel helps diagnose and evaluate connective tissue disease. Instruct the patient to fast for 12 hours before the tests. Tell the patient the tests require one or more blood samples.

Procedure   Perform a venipuncture, and collect each sample in a 3-ml *red-top* tube. Send the samples to the laboratory immediately. If the disease activity assessment assay can't be performed within 4 hours of collection, the serum must be separated from the clot and frozen at –94° F (–70° C) until the test can be done.

Findings   The connective tissue disease screen, which includes a test for antinuclear antibodies (ANA) and rheumatoid factor screen and titer, is useful in the initial evaluation of patients with suspected immune-mediated inflammatory disease. The connective tissue disease autoantibody panel identifies the specific autoantibodies detected by the ANA test. Immunoglobulin G antibodies to double-stranded deoxyribonucleic acid (DNA) occur in SLE; antibodies to extractable nuclear antigens are found in SLE and other connective tissue diseases. The connective tissue disease activity assessment monitors exacerbations of SLE.

Implications of results   See *Connective tissue disease panel and test results*, for clinical conditions associated with abnormal results.

Post-test care   If a hematoma develops at the venipuncture site, applying warm soaks eases discomfort.

Connective tissue disease panel and test results

Test	Normal results	Abnormal results
Screening test ANA (antinuclear antibodies)	Negative	Positive in 60% to 90% of patients with systemic lupus erythematosus (SLE), and many normal people
RF (rheumatoid factor screen)	Nonreactive	Positive in > 75% of patients with rheumatoid arthritis, and many healthy persons
Autoantibody panel ENA (extractable nuclear antigen):		
RNP (ribonucleoprotein antigen)	Negative	Positive in mixed connective tissue disease
Sm (Smith antigen)	Negative	Positive in SLE
SS-A (Sjögren's syndrome antibody A)	Negative	Positive in SLE, Sjögren's syndrome, and congenital complete heart block
SS-B (Sjögren's syndrome antibody B)	Negative	Positive in Sjögren's syndrome and SLE
ds-DNA (double-stranded DNA)	< 70 units	A rise in titer may indicate increased disease activity
Activity assessment ds-DNA	< 70 units	Positive in 60% of SLE patients during active disease
CH$_{50}$ (total complement)	25 to 70 units	Depressed levels of complement occur during active inflammation in SLE

Interfering factors
- False-low total complement (CH$_{50}$) values can result from a delay in testing or from improper storage of specimens.
- The following drugs can cause false-positive results for ANA: chlorpromazine, phenytoin, ethosuximide, hydralazine, methyldopa, oral contraceptives, isoniazid, procainamide, and trimethadione.

Coombs' antibody screening test, indirect

Indirect antiglobulin test, screen for atypical antibodies

This test detects circulating antibodies in the patient's serum. The patient's serum is added to group O red blood cells (RBCs) of known antigen profiles. After an incubation period, the cells are washed to remove any unbound serum antibody. An antiglobulin (Coombs') serum is then added, and the cells are centrifuged. Agglutination or hemolysis occurs if the patient's serum contains an antibody to one or more antigens on the reagent RBCs.

The antibody screening test detects the most common clinically significant circulating antibodies. Occasionally, an antibody titer may be too low for detection, yielding a false-negative reaction. If an antibody is detected, it should be identified before a blood transfusion to prevent a hemolytic transfusion reaction.

Purpose
- To detect circulating antibodies to RBC antigens in the recipient's or donor's serum before transfusion
- To determine the presence of an atypical antibody in maternal blood capable of causing hemolytic disease of the newborn (HDN)
- To evaluate the need for $Rh_o(D)$ immune globulin administration
- To aid diagnosis of acquired hemolytic anemia

Patient preparation
Explain to the prospective blood recipient that the antibody screening test is a routine test performed before a blood transfusion to assess compatibility. If the test is being performed because the patient is anemic, explain that it helps identify the specific type of anemia. Inform the patient that the test requires a blood sample.

Check the patient's history for recent administration of blood, dextran, or I.V. contrast media. Any previous history of transfusion reaction, identified atypical antibody, delivery of an neonate with hemolytic disease of the newborn (HDN), or prior pregnancy should be noted on the Blood Bank laboratory slip.

Procedure
Verify the patient's identity. Perform a venipuncture, and collect the sample in a 10-ml *red-top* tube.

Handle the sample gently to prevent hemolysis. The sample must be completely and properly labeled at the patient's bedside to prevent clerical error or specimen misidentification.

Send the sample to the laboratory immediately. (The antibody screening must be done within 48 hours after the sample is drawn.)

Findings

Normally, agglutination does not occur, indicating that the patient's serum contains no circulating antibodies.

Implications of results

A positive result indicates the presence of one or more circulating antibodies to RBC antigens. Such a reaction may result in donor and recipient incompatibility.

A positive result in a pregnant patient with Rh-negative blood may indicate the presence of anti-D antibodies (antibodies to the Rh factor) from previous exposure during a prior pregnancy with an Rh-positive fetus or recent prophylactic administration of human $Rh_o(D)$ immune globulin.

A positive result should alert the clinician to the possibility that the fetus may develop HDN. As a result, repeated testing throughout the patient's pregnancy is performed to screen for the development of circulating antibodies. If a patient has a positive antibody screening test, tell her to inform her health care providers before a blood transfusion, and to wear a medical identification bracelet.

Post-test care

If a hematoma develops at the venipuncture site, applying warm soaks eases discomfort.

Interfering factors

- Previous administration of blood, dextran, or I.V. contrast media causes aggregation that resembles agglutination.
- Hemolysis caused by excessive agitation of the sample may interfere with accurate determination of test results.
- If a patient has received blood transfusions within the past 3 months, antibodies to this donor blood may develop and interfere with the patient's compatibility testing.

Coombs' antiglobulin test
Direct antiglobulin test, direct Coombs' test

The Coombs' antiglobulin test detects the presence of immunoglobulins (antibodies), or serum complement components that have coated red blood cells (RBCs) within the patient's circulation (in vivo). These coated RBCs may be either the patient's own cells, as occurs in autoimmune hemolytic anemia or hemolytic disease of the newborn (HDN), or be transfused donor cells, as occurs in hemolytic transfusion reactions.

In this one-stage test, RBCs are washed to remove all unbound serum proteins, and Coombs' antiglobulin reagent is added. If immunoglobulin or complement is present on the RBCs, agglutination occurs.

Purpose	• To diagnose HDN • To investigate hemolytic transfusion reactions • To aid diagnosis of hemolytic anemias, which may result from an autoimmune reaction or as an adverse reaction to certain drugs
Patient preparation	Explain to the parents that this test helps diagnose HDN. If the patient is suspected of having hemolytic anemia, explain that the test will help to identify whether the anemia is autoimmune in origin. Inform the adult patient that fasting is not required and that the test requires a blood sample.
Procedure	Verify the patient's identity. For an adult, perform a venipuncture, and collect the sample in either a *lavender-top* or *red-top* tube. (Check with your laboratory for its preference.) For a neonate, draw 5 ml of umbilical cord blood into a *red-top* or *lavender-top* tube after the cord is clamped and cut, or perform a heelstick and collect several capillary tubes. Handle the sample gently to prevent hemolysis. The sample must be completely and properly labeled at the patient's bedside to prevent clerical error or specimen misidentification. Send the specimen to the laboratory immediately. Do not refrigerate the specimen because this may cause a false-positive result. The test must be performed within 24 hours after the sample is drawn. On the laboratory slip, provide a history of recent blood transfusions, medication history, his-

tory of previous pregnancy, or delivery of a child with HDN.

Findings   A negative test in which neither antibodies nor complement appears on the RBCs is normal.

Implications of results   A positive test on umbilical cord blood indicates that maternal antibodies have crossed the placenta and have coated fetal RBCs, causing HDN. The specificity of maternal antibodies should be identified, and blood for neonatal transfusion must lack the corresponding antigen.

A positive direct antiglobulin test in a patient who has recently received a blood transfusion indicates that the patient is developing alloantibodies (atypical serum antibodies) against foreign RBC antigens; the donor cells within the patient's circulation are coated with antibody or complement. These donor cells will be destroyed, causing a hemolytic transfusion reaction. The atypical antibody should be identified and, as in HDN, all further blood for transfusion must lack the corresponding antigen.

A positive test result may indicate warm immune hemolytic anemia, either primary (idiopathic) or secondary to another disease, such as lymphoma, systemic lupus erythematosus, cold hemagglutinin disease, and paroxysmal nocturnal hemoglobinuria. Infections, such as mononucleosis, and some types of viral pneumonia can also produce a positive result.

A positive test result may also follow use of many drugs, including quinidine, methyldopa, cephalosporins, sulfonamides, chlorpromazine, ethosuximide, hydralazine, isoniazid, levodopa, mefenamic acid, melphalan, penicillin, procainamide, rifampin, streptomycin, and tetracyclines. A positive direct antiglobulin test following drug therapy does not always indicate that immune hemolysis is occurring in vivo. If a drug does cause hemolytic anemia, it should be discontinued.

Post-test care   If a hematoma develops at the venipuncture site, applying warm soaks eases discomfort.

Interfering factors   • Hemolysis caused by excessive agitation of the sample or poor venipuncture technique may interfere with accurate determination of test results.

• Refrigeration of blood collected in a *red-top* tube results in nonspecific binding of serum complement components. The cold will cause a false-positive test.

Copper reduction test
Clinitest

The copper reduction test measures the concentration of reducing substances in the urine through their reaction with a commercially prepared tablet such as Clinitest, an agent that reacts to glucose and to other reducing substances (mostly sugars). This test is most valuable for providing a simple, at-home method for monitoring the diabetic patient's urine sugar level.

Purpose
• To detect glycosuria and galactosuria
• To screen for diabetes mellitus and pentosuria (monosaccharides in urine)
• To monitor urine glucose levels during insulin therapy, after determination that the sugar in the urine is glucose

Patient preparation
Explain that this test determines urine sugar level. Teach the patient who has recently been diagnosed as diabetic how to perform the Clinitest tablet test. Have the patient void; then give him a drink of water. After 30 to 45 minutes, collect a second-voided urine specimen. Instruct the patient not to contaminate the specimen with toilet tissue or stool.

Check the patient's history for medications that may interfere with the test results.

Equipment
Specimen container, 10-ml test tube, medicine dropper, Clinitest tablets, Clinitest color chart

Procedure
After collecting a second-voided specimen, perform the five-drop Clinitest tablet test: Hold the medicine dropper vertically, and instill five drops of urine from the specimen container into the test tube. Rinse the dropper with water, and add 10 drops of water to the test tube. Add one Clinitest tablet, and observe the color change, especially during effervescence — the pass-through phase. Wait 15 seconds after effervescence subsides, and gently agitate the test tube. If color develops at the 15-second interval, read the color against the Clini-

test color chart, and record the results. Ignore any changes that develop after 15 seconds.

If rapid color changes occur in the pass-through phase of the five-drop test, record the results as over 2% without comparison to the color chart. Or, perform a two-drop Clinitest tablet test: Hold the medicine dropper vertically, and instill two drops of urine into the test tube. Flush urine residue from the dropper with water, then add 10 drops of water to the test tube. Add one Clinitest tablet, and observe the color change during the pass-through phase. Wait 15 seconds after effervescence stops; compare the color with the appropriate color reference chart, and record the results.

Rapid color changes (bright orange to dark brown or green-brown) in the pass-through phase in a five-drop Clinitest reaction indicate glycosuria of 2% or more; in a two-drop Clinitest reaction, glycosuria up to 5% can be measured.

Precautions
- Ensure that hands are dry when handling Clinitest tablets and avoid contact with eyes, mucous membranes, GI tract, and clothing because sodium hydroxide and moisture produce caustic burns.
- Store tablets in a well-marked, childproof bottle to prevent accidental ingestion.
- Don't use discolored tablets (dark blue). The normal color of fresh tablets is light blue with darker blue flecks.
- During effervescence, hold the test tube near the top to avoid burning your hand; it becomes boiling hot.

Findings
Normally, no glucose is present in urine.

Implications of results
Glycosuria occurs in diabetes mellitus; adrenal and thyroid disorders; hepatic and central nervous system diseases; Fanconi's syndrome; and other conditions involving low renal threshold, toxic renal tubular disease, heavy metal poisoning, glomerulonephritis, nephrosis, pregnancy, and total parenteral nutrition; with administration of large amounts of glucose and some drugs, such as asparaginase, corticosteroids, carbamazepine, ammonium chloride, thiazide diuretics, dextrothyroxine, large amounts of nicotinic acid, lithium carbonate, and prolonged use of phenothiazines.

Reducing substances that give false-positive results		
Aminosalicylic acid	Fructose	Nalidixic acid
Ascorbic acid	Galactose	Nitrofurantoin
Cephalosporins	Glucuronic acid	Penicillin G
Chloral hydrate	Isoniazid	Probenecid
Chloramphenicol	Ketone bodies	Salicylates
Creatinine	Lactose	Tetracycline
Cystine	Levodopa	Uric acid
Formaldehyde	Maltose	

Post-test care Provide written guidelines and a flow sheet to help the patient record the Clinitest results and monitor insulin therapy at home.

Interfering factors
- Large doses of cephalosporins, penicillin, nalidixic acid, ascorbic acid, and probenecid may produce false-positive results. Tetracycline and ascorbic acid may produce false-positive or false-negative results, depending on the test method. See also Urinalysis (UA), Routine for medications that may affect urine glucose levels.
- Presence of reducing substances other than glucose may influence test results. (See *Reducing substances that give false-positive results*.)
- Failure to detect the pass-through phenomenon or to use the correct reference chart for color comparison of the specimen may influence test results.
- Low renal threshold for glucose may alter test results.
- Failure to use whole or fresh Clinitest tablets or to keep tablet container tightly closed to prevent absorption of light or moisture may interfere with accurate determination of test results.
- Failure to use freshly voided urine or to flush urine residue from the medicine dropper may affect test results.

Copper, urine

This test measures the urine level of copper, an essential trace element and a component of several metalloenzymes and proteins necessary for hemoglobin synthesis and oxidation reduction. Urine normally contains only a small amount of free copper; only trace amounts of free copper exist in plasma. Most copper in plasma is bound to and transported by an alpha$_2$-globulin (plasma protein) called ceruloplasmin. When copper is unbound, the ions can inhibit many enzyme reactions, resulting in copper toxicity.

Determination of urine copper levels is frequently used to detect Wilson's disease, a rare, inborn metabolic error, most common among persons of eastern European Jewish, southern Italian, or Sicilian ancestry. Wilson's disease is marked by decreased ceruloplasmin, increased urinary excretion of copper, and accumulation of copper in the interstitial tissues of the liver and brain. The cause of this disorder is unclear. Early detection and treatment (low-copper diet and D-penicillamine) are vital to prevent irreversible changes, such as nerve tissue degeneration and cirrhosis of the liver.

Purpose	• To detect Wilson's disease, Menkes' (kinky hair) syndrome, or copper toxicity • To screen infants with family histories of Wilson's disease
Patient preparation	Explain that this test determines the amount of copper in urine. Inform the patient that the test requires a 24-hour urine specimen, and, if it's to be collected at home, describe the proper collection technique. Tell the patient not to contaminate the urine specimen with toilet tissue or stool.
Procedure	Collect a 24-hour urine specimen in a plastic urine container.
Values	Normal urinary excretion of copper is 15 to 60 µg/day (0.22 to 0.9 µmol/day).
Implications of results	Elevated urine copper levels usually indicate Wilson's disease (a liver biopsy helps establish this diagnosis). High copper levels may also occur in Menkes' syndrome and copper toxicity. Low levels

of copper in the patient's urine indicate a copper nutritional deficiency.

Post-test care   None

Interfering   • Failure to collect all urine during the test period
factors   may alter test results.
             • Administration of D-penicillamine (rarely given
               before diagnosis) causes elevated urine levels of
               copper.
             • Allowing the specimen to come in contact with
               metal or stool may interfere with the results.

Cortisol, plasma

Cortisol — the principal glucocorticoid secreted by the zona fasciculata of the adrenal cortex, primarily in response to adrenocorticotropic hormone (ACTH) stimulation — helps metabolize nutrients, mediate physiologic stress, and regulate the immune system. Cortisol secretion normally follows a diurnal pattern: levels rise during the early morning hours and peak around 8 a.m., then decline to extremely low levels in the evening and during the early phase of sleep. Production of this hormone is influenced by physical or emotional stress, which activates ACTH. Thus, intense heat or cold, infection, trauma, exercise, obesity, and debilitating disease influence cortisol secretion.

This immunoassay, a quantitative analysis of plasma cortisol levels, is usually ordered for patients with signs of adrenal dysfunction, but dynamic tests, suppression tests for hyperfunction, and stimulation tests for hypofunction are generally required for confirmation of diagnoses. (For additional information, see Dexamethasone Suppression Test and ACTH, Rapid-Stimulation Test.)

Purpose   To aid diagnosis of Cushing's disease, Cushing's syndrome, Addison's disease, and secondary adrenal insufficiency

Patient   Explain that this test helps determine if the patient's
preparation   symptoms are caused by improper hormonal secretion. Instruct the patient to maintain a normal salt diet (2 to 3 g/day) for 3 days before the test and to fast and limit physical activity for 10 to 12 hours before the test. Tell the patient the test requires a blood sample.

Withhold all medications that may interfere with plasma cortisol levels, such as estrogens, androgens, and phenytoin, for 48 hours before the test. If the patient is receiving corticosteroid therapy, note this on the laboratory slip, as well as any other medications that must be continued.

The patient should be relaxed and recumbent for at least 30 minutes before the test.

Procedure
: Between 6 a.m. and 8 a.m., perform a venipuncture. Collect the sample in a *green-top* (heparinized) tube, label appropriately, and send to the laboratory immediately. For diurnal variation testing, draw another sample between 4 p.m. and 6 p.m. Collect it in a *green-top* tube, label appropriately, and send to the laboratory immediately.

Handle the sample gently to prevent hemolysis. Record the collection time on the laboratory slip.

Values
: Normally, plasma cortisol levels range from 7 to 28 mcg/dl (190 to 760 nmol/L) in the morning, and from 2 to 18 mcg/dl (50 to 490 nmol/L) in the afternoon. (The afternoon level is usually half the morning level.)

Implications of results
: Increased plasma cortisol levels may indicate adrenocortical hyperfunction in Cushing's disease (a rare disease caused by basophilic adenoma of the pituitary gland) or in Cushing's syndrome (glucocorticoid excess from any cause). In most patients with Cushing's syndrome, the adrenal cortex tends to secrete independently of any natural rhythm. Thus, absence of diurnal variation in cortisol secretion is a significant finding in almost all patients with Cushing's syndrome; in these patients, little difference in values is found between morning samples and those taken in the afternoon. Diurnal variations may also be absent in otherwise healthy persons who are under emotional or physical stress.

Decreased cortisol levels may indicate primary adrenal hypofunction (Addison's disease), most often caused by idiopathic glandular atrophy (a presumed autoimmune process). Tuberculosis, fungal invasion, and hemorrhage can cause adrenocortical destruction. Low cortisol levels resulting from secondary adrenal insufficiency may occur in conditions of impaired ACTH secretion, such as hypophysectomy, postpartum pituitary necrosis, craniopharyngioma, or chromophobic adenoma.

Post-test care
- If a hematoma develops at the venipuncture site, applying warm soaks eases discomfort.
- The patient may resume diet and medications that were discontinued before the test.

Interfering factors
- Failure to observe restrictions of diet, medications, or physical activity may interfere with accurate determination of test results. Plasma cortisol levels are falsely elevated by estrogens (during pregnancy or in oral contraceptives), which increase plasma proteins that bind with cortisol. Obesity, stress, or severe hepatic or renal disease may also increase these levels. Plasma cortisol levels may be decreased by androgens and phenytoin, which decrease cortisol-binding proteins.
- Radioactive scan performed within 1 week before the test may influence the results.
- Hemolysis caused by excessive agitation of the sample may interfere with accurate determination of test results.

Cortisol, urine-free

This test measures urine levels of the portion of cortisol not bound to the corticosteroid-binding globulin transcortin. It is one of the best diagnostic tools for detecting Cushing's syndrome. The major glucocorticoid secreted by the adrenal cortex in response to adrenocorticotropic hormone (ACTH) stimulation, cortisol helps regulate fat, carbohydrate, and protein metabolism; it also helps promote glyconeogenesis, anti-inflammatory response, and cellular permeability. Only about 10% of this hormone is unbound and physiologically active; this small portion is known as free cortisol. Urine-free cortisol concentrations increase significantly when the cortisol secreted exceeds the binding capacity of transcortin, which is normally almost saturated.

Assays of free cortisol levels in a 24-hour urine specimen — unlike a single measurement of plasma cortisol — reflect cumulative secretion levels instead of diurnal variations. Concurrent measurements of plasma cortisol and ACTH, with urine 17-hydroxycorticosteroids and the dexamethasone suppression test, may be used to confirm diagnosis.

Purpose   To aid diagnosis of Cushing's syndrome

Patient preparation
Explain that this test helps evaluate adrenal gland function. Advise the patient to maintain food and fluid intake before the test, but to avoid stressful situations and excessive physical exercise during the collection period. Inform the patient that the test requires collection of a 24-hour urine specimen, and teach the proper collection technique.

Check the patient's recent drug history for medications (such as those listed below) that may interfere with test results and restrict such medications before the test.

Procedure
Collect a 24-hour urine specimen in a bottle containing a preservative to keep the specimen at a pH of 4.0 to 4.5. Refrigerate the specimen or place it on ice during the collection period.

Values
Normally, free cortisol values range from 24 to 108 mcg/day (60 to 300 nmol/day).

Implications of results
Elevated free cortisol levels may indicate Cushing's syndrome resulting from adrenal hyperplasia, adrenal or pituitary tumor, or ectopic ACTH production. Hepatic disease and obesity, which can raise plasma cortisol levels, generally don't appreciably affect urine levels of free cortisol.

This test is designed to screen for excessive secretion of free cortisol. Low levels have little diagnostic significance and don't necessarily indicate adrenocortical hypofunction.

Post-test care
The patient may resume normal activity restricted during the test and medications discontinued before the test.

Interfering factors
- Corticosteroid therapy and medications such as reserpine, phenothiazines, morphine, and amphetamines may elevate free cortisol levels.
- Failure to collect all urine during the test period or to store the specimen properly will interfere with accurate determination of test results.
- Failure to observe drug restrictions may interfere with accurate determination of test results.

C-reactive protein

Usually present only in very low levels in the sera of healthy persons, C-reactive protein (CRP) is an acute-phase reactant produced by the liver and excreted into the bloodstream during the acute phase of inflammation of any cause. CRP was initially discovered in the sera of patients with pneumococcal pneumonia, where it was shown to react with the C-mucopolysaccharide of the bacterial capsule — hence the name C-reactive protein. The major function of CRP is its interaction with the complement system.

Antiserum is used to detect CRP in several immunoassays — radioimmunoassay, capillary precipitation, gel diffusion, and latex agglutination. Although the presence of CRP strongly suggests active inflammation, the test is nonspecific for any disorder. Nevertheless, early detection of inflammation allows prompt treatment, possibly with anti-inflammatory agents, to prevent tissue damage from the disorder.

Purpose
- To detect inflammatory disease, such as rheumatoid arthritis and rheumatic fever
- To monitor response to therapy, especially in acute rheumatic fever and rheumatoid arthritis

Patient preparation
Explain that this test detects generalized inflammation. This test is a nonspecific method used to evaluate the severity and course of inflammatory diseases, and to monitor the effectiveness of treatment. Tell the patient the test requires a blood sample, but no fasting.

Procedure
Perform a venipuncture, and collect the sample in a 7-ml *red-top* tube.

Values
Normal test value is less than 0.8 mg/dl.

Implications of results
The presence of CRP in serum indicates an acute inflammatory condition (tissue reaction to injury resulting from infectious or noninfectious causes), and an elevation in CRP levels usually occurs before the erythrocyte sedimentation rate rises. CRP disappears when treatment with corticosteroids or salicylates suppresses inflammation. A positive test for CRP commonly occurs in bacterial infections, such as tuberculosis and pneumococcal pneumonia, and in many noninfectious inflammatory conditions, such as acute rheumatic fever, acute rheumatoid arthritis, systemic lupus erythematosus, malignancy, and myocardial infarction.

Positive CRP occurs during the last half of pregnancy and also accompanies the use of oral contraceptives.

Post-test care
- If a hematoma develops at the venipuncture site, applying warm soaks eases discomfort.
- The patient may resume a normal diet.

Interfering factors
Pregnancy, ingestion of oral contraceptives, or use of an intrauterine device may cause positive test results through production of CRP because of tissue stress.

Creatine, serum

This test measures serum levels of creatine, an end product of protein metabolism. Creatine is formed in the liver, kidneys, small intestinal mucosa, and pancreas, and is distributed to muscle tissues, where it combines with phosphate to form phosphocreatine — a high-energy compound. In the anaerobic stage of muscle contraction, this compound is enzymatically cleaved, and some creatine enters the bloodstream, normally in an amount proportional to the body's muscle mass. However, muscular diseases may greatly increase the amount of creatine released into the blood. Creatine levels are usually measured by the difference in creatinine before and after conversion to creatinine by heat.

Purpose
To aid diagnosis of muscular diseases, including muscular dystrophies

Patient preparation
Explain the purpose of this test and that the test requires a blood sample. Instruct the patient to restrict food, fluids, and exercise for approximately 12 hours before the test. Check the patient's medication history for recent use of drugs that may influence creatine levels. If such medications must be continued, note this on the laboratory slip.

Procedure
Perform a venipuncture, and collect the sample in a 10- to 15-ml *red-top* tube. Handle the sample gently to prevent hemolysis, and send the specimen to the laboratory immediately.

Values
: Creatine values in males normally range from 0.2 to 0.6 mg/dl (10 to 50 μmol/L); in females, from 0.6 to 1 mg/dl (50 to 80 μmol/L).

Implications of results
: Greatly increased serum creatine levels follow necrosis or atrophy of skeletal muscle, as in trauma, amyotrophic lateral sclerosis, dermatomyositis, and the progressive muscular dystrophies. Creatine levels may also rise above normal in hyperthyroidism and pregnancy, and after excessive dietary intake of protein.

Post-test care
: • If a hematoma develops at the venipuncture site, applying warm soaks eases discomfort.
  • The patient may resume withheld medications.

Interfering factors
: • Testosterone therapy increases creatine synthesis by the liver and can therefore elevate serum creatine levels.
  • Hemolysis caused by excessive agitation of the sample may alter test results.

Creatine kinase

Creatine kinase (CK), formerly known as creatine phosphokinase (CPK) is an enzyme that catalyzes the phosphorylation of creatine by adenosine triphosphate in muscle cells and brain tissue. Because of its intimate role in energy production, CK reflects normal tissue catabolism; an increase above normal serum levels indicates trauma to cells with high CK content. CK may be separated into three isoenzymes with distinct molecular structures: CK-BB, CK-MB, and CK-MM. CK-BB is found primarily in brain tissue; CK-MB, in cardiac muscle (a small amount also appears in skeletal muscle); and CK-MM, in skeletal muscle.

An assay of total serum CK was once widely used to detect acute myocardial infarction (MI), but elevated serum CK levels caused by skeletal muscle damage reduce the test's specificity for this disorder. Fractionation and measurement of CK isoenzymes is rapidly replacing use of total CK to accurately localize the site of increased tissue destruction.

Purpose
: • To detect and diagnose acute MI and reinfarction (CK-MB primarily used)

- To evaluate possible causes of chest pain and to monitor the severity of myocardial ischemia after cardiac surgery, cardiac catheterization, or cardioversion (CK-MB primarily used)
- To detect skeletal muscle disorders that are not of neurogenic origin, such as Duchenne's muscular dystrophy (total CK primarily used), and early dermatomyositis

Patient preparation

Explain the purpose of this test, and that multiple blood samples are required to detect fluctuations in serum levels. The patient need not restrict food or most fluids before the test. The patient who is being evaluated for skeletal muscle disorders should avoid exercising for 24 hours before the test.

Withhold alcohol, aminocaproic acid, and lithium before the test. If these substances must be continued, note this on the laboratory slip.

Procedure

Perform a venipuncture, and collect the sample in a 7-ml *red-top* tube. Handle the collection tube gently to prevent hemolysis, and send the sample to the laboratory immediately (CK activity diminishes significantly after 2 hours at room temperature).

Precautions

- Draw the sample before or within 1 hour of I.M. injections, as muscle trauma raises total CK levels.
- Obtain the sample on schedule. Note on the laboratory slip the time the sample was drawn and the hours elapsed since onset of chest pain.

Values

Total CK values determined by the most commonly performed assay range from 40 to 175 U/L (0.67 to 2.9 μkat/L in males; in females, from 25 to 140 U/L (0.42 to 2.3 μkat/L). *Note:* different methods give different ranges. Typical ranges for isoenzyme levels are as follows: CK-BB, undetectable; CK-MB, undetectable to 7 U/L; CK-MM, 5 to 70 U/L.

Implications of results

CK-MM constitutes over 99% of total CK normally present in serum. Detectable CK-BB isoenzyme may indicate brain tissue injury, certain widespread malignant tumors, severe shock, or renal failure. However, such elevations don't confirm a specific diagnosis.

CK-MB isoenzyme greater than 5% of total CK (or more than 10 U/L) suggests MI, especially if the ratio of isoenzyme lactate dehydrogenase$_1$ to lactate dehydrogenase$_2$ (LD_1:LD_2) is greater than 1 (flipped LD). In acute MI and following cardiac surgery, the CK-MB level begins to rise in 2 to 4 hours, peaks in 12 to 24 hours, and usually returns to normal in 24 to 48 hours; persistent elevations or increasing levels indicate ongoing myocardial damage. Total CK levels follow roughly the same pattern but rise slightly later. CK-MB levels don't rise in congestive heart failure or during angina pectoris not accompanied by myocardial cell necrosis (not all investigators agree on this, however). Serious skeletal muscle injury that occurs in certain muscular dystrophies, polymyositis, and severe myoglobinuria may produce mild CK-MB elevation because a small amount of this isoenzyme is present in some skeletal muscles.

Rising CK-MM values follow skeletal muscle damage from trauma, such as surgery and I.M. injections, or from diseases, such as dermatomyositis and muscular dystrophy (values may be 50 to 100 times normal). A moderate rise in CK-MM levels develops in patients with hypothyroidism; sharp elevations occur with muscular activity caused by agitation, such as an acute psychotic episode.

Total CK levels may be elevated in patients with severe hypokalemia, carbon monoxide poisoning, malignant hyperthermia, postconvulsions, alcoholic cardiomyopathy, and, occasionally, in those who have suffered pulmonary or cerebral infarctions.

Post-test care
- If a hematoma develops at the venipuncture site, applying warm soaks eases discomfort.
- The patient may resume medications discontinued before the test.

Interfering factors
- Hemolysis caused by excessive agitation of the sample may affect CK levels.
- Failure to send the sample to the laboratory immediately or to refrigerate the serum if testing will be delayed for more than 2 hours may hinder accurate determination of CK levels.
- Failure to draw the samples at the scheduled time, missing peak levels, may interfere with accurate determination of test results.
- Halothane and succinylcholine, alcohol, lithium, and large doses of aminocaproic acid reportedly cause elevated CK levels. Intramuscular injections, cardioversion, invasive diagnostic procedures, surgery, trauma, recent vigorous exercise

or muscle massage, and severe coughing also increase total CK values.

Creatinine, serum

A quantitative analysis of serum creatinine levels, this test provides a more sensitive measure of renal damage than blood urea nitrogen levels, because renal impairment is virtually the only cause of creatinine elevation. Creatinine is a nonprotein end product of creatine metabolism. Similar to creatine, creatinine appears in serum in amounts proportional to the body's muscle mass; unlike creatine, it is easily excreted by the kidneys, with minimal or no tubular reabsorption. Creatinine levels therefore are directly related to the glomerular filtration rate. Because creatinine levels normally remain constant, elevated levels usually indicate diminished renal function.

Purpose	• To assess renal glomerular filtration • To screen for renal damage
Patient preparation	Explain that this test evaluates kidney function. Inform the patient that the test requires a blood sample. Instruct him to restrict food and fluids for approximately 8 hours before the test. Check the patient's history for any medications that may interfere with test results.
Procedure	Perform a venipuncture, and collect the sample in a 10- to 15-ml *red-top* tube. Send the sample to the laboratory immediately.
Values	Creatinine concentrations in males normally range from 0.8 to 1.2 mg/dl (60 to 90 µmol/L); in females, from 0.6 to 0.9 mg/dl (45 to 70 µmol/L).
Implications of results	Elevated serum creatinine levels generally indicate renal disease that has damaged 50% or more of the nephrons. Elevated creatinine levels may also be associated with gigantism and acromegaly.
Post-test care	If a hematoma develops at the venipuncture site, applying warm soaks eases discomfort.
Interfering factors	• Ascorbic acid, barbiturates, and diuretics may raise serum creatinine levels.

- Sulfobromophthalein or phenolsulfonphthalein given within the previous 24 hours can elevate creatinine levels if the test is based on the Jaffé reaction.
- Patients with exceptionally large muscle masses, such as athletes, may have above-average creatinine levels, even in the presence of normal renal function.

Creatinine, urine

This test measures urine levels of creatinine, the chief metabolite of creatine. Produced in amounts proportional to total body muscle mass, creatinine is removed from the plasma primarily by glomerular filtration and is excreted in the urine. Because the body doesn't recycle it, creatinine has a relatively high, constant clearance rate, making it an efficient indicator of renal function. However, the creatinine clearance test, which measures both urine and plasma creatinine clearance, is a more precise index than this test.

Purpose
- As part of the creatinine clearance test
- To check the accuracy of 24-hour urine collection, based on the relatively constant levels of creatinine excretion

Patient preparation
Explain that this test helps evaluate kidney function. Advise the patient to avoid eating an excessive amount of meat before the test, and to avoid strenuous physical exercise during the collection period. Tell him the test usually requires a 24-hour urine specimen, and teach the proper collection technique.

Check the patient's medication history for drugs that may affect creatinine levels. As appropriate, restrict such medications before the test.

Procedure
Collect a 24-hour urine specimen in a specimen bottle that contains a preservative to prevent the degradation of creatinine.

Refrigerate the specimen or keep it on ice during the collection period. When the collection is completed, send the specimen to the laboratory immediately.

Values   Normally, urine creatinine levels range from 1 to 1.9 g/day (7 to 14 mmol/day) for males, and from 0.8 to 1.7 g/day (6 to 13 mmol/day) for females.

Implications of results   Decreased urine creatinine levels may result from impaired renal perfusion (associated with shock, for example) or from renal disease caused by urinary tract obstruction. Chronic bilateral pyelonephritis, acute or chronic glomerulonephritis, and polycystic kidney disease may also depress creatinine levels. Increased urine creatinine levels generally have little diagnostic significance.

Post-test care   The patient may resume medications discontinued before the test.

Interfering factors

- Medications that may affect urine creatinine levels include corticosteroids, gentamicin, tetracyclines, diuretics, and amphotericin B.
- Failure to observe pretest restrictions, to collect all urine during the test period, or to store the specimen properly may interfere with accuracy of test results.

Creatinine clearance

Creatinine, an anhydride of creatine, is formed and excreted in constant amounts by an irreversible reaction, and is the main end product of creatine. Creatinine production is proportional to total muscle mass and is relatively unaffected by normal physical activity, diet, or urine volume.

An excellent diagnostic indicator of renal function, the creatinine clearance test determines how efficiently the kidneys are clearing creatinine from the blood. The rate of clearance is expressed in terms of the volume of blood (in milliliters) that can be cleared of creatinine in 1 minute (see *Calculating creatinine clearance,* page 206).

A final adjustment must be made to allow for renal parenchymal mass, which differs in each patient. To do this, the clearance rate established in the above equation is multiplied by 1.73 divided by surface area in square meters. Creatinine levels become abnormal when more than 50% of the total nephron units have been damaged.

Purpose

- To assess renal function (primarily glomerular filtration)

Calculating creatinine clearance

Clearance refers to renal capacity to remove various substances from the plasma. Although plasma clearance values of certain substances (inulin, creatinine) can parallel their glomerular filtration rate, tubular reabsorption and secretion of other measured substances (sodium and phosphate) reflect a combination of glomerular and tubular filtration.

To calculate plasma clearance for creatinine, use the formula:

$$\text{Creatinine clearance (ml/min)} = \frac{\text{Urine concentration (mg/dl)} \times \text{Urine volume (ml/min)}}{\text{Plasma concentration } (mg/dl)} \times \frac{1.73\,\text{m}^2}{\text{body surface area (m}^2)}$$

- To monitor progression of renal insufficiency

Patient preparation

Explain that this test evaluates kidney function. Advise the patient to avoid eating an excessive amount of meat before the test, and to avoid strenuous physical exercise during the collection period. Tell the patient the test requires a timed urine specimen, and describe how the urine specimen will be collected. Explain that the test requires at least one blood sample, but more than one venipuncture may be necessary.

Check the patient's medication history for drugs that may affect creatinine clearance. As appropriate, restrict these medications before the test.

Procedure

Collect a timed urine specimen at 2, 6, 12, or 24 hours in a bottle containing a preservative to prevent degradation of the creatinine.

Perform a venipuncture anytime during the collection period, and collect the sample in a 7-ml *red-top* tube.

Refrigerate the urine specimen or keep it on ice during the collection period. When the collection is completed, send the specimen to the laboratory immediately.

Values

For males (age 20), normal creatinine clearance is 90 ml/minute/1.73 m² (1.50 ml/second/1.73 m²) of body surface; for females (age 20), 84 ml/minute/1.73 m² (2.04 ml/second/1.73 m²). For older patients, concentrations normally decrease by 6 ml/minute/decade.

Implications of results

Low creatinine clearance may result from reduced renal blood flow (associated with shock or renal artery obstruction), acute tubular necrosis, acute or chronic glomerulonephritis, advanced bilateral chronic pyelonephritis, advanced bilateral renal lesions (as in polycystic kidney disease, renal tuberculosis, and malignancy), or nephrosclerosis. Congestive heart failure and severe dehydration may also cause creatinine clearance to fall below normal.

High creatinine clearance rates have no diagnostic significance.

Post-test care

- If a hematoma develops at the venipuncture site, applying warm soaks eases discomfort.
- The patient may resume medications, normal diet, and activity discontinued before the test.

Interfering factors

- Medications that may affect creatinine clearance include amphotericin B, thiazide diuretics, furosemide, and aminoglycosides.
- A high-protein diet before the test and strenuous physical exercise during the collection period may increase creatinine excretion.
- Failure to observe pretest restrictions, to collect all urine during the test period, or to store the specimen properly may interfere with accurate test results.

Crossmatching

Crossmatching is performed to determine compatibility or incompatibility between the donor's and the recipient's blood. It's the best antibody detection test available for avoiding lethal transfusion reactions. After the donor's and the recipient's ABO and Rh types are determined, ABO- and Rh-compatible donor units are selected for crossmatching. The donor's red blood cells (RBCs) are tested with the recipient's serum to determine compatibility. They are considered compatible if the recipient's serum has no antibodies that would destroy the transfused cells, causing a hemolytic reaction.

Blood is always crossmatched before transfusion, except in extreme emergencies, such as severe trauma or massive hemorrhage. Crossmatching may take from 20 minutes to 1 hour, depending upon the methodology used by the laboratory. An abbreviated (10-minute) crossmatch may be acceptable in emergencies. In such emergencies, uncrossmatched group O red blood cells (universal donor) may be temporarily transfused while blood typing and crossmatching are being performed. Generally, it's acceptable to transfuse O positive units to all males or females beyond child-bearing age. O negative blood should be transfused to females of child-bearing age until blood typing is performed to prevent possible Rh sensitization. An emergency transfusion must proceed with special awareness of the complications that may arise because of incomplete typing and crossmatching. After crossmatching, compatible units of blood are labeled, and a compatibility record is completed.

Purpose	To serve as the final check for compatibility between the donor's blood and the recipient's blood
Patient preparation	Explain that this test is used to identify blood for transfusion that correctly matches the patient's own to prevent a transfusion reaction. Inform the patient that the test requires a blood sample.

Check the patient's history for recent administration of blood, dextran, or I.V. contrast media.

Procedure	Verify the patient's identity. Perform a venipuncture, and collect the sample in a 10-ml *red-top* tube. ABO typing, Rh typing, and crossmatching can be performed on the same specimen.

Handle the sample gently to prevent hemolysis. Because hemolysis is used as a sign of blood incompatibility, grossly hemolyzed specimens are not considered acceptable for testing. The specimen must be completely and properly labeled at the patient's bedside to prevent clerical error or specimen misidentification.

The laboratory slip should include any history of transfusions, previous transfusion reaction, previously identified antibody, pregnancies, drug therapy, and the amount and type of blood component desired.

Send the sample to the laboratory immediately. (Crossmatching must be performed on the sample within 48 hours.)

Precautions   If more than 48 hours have elapsed since the previous transfusion, previously crossmatched donor
blood must be recrossmatched with a new recipient
serum sample. This is required because the patient
may develop alloantibodies (atypical antibodies) as
a result of prior transfusions. These antibodies can
cause subsequent incompatible crossmatches.

Findings   Absence of agglutination or hemolysis indicates
compatibility between the donor's and the recipient's blood, which means the transfusion of donor
blood *can* proceed.

Implications of   A *positive* crossmatch indicates incompatibility be-
results   tween the donor's blood and the recipient's blood,
which means the donor's blood can't be transfused
to the recipient. The signs of a positive crossmatch
are agglutination (clumping) or hemolysis when
the donor's RBCs and the recipient's serum are correctly mixed and incubated. Agglutination and hemolysis indicate an undesirable antigen-antibody
reaction. If an incompatible crossmatch is detected,
the causative antibody must be identified before the
transfusion. The patient must receive blood that
lacks the corresponding antigen for all subsequent
transfusions, or a hemolytic transfusion reaction
will occur. It will require additional time to find compatible blood for these patients, and these patients'
transfusion needs should be anticipated to allow the
Blood Bank adequate time for donor screening.

A *negative* crossmatch — the absence of agglutination or hemolysis — indicates probable compatibility between the donor's blood and the recipient's
blood, which means the transfusion of donor blood
can proceed. It doesn't guarantee a safe transfusion, but it's the best method available to prevent an
acute hemolytic reaction. Transfusion reactions
can occur because of other factors in the donor's
blood that cannot be tested for in the crossmatch,
such as serum proteins and white blood cell and
platelet antigens.

Post-test care   If hematoma develops at the venipuncture site, applying warm soaks eases discomfort.

Interfering   • Previous administration of dextran or I.V. con-
factors   trast media causes aggregation resembling agglutination. Previous blood administration may

produce antibodies to the donor blood that may interfere with compatibility testing.
- Hemolysis caused by excessive agitation of the sample interferes with accurate determination of test results.
- High serum protein levels can cause false-positive agglutination reactions.

Cryoglobulins

Cryoglobulins are abnormal serum proteins that precipitate at low laboratory temperatures (39.2° F [4° C]) and redissolve after being warmed. Their presence in the blood (cryoglobulinemia) is usually associated with immunologic disease but can also occur in the absence of known immunopathology. Cryoglobulinemia occurs in three forms: Type I, which involves the reaction of a single monoclonal immunoglobulin; Type II, with two or more immunoglobulins, one of which is monoclonal; and Type III, in which both components are polyclonal immunoglobulins. If patients with cryoglobulinemia are subjected to cold, they may experience Raynaud-like symptoms (pain, cyanosis, and coldness of fingers and toes), which generally result from precipitation of cryoglobulins in cooler parts of the body. In some patients, for example, cryoglobulins may precipitate at temperatures as high as 86° F (30° C); such temperatures are possible in some peripheral blood vessels.

The cryoglobulin test involves refrigerating a serum sample at 39.2° F (4° C) for at least 72 hours and observing for formation of a heat-reversible precipitate. Such a precipitate requires further study by immunoelectrophoresis or double diffusion, to identify cryoglobulin components.

Purpose
- To detect cryoglobulinemia in patients with Raynaud-like vascular symptoms
- To aid diagnosis of certain diseases, including collagen disorders, malignant diseases, and certain infections

Patient preparation

Explain that this test, which requires a blood sample, detects antibodies in blood that may cause sensitivity to low temperatures. Instruct the patient to fast for 4 to 6 hours before the test.

Cryoglobulin levels in associated diseases

Type of cryoglobulin	Serum level	Diseases
Type I **Monoclonal cryoglobulin**	> 5 mg/ml	• Myeloma • Waldenström's macroglobulinemia • Chronic lymphocytic leukemia
Type II **Mixed cryoglobulin**	> 1 mg/ml	• Rheumatoid arthritis • Sjögren's syndrome • Mixed essential cryoglobulinemia
Type III **Mixed polyclonal cryoglobulin**	> 1 mg/ml (50% below 80 mcg/ml)	• Systemic lupus erythematosus • Rheumatoid arthritis, Sjögren's syndrome • Infectious mononucleosis • Cytomegalovirus infections • Acute viral hepatitis • Chronic active hepatitis • Primary biliary cirrhosis • Poststreptococcal glomerulo-nephritis • Infective endocarditis • Hansen's disease • Kala-azar • Tropical splenomegaly syndrome

Procedure   Perform a venipuncture, and collect the sample in a prewarmed 10-ml *red-top* tube. Warm the syringe and collection tube to 98.6° F (37° C) before the venipuncture and keep it at that temperature to prevent loss of cryoglobulins. Send the sample to the laboratory immediately.

Findings   Normally, serum is negative for cryoglobulins.

Implications of results   *Cryoglobulin levels in associated diseases* indicates expected serum levels and diseases associated with the three types of cryoglobulinemia. Although the presence of cryoglobulins in the blood confirms cryoglobulinemia, this finding doesn't always indicate clinical disease.

Post-test care
- The patient may resume usual diet.
- If the test is positive for cryoglobulins, tell the patient to avoid cold temperatures or contact with cold objects.

- If a hematoma develops at the venipuncture site, applying warm soaks eases discomfort.
- Observe for signs of intravascular coagulation (decreased color and temperature in distal extremities, and increased pain).

Interfering factors
- Failure to adhere to dietary restrictions may interfere with accurate determination of test results.
- Failure to maintain the sample at 98.6° F (37° C) before centrifugation may cause loss of cryoglobulins.
- Reading the sample before the end of the 72-hour precipitation period may cause test results to be reported incorrectly because some cryoglobulins take several days to precipitate.

Cryptococcus antigen, serum or cerebrospinal fluid

This test detects cryptococcal antigen in serum or cerebrospinal fluid (CSF) by latex agglutination. *Cryptococcus neoformans*, a yeastlike fungus that is prevalent worldwide, causes a severe infection that characteristically causes fever, headache, dizziness, ataxia, somnolence, and cough. When it involves the central nervous system, this infection is invariably fatal if untreated; it's associated with a 25% mortality rate despite treatment with antimycotic therapy. About 50% of patients who develop this infection have a predisposing condition such as Hodgkin's or other malignant lymphoma, sarcoidosis, or acquired immunodeficiency syndrome, or are currently taking corticosteroids.

Purpose
To detect infection caused by *C. neoformans*

Patient preparation
Explain the purpose of this test, and inform the patient that the test requires a sample of blood or spinal fluid.

Procedure
A sample of venous blood or spinal fluid is collected into an appropriate container and sent to the laboratory for testing by latex agglutination, enzyme immunoassay, or indirect fluorescent assay.

Findings
Normal serum or CSF is negative for cryptococcus antigen. Positive results are reported in titer.

Implications of results
When performed on CSF, this test produces a positive result in 95% to 98% of cases of cryptococcal meningitis. A positive serum test occurs in 95% of patients with disseminated meningitis and in approximately 30% of patients without meningitis.

Post-test care
- After lumbar puncture, the patient should remain recumbent and avoid raising his head for 8 hours after the procedure to prevent headache.
- If a hematoma develops at the venipuncture site, applying warm soaks eases discomfort.

Interfering factors
- Rheumatoid factor can cause false-positive results.
- A severely immunocompromised patient may generate no immune response, invalidating test results.
- False-negative results may be caused by very high prozone titers. Dilution of antiserum will result in a positive level.

Cyclic adenosine monophosphate (cAMP)

Formed from adenosine triphosphate by the action of the enzyme adenylate cyclase, the nucleotide cyclic adenosine monophosphate (cAMP) influences the protein synthesis rate within cells. Measurement of urinary excretion of cAMP after I.V. infusion of a standard dose of parathyroid hormone can show renal tubular resistance in a patient with hypoparathyroid symptoms and high levels of parathyroid hormone. Such findings suggest Type I pseudohypoparathyroidism. (Urinary cAMP levels respond normally with Type II pseudohypoparathyroidism because the defect is beyond the level of cAMP generation.) This rare inherited disorder results from tissue resistance to parathyroid hormone, and produces hypocalcemia, hyperphosphatemia, and skeletal and constitutional abnormalities.

This test is contraindicated in patients with high calcium levels (because parathyroid hormone further raises calcium levels). It should be used cautiously in patients receiving digitalis and in those with sarcoidosis or renal or cardiac disease.

Purpose To aid differential diagnosis of pseudohypoparathyroidism

Patient preparation Explain the purpose of this test. Tell the patient the test requires a 15-minute I.V. infusion of parathyroid hormone and collection of a 3- to 4-hour urine specimen.

Perform a skin test to detect a possible allergy to parathyroid hormone; keep epinephrine readily available in case of an adverse reaction. Just before the procedure is performed, instruct the patient not to touch the I.V. or exert pressure on the arm receiving the infusion. Warn the patient that transient discomfort may result from the needle puncture. Advise the patient to report severe burning or swelling at the site.

Equipment Parathyroid hormone (300 units, in refrigerated ampules), vial of sterile water (saline solution causes precipitate to form), urine collection container, to which hydrochloric acid has been added as a preservative

Procedure The patient should empty his bladder before the test begins. Parathyroid hormone is infused over 15 minutes. The start of the infusion is recorded as time zero. If the patient has an indwelling urinary catheter in place, the collection bag should be changed before the collection begins, and the collection bag should be kept on ice.

Collect a urine specimen 3 to 4 hours after infusion. Tell the patient to avoid contaminating the urine specimen with toilet tissue or stool.

Send the specimen to the laboratory immediately; if transport is delayed, refrigerate the specimen.

Values and implications of results A 10- to 20-fold increase (3 to 4 μmol/g creatinine; 0.4 to 0.5 μmol/mmol creatine) in cAMP demonstrates a normal response or hypoparathyroidism. Failure to respond to parathyroid hormone, indicated by normal urinary excretion of cAMP, suggests Type I pseudohypoparathyroidism.

Post-test care • Observe the patient for symptoms of hypercalcemia: lethargy, anorexia, nausea, vomiting, vertigo, and abdominal cramps.

- If a hematoma or irritation develops at the venipuncture site, applying warm soaks eases discomfort.

Interfering factors Contamination or improper storage of the specimen, or failure to acidify the urine with hydrochloric acid may alter test results.

Cystine, urine

This test detects excessive amounts of cystine in the urine of patients with the inherited disease, cystinuria. Cystinuria is also associated with increased urinary excretion of lysine, ornithine, and arginine. The amount of cystine excreted exceeds solubility in urine and leads to formation of urinary tract stones.

Purpose To aid diagnosis of cystinuria

Patient preparation Explain the purpose of this test and inform the patient that the test requires a random urine specimen or a 24-hour urine collection. If necessary, teach the patient the correct procedure for collecting a 24-hour urine specimen.

Procedure Obtain a 20-ml urine specimen, or collect a 24-hour urine specimen into a container with a preservative. Notify the laboratory if the patient is taking penicillamine.

Values Normal result of the qualitative test is negative for cystine. Normal cystine content of a 24-hour urine collection is 2.6 to 13 mg/day (11 to 53 µmol/day) in children under age 7, and 7 to 28 mg/day (28 to 115 µmol/day) in adults and children over age 7.

Implications of results Increased cystine values indicate cystinuria.

Post-test care None

Interfering factor Treatment with penicillamine may interfere with accurate test results.

Cytomegalovirus, rapid monoclonal test

Cytomegalovirus (CMV), a member of the herpesvirus group, can cause systemic infection in congenitally infected infants, and in such immuno-suppressed patients as transplant recipients, patients receiving chemotherapy for neoplastic disease, and in those with acquired immunodeficiency syndrome (AIDS).

In the past, CMV infections were detected in the laboratory by recognizing the distinctive cytopathic effects (CPE) that the virus produced in conventional tube cell cultures. This slow method of CMV detection requires an average of 9 days to develop CPE in the cultures. Alternatively, the shell vial assay (rapid monoclonal test) is based on centrifugal inoculation of specimens onto cell monolayers grown on round cover slips in 1-dram shell vials and the immunologic detection of early products of viral replication with specific monoclonal antibodies after 16 hours' incubation. This assay is based on the availability of a monoclonal antibody specific for the 72 kd protein of CMV synthesized during the immediate early stage of viral replication. Through indirect immunofluorescence, CMV-infected fibroblasts are recognized by their dense, homogeneous staining confined to the nucleus of these cells. Because of the smooth, regular shape of the nucleus and the surrounding nuclear membrane, infected cells are readily differentiated from nonspecific background fluorescence that may be present in some specimens.

Purpose
To obtain rapid laboratory diagnosis of CMV infection, especially in immunocompromised patients who have or are at risk for developing systemic infections caused by this virus

Patient preparation
Explain the purpose of this test, and describe the procedure for collecting the specimen for culture.

Procedure
Specimens should be collected during the prodromal and acute stages of clinical infection to ensure the best chance of detecting CMV. As required by the laboratory, collect a specimen for culture. Each type of specimen requires a specific collection device, as listed below—
Throat: microbiological transport swab

Urine, cerebrospinal fluid: sterile screw-capped tube or vial
Bronchoalveolar lavage tissue: sterile screw-capped jar
Blood: sterile tube with anticoagulant (heparin).

Specimens should be transported to the laboratory as soon as possible after collection. If the anticipated time between collection and inoculation into shell vial cell cultures is longer than 2 to 3 hours, the specimen should be transported at 39.2° F (4° C). Do not freeze the specimen or allow the specimen to become dry.

Findings

CMV can be detected in urine and throat specimens from patients who are asymptomatic. However, the detection of CMV from these sites indicates active, asymptomatic infection, which may alert the clinician to anticipate later symptomatic involvement, especially in immunosuppressed patients. Detection of CMV in specimens of blood, tissue, and bronchoalveolar lavage generally indicates systemic infection and disease.

Implications of results

CMV is a significant cause of morbidity and mortality in immunosuppressed patients, such as patients with AIDS and those who receive organ transplants. An antiviral drug, gancyclovir, is indicated for treatment of CMV retinitis.

Post-test care

None

Interfering factor

Administration of antiviral drugs before collection of the specimen may interfere with detection of CMV.

Cytomegalovirus antibody screen, serum

After primary infection, cytomegalovirus (CMV), establishes latency in blood leukocytes. For an immunocompromised host, CMV can be reactivated from a latent state to produce an active infection. The presence of antibodies to CMV indicates past infection with this virus. CMV-seronegative organ transplant recipients and neonates (especially those born prematurely) are at high risk for active CMV infection if given blood or tissue from a seropositive donor. Antibodies to CMV can be detected by several methods, which include passive hemagglutination, latex agglutination, enzyme immunoassay, and indirect immunofluorescence. The complement fixation test is only 60% sensitive compared to these other assays and should not be used to screen for CMV antibodies. This screen for CMV antibodies is qualitative; it detects the presence of antibody at a single low dilution (for example, 1:5) to identify past infection with the CMV virus. Quantitative methods are designed to be used diagnostically by testing several dilutions of the serum specimen to indicate acute infection with CMV.

Purpose
- To detect past CMV infection in organ transplant donors and recipients
- To detect past CMV infection in immunocompromised patients and especially in premature neonates who receive transfused blood products

Patient preparation
Explain the purpose of this test, and inform the patient (or the parents of the infant) that the test requires a blood sample.

Procedure
Perform a venipuncture to collect 5 ml of sterile blood in a *red-top* tube. Allow the blood to clot for at least 1 hour at room temperature. Handle the sample gently to prevent hemolysis. Transfer the serum to a sterile tube or vial, and send it to the laboratory. If transport must be delayed, store the serum at 39.2° F (4° C) for 1 or 2 days or at −4° F (−20° C) for longer periods to avoid microbial contamination.

Findings
Patients who have never been infected with CMV have no detectable antibodies to the virus (less than 1:5). A serum specimen positive for antibody at this single dilution indicates that the patient has been infected with CMV and that the patient's blood leukocytes contain latent virus capable of being reactivated in an immunocompromised host.

Implications of results
Immunosuppressed patients who lack antibodies to CMV (screening test less than 1:5) should receive blood products or organ transplants from donors who are also seronegative to avoid the morbidity and mortality associated with active infection with this virus. Patients with CMV antibodies (screen-

ing test greater than 1:5) are not provided seroneg-ative blood products.

Post-test care   If a hematoma develops at the venipuncture site, applying warm soaks eases discomfort.

Interfering factors   None

D

Delta-aminolevulinic acid, urine

Using the colorimetric technique, this quantitative analysis of urine delta-aminolevulinic acid (ALA) levels helps diagnose porphyrias, hepatic disease, and lead poisoning. ALA, the basic precursor of the porphyrins, normally converts to porphobilinogen through the action of the enzyme ALA-dehydrase during heme synthesis. Impaired conversion, as in porphyrias and lead poisoning, causes urine ALA levels to rise before other chemical or hematologic changes occur.

Purpose
- To screen for lead poisoning
- To aid diagnosis of porphyrias

Patient preparation
Explain that this test detects abnormal hemoglobin formation. If lead poisoning is suspected, tell the patient or parents that the test helps detect the presence of excessive lead in the body. Inform the patient or parents that the test requires a 24-hour urine specimen but does not require restriction of food or fluids. Teach the patient (or parents) the proper collection technique.

Check the patient's medication history for recent administration of drugs that may alter ALA levels. Review findings with the laboratory to consider restricting medications before the test.

Procedure
Collect a 24-hour urine specimen in a dark bottle containing a preservative (usually glacial acetic acid) to prevent degradation of ALA. During collection, protect the specimen from direct sunlight. If the patient has an indwelling catheter in place, insert the drainage bag in a dark plastic bag.

Refrigerate the specimen or keep it on ice during the collection period. When the collection is completed, send the specimen to the laboratory immediately.

Values
Normally, urine ALA values range from 1.5 to 7.5 mg/day (11 to 57 μmol/day).

Implications of results	Elevated urine ALA levels occur in lead poisoning, acute porphyria, hepatic carcinoma, and hepatitis.
Post-test care	The patient may resume discontinued medications.
Interfering factors	• Barbiturates and griseofulvin cause porphyrins to accumulate in the liver and thus raise urine ALA levels. Vitamin E in pharmacologic doses may lower urine ALA levels. • Failure to observe medication restrictions, to collect all urine during the test period, or to store the specimen properly may interfere with accurate determination of test results.

Deoxyribonucleic acid (DNA) antibodies
Anti-DNA antibodies

This test measures antinative deoxyribonucleic acid (DNA) antibody levels in a serum sample, using radioimmunoassay, immunofluorescence, or a less sensitive technique, such as agglutination, complement fixation, or immunoelectrophoresis. To measure anti-DNA antibodies, a less sensitive test is more specific and may be more useful. Enzyme-linked immunoabsorbent assay (ELISA) is considered the method of choice. For radioimmunoassay, the sample is mixed with radio-labeled native DNA. If antinative DNA antibodies are in the serum sample, they combine with the native DNA, forming complexes that are too large to pass through a membrane filter. If such antibodies are not present, the radiolabeled DNA is able to pass through the filter. The DNA that does not pass through the membrane filter is then counted.

In autoimmune diseases, such as systemic lupus erythematosus (SLE), native DNA is thought to be the antigen that complexes with antibody and complement, and causes local tissue damage where these complexes are deposited. Unlike delta-aminolevulinic acid, anti-DNA is nearly unique to SLE; anti-DNA antibody levels correlate with activity of the disease.

Two different types of anti-DNA antibodies are present in patients with SLE: anti–single-stranded (denatured) DNA and anti–double-stranded (native) DNA. Antibodies to native DNA, however, are more specific for SLE. Determination of these antibodies, with serum complement, also proves useful in monitoring immunosuppressant therapy.

Purpose
- To confirm SLE after a positive antinuclear antibody test
- To monitor response to SLE therapy and disease activity
- To discriminate SLE from drug-induced lupus

Patient preparation
Explain to the patient that this test detects certain antibodies and that test results help determine diagnosis and appropriate therapy; or, when indicated, tell the patient that the test assesses the effectiveness of present treatment. Tell the patient that the test requires a blood sample but does not require restriction of food or fluids.

If the patient is scheduled for a radionuclide scan, make sure the sample is collected before the scan.

Procedure
Perform a venipuncture, and collect the sample in a 7-ml *red-top* tube. (Some laboratories may specify a *lavender-* or *gray-top* tube.) Handle the sample gently to prevent hemolysis.

Values
Normal values are less than 1 mcg of native DNA bound/ml of serum (1 mg/L).

Implications of results
Elevated antinative DNA levels may indicate SLE. A value of 1 to 2.5 mcg/ml (mg/L) suggests a remission phase of SLE or the presence of other autoimmune disorders. A value of 10 to 15 mcg/ml (mg/L) indicates active SLE. Depressed levels following immunosuppressant therapy demonstrate effective treatment of SLE.

Post-test care
If a hematoma develops at the venipuncture site, applying warm soaks eases discomfort.

Interfering factors
- Hemolysis caused by excessive agitation of the sample may interfere with accurate determination of test results.
- Radioactive scan performed within 1 week of collecting the sample may alter the test results.

Dexamethasone suppression test

The dexamethasone suppression test (DST), a standard screening test for Cushing's syndrome, also appears useful in diagnosing major depression and monitoring its treatment. This use is based on the finding that certain patients with major depression have high levels of circulating adrenal steroid hormones. Administration of an oral steroid, such as dexamethasone, suppresses these levels in normal persons, but fails to suppress them in persons with Cushing's syndrome and some forms of depression.

Purpose
- To identify patients with Cushing's syndrome
- To aid diagnosis of some forms of depression

Procedure
The patient is given 1 mg of dexamethasone at 11 p.m.; then, blood samples are drawn at 4 p.m. and 11 p.m. the next day. (More frequent sampling may increase the likelihood of measuring a non-suppressed cortisol peak.)

Patient preparation
Explain the purpose of the test. Inform the patient that the test will require two blood samples that will be drawn after administration of dexamethasone.

Values
A cortisol level of 5 µg/dl (140 nmol/L) or greater indicates failure of dexamethasone suppression.

Implications of results
A normal test result doesn't rule out major depression, but an abnormal test result strengthens a clinically based diagnosis. Failure of suppression occurs in patients with Cushing's syndrome, conditions of severe stress, and depression that is likely to respond to treatment with antidepressants. The DST has proven disappointing in differentiating dysthymic disorder (neurotic depression) from major affective illness (psychotic depression), but may have use in patients with other psychological diagnoses (such as schizoaffective disorder, for example) to establish the need for treatment of coexisting depression.

Post-test care
If a hematoma develops at the venipuncture site, applying warm soaks eases discomfort.

- False-positive results can occur in diabetes mellitus, pregnancy, and situations of severe bodily stress (such as trauma, severe weight loss, dehydration, and acute alcohol withdrawal).
- False-positives can follow use of certain medications, particularly barbiturates or phenytoin, within 3 weeks before the test.

Diazepam, serum

Diazepam is the most commonly prescribed benzodiazepine. The benzodiazepines interact with neuronal gamma-aminobutyric acid (GABA) receptors and enhance synaptic transmission by GABA-ergic neurons. Such enhancement leads to inhibition of nerve impulse conduction in the central nervous system and, by mechanisms not yet fully understood, reduces anxiety. Diazepam also is an effective muscle relaxant and anticonvulsant agent and frequently is the drug of choice in controlling seizures in emergency situations.

Diazepam is metabolized almost exclusively by the liver. One of its major metabolites, nordiazepam (N-desmethyldiazepam), has full anxiolytic activity. Therefore, monitoring of diazepam serum levels must measure nordiazepam as well. Elimination of these drugs is quite slow; diazepam and nordiazepam have half-lives of approximately 2 to 4 days and 4 to 7 days, respectively. Diazepam has a wide therapeutic index; toxicity usually does not occur until serum levels are five to ten times higher than therapeutic levels. Toxic symptoms include muscular weakness, ataxia, and drowsiness. Fatalities from diazepam overdose are rare.

Purpose

- To confirm therapeutic dosage
- To assess patient compliance
- To assess possible abuse of diazepam

Patient
preparation

Explain the purpose of the test and inform the patient that this test requires a blood sample. If the test has legal implications, observe appropriate guidelines and institutional policies.

Procedure

Perform a venipuncture, and obtain a blood sample. The test requires 3 ml of serum collected into a *red-top* tube. Because the extended half-lives of diazepam and nordiazepam tend to minimize serum fluctuations during the dosing intervals, collection time relative to dose is less critical than with other drugs.

Values

Therapeutic range: concentrations of diazepam range from 0.2 to 0.8 μg/ml (0.7 to 2.8 μmol/L); of nordiazepam, from 0.2 to 1.0 μg/ml (0.7 to 3.5 μmol/L); and of the total, diazepam and nordiazepam from 0.4 to 1.8 μg/ml (1.4 to 6.3 μmol/L).

Implications of results

Total benzodiazepines concentrations greater than 2.5 μg/ml (8.7 μmol/L) produce sedation; concentrations greater than 5.0 ug/ml (17 μmol/L) are toxic.

Post-test care

If a hematoma develops at the venipuncture site, applying warm soaks eases discomfort.

Interfering factors

None

Digitalis glycosides, serum

This radioimmunoassay for monitoring digitalis glycoside therapy is especially useful for elderly patients or those with renal or hepatic disease. After oral administration of digitalis glycosides, the serum cardiac glycoside level rises rapidly but drops sharply as the drug enters the myocardium and other tissues. Toxicity usually results from hepatic or renal dysfunction, hypokalemia, hypothyroidism, severe hypoxic heart or respiratory disease, and from variations in patient response rather than excessive dosage. Although digoxin and digitoxin assays are highly accurate (generally within 3% to 6% of true serum concentration), serum levels may not always correlate with the clinical state.

Purpose

- To monitor therapeutic levels of digitalis glycosides
- To check for toxicity suspected from history or after onset of symptoms, such as headache, drowsiness, anorexia, nausea, vomiting, diarrhea, yellow vision, generalized weakness, hypotension, delirium, slow and irregular pulse, or cardiac arrhythmias
- To assess compliance

Patient preparation

Explain that this test helps determine the most effective drug dosage. Inform the patient that the test requires a blood sample.

Check the patient's recent medication history to ensure that the test is ordered for the appropriate digitalis glycoside.

Procedure

Perform a venipuncture, and collect a trough-level sample in a 7-ml *red-top* tube. Note on the laboratory slip the specific digitalis glycoside being monitored; the date, time, amount, and route of administration of the last dose; and the time of sample collection. For this test, the blood sample should be drawn just before the next dose. Ideally, this is 4 to 10 hours after the last dose of digitoxin or 6 to 8 hours after the last dose of digoxin. Observe the same time span between drug administration and sample collection in serial testing.

Send the sample to the laboratory promptly.

Values

Therapeutic and toxic serum levels of digoxin and digitoxin vary (see *Blood levels of digitalis glycosides*).

Implications of results

Serum values at 3.0 µg/ml (3.9 µmol/L) or higher are commonly associated with symptoms of digoxin toxicity. In children, toxic concentrations may be higher. However, serum digitalis glycoside levels must be considered in relation to the patient's current clinical status, past levels and status, and renal function tests. Some patients with supraventricular arrhythmias don't exhibit symptoms of toxicity even though they require high digitalis glycoside dosages to control ventricular rate.

Post-test care

If a hematoma develops at the venipuncture site, applying warm soaks eases discomfort.

Interfering factors

- Absorption of digitoxin and digoxin is decreased by aminosalicylic acid, antacids, cholestyramine, colestipol, kaolin-pectin, and neomycin.
- Phenobarbital, phenytoin, cholestyramine, and phenylbutazone suppress digitoxin levels; quinidine and verapamil (and possibly other calcium channel blocking agents) raise digoxin levels; spironolactone interferes with the test, producing false elevations.
- Drugs that deplete body extracellular potassium levels predispose the patient to toxicity.

Blood levels of digitalis glycosides

Drug	Peak time	Steady state (without loading dose)	Therapeutic levels	Toxic levels
Digoxin	6 to 8 hours P.O. 4 to 6 hours I.M. 1 to 5 hours I.V.	7 days *	0.5 to 2 ng/ml	<2 ng/ml
Digitoxin	4 to 12 hours	21 to 28 days	20 to 35 ng/ml	<40 to 45 ng/ml

Digoxin and digitoxin, the two most commonly used digitalis glycosides, have similar clinical effects but are metabolized differently: digoxin is eliminated primarily through the kidneys, whereas digitoxin is primarily metabolized in the liver and excreted in feces. Consequently, renal dysfunction can cause digoxin toxicity; hepatic dysfunction can cause digitoxin toxicity. Moreover, toxicity may result from hypokalemia, hypothyroidism, and from heart and respiratory disease. With either drug, toxicity isn't necessarily dose-related.

Higher therapeutic plasma concentrations of these drugs may be necessary for patients with supraventricular tachycardias or atrial fibrillation than for patients with heart failure.

*Assuming normal renal function

- Testing before steady state is achieved produces misleading findings.
- Plasma levels drawn earlier than 6 hours after the last dose may show higher digoxin levels than those present after the drug distributes into the tissues.
- Concurrent treatment with spironolactone causes falsely elevated test results.
- Patients poisoned with digitalis glycosides who are given digoxin immune FAB show a dramatic increase in digoxin blood levels, because of the presence of bound digoxin.
- Testing for the wrong digitalis glycoside — such as digitoxin rather than digoxin — results in erroneous findings.

Drug abuse survey

Laboratory testing to detect illicit drugs, alcohol, or other toxins may be done for various clinical or forensic reasons. An emergency screening is often ordered for a rule-out diagnosis in an unconscious or seriously impaired patient or to identify the types and amounts of substances ingested in an over-dose. Drug screening is also an important part of inpatient and outpatient drug abuse treatment, helping to guide and evaluate the success of treatment.

Most often, however, drug screening is done for forensic reasons — for example, to confirm a law enforcement officer's or employer's probable suspicion of an individual's drug use or to find out if drugs or alcohol may have been a contributing factor in an accident. More and more commonly, employers are now requesting drug screening as part of a routine preemployment physical examination. Despite the controversy this practice generates, employers defend it as necessary to protect themselves from the costs and liabilities associated with employee drug and alcohol abuse. Certain government agencies, such as the Department of Transportation, have regulations either requiring or strongly recommending preemployment drug screening for all prospective employees. Some businesses and agencies also require periodic drug testing for their existing employees.

Along with controversy regarding an individual's right to privacy and the need for strict confidentiality of test results, arguments against routine drug screening center on the unreliability of current methods and the difficulty of obtaining accurate results. The use of confirming tests for all initially positive specimens dramatically improves accuracy and reduces the chance of false-positive results. The best laboratory confirmation procedure is gas chromatography-mass spectrometry (GCMS); GCMS removes any potential interfering factors, such as other drugs, food, and vitamins.

Urine is the specimen of choice for most routine drug screening. But the presence of drugs in urine does not always adequately reflect impairment or intoxication and is a generally poor indicator of time of ingestion (see *Detection time for drugs in urine*). Measurement of serum concentrations more accurately determines the degree of overdose and guides emergency treatment.

Purpose
To detect harmful or illicit drugs for medical or forensic purposes

Patient preparation
Explain this procedure to the patient. If urine screening is scheduled, tell the patient that the test requires a urine specimen. If the patient will be per-

Detection time for drugs in urine

Drug	Maximum detection time after ingestion
Alcohol (ethyl)	3 to 10 hours
Amphetamines	24 to 48 hours
Barbiturates • Secobarbital • Phenobarbital	24 hours 2 to 6 weeks
Benzodiazepines • Prescription doses • High-level abuse	3 to 5 days 6 weeks
Cocaine	1 to 5 hours
Cocaine metabolites	2 to 4 days
Codeine	1 to 2 days
Heroin (as morphine)	1 to 2 days
Hydromorphone	1 to 2 days
Methadone	2 to 3 days
Morphine	1 to 2 days
Phencyclidine (PCP)	1 to 8 days
Propoxyphene	6 hours
Propoxyphene metabolites	6 to 48 hours
Tetrahydrocannabinol (THC) metabolites • One-time use • Thrice weekly use • Daily use • Heavy use	2 days 2 weeks 3 to 6 weeks 6 to 11 weeks

forming specimen collection, teach the correct way to collect a random urine specimen. Explain that collection is monitored to guard against specimen tampering.

For serum screening, tell the patient that the test requires a blood sample.

If the screening is being performed for forensic purposes, make sure that the patient or a responsible family member has signed a consent form. Obtain the patient's recent medication history, including doses, times, and routes of administration.

Procedure For urine screening, a random specimen is usually collected by the patient. An unconscious or seriously intoxicated patient may have to be catheterized to obtain a specimen. Most laboratories require a minimum specimen of 10 ml of urine; some may require up to 50 ml. A "second-catch" specimen may be used to screen for alcohol.

If supervising specimen collection, take precautions to prevent the patient from altering or substituting a specimen. If possible, have the patient put on a gown and remove access to clothing or personal effects and to a source of water — warm water in particular — with which he can dilute a specimen. (You can detect dilution with cold water simply by feeling the specimen container.)

Immediately seal the urine collection container to prevent air infiltration and contamination. Promptly send the specimen to the laboratory, or refrigerate it if storage is necessary. To obtain a serum sample, perform a venipuncture, and collect the sample in a 10-ml *red-top* tube. For blood alcohol screening, collect the sample in a *gray-top* tube containing sodium fluoride and potassium oxalate; be sure to prepare the venipuncture site with an alcohol-free sponge. Handle the serum sample gently to prevent hemolysis, and send it to the laboratory immediately or refrigerate it.

Make sure that all specimens are properly and completely labeled and secured for transportation to the laboratory. For employee or forensic screening, maintain a strict *chain of custody* to prevent tampering and ensure accurate results. This chain of custody, recorded on a form that accompanies the specimen at all times, provides a written record of every person responsible for handling the specimen from collection through laboratory analysis. If possible, use tamper-evident seals on all specimen containers as a further safeguard.

Findings The normal result of a drug screening is no drugs detected, or negative. Many persons have moderate-to-high levels of legal substances, such as nicotine and caffeine. But most drug screening reports omit this information unless it is specifically requested.

Because it is so rapidly metabolized and excreted, alcohol is difficult to detect on routine drug screening. Even chronic alcoholics often test negative.

Implications of results

By speeding diagnosis and guiding intervention, results of an emergency drug screening often literally make the difference between life and death.

Serious issues — including privacy, confidentiality, and accuracy of test results and their interpretations — surround forensic and employee drug screening. When caring for a patient undergoing such screening, ensuring the confidentiality of test results is a major responsibility. Take steps to ensure that only authorized persons receive the test results. Also verify that positive results have been confirmed by a second laboratory technique to ensure accuracy.

Post-test care

None

Interfering factors

- Overdilution of specimens can produce false-negative results.
- Positive results for opiates may result from heavy ingestion of poppy seeds before testing, and false-positive results for amphetamines may result from use of medications that contain pseudo-ephedrine, phenylpropanolamine, or related drugs. Confirmation with GCMS eliminates such misleading results.

Duodenal contents, culture

This test requires duodenal intubation, aspiration of duodenal contents, and cultivation of any microbes present to isolate and identify a duodenal or biliary pathogen. Occasionally, a specimen may be obtained during surgery, such as a cholecystectomy. Duodenal contents (pancreatic and duodenal enzymes and bile) are normally almost sterile, but are subject to infection by many pathogens, such as *Escherichia coli, Staphylococcus aureus,* and *Salmonella,* as well as *Giardia lamblia, Strongyloides stercoralis,* and many other parasites. Such microbial infection of the biliary tract and duodenum can result in duodenitis, cholecystitis, or cholangitis.

Purpose

- To detect infection of the biliary tract and duodenum; to differentiate between such infection and gallstones

- To rule out infection as the cause of persistent GI symptoms (epigastric pain, nausea, vomiting, and diarrhea)

Patient preparation

Explain that this test helps to determine the cause of GI symptoms. Instruct the patient to restrict food and fluids for 12 hours before the test.

Describe the intubation procedure and assure the patient that although this procedure is uncomfortable, it isn't dangerous. Explain that passage of the tube may make him gag, but following the examiner's instructions about proper positioning, breathing, swallowing, and relaxing will minimize discomfort. Encourage the patient to empty his bladder before the procedure, to increase his general comfort.

Equipment

Double-lumen tube with olive tip, water-soluble jelly, 30-ml sterile syringe, emesis basin, sterile specimen container, ½″ (1.2 cm) adhesive tape

Procedure

After the nasoenteric tube is inserted, the patient is placed in a left lateral decubitus position, with feet elevated, to allow peristalsis to move the tube into the duodenum. The pH of a small amount of aspirated fluid determines tube position: if the tube is in the stomach, pH is lower than 7.0; if the tube is in the duodenum, pH is higher than 7.0.

Correct position of the tube can also be confirmed by fluoroscopy. After position is confirmed, duodenal contents are aspirated.

Collect the specimen for culture before antibiotic therapy begins. Occasionally, a specimen for culture of duodenal contents is obtained during duodenoscopy.

Transfer the specimen to a sterile container, and label it with the patient's name and room number, physician's name, date and time of collection, and send the specimen to the laboratory immediately.

Precautions

Duodenal intubation is contraindicated in conditions such as acute pancreatitis; acute cholecystitis; esophageal varices, stenosis, diverticula or malignant neoplasms; recent severe gastric hemorrhage; aortic aneurysm; congestive heart failure; or myocardial infarction.

Findings

Normally, a duodenal contents culture contains small amounts of polymorphonuclear leukocytes and epithelial cells with no pathogens. The bacterial count is usually less than 100,000, and parasites are absent.

Implications of
results

Generally, bacterial counts of 100,000 or more, or the presence of pathogens, such as *Salmonella,* in any number indicates infection. Sensitivity testing may be required. Numerous polymorphonuclear leukocytes, copious mucous debris, and bile-stained epithelial cells in the bile fluid suggest inflammation of the biliary tract; many segmented neutrophils and exfoliated epithelial cells suggest inflammation of the pancreas, the duodenum, or bile ducts. The presence of bile sand indicates cholelithiasis or calculi in the biliary tract. Differential diagnosis requires further testing, including oral or I.V. cholecystography; white blood cell count; cholangiography, measurement of serum bilirubin, alkaline phosphatase, serum amylase, and urine urobilinogen; and culture of surgical material.

Post-test care

- After duodenal intubation or duodenoscopy, observe the patient carefully for signs of perforation from the tube's passage, such as dysphagia, epigastric or shoulder pain, dyspnea, or fever.
- After the duodenoscopy, monitor vital signs until the patient is stable. The patient should be kept on bed rest with the side rails up until he is fully alert.
- The patient may resume discontinued diet.

Interfering
factors

- Failure to observe a 12-hour fast can dilute the specimen, which decreases the bacterial count.
- Improper collection technique can contaminate the specimen.

Duodenal parasites test

This test evaluates duodenal contents for the presence of parasites in a specimen obtained by duodenal intubation and aspiration or by the string test (capsule test). Such parasites include trophozoites of *Giardia lamblia;* the larvae of *Strongyloides stercoralis;* or the larvae of *Necator americanus* or *Ancylostoma duodenale.* This test can also detect ova of the liver flukes *Clonorchis sinensis* and *Fasciola hepatica* in the biliary tract. (Liver fluke infections are rare in North America.)

Note: Examination of duodenal contents for ova and parasites is performed only in a symptomatic patient with negative stool examinations.

Purpose To detect parasitic infection when stool examinations are negative

Patient preparation Explain that this test detects parasitic infection of the GI tract. Instruct the patient to restrict food and fluids for 12 hours before the test. If the test will be done with a nasoenteric tube, warn the patient that the tube's passage may cause gagging, but emphasize that following the examiner's instructions about positioning, breathing, and swallowing will minimize discomfort. Just before the procedure, instruct the patient to empty his bladder.

Equipment Double-lumen nasoenteric tube with olive tip (or weighted gelatin capsule with string attached, for string test), water-soluble jelly, 30-ml sterile syringe, emesis basin, sterile specimen container, adhesive tape (½″ [1.2 cm] wide)

Procedure *Using a nasoenteric tube:* After the nasoenteric tube is inserted, place the patient in a left lateral decubitus position, with his feet elevated, to allow peristalsis to move the tube into the duodenum. The pH of a small amount of aspirated fluid determines tube position: if the tube is in the stomach, pH is lower than 7.0; if the tube is in the duodenum, pH is higher than 7.0. Correct positioning of the tube can also be determined by fluoroscopy. After position of the tube is confirmed, residual duodenal contents are aspirated. Transfer the entire specimen to a sterile container; label it appropriately.

Using a weighted gelatin capsule with string: Tape the free end of the string to the patient's cheek. Then, instruct him to swallow the capsule (on the other end of the string) with water. Leave the string in place for 4 hours; then pull it out gently and place it in a sterile container. Label the container appropriately.

When possible, obtain the specimen before the start of drug therapy.

Send the specimen to the laboratory immediately, because detection may rest on observing the parasite's motility.

Precautions
- Duodenal intubation is contraindicated during pregnancy or for patients with acute cholecystitis; acute pancreatitis; esophageal varices, stenosis, diverticula, or malignant neoplasms; recent severe gastric hemorrhage; aortic aneurysm; or congestive heart failure.
- Withdraw the tube slowly (6″ to 8″ [15 to 20 cm] every 10 minutes) to the esophagus; then clamp the tube and remove it quickly. *Never* force the tube.

Findings
Normally, no ova or parasites appear.

Implications of results
The presence of *G. lamblia* indicates giardiasis; *S. stercoralis* suggests strongyloidiasis; and *A. duodenale* and *N. americanus* imply hookworm disease. The presence of *C. sinensis* and *F. hepatica* signifies infections in the bile ducts.

Post-test care
- Provide mouth care, and offer water.
- Monitor the patient carefully for signs of perforation, such as dysphagia or fever.
- The patient may resume a normal diet.

Interfering factors
- Failure of the patient to observe the 12-hour fast can dilute the specimen.
- Delay in sending the specimen may interfere with detection of parasites.
- Previous drug therapy may decrease the number of parasites in the specimen.

D-xylose absorption

One of the most important tests for malabsorption, D-xylose absorption evaluates patients with symptoms of malabsorption, such as weight loss and generalized malnutrition, weakness, and diarrhea. In this test, the patient ingests a standard dose of D-xylose — a pentose sugar that's absorbed in the small intestine without the aid of pancreatic enzymes, passed through the liver without being metabolized, and excreted in the urine. Because of its absorption in the small intestine without digestion, measurement of D-xylose in the urine and blood indicates the absorptive capacity of the small intestine. Normally, blood levels of D-xylose peak 2 hours after ingestion, and 80% to 95% of the dose is excreted in 5 hours; the remaining dose, in 24 hours.

To ensure accurate results, the test requires the patient to fast, to remain in bed during the specimen collection period, and to have adequate renal function for the absorption and excretion of D-xylose.

Purpose
- To aid differential diagnosis of malabsorption
- To determine the cause of malabsorption syndrome

Patient preparation

Explain to the patient that this test helps evaluate digestive function by analyzing blood and urine specimens after ingestion of a sugar solution. Advise him to fast overnight before the test. The patient must abstain from all food and fluids and remain in bed during the test because activity affects test results. Inform the patient that the test requires several blood samples and that all his urine will be collected for 5 or 24 hours. Tell the patient not to contaminate the urine specimens with toilet tissue or stool.

As ordered, withhold aspirin and indomethacin, which alter test results, and record any medications the patient is taking on the laboratory slip.

Procedure

Perform a venipuncture to obtain a fasting blood sample, and collect the sample in a 10-ml *red-top* tube. Then, collect a first-voided morning urine specimen. Label these specimens, and send them to the laboratory immediately to serve as a baseline.

Give the patient 25 g of D-xylose dissolved in 8 oz (240 ml) water, followed by an additional 8 oz (240 ml) of water. If the patient is a child, administer 0.5 g of D-xylose/lb body weight, up to 25 g. Record the time of D-xylose ingestion.

In an adult, draw a blood sample 2 hours after D-xylose ingestion; in a child, after 1 hour. Collect the sample in a 10-ml *red-top* tube (or a 10-ml *gray-top* tube if the sample won't be tested immediately). Occasionally, a 5-hour sample may be drawn to support the findings of the 1- or 2-hour sample. Collect and pool all urine during the 5 or 24 hours following D-xylose ingestion.

Be sure to collect all urine, and refrigerate the specimen during the collection period. At the end of the collection period, send the urine specimen to the laboratory immediately.

Handle the blood collection tubes gently to prevent hemolysis.

Precautions   To determine the length of the collection period,
                  consider that patients aged 65 and older, or those
                  with borderline or elevated creatinine levels tend to
                  have low 5-hour urine levels but normal 24-hour
                  levels.

Values   The following are normal values for the D-xylose
                  absorption test —
                  Children: blood concentration, greater than 30
                  mg/dl (2.0 mmol/L) in 1 hour; urine, 16% to 33% of
                  ingested D-xylose excreted in 5 hours
                  Adults under age 65: blood concentration, 25 to 40
                  mg/dl (1.7 to 2.7 mmol/L) in 2 hours; urine, more
                  than 4 g in 5 hours
                  Adults aged 65 and older: blood concentration, 25 to
                  40 mg/dl (1.7 to 2.7 mmol/L) in 2 hours; urine,
                  more than 3.5 g excreted in 5 hours and more than
                  5 g excreted in 24 hours.

Implications of   Depressed blood and urine D-xylose levels most
results   commonly result from malabsorptive disorders af-
                  fecting the proximal small intestine, such as sprue
                  and celiac disease. However, depressed levels may
                  also result from regional enteritis involving the jeju-
                  num, Whipple's disease, multiple jejunal diver-
                  ticula, myxedema, diabetic neuropathic diarrhea,
                  rheumatoid arthritis, alcoholism, severe conges-
                  tive heart failure, and ascites.

Post-test care   • If a hematoma develops at the venipuncture site,
                    applying warm soaks eases discomfort.
                  • Monitor for abdominal discomfort or mild diar-
                    rhea caused by D-xylose ingestion.
                  • The patient may resume medications and diet
                    discontinued before the test.

Interfering   • Failure to adhere to restrictions of diet and activ-
factors   ity affects absorption of D-xylose.
                  • Aspirin decreases D-xylose excretion by the kid-
                    neys; indomethacin depresses its intestinal ab-
                    sorption.
                  • Failure to obtain a complete urine specimen or to
                    collect blood samples at designated times inter-
                    feres with accurate testing.
                  • Intestinal overgrowth of bacteria or renal reten-
                    tion or insufficiency may cause depressed urine
                    levels.

E

Epstein-Barr virus antibodies

Epstein-Barr virus (EBV), a member of the herpes-virus group, is the causative agent of heterophile-positive infectious mononucleosis, Burkitt's lymphoma, and nasopharyngeal cancer. Although the virus does not replicate in standard cell cultures, most EBV infections can be recognized by testing the patient's serum for heterophile antibodies, which usually appear within the first 3 weeks of illness and then decline rapidly within a few weeks. (See Infectious Mononucleosis Screening Test.) In about 10% of adults and a larger percentage of children, the monospot test is negative despite primary infection with EBV. Furthermore, EBV has been associated with lymphoproliferative processes in immunosuppressed persons. These disorders occur with reactivated rather than primary EBV infections and therefore are also monospot-negative. Alternatively, EBV-specific antibodies, which develop into several antigens of the virus during active infection, can be measured with a high level of sensitivity and specificity by indirect immuno-fluorescence tests. The test profile results of immunoglobulins G, M, and A (IgG, IgM, and IgA) antibodies directed to the EBV antigens, viral capsid antigen (VCA) and Epstein-Barr nuclear antigen (EBNA), can help determine whether the patient had a recent or remote past infection caused by EBV.

Purpose
- To provide a laboratory diagnosis of heterophile (or monospot) negative cases of infectious mononucleosis
- To determine the antibody status to EBV of immunosuppressed patients with lymphoproliferative processes

Patient preparation
Explain the purpose of this test, and inform the patient that the test requires a blood sample.

Procedure
Perform a venipuncture to collect 5 ml of sterile blood in a *red-top* tube. Allow the blood to clot for at least 1 hour at room temperature. Handle the sam-

ple gently to prevent hemolysis. Transfer the serum to a sterile tube or vial, and send it to the laboratory. If transfer must be delayed, store the serum at 39.2° F (4° C) for 1 or 2 days, or at –4° F (–20° C) for longer periods to prevent bacterial contamination.

Findings
Sera from patients who have never been infected with EBV will have no detectable antibodies to the virus measured by either the monospot or indirect immunofluorescence test. The monospot test is positive only during the acute phase of infection with EBV; the indirect immunofluorescence test for VCA and EBNA will detect and discriminate between acute and past infection with the virus. For the profile of test results and their clinical implications, see *Clinical implications of antibody response*.

Implications of results
EBV infection can be ruled out if no antibodies to EBV antigens are detected in the indirect immunofluorescence test. A positive monospot test or an indirect immunofluorescence test that is either IgM-positive or EBNA-negative indicates acute EBV infection. However, a monospot-negative result does not necessarily rule out acute or past infection with EBV. Conversely, IgG class antibody to

Clinical implications of antibody response

Antigen	Acute infectious mono- nucleosis	Remote Epstein- Barr virus infection	Burkitt's lymphoma	Naso- pharyngeal cancer
VCA* ***Antibody class***				
IgM	+++	–	–	–
IgG	+++	++	++++	+++
IgA				++
Epstein-Barr nuclear antigen	–	++	++	++
Heterophile antibody (mono- spot)	++++	–	–	–

Key: + antibody titer   *Viral capsid antigen
       – negative for antibody

VCA and EBNA antigens (IgM-negative) indicates remote (more than 2 months) infection with EBV. Recognize that most cases of monospot-negative infectious mononucleosis are caused by cytomegalovirus infections.

Post-test care
If a hematoma develops at the venipuncture site, applying warm soaks eases discomfort.

Interfering factors
None

Erythrocyte count
Red blood cell count

This test reports the number of red blood cells (RBCs) found in a microliter (cubic millimeter) of whole blood, and is included in the complete blood count. RBCs are now always counted with electronic devices. (Manual hemocytometer counts are now regarded as unacceptably error-prone.) The RBC count itself provides no qualitative information regarding the size, shape, or concentration of hemoglobin within the corpuscles but may be used to calculate two erythrocyte indices: mean corpuscular volume (MCV) and mean corpuscular hemoglobin (MCH).

Purpose
• To supply figures for computing the erythrocyte indices, which reveal RBC size and hemoglobin content
• To support other hematologic tests in diagnosis of anemia and polycythemia

Patient preparation
Explain to the patient that this test evaluates the number of RBCs to detect suspected blood disorders. Inform the patient that this test requires a blood sample. If the patient is a child, explain to the parents (and to the child if he is old enough to understand) that a small amount of blood will be drawn from a finger or earlobe.

Procedure
For adults and older children, draw venous blood into a 7-ml *lavender-top* tube. For younger children, collect capillary blood in a microcapillary tube.

Completely fill the collection tube, and invert it gently several times to mix the sample and the anticoagulant. Handle the sample gently to prevent hemolysis.

Values   Normal RBC values vary, depending on age, sex, sample, and geographic location. In adult males, red cell counts range from 4.5 to 6.2 million/μliter (4.5 to 6.2 × 10^{12}/L) of venous blood; in adult females, 4.2 to 5.4 million/μliter (4.2 to 5.4 × 10^{12}/L) of venous blood; in children, 4.6 to 4.8 million/μliter (4.6 to 4.8 × 10^{12}/L) of venous blood. In full-term infants, values range from 4.4 to 5.8 million/μliter (4.4 to 5.8 × 10^{12}/L) of capillary blood at birth; fall to 3 to 3.8 million/μliter (3.0 to 3.8 × 10^{12}/L) at age 2 months; and increase slowly thereafter. Values are generally higher in persons living at high altitudes.

Implications of results   An elevated RBC count may indicate primary or secondary polycythemia, or dehydration; a depressed count may indicate anemia, fluid overload, or recent hemorrhage. Further tests, such as stained cell examination, hematocrit, hemoglobin, red cell indices, and white cell studies, are needed to confirm diagnosis.

Post-test care   If a hematoma develops at the venipuncture site, applying warm soaks eases discomfort.

Interfering factors   The following factors may interfere with accurate determination of test results:

- failure to use the proper anticoagulant in the collection tube and to adequately mix the sample and anticoagulant
- hemolysis caused by excessive agitation of the sample
- hemoconcentration caused by prolonged tourniquet constriction
- hemodilution caused by drawing the sample from the same arm that is being used for I.V. infusion of fluids
- high white cell count, which falsely elevates red cell count in semiautomated and automated counters
- diseases that cause RBCs to agglutinate or form rouleaux, which falsely decreases red cell count.

Erythrocyte distribution, fetal-maternal

Some exchange of red blood cells (RBCs) from fetal to maternal circulation occurs during most spontaneous or elective abortions during the last half of pregnancy and during most normal deliveries. Usually, the amount of blood transferred is minimal and of no clinical significance. But transfer of significant amounts of blood from an Rh-positive fetus to an Rh-negative mother can result in maternal immunization to the $Rh_o(D)$ antigen and the development of anti-D antibody in maternal circulation. During subsequent pregnancy, the maternal immunization subjects an Rh-positive fetus to potentially fatal hemolysis and erythroblastosis fetalis.

To prevent maternal $Rh_o(D)$ immunization, Rh_o immune globulin (anti-D) is given to an unsensitized Rh-negative mother after amniocentesis, abortion, or rupture of an ectopic pregnancy, prophylactically during the 28th and 29th week of gestation, and shortly after the birth of an Rh-positive infant. The amount of $Rh_o(D)$ immune globulin needed depends on the volume of fetal blood transferred. This test measures the number of fetal RBCs in maternal circulation to allow calculation of the $Rh_o(D)$ immune globulin dosage needed for protection.

This test usually employs a modification of the Kleihauer-Betke technique and requires a postpartum maternal blood specimen. A blood smear is then prepared and fixed in alcohol, immersed in an acidic buffer of pH 3.2, and then stained. This technique is based on the fact that fetal hemoglobulin is resistant to acid elution, whereas normal adult hemoglobin is not. The adult cells lose their hemoglobin and appear as pale ghost cells, while fetal cells retain their hemoglobin and appear red, allowing a visual identification of the two cell types. Two thousand adult cells are counted, and the number of fetal cells observed is recorded. The percentage of fetal cells is determined, and the total volume of fetal-maternal hemorrhage can then be calculated.

Purpose
- To detect and quantify the extent of fetal-maternal hemorrhage
- To determine the amount of $Rh_o(D)$ immune globulin needed to prevent maternal immunization to the $Rh_o(D)$ antigen

Patient preparation
Explain to the patient that this test is used to determine the amount of Rh_o immune globulin she needs to protect future infants from complications resulting from Rh incompatibility. Tell her that she needn't restrict food or fluids before the test and that the test requires a blood sample.

Procedure
Verify the patient's identity. Perform a venipuncture, and collect at least 1 ml of blood in a *lavender-top* or *red-top* tube. The specimen must be properly labeled. The specimen must be collected postpartum; and testing must be completed within 72 hours of delivery.

Findings
Normal maternal whole blood contains no fetal RBCs.

Implications of results
An elevated fetal RBC volume in maternal circulation may necessitate administration of additional $Rh_o(D)$ immune globulin. One vial (a 1 ml dose) is sufficient to cover fetal-to-maternal bleeding of 30 ml of whole blood. $Rh_o(D)$ immune globulin must be administered within 72 hours of amniocentesis, abortion, ruptured ectopic pregnancy, or delivery to ensure adequate protection from Rh immunization. However, the presence of anti-D in maternal serum does not always preclude the antenatal or postpartum administration of $Rh_o(D)$ immune globulin; low levels of anti-D may be present in maternal serum for a few months following administration. Include any information regarding prior $Rh_o(D)$ immune globulin administration on the patient history and the Blood Bank request form.

Post-test care
If a hematoma develops at the venipuncture site, applying warm soaks eases discomfort.

Interfering factors
- Hemolysis caused by improper temperature control, excessive agitation of the sample, or poor phlebotomy technique may interfere with accurate determination of test results.
- Sample analysis done after 72 hours of collection may yield inaccurate results.
- Adult patients with hemoglobinopathies that result in the production of elevated amounts of fetal hemoglobin will have falsely elevated results in this test.

Erythrocyte indices
Red cell indices

Using the results of the red blood cell (RBC) count, hematocrit, and total hemoglobin tests, the red cell indices provide important information about the size, hemoglobin weight of an average RBC, and the average hemoglobin concentration in RBCs. The indices include mean corpuscular volume (MCV), mean corpuscular hemoglobin (MCH), and mean corpuscular hemoglobin concentration (MCHC).

MCV, the ratio of hematocrit (packed cell volume) to the RBC count, expresses the average size of the erythrocytes and indicates whether they are undersized (microcytic), oversized (macrocytic), or normal (normocytic). MCH, the hemoglobin to RBC ratio, gives the weight of hemoglobin in an average red cell. MCHC, the ratio of hemoglobin to hematocrit, defines the concentration of hemoglobin in 100 ml of packed RBCs. It helps distinguish normally colored (normochromic) RBCs from paler (hypochromic) RBCs.

Purpose To aid diagnosis and classification of anemias

Patient preparation Explain that this test helps detect anemia. Tell the patient the test requires a blood sample.

Procedure Perform a venipuncture, and collect the sample in a 7-ml *lavender-top* tube. Completely fill the collection tube, and invert it gently several times to adequately mix the sample and anticoagulant. Handle the sample gently to prevent hemolysis.

Values The range of normal red cell indices is as follows —
MCV: 84 to 99 μm^3 (84 to 99 fL)
MCH: 26 to 32 pg
MCHC: 30% to 36% (30 to 36 g/dl).

Implications of results The red cell indices aid in classification of anemias. Low MCV and MCHC indicate microcytic, hypochromic anemias caused by iron deficiency anemia, pyridoxine-responsive anemia, and thalassemia. A high MCV suggests macrocytic anemias caused by megaloblastic anemias, caused by folic acid or vitamin B_{12} deficiency, inherited disorders of DNA synthesis, or reticulocytosis. Because MCV reflects the average volume of many cells, a value within the normal range can encompass RBCs of various sizes, from microcytic to macrocytic.

Post-test care If a hematoma develops at the venipuncture site, applying warm soaks eases discomfort.

Interfering factors The following factors may interfere with accurate determination of test results:
- failure to use the proper anticoagulant in the collection tube, and to adequately mix the sample and anticoagulant
- hemolysis caused by excessive agitation of the sample
- hemoconcentration caused by prolonged tourniquet constriction
- high white cell count, which causes a false-high RBC count in semiautomated and automated counters, invalidates MCV and MCH results
- falsely elevated hemoglobin values invalidate MCH and MCHC results
- diseases that cause RBCs to agglutinate or form rouleaux falsely decrease RBC count and invalidate test results.

Erythrocyte sedimentation rate (ESR)
Sed rate

The erythrocyte sedimentation rate (ESR) measures the time required for erythrocytes in a whole blood sample to settle to the bottom of a vertical tube. As the red cells descend in the tube, they displace an equal volume of plasma upward, which retards the downward progress of other settling blood elements. Factors affecting ESR include red cell volume, surface area, density, aggregation, and surface charge. Plasma proteins (notably fibrinogen and globulin) encourage aggregation, increasing ESR.

The ESR is a sensitive but nonspecific test that is frequently the earliest indicator of disease when other chemical or physical signs are normal. It often is increased in widespread inflammatory disorders caused by infection or autoimmune disorders; such elevations may be prolonged in localized inflammation and malignant disease.

Purpose • To monitor inflammatory or malignant disease

- To aid detection and diagnosis of occult disease, such as tuberculosis, tissue necrosis, or connective tissue disease

Patient preparation

Explain that this test evaluates the condition of the blood. Inform the patient that the test requires a blood sample.

Procedure

Perform a venipuncture, and collect the sample in a 7-ml *lavender-top*, 4.5-ml *black-top*, or 4.5-ml *blue-top* tube, depending on laboratory preference.

Completely fill the collection tube, and invert it gently several times to adequately mix the sample and the anticoagulant.

Because prolonged standing decreases the ESR, after examining the sample for clots or clumps, send it to the laboratory immediately (it must be tested within 2 hours).

Values

Normal sedimentation rates range from 0 to 20 mm/hour; rates gradually increase with age.

Implications of results

The ESR rises in pregnancy, acute or chronic inflammation, tuberculosis, paraproteinemias (especially multiple myeloma and Waldenström's macroglobulinemia), rheumatic fever, rheumatoid arthritis, and some malignancies. Anemia also tends to raise ESR, because less upward displacement of plasma occurs to retard the relatively few sedimenting RBCs. Polycythemia, sickle cell anemia, hyperviscosity, or low plasma protein level tends to depress ESR.

Post-test care

If a hematoma develops at the venipuncture site, applying warm soaks eases discomfort.

Interfering factors

- Failure to use the proper anticoagulant in the collection tube, to adequately mix the sample and anticoagulant, and to send the sample to the laboratory immediately may interfere with accurate determination of test results.
- Hemolysis caused by excessive agitation of the sample may affect the sedimentation.
- Prolonged tourniquet constriction may cause hemoconcentration.

Erythrocyte survival time
Red blood cell survival time

Normally, red blood cells (RBCs) are only destroyed when they reach senility. However, in hemolytic diseases, RBCs of all ages are randomly destroyed, resulting in anemia. This test measures the survival time of circulating RBCs and detects sites of abnormal RBC sequestration and destruction, aiding evaluation of unexplained anemia.

Survival time is measured by labeling a random sample of the patient's own RBCs with radioactive sodium chromate chromium 51 (^{51}Cr). The ^{51}Cr quickly crosses RBC membranes and binds to hemoglobin. This labeled group of RBCs is then injected back into the patient. Serial blood samples measure the percentage of labeled cells per unit volume over 3 to 4 weeks, until 50% of the cells have disappeared. A normal RBC survives about 120 days (half-life of 60 days); the ^{51}Cr-labeled RBCs have a shorter half-life (25 to 30 days) because about 1% of senescent RBCs are removed from the circulation each day and about 1% of ^{51}Cr is spontaneously eluted from the labeled RBCs each day.

During the test period, a gamma camera scans the body for sites of abnormally high radioactivity, which indicate sites of excessive RBC sequestration and destruction. Other tests performed with the RBC survival time test may include spot-checks of the stool to detect GI blood loss; hematocrit; blood volume studies; and radionuclide iron uptake and clearance tests to aid differential diagnosis of anemia.

Purpose
- To help evaluate unexplained anemia, particularly hemolytic anemia
- To identify sites of abnormal RBC sequestration and destruction

Patient preparation
Explain that this test helps identify the cause of anemia; that the test involves labeling a blood sample with a radioactive substance; and that it requires regular blood samples at 3-day intervals for 3 to 4 weeks. Reassure the patient that the small amount of radioactive substance used is harmless.

Procedure
A 30-ml blood sample is drawn and mixed with 100 millicuries (mCi) of ^{51}Cr for an adult; less for a child. After an incubation period, the mixture is in-

jected intravenously into the patient. A blood sample is drawn 30 minutes after injection to determine blood and RBC volumes.

A 6-ml sample is collected in a *green-top* tube after 24 hours; follow-up samples are collected at 3-day intervals for 3 to 4 weeks. (The interval between samples may vary, depending on the laboratory.) To avoid error from physical decay of the ^{51}Cr, each sample is measured with a scintillation well counter on the day it's drawn. Radioactivity per ml of RBCs is calculated; these values are then plotted to determine mean RBC survival time. Simultaneous gamma camera scans of the precordium, sacrum, liver, and spleen detect radioactivity at sites of excess RBC sequestration. A hematocrit is done on a small portion of each blood sample to check for blood loss.

Precautions
- This test is contraindicated during pregnancy, because it exposes the fetus to radiation.
- Because excess blood loss can invalidate test results, this test is usually contraindicated for a patient with active bleeding or poor clotting function. However, if the test is necessary for a patient with poor clotting function, observe the venipuncture sites carefully for signs of hemorrhage.
- The patient should not receive blood transfusions during the test period and should not have blood samples drawn for other tests.

Findings
Normal half-life for RBCs labeled with ^{51}Cr is 25 to 35 days. Normal gamma camera scans reveal slight radioactivity in the spleen, liver, and sometimes the bone marrow.

Implications of results
Decreased RBC survival time indicates a hemolytic disease, such as chronic lymphocytic leukemia, congenital nonspherocytic hemolytic anemia, hemoglobin C disease, hereditary spherocytosis, idiopathic acquired hemolytic anemia, paroxysmal nocturnal hemoglobinuria, elliptocytosis, pernicious anemia, sickle cell anemia, sickle cell hemoglobin C disease, or hemolytic-uremic syndrome. If hemolytic anemia is diagnosed, additional tests using cross transfusion of labeled RBCs can determine if anemia results from an intrinsic RBC defect or an extrinsic factor.

A gamma camera scan that detects a site of excess RBC sequestration provides direction for treat-

ment. For example, abnormally high RBC sequestration in the spleen may require a splenectomy.

Post-test care   If a hematoma develops at the venipuncture site,
applying warm soaks eases discomfort.

Interfering   • Dehydration, overhydration, or blood loss (from
factors   hemorrhage or blood samples drawn for other
                tests) can change the circulating RBC volume
                and invalidate test results.
              • Blood transfusions during the test period alter
                the proportion of labeled RBCs to total RBCs,
                thus altering results.

Erythrocyte total porphyrins
Erythropoietic porphyrins

This test measures total erythrocyte porphyrins —
mostly protoporphyrin, but also coproporphyrin
and uroporphyrin. Porphyrins are pigments that exist in all protoplasm and are needed for energy storage and use. Protoporphyrin, coproporphyrin, and
uroporphyrin are produced during heme biosynthesis. Small amounts of these porphyrins or their
precursors normally appear in blood, urine, and feces. Production and excretion of porphyrins or
their precursors increase in porphyrias, disorders
of porphyrin metabolism, erythropoietic or hepatic.
This test detects erythropoietic porphyrias.

After an initial screening test for total porphyrins,
quantitative fluorometric analysis can identify specific porphyrins and suggest specific disorders.

Purpose   • To aid diagnosis of congenital or acquired eryth-
             ropoietic porphyrias
           • To help confirm diagnosis of disorders affecting
             red blood cell (RBC) activity

Patient   Explain that this test helps detect blood cell disor-
preparation   ders. Instruct the patient to fast (allowing only water) for 12 to 14 hours before the sample is drawn.

Procedure   Perform a venipuncture, and collect the sample in
a 5-ml or larger *green-top* tube. Label the sample,
place it on ice, and send it to the laboratory promptly. Handle the sample gently to prevent hemolysis.

Values
Total porphyrin levels range from 16 to 60 µg/dl (0.30 to 1.08 µmol/L) of packed RBCs. Protoporphyrin levels range from 16 to 60 µg/dl (0.30 to 1.08 µmol/L); coproporphyrin and uroporphyrin levels are each below 2 µg/dl (0.03 µmol/L).

Implications of results
Elevated protoporphyrin levels may indicate erythropoietic protoporphyria, infection, increased erythropoiesis, thalassemia, sideroblastic anemia, iron deficiency anemia, or lead poisoning. Elevated coproporphyrin levels may indicate congenital erythropoietic porphyria, erythropoietic protoporphyria or coproporphyria, and sideroblastic anemia. Elevated uroporphyrin levels typically suggest congenital erythropoietic porphyria or erythropoietic protoporphyria.

Post-test care
If a hematoma develops at the venipuncture site, applying warm soaks eases discomfort.

Interfering factors
Hemolysis of the sample or failure to observe dietary restrictions may alter test results.

Estrogen or progesterone receptor assay, tissue

Estrogen receptors are cellular proteins that bind estradiol in the first step of a cellular response. They can be detected by radiologic assay.

Measuring estrogen and progesterone receptors in tissue samples of mammary carcinoma is useful to evaluate potential responsiveness to endocrine therapy. Significant estrogen receptor values are present in up to 77% of primary tumors, and 66% of metastatic tumors. Approximately 55% of receptor-positive tumors respond to endocrine therapy.

Purpose
To evaluate estrogen binding of tissue cytosol

Patient preparation
Explain the purpose of this test, and inform the patient about the specimen and method of collection.

Procedure
The test requires a specimen of 200 mg to 500 mg quick-frozen (not fixed) tumor material for assay. The laboratory provides specific guidelines and materials for transport of the required tissue specimen.

Values
The test result is reported as negative if tissue binding is undetectable (less than 3 fmol/mg cytosol protein). The result is positive if estrogen or progesterone binding is more than 3 fmol/mg cytosol protein.

Implications of results
Estrogen-receptor-negative tumors rarely respond to endocrine therapy.

Post-test care
As appropriate, counsel patient regarding implications of test results.

Interfering factor
An inadequate tissue sample or incorrect preparation of the tissue sample may prevent accurate determination of test results.

Estrogens, serum

Estrogens (and progesterone) are secreted by the ovaries under the influence of the pituitary gonadotropins, follicle-stimulating hormone (FSH) and luteinizing hormone (LH). Estrogens — in particular, estradiol, which is the most potent estrogen — interact with the hypothalamic-pituitary axis through both negative and positive feedback mechanisms. Slowly rising or sustained high levels inhibit secretion of FSH and LH (negative feedback), but a rapid rise in estrogen that occurs just before ovulation seems to stimulate LH secretion (positive feedback).

This radioimmunoassay measures serum levels of estradiol, estrone, and estriol (the only estrogens that appear in serum in measurable amounts) and has diagnostic significance in evaluating female gonadal dysfunction. Tests of hypothalamic-pituitary function may be required to confirm diagnosis.

Purpose
• To determine sexual maturation and fertility
• To aid diagnosis of gonadal dysfunction: precocious or delayed puberty, menstrual disorders (especially amenorrhea), or infertility
• To determine fetal well-being
• To aid diagnosis of tumors known to secrete estrogen

Patient preparation
Explain to the patient that this test helps determine if secretion of female hormones is normal and that the test may be repeated during the various phases

of the menstrual cycle. Tell her she needn't restrict food or fluids before the test and that the test requires a blood sample. Withhold all steroid and pituitary-based hormones (including estrogens and progestogen). If these medications must be continued, note this on the laboratory slip.

Procedure Perform a venipuncture, and collect the sample in a 10-ml *red-top* tube.

To prevent hemolysis, handle the sample gently. Send it to the laboratory immediately for centrifugation.

If the patient is premenopausal, indicate the phase of her menstrual cycle on the laboratory slip.

Values Normal serum estrogen levels for premenopausal females vary widely during the menstrual cycle —
1 to 10 days: 24 to 68 pg/ml (90 to 250 pmol/L)
11 to 20 days: 50 to 186 pg/ml (180 to 690 pmol/L)
21 to 30 days: 73 to 149 pg/ml (270 to 550 pmol/L).

Serum estrogen levels in males range from 12 to 34 pg/ml (40 to 120 pmol/L). In girls age 6 and older, levels rise gradually to adult female values. In children under age 6, the normal range of serum estrogen is 3 to 10 pg/ml (10 to 40 pmol/L).

Implications of results Decreased estrogen levels may indicate primary hypogonadism, or ovarian failure, as in Turner's syndrome or ovarian agenesis; secondary hypogonadism, as in hypopituitarism; or menopause. Abnormally high levels can occur with estrogen-producing tumors, in precocious puberty, or in severe hepatic disease, such as cirrhosis, that prevents clearance of plasma estrogens. High levels may also result from congenital adrenal hyperplasia (increased conversion of androgens to estrogen).

Post-test care • If a hematoma develops at the venipuncture site, applying warm soaks eases discomfort.
• The patient may resume medications discontinued before the test.

Interfering factors • Pregnancy and pretest use of estrogens (oral contraceptives) can increase serum estrogen levels. Clomiphene, an estrogen antagonist, can decrease serum estrogen levels. Ingestion of steroids or pituitary-based hormones can alter test results. For example, dexamethasone may suppress adrenal androgen secretion.

- Hemolysis caused by excessive agitation of the sample may interfere with accurate determination of test results.

Estrogens, total urine

This test is a quantitative analysis of total urine levels of estradiol, estrone, and estriol — the major estrogens present in significant amounts in urine. In females who are past puberty, these estrogens are secreted by the theca interna cells of the ovarian follicle and by the corpus luteum; in pregnancy, by the placenta; and after menopause, primarily by the adrenal glands. In males, two-thirds of estradiol and of estrone are derived from testosterone; the remaining third of estradiol and smaller quantities of estrone are secreted by the testes. In both sexes, the liver, which oxidizes or converts hormones to glucuronide and sulfate conjugates, is the major organ of estrogen metabolism.

Clinical indications for this test include tumors of ovarian, adrenocortical, or testicular origin. A common method for measuring total urine estrogen levels involves purification by gel filtration, followed by spectrophotofluorometry. Supplementary tests that may provide further information about ovarian function include cytologic examination of vaginal smears, measurement of urine levels of pregnanediol and follicle-stimulating hormone, and evaluation of response to an injection of progesterone.

Purpose

- To evaluate ovarian activity and help determine the cause of amenorrhea and female hyperestrogenism
- To aid diagnosis of testicular tumors
- To assess fetoplacental status

Patient preparation

Explain to the female patient that this test helps evaluate ovarian function; to the patient who is pregnant that this test helps evaluate fetal development and placental function; and to the male patient that this test helps evaluate testicular function. Inform all patients that the test requires collection of a 24-hour urine specimen, and that no pretest restrictions of food or fluids are necessary. If the 24-hour specimen is to be collected at home, teach the patient the proper collection technique. Check the patient's medication history for use of drugs that may influence estrogen levels.

Procedure   Collect a 24-hour specimen in a bottle containing a preservative to keep the specimen at a pH of 3.0 to 5.0. If the patient is pregnant, note the approximate week of gestation on the laboratory slip. If the patient is a nonpregnant female, note the stage of her menstrual cycle.

Refrigerate the specimen or keep it on ice during the collection period.

Values   In nonpregnant females, total urine estrogen levels rise and fall during the menstrual cycle, peaking shortly before midcycle, decreasing immediately following ovulation, increasing through the life of the corpus luteum, and decreasing greatly as the corpus luteum degenerates and menstruation begins.

Normal values for nonpregnant females are as follows—
Preovulatory phase: 5 to 25 mcg/day (15 to 85 nmol/day)
Ovulatory phase: 24 to 100 mcg/day (80 to 350 nmol/day)
Luteal phase: 12 to 80 mcg/day (40 to 280 nmol/day).

In postmenopausal females, values are less than 10 mcg/day (40 nmol/day); in males, from 4 to 25 mcg/day (10 to 80 nmol/day).

Implications of results   Decreased total urine estrogen levels may reflect ovarian agenesis, primary ovarian insufficiency (caused by Stein-Leventhal syndrome, for example), or secondary ovarian insufficiency (caused by pituitary or adrenal hypofunction, or metabolic disturbances).

Elevated total estrogen levels in nonpregnant females may indicate tumors of ovarian or adrenocortical origin, adrenocortical hyperplasia, or a metabolic or hepatic disorder. In males, elevated total estrogen levels are associated with testicular tumors.

Elevated total urine estrogen levels are normal during pregnancy; serial determinations should show a rising titer.

Post-test care   The patient may resume medications withheld before the test.

Interfering factors   • Drugs that may influence total urine estrogen levels include steroids (estrogens, progesterone, and high-dose corticosteroids), methenamine mandelate, phenazopyridine hydrochloride, phenothiazines, tetracyclines, phenolphthalein, ampicillin, meprobamate, senna, cascara sagrada, and hydrochlorothiazide.

- Failure to collect all urine during the 24-hour period and to refrigerate the specimen or keep it on ice, and improper pH control may affect test results.

Ethanol, blood

This quantitative test uses gas chromatography or microdiffusion to measure the blood ethanol level. This assay determines the degree of ethanol intoxication, for use in medicolegal procedures, or rules out intoxication in a person who is comatose. Although the degree of intoxication can be measured using a breath or urine specimen, medicolegal tests in the United States require a blood sample because the findings are more specific.

About 80% of ingested ethanol is absorbed in the jejunum, and 20% is absorbed in the stomach. When the stomach is empty, about 50% of ethanol is absorbed within 15 minutes, and peak levels are reached in 40 to 70 minutes (food in the stomach slows absorption). About 90% of ethanol reaches the liver, where alcohol dehydrogenase converts it to acetaldehyde, which then metabolizes to water and carbon dioxide. The remaining 10% is excreted unchanged in breath, sweat, and urine.

Purpose
- To rule out alcohol intoxication in a person who is comatose
- To evaluate the degree of ethanol intoxication, for medicolegal purposes
- To monitor ethanol levels when used as an antidote to methanol poisoning

Patient preparation
Explain to the patient and his family that this test determines the amount of ethanol in the blood. Tell him the test requires a blood sample.

If the test is being performed for medicolegal purposes, make sure that the patient or a responsible family member has signed a consent form. Check the patient's recent medication history for the time and amount of ethanol ingestion as well as for dosage of other drugs being used.

Clinical effects of ethanol

Ethanol's clinical effects vary widely, depending on such factors as the patient's body weight, nutritional status, and rate of ingestion. Also, the type of alcohol affects the clinical state because the oil and sugar content raise the ethanol level. The following chart estimates ethanol's effects on a 160-pound person drinking whiskey at a rate of 3 oz/hour.

Quantity consumed	Blood ethanol level		Clinical effect
	% wt/vol	mg/dl	
3 oz (90 ml)	0.05	50	Sedation and tranquility
6 oz (180 ml)	0.10	100	Lack of coordination, slurred speech, slow mental response
12 oz (360 ml)	0.20	200	Obvious intoxication, disturbed equilibrium, poor color perception
15 oz (450 ml)	0.30	300	Unconsciousness, tremors, sweating, and vomiting
24 oz (720 ml)	0.40	400	Deep coma, which may be irreversible
30 oz (900 ml)	0.50	500	Death

Procedure After cleaning the venipuncture site with benzalkonium chloride (aqueous 1:75 dilution) or povidone-iodine solution, perform a venipuncture, and collect the sample in a 7-ml *red-top* tube. Send the sample to the laboratory immediately, or refrigerate it.

Precautions
- Don't clean the venipuncture site with alcohol or tincture of iodine because these interfere with test results.
- For a medicolegal test, observe appropriate precautions.

Values For intoxicating and lethal alcohol levels, see *Clinical effects of ethanol*.

Implications of results The overall effect of ethanol is central nervous system (CNS) depression. Values listed in the chart apply primarily to acute toxicity, and treatment is based on confirmation of toxicity. Acute toxicity can also result from inhaling ethanol fumes in an industrial setting, such as a distillery.

Chronic alcoholics tolerate much higher (even lethal) levels, metabolizing ethanol to acetaldehyde in half the normal time. The resultant high acetaldehyde levels may cause liver damage.

Ethanol levels have medicolegal implications.

Post-test care
If a hematoma develops at the venipuncture site, applying warm soaks eases discomfort.

Interfering factors
• Blood ethanol levels are elevated by chloral hydrate and glutethimide. False elevations of the specimen's ethanol level can follow contamination by alcohol or tincture of iodine at the venipuncture site.
• Both ethanol and barbiturates are metabolized in the microsomal enzyme system. When taken together, they produce high blood levels, with greatly increased CNS depression.

Euglobulin lysis time

This test measures the interval between clot formation and dissolution in the euglobulin (acid-insoluble) fraction of plasma. In the laboratory, a blood sample is acidified, the euglobulins precipitated, redissolved, then mixed with calcium and thrombin to form a clot. The time required for this clot to lyse is recorded.

Purpose
• To assess systemic fibrinolysis
• To help detect abnormal fibrinolytic states

Patient preparation
Explain that this test evaluates the blood clotting mechanism. Tell the patient the test requires a blood sample.

Procedure
Perform a venipuncture. Collect a 4.5-ml sample in a *blue-top* tube. Mix the sample and anticoagulant thoroughly. Then pack the sample in ice, and send it to the laboratory immediately.

Precautions
When drawing the sample, be careful not to rub the area over the vein too vigorously, to pump the fist excessively, or to leave the tourniquet in place too long. Avoid excessive probing during the venipuncture; handle the sample gently.

Findings
The normal lysis time is at least 2 hours.

Implications of results	A clot lysis within 1 hour indicates accelerated fibrinolysis. In pathologic fibrinolysis, lysis time may be as brief as 5 to 10 minutes.
Post-test care	If a hematoma develops at the venipuncture site, applying warm soaks eases discomfort.
Interfering factors	• Prolonged tourniquet constriction, vigorous vein preparation, or excessive pumping of the fist shortens lysis time. • Failure to determine deficient fibrinogen levels before performing this test will falsely shorten lysis time. • Hemolysis caused by excessive probing during venipuncture or by excessive agitation of the sample may alter test results. • Failure to follow appropriate precautions for the type of collection tube used may impair accuracy of results. • Depressed fibrinogen levels (less than 100 mg/dl) can shorten lysis time.

Extractable nuclear antigen antibodies

Ribonucleoprotein antibodies, anti-Sm antibodies, Sjögren's antibodies

Extractable nuclear antigen (ENA) is a complex of at least two and possibly three antigens. One of these — ribonucleoprotein (RNP) — is susceptible to degradation by ribonuclease. The second — Smith (Sm) antigen — is an acidic nuclear protein that resists ribonuclease degradation. The third antigen sometimes included in this group — Sjögren's syndrome B (SS-B; or La, Ha) antigen — forms a precipitate when antibody is present. Antibodies to these antigens are associated with certain autoimmune disorders.

Tests to detect ENA antibodies help differentiate autoimmune disorders with similar signs and symptoms. The RNP antibody test detects RNP autoantibodies, which are associated with systemic lupus erythematosus (SLE), mixed connective tissue disease, progressive systemic sclerosis, and other rheumatic disorders. This test aids in the differential diagnosis of systemic rheumatic disease and is a useful follow-up test for collagen vascular autoimmune disease. The anti-Sm antibody test detects

Sm autoantibodies, which are a specific marker for SLE; positive results are thus highly diagnostic of SLE. This test also helps monitor collagen vascular autoimmune disease. The Sjögren's antibody test detects the SS-B autoantibodies produced in Sjögren's syndrome, an immunologic abnormality sometimes associated with rheumatoid arthritis and SLE. However, this test is not diagnostic for Sjögren's syndrome. RNP and Sm autoantibodies can also be detected by immunodiffusion, counterimmunoelectrophoresis, or enzyme immunoassay.

To perform these tests, red blood cells from sheep are sensitized with ENA extracted from rabbit thymus and then incubated with serum samples; ENA antibodies present in the serum will agglutinate the cells. If the serum sample shows agglutination, differential double immunoassays are done to determine which antibodies are present. Anti-ENA tests are most useful with anti-DNA, serum complement, and antinuclear antibody tests.

Purpose
- To aid differential diagnosis of autoimmune disease
- To distinguish between anti-RNP antibodies (common in mixed connective tissue disease)
- To screen for anti-RNP antibodies (common in mixed connective tissue disease)
- To screen for anti-Sm antibodies (common in SLE)
- To support diagnosis of collagen vascular autoimmune diseases
- To monitor response to therapy

Patient preparation
Explain that this test detects certain antibodies and that test results help determine diagnosis and treatment; or, when indicated, explain that the test assesses the effectiveness of treatment. Tell the patient that the test requires a blood sample.

Procedure
Perform a venipuncture, and collect the sample in a 7-ml *red-top* tube. Send the sample to the laboratory immediately.

Findings
Normally, serum is negative for anti-RNP, anti-Sm, and SS-B antibodies.

Implications of results
The presence of anti-Sm antibodies is highly diagnostic of SLE. A high level of anti-RNP antibodies

with a low titer of anti-Sm antibodies suggests mixed connective tissue disease. Although SS-B antibodies are associated with primary Sjögren's syndrome, their presence is not considered diagnostic of this disorder; however, a positive test for SS-B antibodies mandates further testing.

Post-test care
- Check the venipuncture site carefully for signs of infection. Keep a clean, dry bandage over the site for at least 24 hours.
- If a hematoma develops at the venipuncture site, applying warm soaks eases discomfort.

Interfering factor

Failure to send the sample to the laboratory immediately may interfere with accurate determination of test results.

F

Febrile agglutination tests

Bacterial infections (such as tularemia, brucellosis, and the disorders caused by salmonella) and rickettsial infections (such as Rocky Mountain spotted fever and typhus) sometimes cause puzzling fevers (fever of undetermined origin [FUO]). In these infections and others in which microorganisms are difficult to isolate from blood or excreta, febrile agglutination tests can provide important diagnostic information.

The Weil-Felix reaction for rickettsial disease, Widal's test for *Salmonella*, and tests for brucellosis and tularemia are essentially the same. In these tests, a serum sample is mixed with a few drops of prepared antigens in normal saline solution on a slide; the reaction is observed with the unaided eye. If agglutination occurs, antigen is added to serial dilutions of the patient's serum. Antibody titer is expressed as the reciprocal of the last dilution showing visible agglutination.

The Weil-Felix reaction establishes rickettsial antibody titers. Unlike other febrile agglutination tests, the Weil-Felix reaction doesn't use the causal agent as the antigen, but uses instead three forms of *Proteus* antigens (OX-19, OX-2, and OX-K) that cross-react with the various strains of rickettsiae. Other methods for detecting rickettsial infections include complement fixation, indirect fluorescent assay, and enzyme-linked immunosorbent assay.

In *Salmonella* infection — gastroenteritis and extraintestinal focal infections, both caused by *Salmonella enteritidis*, and in enteric (typhoid) fever, caused by *S. typhosa* — the *Salmonella* organism presents flagellar (H) and somatic (O) antigens; Widal's test establishes their titers. Antibodies that agglutinate with H antigens form coarse, unstable aggregates that return to solution easily; those that agglutinate with O antigens form finer, more stable aggregates. The O antigens are considered more specific for *Salmonella* than for H antigens. A third antigen — Vi, or envelope, antigen — may indicate typhoid carrier status, which often tests negative for H and O antigens, but results so far have been difficult to standardize. Widal's test isn't recommended for diagnosing *Salmonella* gastroenteritis because symptoms subside before the titer rises.

Slide-agglutination and tube dilution tests, using killed suspensions of the disease organisms as antigens, establish titers for the gram-negative coccobacilli *Brucella* and *Francisella tularensis*, which cause brucellosis and tularemia, respectively.

Purpose
- To support clinical findings in diagnosis of disorders caused by *Salmonella*, rickettsiae, *F. tularensis*, or *Brucella* organisms in which isolation from the blood or excreta is difficult
- To identify the cause of FUO

Patient preparation

Explain to the patient that this test detects and measures antibodies to microorganisms that may cause fever and other symptoms. Inform him that he needn't restrict food or fluids before the test and that the test requires a blood sample.

Explain that this test may require a series of blood samples to detect a titer pattern that is characteristic of the suspected disorder. Reassure the patient that a positive titer only suggests a disorder.

If the patient is receiving antibiotics, note on the laboratory slip when such therapy began.

Procedure

Perform a venipuncture, and collect the sample in a 7-ml *red-top* tube. Send samples to the laboratory immediately.

Precautions

Use standard hospital isolation procedures when collecting and handling samples. Send samples to the laboratory immediately.

Values

Normal dilutions are as follows —
Salmonella antibody: < 1:80
Brucellosis antibody: < 1:80
Tularemia antibody: < 1:40
Rickettsial antibody: < 1:40.

Implications of results

Observed rise and fall of titers are crucial for detecting active infection. If this is not possible, certain titer levels can suggest the disorder.

The Weil-Felix reaction is positive for rickettsiae (Rocky Mountain spotted fever; typhus [murine, scrub, epidemic, or recrudescent]) with antibodies to *Proteus* appearing 6 to 12 days after infection; titers peak in 1 month and usually drop to negative in 5 or 6 months. However, this test cannot be used for diagnosing rickettsialpox or Q fever, because the antibodies of these diseases don't cross-react with *Proteus* antigens; the test shows positive titers in *Proteus* infections and, in such cases, is nonspecific for rickettsiae.

In *Salmonella* infection (typhoid and paratyphoid), H and O agglutinins usually appear in serum after 1 week, and titers continue to rise for 3 to 6 weeks. O agglutinins usually fall to insignificant levels in 6 to 12 months. H agglutinin titers may remain elevated for several years.

In brucellosis, titers usually rise after 2 or 3 weeks, and reach their highest levels between 4 and 8 weeks; nevertheless, absence of *Brucella* agglutinins doesn't rule out brucellosis. In tularemia, titers usually become positive in the second week of infection, exceed 1:320 by the third week, peak in 4 to 7 weeks, and usually decline gradually 1 year after recovery.

For all febrile agglutinins, a fourfold increase in titers is strong evidence of infection.

Post-test care

- If a hematoma develops at the venipuncture site, applying warm soaks eases discomfort.
- In FUO and suspected infection, consider that isolation may be necessary.

Interfering factors

- Failure to send the sample to the laboratory immediately may affect the accuracy of test results.
- Vaccination or continuous exposure to bacterial or rickettsial infection (resulting in immunity) causes high titers.
- Many antibodies cross-react with bacteria that cause other infectious diseases. For example, tularemia antibodies cross-react with *Brucella* antigens.
- Immunodeficient patients may show infectious symptoms but be unable to produce antibodies. In such cases, titers remain negative, even during infection.
- Patients receiving antibiotic therapy show depressed titers early in the course of the disorder.
- Patients with elevated immunoglobulin levels caused by hepatic disease, or those who use drugs excessively, often have high *Salmonella* titers.
- Patients who have had skin tests with *Brucella* antigen may show elevated *Brucella* titers.

- In patients with *Proteus* infections, positive Weil-Felix titers are nonspecific for rickettsial disease.

Fecal occult blood

Fecal occult blood can be detected by chemical tests for hemoglobin, such as the guaiac or orthotoluidine test. Because small amounts of blood (2 to 2.5 ml/day) normally appear in the feces, tests for occult blood are designed to detect quantities larger than this. These tests are indicated in patients whose clinical symptoms and preliminary blood studies suggest GI bleeding. However, further tests are required to pinpoint the origin of the bleeding. Stool color correlates roughly with the site of bleeding; for example, melena usually results from hemorrhage in the esophagus or stomach. Gastric juices act to digest this blood, blackening it. Melena may also result from hemorrhage in the jejunum or ileum, provided its passage through the intestine is slow. Dark maroon stools result from hemorrhage beyond the ligament of Treitz.

Purpose
- To detect GI bleeding
- To aid early diagnosis of colorectal cancer

Patient preparation
Explain that this test helps detect abnormal GI bleeding. Instruct the patient to maintain a high-fiber diet and to avoid eating red meats, poultry, fish, turnips, and horseradish for 48 to 72 hours before the test and throughout the collection period. Explain that the test requires collection of three stool specimens.

As ordered, withhold iron preparations, bromides, iodides, rauwolfia derivatives, indomethacin, colchicine, salicylates, phenylbutazone, steroids, and ascorbic acid for 48 hours before the test and also during it. If these medications must be continued, note this on the laboratory slip.

Procedure
Collect three stool specimens. Testing can take place immediately or in the laboratory.

For immediate testing, first place a small amount of stool on a piece of filter paper. Then, add two drops each of tap water, glacial acetic acid, 1:60 solution of gum guaiac in 95% ethyl alcohol, and 3% hydrogen peroxide, *or* two drops each of 0.2% orthotolidin and 0.3% hydrogen peroxide. Mix thoroughly with a tongue blade. Note the color immediately, and check it again after 5 minutes.

Be sure to obtain specimens from two different areas of each stool, to allow for variance in distribution of blood.

Precautions
- Instruct the patient to avoid contaminating the stool specimen with toilet tissue or urine.
- Send the specimen to the laboratory or perform the test immediately.

Findings
Normally, less than 2.5 ml of blood is present, resulting in a green reaction.

Implications of results
A dark blue reaction that appears within 5 minutes indicates that the test is positive for occult blood; a strongly positive reaction within 3 to 4 minutes is always abnormal. A faint blue reaction is weakly positive and isn't necessarily abnormal. A positive test indicates GI bleeding, which may result from many disorders, such as varices, peptic ulcer, cancer, ulcerative colitis, dysentery, or hemorrhagic disease. This test is particularly important for early diagnosis of colorectal cancer because 80% of persons with this type of cancer demonstrate positive results. Further tests, such as barium swallow, analyses of gastric contents, and endoscopy, are necessary to further define the site and extent of bleeding.

Post-test care
The patient may resume a normal diet and medications restricted before the test.

Interfering factors
- Failure to observe dietary restriction, to test the specimen immediately, or to send it to the laboratory immediately may affect test results.
- Bleeding may result from use of iron preparations, bromides, rauwolfia derivatives, indomethacin, colchicine, phenylbutazone, or steroids.
- Ingestion of ascorbic acid (vitamin C) can interfere with accurate testing by producing normal test results even in the presence of significant bleeding.
- Ingestion of 2 to 5 ml of blood, such as from bleeding gums, can cause abnormal results.

Ferritin, serum

Ferritin, a major iron-storage protein found in reticuloendothelial cells, normally appears in small quantities in serum. In healthy adults, serum ferritin levels are directly related to the amount of available iron stored in the body and can be measured accurately by immunoassay. Unlike many other blood studies, the serum ferritin test isn't affected by moderate hemolysis of the sample or by any known drugs.

Purpose
- To screen for iron deficiency and iron overload
- To measure iron storage
- To distinguish between iron deficiency (a condition of low iron storage) and chronic inflammation (a condition of normal storage)

Patient preparation
Explain to the patient that this test assesses the available iron stored in the body. Inform him that he needn't restrict food, fluids, or medications before the test and that the test requires a blood sample. Review the patient's history for recent transfusion.

Procedure
Perform a venipuncture, and collect the sample in a 10-ml *red-top* tube.

Values
Normal serum ferritin values vary with age. According to the Mayo Medical Laboratories, serum ferritin levels range as follows—
Males: 20 to 300 ng/ml (µg/L)
Females: 20 to 120 ng/ml (µg/L)
Children aged 6 months to 15 years: 7 to 140 ng/ml (µg/L)
Infants aged 2 to 5 months: 50 to 200 ng/ml (µg/L)
Infants aged 1 month: 200 to 600 ng/ml (µg/L)
Neonates: 25 to 200 ng/ml (µg/L).

Implications of results
High serum ferritin levels may indicate acute or chronic hepatic disease, iron overload, leukemia, acute or chronic infection or inflammation, Hodgkin's disease, or chronic hemolytic anemias; in these disorders, iron stores in the bone marrow may be normal or significantly increased. Serum ferritin levels are characteristically normal or slightly elevated in those patients who have chronic renal disease. Normal or high serum ferritin levels do not exclude iron deficiency in the presence of

these elevating factors. Low serum ferritin levels reliably indicate chronic iron deficiency.

Post-test care
If a hematoma develops at the venipuncture site, applying warm soaks eases discomfort.

Interfering factor
Recent transfusion may cause elevated serum ferritin levels.

Fibrin degradation products (FDP)

Fibrin breakdown products (FBP), fibrin split products (FSP)

After a fibrin clot forms in response to vascular injury, the fibrinolytic system acts to prevent excessive clotting by converting plasminogen into the fibrin-dissolving enzyme plasmin. Plasmin breaks down fibrin and fibrinogen into fragments, or split products, known as X, Y, D, and E, in order of decreasing molecular weight. These products may combine with fibrin monomers to prevent polymerization; that is, the fragments retain some anticoagulant activity. An excess of such products in circulation is seen in abnormally active fibrinolysis and in coagulation disorders, such as disseminated intravascular coagulation (DIC).

Fibrinogen degradation products (FDP) are commonly detected by an immunoprecipitation reaction. Serum (clotted with excessive thrombin, with fibrinolytic inhibitors added) is mixed on a slide with latex particles coated with antibodies to FDP. These products adhere in clumps if fibrin or fibrinogen degradation products are present in serum. Immunoassays also may be used to detect FDP, but are more time-consuming.

Purpose
• To detect FDP in the circulation
• To help diagnose DIC and distinguish it from other coagulation disorders

Patient preparation
Explain to the patient that this test helps determine if his blood clots normally. Inform him that he needn't restrict food or fluids before the test and that the test requires a blood sample. Check the patient's history for use of medications that may interfere with accurate determination of test results.

Procedure — Perform a venipuncture, and draw 2 ml of blood into a plastic syringe. Draw the sample, using special tubes that contain thrombin and fibrinolytic inhibitors. Gently invert the collection tube several times to mix the contents adequately; don't shake the tube vigorously or hemolysis may result. The blood clots within 2 seconds and must then be immediately sent to the laboratory and incubated at 98.6° F (37° C) for 30 minutes before testing proceeds, to ensure that all of the fibrinogen is removed.

Values — In a screening assay, serum contains less than 10 mcg/ml (mg/L) of FDP. A quantitative assay shows normal levels of less than 3 mcg/ml (mg/L).

Implications of results — FDP levels rise in primary fibrinolytic states and in DIC. Elevations are also seen postoperatively and in acute thrombosis, liver disease, obstetric problems (abruptio placentae, intrauterine death, and preeclampsia), burns, and sunstroke. FDP levels usually exceed 100 mcg/ml (mg/L) in active renal disease or renal transplant rejection.

Post-test care — If a hematoma develops at the venipuncture site, applying warm soaks eases discomfort.

Interfering factors —
• Pretest administration of heparin causes false-positive results.
• Fibrinolytic drugs, such as urokinase and streptokinase, may increase FDP levels.
• Failure to fill the collection tube completely, to mix the sample and anticoagulant adequately, or to send the sample to the laboratory immediately may interfere with the accurate test results.
• Hemolysis caused by excessive agitation of the sample may alter test results.

Fibrinogen, plasma

Fibrinogen (factor I), a plasma protein originating in the liver, isn't normally present in serum; it is converted to insoluble fibrin by thrombin during clotting. Because fibrin is a necessary part of a blood clot, fibrinogen deficiency can produce mild-to-severe bleeding disorders. When fibrinogen levels drop below 100 mg/dl, accurate interpretation of all coagulation tests having a fibrin clot as an end point is difficult.

Fibrinogen levels can be measured using clot-based assays (Clauss) or immunologic, nephelometric, or quantitative methods (measuring the amount of clottable protein). Most laboratories use the Clauss method, in which diluted plasma is clotted with thrombin. The time it takes for a clot to form is recorded and read, according to a standard curve. Some automatic coagulation instruments use a nephelometric technique.

Purpose
To aid the diagnosis of suspected bleeding disorders

Patient preparation
Explain to the patient that this test helps determine if his blood clots normally. Inform him that he needn't restrict food or fluids before the test and that a blood sample is required. Check the patient's history for use of heparin and oral contraceptives. Note such drugs on the laboratory slip.

Procedure
Perform a venipuncture, and collect the sample in a 7-ml *blue-top* tube. If the patient is receiving heparin therapy, notify the laboratory; such therapy requires use of a different reagent. Completely fill the collection tube, invert it gently several times, and send it immediately or place it on ice. To prevent hemolysis, avoid excessive probing during venipuncture and excessive agitation of the sample.

Values
Fibrinogen levels normally range from 195 to 365 mg/dl (1.9 to 3.6 g/L).

Implications of results
Depressed fibrinogen levels may indicate congenital afibrinogenemia; hypofibrinogenemia or dysfibrinogenemia; disseminated intravascular coagulation; fibrinolysis; or severe hepatic disease. Low levels may also follow obstetric complications or trauma. Elevated levels may be observed in inflammatory or malignant disorders or during pregnancy.

Prolonged activated partial thromboplastin time, coagulation time, prothrombin time, or thrombin time also suggests a fibrinogen deficiency.

Post-test care
If a hematoma develops at the venipuncture site, applying warm soaks eases discomfort.

Interfering factors

- Fibrinogen levels may also be elevated during pregnancy (third trimester) and in postoperative patients.
- Hemolysis caused by traumatic venipuncture or excessive agitation of the sample may affect test results.
- Failure to fill the collection tube completely, to mix the sample and anticoagulant adequately, to send the sample to the laboratory promptly, or to place it on ice may interfere with accurate test results.

Flecainide, serum

This quantitative analysis uses either capillary gas chromatography with electron capture detection or liquid chromatography with fluorescent detection to measure serum levels of flecainide acetate. An oral antiarrhythmic drug used for suppression of premature ventricular contractions, flecainide is classified as a class 1C antiarrhythmic, with properties including increased refractory time; slowed atrial, nodal, and ventricular conduction; and prolonged PR interval and QRS complex on electrocardiography (ECG). Measuring serum flecainide concentration detects subtherapeutic, therapeutic, and potentially toxic doses during initial dose titration and ongoing therapy.

Purpose

- To monitor therapeutic levels of flecainide
- To detect flecainide toxicity and monitor its treatment

Patient preparation

Explain to the patient that this test helps determine the safest and most effective dosage of flecainide. Tell him he needn't restrict food or fluids before the test and that the test requires a blood sample. Before sample collection, obtain a complete medication history.

Procedure

Perform a venipuncture, and collect a trough-level or peak-level sample, as ordered, in a *red-, green-,* or *lavender-top* tube, as directed by the testing laboratory. Record the date and time of the last dose of flecainide and the time of sample collection on the laboratory slip. Handle the specimen gently to prevent hemolysis, and send it to the laboratory immediately.

Values

The therapeutic range for serum flecainide is 0.2 to 1.0 µg/ml (0.5 to 2.3 µmol/L), reported as flecainide acetate. The toxic level is over 1.0 µg/ml (2.3 µmol/L).

Implications of results

Trough levels guide adjustment of therapeutic dosage; peak levels detect toxicity and monitor its treatment. Therapeutic effectiveness of flecainide is more likely when serum concentration is within the therapeutic range; if control of arrhythmia isn't achieved by therapeutic dosage, another antiarrhythmic agent should be considered. Serum concentration at the upper end of the therapeutic range is more likely to produce side effects such as cardiac conduction disturbances and reduction of left ventricular function; thus, the lowest effective dose should be prescribed for long-term therapy.

Because serum flecainide levels correlate well with ECG interval prolongation, both baseline and 24-hour continuous ECGs help guide drug therapy.

A patient with a serum flecainide level in the toxic range requires immediate assessment for dangerous ECG interval prolongation and slowed conduction, evaluation of left ventricular function (especially in the presence of congestive heart failure), and neurologic assessment for typical adverse effects such as dizziness, paresthesias, and tremor. Serious toxic effects can be minimized by immediately reducing the dose when concentration reaches the lower limit of the toxic range.

Post-test care

If a hematoma develops at the venipuncture site, applying warm soaks eases discomfort.

Interfering factor

Hemolysis caused by excessive agitation of the sample can interfere with accurate determination of test results.

Fluorescent treponemal antibody test

The fluorescent treponemal antibody absorption (FTA-ABS or FTA) test uses indirect immunofluorescence to detect antibodies to the cause of syphilis — the spirochete *Treponema pallidum* — in serum. In this test, prepared *T. pallidum* is fixed on a slide, and the patient's serum is added, after addition of an absorbed preparation of Reiter treponema. This addition to the test serum prevents interference by antibodies from nonsyphilitic treponemas; Reiter treponema combines with most nonsyphilitic antibodies, making the FTA-ABS test specific for *T. pallidum.*

If syphilitic antibodies are present in the test serum, they will coat the treponemal organisms. The slide is then stained with fluorescein-labeled antiglobulin. This antiglobulin attaches to the coated spirochetes, which fluoresce when viewed under a microscope with ultraviolet light.

Although the FTA-ABS test is generally performed on a serum sample to detect primary or secondary syphilis, it requires a cerebrospinal fluid (CSF) specimen to detect tertiary syphilis. Because antibody levels remain constant for long periods, the FTA-ABS test is not recommended for monitoring response to therapy.

Purpose
- To confirm primary or secondary syphilis
- To verify syphilis as the cause of suspected false-positive results of Venereal Disease Research Laboratory tests

Patient preparation
Explain the purpose of this test. Inform the patient that he needn't restrict food or fluids before the test and that the test requires a blood sample.

Procedure
Perform a venipuncture, and collect the sample in a 7-ml *red-top* tube. Handle the sample gently to prevent hemolysis.

Findings
Normally, reaction to the FTA-ABS test is negative (no fluorescence).

Implications of results
The presence of treponemal antibodies in the serum — a reactive test result — does not indicate the stage or the severity of syphilitic infection. (However, the presence of these antibodies in CSF is strong evidence of tertiary neurosyphilis.) Elevated antibody levels appear in 80% to 90% of patients with primary syphilis and in 100% of patients with secondary syphilis. Higher antibody levels persist for several years, with treatment or without treatment.

The absence of treponemal antibodies — a nonreactive test — doesn't necessarily rule out syphilis. *T. pallidum* causes no detectable immunologic changes in the blood for 14 to 21 days after initial infection. Organisms may be detected earlier by examining suspicious lesions with a dark-field microscope. Low antibody levels or other nonspecific factors produce borderline findings. In such cases, repeated testing and a thorough review of the patient's history may be productive.

False positive results occasionally occur in elderly persons; in patients with systemic lupus erythematosus (SLE), genital herpes, or increased or abnormal globulins; or those who are pregnant. In addition, the FTA-ABS test doesn't always distinguish between *T. pallidum* and certain other treponemas, such as those that cause pinta, yaws, and bejel.

Post-test care
- If a hematoma develops at the venipuncture site, applying warm soaks eases discomfort.
- If the test is reactive, explain the nature of syphilis, and stress the importance of proper treatment and the need to find and treat the patient's sexual contacts. If appropriate, provide additional information about syphilis and how it is spread; emphasize the need for antibiotic therapy. Also, prepare the patient for inquiries from public health authorities.
- If the test is nonreactive or findings are borderline but syphilis has not been ruled out, instruct the patient to return for follow-up testing; explain that inconclusive results don't necessarily indicate absence of the disease.

Interfering factors
- Hemolysis caused by excessive agitation of the sample may alter test results.
- SLE or other immune complex diseases may cause false-positive results.

Folic acid, serum
Pteroylglutamic acid, folacin, serum folate

A quantitative analysis of serum folic acid levels by radioisotopic assay of competitive binding, this test is often performed concomitantly with serum vitamin B_{12} determinations. Like vitamin B_{12}, folic acid is a water-soluble vitamin that influences hematopoiesis, deoxyribonucleic acid synthesis, and overall body growth. The parent compound of folate vitamins, folic acid is biologically inactive and requires enzymatic breakdown in the small intestine for absorption into the bloodstream. Once in the bloodstream, folic acid is rapidly absorbed into the tissues. A normal diet supplies folic acid in liver, kidney, yeast, fruits, leafy vegetables, eggs, and milk. Because the body stores only small amounts of folic acid (mostly in the liver), inadequate dietary intake causes a deficiency, especially during pregnancy, when the metabolic demand for folic acid rises. Because of folic acid's vital role in hematopoiesis, the usual indication for this test is a suspected hematologic abnormality.

Purpose
- To aid diagnosis of megaloblastic and macrolytic anemia
- To detect folate deficiency
- To monitor folate therapy
- To assess folate stores in pregnancy

Patient preparation
Explain to the patient that this test determines the folic acid level in the blood. Instruct him to observe an overnight fast before the test. Tell him the test requires a blood sample. Check the patient's medication history for drugs that may affect test results.

Procedure
Perform a venipuncture, and collect the sample in a 7-ml *red-top* tube. Handle the sample gently to prevent hemolysis and send it to the laboratory immediately.

Values
Normally, serum folic acid values range from 2 to 10 ng/ml (4 to 22 nmol/L).

Implications of results
Low serum levels (less than 2 ng/ml [4 nmol/L]) may indicate hematologic abnormalities, such as anemia (especially megaloblastic anemia), leukopenia, and thrombocytopenia. The Schilling test is often performed to rule out vitamin B_{12} deficiency, which also causes megaloblastic anemia (pernicious anemia). Decreased folic acid levels can also result from hypermetabolic states (such as hyperthyroidism), inadequate dietary intake, chronic alcoholism, small-bowel malabsorption syndrome, or pregnancy.

High serum levels (more than 20 ng/ml) may indicate excessive dietary intake of folic acid or folic acid supplements. Folate levels are high in patients with vitamin B_{12} deficiency, because vitamin B_{12} is necessary for the incorporation of folate into tissue cells. This vitamin is nontoxic in humans, even when taken in large doses.

Post-test care
- If a hematoma develops at the venipuncture site, applying warm soaks eases discomfort.
- The patient may resume his diet.

Interfering factors
- Alcohol and phenytoin interfere with folic acid absorption and lower serum folic acid. Pyrimethamine can induce folate deficiency and low folic acid levels.
- Hemolysis caused by excessive agitation of the sample may alter test results.
- Exposure to light will cause folate to disintegrate.
- Oral contraceptives may decrease folate levels.

Follicle-stimulating hormone (FSH), serum

This test of gonadal function, performed more often on females than on males, measures plasma follicle-stimulating hormone (FSH) levels by radioimmunoassay and is usually vital to infertility studies. However, the test's overall diagnostic significance often depends on the results of related hormone tests (for luteinizing hormone, estrogen, or progesterone, for example). A glycoprotein secreted by the anterior pituitary, FSH stimulates gonadal activity in both sexes. In females, FSH spurs development of primary ovarian follicles into graafian follicles for ovulation. Secretion fluctuates rhythmically during the menstrual cycle, peaking at ovulation. In males, continuous secretion of FSH (and testosterone) stimulates and maintains spermatogenesis. Plasma levels fluctuate widely in females, and to obtain a true baseline level, daily testing may be necessary (for 3 to 5 days), or multiple samples can be drawn on the same day.

Purpose
- To aid diagnosis of infertility and disorders of menstruation, such as amenorrhea
- To aid diagnosis of precocious puberty in girls (before age 9) and in boys (before age 10)
- To aid differential diagnosis of hypogonadism

Patient preparation
Explain to the patient that this test helps determine if her hormonal secretion is normal. Inform her that she needn't fast or limit physical activity before the test and that it requires a blood sample. For 48 hours before the test, withhold medications, such as estrogens or progestogen, that may interfere

with accuracy of results. If these medications must be continued, note this on the laboratory slip.

Make sure the patient is relaxed and recumbent for 30 minutes before the test.

Procedure
Perform a venipuncture, preferably between 6 a.m. and 8 a.m., using a 7-ml *red-top* collection tube, and send the sample to the laboratory immediately. Handle the sample gently to prevent hemolysis.

If the patient is a female, indicate the date of her last menstrual cycle on the laboratory slip. If she is menopausal, note this on the laboratory slip.

Values
Reference values vary greatly, depending on the patient's age and stage of sexual development, and — for a female — the phase of her menstrual cycle. For menstruating females, approximate values are as follows—
Follicular phase: 5 to 20 mIU/ml (U/L)
Midcycle peak: 15 to 30 mIU/ml (U/L)
Luteal phase: 5 to 15 mIU/ml (U/L).

Approximate values for adult males are 5 to 20 mIU/ml (U/L); for menopausal women, 50 to 100 mIU/ml (U/L).

Implications of results
Decreased FSH levels may cause male or female infertility: aspermatogenesis in males and anovulation in females. Low FSH levels may indicate secondary hypogonadotropic states, which can result from anorexia nervosa, panhypopituitarism, or hypothalamic lesions.

High FSH levels in females may indicate ovarian failure associated with Turner's syndrome (primary hypogonadism). Elevated levels may occur in patients with precocious puberty (idiopathic or with central nervous system lesions) and in post-menopausal women. In males, abnormally high FSH levels may indicate destruction of the testes (from mumps orchitis or X-ray exposure), testicular failure, seminoma, or male climacteric. Congenital absence of the gonads and early-stage acromegaly may cause FSH levels to rise in both sexes.

Post-test care
• If a hematoma develops at the venipuncture site, applying warm soaks eases discomfort.
• The patient may resume medications that were discontinued before the test.

Interfering factors

- Failure to observe restriction of medications may hinder accurate determination of test results. Ovarian steroid hormones, such as estrogen or progesterone, and related compounds may, through negative feedback, inhibit secretion of hormones from the pituitary gland and hypothalamus; phenothiazines (such as chlorpromazine) may exert a similar effect.
- Radioactive scan performed within 1 week before the test may affect results.
- Hemolysis caused by excessive agitation of the sample may interfere with accurate determination of test results.

Fragile X syndrome, chromosome and molecular analysis, blood

Fragile X syndrome is an X-linked disorder that affects primarily males and is associated with mental retardation, large ears, loose connective tissue, and large testes. The observation of a fragile site near the end of the long arm of an X chromosome at band Xq27.3 is considered evidence for the syndrome. Because special culture procedures are necessary to show fragile X chromosomes, it is important to inform the cytogenetic laboratory that the patient may have the fragile X syndrome.

A molecular method using a polymerase chain reaction or Southern blot analysis amplification of a $p(CCG)_n$ trinucleotide repeat can detect fragile X syndrome at the untranslated 5' end of the FMR1 gene. Because this method does not rule out chromosome abnormalities, most laboratories now test patients suspected of having fragile X syndrome with both cytogenetic and molecular methods.

Purpose

- To help diagnose fragile X syndrome
- To detect female carriers of the fragile X chromosome
- To identify male and female carriers of FMR1 mutations (with the molecular method)

Patient preparation

Explain the purpose of this test and that the test requires a blood specimen. This test is best performed or interpreted by clinical geneticists or physicians familiar with the fragile X syndrome. Because the interpretation of the results may be difficult, specific counseling of patients and their relatives is appropriate and may be complicated.

Procedure

For cytogenetic studies, draw 7.0 ml of peripheral blood into a 10-ml, *green-top* (heparinized), sterile vacuum blood specimen tube. Invert the tube several times to mix the blood and anticoagulant. Handle the sample gently to prevent hemolysis or clotting. Label the vial carefully and send the specimens immediately at ambient temperature to a cytogenetic laboratory. The laboratory will use special procedures to enhance the expression of fragile X chromosomes. Most laboratories use at least two different fragile X expression systems to improve the sensitivity of the test.

For molecular studies, draw peripheral blood into a 10-ml, *lavender-top* (EDTA), sterile vacuum blood specimen tube. Invert several times to mix the blood.

Values

Fragile X syndrome is inherited; therefore, each cell in patients with this disorder contains a fragile X chromosome. However, the cytogenetic method is not perfect and detects fragile X chromosomes in only some cells. Most laboratories examine 50 to 100 cells from males and 100 to 200 cells from females. The proportion of cells with an apparent fragile X varies among patients, but to confirm diagnosis of fragile X syndrome, most cytogeneticists require 4% or more of the cells to show the fragile X chromosomes (the incidence usually is 20% to 40%). In carrier females, the incidence of fragile X chromosomes is usually much lower and is usually undetectable.

The molecular method can identify premutations not typically associated with mental retardation, or full mutation resulting in the fragile X syndrome. If the $p(CGG)_n$ repeat is less than 45, the result is normal; if 50 to 199, a partial mutation; if greater than 200, a full mutation.

Implications of results

Patients whose tests are positive for fragile X chromosomes in more than 4% of their cells are considered to have fragile X syndrome. In males, the proportion of fragile X positive cells is probably not associated with the severity of disease. Patients whose tests are negative for the fragile X chromosome are unlikely to have fragile X syndrome, but some exceptions are known. The results of molecular testing are more accurate, but false-negative results do occur.

Post-test care   Regardless of the test result, genetic counseling is appropriate to explain the clinical significance of the findings. If the test result is fragile X positive, additional testing of other members of the patient's family may be necessary. If the result is fragile X negative, the patient may not have the fragile X syndrome, or invalidating factors may have interfered with the test. Some patients may have a chromosome abnormality other than fragile X or another genetic disorder.

Interfering factors
- Failure to use the proper anticoagulant or to mix the sample and the anticoagulant adequately may interfere with accurate test results.
- With the cytogenetic method, the proportion of fragile X positive cells is lower in some older patients than it is in younger patients. Thus, the patient's age may affect the study's accuracy.
- With the cytogenetic method, female carriers of fragile X usually do not show fragile X chromosomes. When they do, the proportion of positive cells can be low and difficult to detect.

Free fatty acids
Nonesterified fatty acids

This test measures blood levels of free (nonesterified) fatty acids. Free fatty acids (FFAs), essential components of lipoproteins and triglycerides, account for 2% to 5% of all lipids in the plasma, and are bound to albumin as they travel in the circulation. Formed by synthesis within cells or by the breakdown of lipoproteins and triglycerides, fatty acids are released from adipose tissue when stimulated by hormones, usually during periods of fasting, anxiety, or physical exertion. The most common causes of elevated FFA levels are uncontrolled diabetes, prolonged fasting, or malnutrition. Elevated FFA levels in turn stimulate hormones, including epinephrine, norepinephrine, corticotropin, glucagon, growth hormone, thyroxine, and cortisol. Elevated levels of FFAs, from whatever source, are typically cleared from the blood by the liver and then converted into various lipoproteins, especially very low-density lipoprotein (VLDL). Therefore, disorders marked by excessive fatty acids are usually marked as well by excessive VLDL. The latter, released into the blood, causes secondary hyperlipoproteinemia. Stimuli that raise FFA levels usually also raise serum triglyceride levels and alter lipoprotein levels.

Purpose
• To aid diagnosis of suspected malnutrition
• To aid diagnosis of secondary hyperlipoproteinemia

Patient preparation

Explain the purpose of the test. Instruct the patient to fast after midnight and to abstain from alcohol for 24 hours before this test. Tell him the test requires a blood sample.

Check the patient's recent medication history for use of heparin, aspirin, antilipemics, glucose, hypoglycemic agents, thyroglycemic agents, thyroxine, neomycin, streptozocin, amphetamines, some tranquilizers and antidepressants, catecholamines, reserpine, caffeine, and nicotine, which may interfere with accurate determination of test results.

Procedure

Encourage the patient to relax before the test because the secretion of epinephrine associated with stress elevates FFA levels. Perform a venipuncture, and collect the sample in a 10- to 15-ml *red-top* tube.

Precautions

Send the sample to the laboratory immediately because serum triglycerides break down rapidly and increase FFA levels.

Values

Normally, serum FFA levels range from 8 to 20 mg/dl (80 to 200 mg/L).

Implications of results

Elevated levels of FFAs are associated with diabetes, acute fasting or starvation, or pheochromocytoma. Increased levels are also associated with hyperthyroidism, acute alcohol intoxication, chronic hepatitis, and acute renal failure. Elevated levels associated with elevated VLDL may indicate secondary hyperlipoproteinemia.

Post-test care

Patient may resume diet and activity restricted before the test.

Interfering factors

• Ingestion of alcohol within 24 hours of the test may falsely elevate FFA values.

- Failure to follow diet restrictions may alter test results.
- Recent use of amphetamines, corticotropin, cortisone, epinephrine, norepinephrine, growth hormone, growth hormone, thyroid stimulating hormone, thyroxine, chlorpromazine, isoproterenol, reserpine, tolbutamide, or caffeine may cause elevated FFA levels.
- Use of aspirin, clofibrate, glucose, insulin, neomycin, or streptozocin may cause decreased FFA levels.

Fungal serology

To detect fungal infection, these tests, which use complement fixatives, immunodiffusion, and agglutination methods, identify antibodies to blastomycosis, coccidioidomycosis, histoplasmosis, aspergillosis, and sporotrichosis cryptococcosis antigen. Although cultures are usually performed to diagnose mycoses by identifying the causative organism, occasionally serologic tests provide the sole evidence for mycosis.

Purpose
- To rapidly detect the presence of antifungal antibodies, aiding the diagnosis of mycoses
- To monitor effectiveness of therapy for mycoses

Patient preparation
Explain to the patient that this test aids diagnosis of certain fungal infections. If appropriate, explain that this test monitors response to therapy and that it may be necessary to repeat the test during his illness. Instruct him to restrict food and fluids for 12 to 24 hours before the test and tell him the test requires a blood sample.

Procedure
Perform a venipuncture, and collect the sample in a 10-ml sterile *red-top* tube. Send the sample to the laboratory immediately. If transport to the laboratory is delayed, store the sample at 39.2° F (4° C).

Findings
Depending on the test method, a negative finding, or normal titer, usually indicates the absence of mycosis.

Implications of results
Serum test methods for fungal infections, pages 282 and 283, summarizes the clinical significance of abnormal serologic test values for specific organisms.

Serum test methods for fungal infections

Disease and normal values	Clinical significance of abnormal results
Blastomycosis	
Complement fixation: titers < 1:8	Titers ranging from 1:8 to 1:16 suggest infection; titers > 1:32 denote active disease. A rising titer in serial samples taken every 3 to 4 weeks indicates disease progression; a falling titer indicates regression. This test has limited diagnostic value because of the high percentage of false-negative results.
Immunodiffusion: negative	A more sensitive test for blastomycosis; detects 80% of infected persons.
Coccidioidomycosis	
Complement fixation: titers < 1:2	Most sensitive test for this fungus. Titers ranging from 1:2 to 1:4 suggest active infection; titers > 1:16 usually denote active disease. Test may remain negative in mild infections.
Immunodiffusion: negative	Most useful for screening, followed by complement fixation test for confirmation.
Precipitin: titers < 1:16	Good screening test; titers > 1:16 usually indicate infection; 80% of infected persons show positive titers by 2 weeks; most revert to negative by 6 months. Early primary disease is shown by positive precipitin and negative complement fixation test. A positive complement fixation and negative precipitin test indicate chronic disease.
Histoplasmosis	
Complement fixation: (histoplasmin): titers < 1:8	Titers ranging from 1:8 to 1:16 suggest infection; titers > 1:32 indicate active disease. Antibodies generally appear 10 to 21 days after initial infection. Test is positive in 10% to 15% of cases.
Complement fixation (yeast): titers < 1:18	More sensitive than histoplasmin complement fixation test; gives positive results in 75% to 80% of cases. (Both histoplasmin and yeast antigens are positive in 10% of cases.) A rising titer in serial samples taken every 2 to 3 weeks indicates progressive infection; a decreasing titer indicates regression. Titers ranging from 1:8 to 1:16 suggest infection; titers > 1:32 indicate active disease.
Immunodiffusion (histoplasmin): negative	Appearance of both H and M bands indicates active infection. If the M band appears first and lasts longer than the H band, the infection may be regressing. The M band alone may indicate early infection, chronic disease, or a recent skin test.
Aspergillosis	
Complement fixation: titer < 1:8	Titers > 1:8 suggest infection; 70% to 90% of patients with known pulmonary aspergillosis or aspergillus allergy present antibodies, and so do about 5% of the general population. This test is ambiguous in detecting invasive aspergillosis because patients with this disease may or may not have antibodies; biopsy is required.

(continued)

Serum test methods for fungal infections *(continued)*	
Disease and normal values	**Clinical significance of abnormal results**
Aspergillosis *(continued)* Immunodiffusion: negative	One or more precipitin bands suggest infection; precipitins appear in 95% of patients with pulmonary fungus balls and in 50% of those with allergic bronchopulmonary disorders. The number of bands is related to complement fixation titers; the more precipitin bands, the higher the titer.
Sporotrichosis Agglutination: titers < 1:40	Titers > 1:80 usually indicate active disease. The test usually is negative in cutaneous infections, positive in extracutaneous infections.
Cryptococcosis Latex agglutination for crytococcal antigen: negative	About 90% of patients with cryptococcal meningoencephalitis present capsular antigen in cerebrospinal fluid (CSF). (Serum is less frequently positive than is CSF.) A culture is definitive because false-positive results do occur. (Presence of rheumatoid factor may cause a positive reaction.) Serum antigen tests are positive in 33% of patients with pulmonary cryptococcosis; biopsy is usually required.

Post-test care
- If a hematoma develops at the venipuncture site, applying warm soaks eases discomfort.
- Patient may resume normal diet.

Interfering factors
- Some antigens, such as the blastomycosis and histoplasmosis antigens, may cross-react to produce false-positive results or high titers.
- Recent skin testing with fungal antigens may elevate titers.
- Many patients with mycoses are immunosuppressed because of a primary disease, such as human immunodeficiency virus, or because of therapeutically induced immunosuppression, further depressing the immune system and causing low titers or false-negative test results.
- Failure to send a sterile sample to the laboratory immediately or to store the sample properly if transport is delayed may interfere with accurate determination of test results.
- A nonfasting specimen may alter test results.

G

Galactose-1-phosphate uridyl transferase, red blood cells

Galactosemia, a disorder reflecting an inborn error of metabolism, results from the congenital inability to metabolize galactose to glucose at the diphosphonucleotide level. The reaction product, uridine diphosphate galactose (UDP-galactose), is used for synthesis of glycolipids, glycoproteins, and other galactose-containing complex polysaccharides. The enzyme galactose-1-phosphate uridyltransferase (GALT) is encoded on chromosome 9, and galactosemia is transmitted by autosomal recessive inheritance. Galactosemia is associated with cataracts, hepatic and renal disease, and other widespread tissue damage; it usually occurs in infants and children. Heterozygous carriers of galactosemia commonly show transferase activities intermediate between that of normal persons and of those with galactosemia. Because galactosemia may also result from deficiency of other enzymes, measurement of GALT will not identify all cases of galactosemia.

Purpose
To aid diagnosis of genetic galactosemia resulting from deficiency of galactose-1-phosphate uridyltransferase

Patient preparation
Explain the purpose of this test and inform the patient that the test will require a blood sample.

Procedure
Collect a blood sample in a *green-top* tube or a *blue-* or *yellow-top* tube. For microcollection, blood is collected in heparinized 0.5-ml microcentrifuge tubes.

GALT is stable in heparin at 39.2° F (4° C) for up to 4 weeks. Reportedly, GALT remains unchanged when stored in sterile heparinized containers at room temperature for as long as 14 days.

The test requires a minimum of 0.5 ml of heparinized blood, but 1 to 2 ml of blood is preferred. Samples should be sent to the laboratory in such a way as to preserve red cells in their native state. Frozen samples cannot be analyzed readily.

Precautions   Because this test is most often performed on neonates, a minimal amount of blood should be drawn.

Values   Red blood cell levels in normal individuals range
from 18.5 to 28.5 U/g hemoglobin.

Implications of   GALT deficiency requires immediate restriction of
results   the patient's intake of galactose. Low levels of
GALT activity do not always indicate galactosemia.
Residual activity in some variants apparently is sufficient to metabolize the usual intake level of galactose. These variants can be further identified by
special electrophoresis and perhaps soon by deoxyribonucleic acid analysis.

Post-test care   • Immediately after venipuncture, apply pressure
to the site, and wrap the arm with a bandage.
• If a hematoma develops at the venipuncture site,
applying warm soaks eases discomfort.

Interfering   Because this assay is performed on red cell lysates,
factor   any condition that can damage the whole red cells
before isolation and washing will make this analysis
difficult or impossible.

Gamma-glutamyl transpeptidase (GGT), serum

Gamma-glutamyl transpeptidase (GGT) is most
commonly elevated in hepatobiliary disease. This
enzyme is extremely sensitive to drug induction
and thus is often used to detect recent alcohol ingestion, which is important in determining compliance with treatment of alcoholism. GGT is more
sensitive than alkaline phosphatase in predicting
cholestatic processes and neoplastic liver disease.
However, GGT's sensitivity to induction by drugs is
problematic in regard to specificity.

Purpose   • To aid diagnosis of obstructive jaundice in neoplastic liver disease and detection of recent alcohol consumption
• When used with alkaline phosphatase, to suggest
the source of elevated serum alkaline phosphatase levels

Patient   Explain the purpose of this test. Inform the patient
preparation   that the test requires the collection of a blood sam-

ple and fasting before collection of the sample. Ask the patient about the intake of medications or alcohol, which can cause GGT elevation. Note the prior use of drugs or alcohol on the laboratory slip.

Procedure
Perform a venipuncture and collect a 0.5-ml sample of blood into a container without anticoagulant and send to the laboratory promptly. There, after centrifuging of the clotted blood for 10 minutes at 2,000 rpms, the serum is separated. If transport must be delayed, the sample may be refrigerated for up to 4 days or kept frozen at $-40°$ F $(-40°$ C) for up to 1 month and still maintain the original activity.

Precautions
Because GGT is used to monitor liver disease, the possibility of a transmissible agent should be carefully considered and requires the usual safety precautions, including gloves.

Values
The normal range for GGT varies considerably with age in males but is not affected in females. The normal range in males between ages 18 and 50 is 10 to 39 U/L. In older males, it ranges from 10 to 48 U/L. The normal range in females is 6 to 29 U/L.

Implications of results
Usually, elevated GGT levels signal a cholestatic liver process. Alternatively, elevated GGT levels occur within 24 hours of significant alcohol ingestion. When both alkaline phosphatase and GGT levels are elevated, the source of the alkaline phosphatase is most likely the liver.

Post-test care
If a hematoma develops at the venipuncture site, applying warm soaks eases discomfort.

Interfering factor
Because the normal biological response to numerous drugs is an elevation of GGT via induction of microsomal enzymes, this should be considered whenever an elevation of this enzyme occurs in patients receiving therapeutic drugs.

Gastric culture

This test requires aspiration of gastric contents and cultivation to identify mycobacterial infection. It's performed in conjunction with a chest X-ray and a purified protein derivative (PPD) skin test, and is especially useful when a sputum specimen can't be obtained by expectoration or nebulization.

Purpose

To aid diagnosis of mycobacterial infections

Patient preparation

Explain that gastric culture helps diagnose tuberculosis. If appropriate, instruct the patient to fast for 8 hours before the test. Tell the patient that the same procedure may be performed on three consecutive mornings. Instruct the ambulatory patient to remain in bed each morning until specimen collection has been completed, to prevent premature emptying of stomach contents.

Describe the procedure. Tell the patient that the nasogastric (NG) tube may cause gagging but passes more easily if he relaxes and follows instructions about breathing and swallowing. Just before the procedure, obtain baseline heart rate and rhythm, and place the patient in high Fowler's position.

Inform the patient that test results may take several weeks because acid-fast bacteria generally grow slowly. Check the history for recent antibiotic therapy.

Equipment

Water-soluble lubricant, sterile water, size 16 or 18 French disposable plastic NG tube, 50-ml sterile syringe, sterile specimen container, sterile gloves, emesis basin, stethoscope, clamp (if necessary)

Procedure

Perform NG intubation when the patient awakens and obtain gastric washings. Clamp the tube before removing quickly. Note recent antibiotic therapy on the laboratory slip, along with the site and time of collection, the patient's name, and other identifying information.

If possible, obtain the specimens before the start of antibiotic therapy.

Handle the NG tube with gloved hands, and dispose of all equipment carefully to prevent staff contamination.

Send the specimens to the laboratory immediately. Be sure the specimen container is tightly capped. Wipe the outside of the container with disinfectant, and send it to the laboratory upright in a plastic bag.

Precautions

• Gastric intubation is contraindicated in conditions such as esophageal disorders (varices, stenosis, diverticula), malignant neoplasms, recent severe gastric hemorrhage, aortic aneurysm, congestive heart failure, and myocardial infarction.

- Watch for signs that the tube has entered the trachea — coughing, cyanosis, or gasping.
- *Never* inject water into an NG tube unless you're sure the tube is correctly placed in the patient's stomach. During lavage, use sterile, distilled water to decrease risk of contamination with saprophytic mycobacteria.
- Because some patients develop arrhythmias during this procedure, monitor the pulse rate for irregularities.

Findings Normally, the culture specimen is negative for pathogenic mycobacteria.

Implications of results Isolation and identification of the organism *Mycobacterium tuberculosis* indicates the presence of active tuberculosis; other species of *Mycobacterium,* such as *M. bovis, M. kansasii,* and *M. avium-intracellulare* complex, may cause pulmonary disease that is clinically indistinguishable from tuberculosis. Treatment of these mycobacterial diseases may be difficult and commonly requires sensitivity studies to determine effective antibiotic therapy.

Post-test care
- The patient may resume normal diet and medications discontinued before the test.
- Instruct the patient to prevent bleeding by not blowing the nose for at least 4 to 6 hours.

Interfering factors
- Failure to observe an 8-hour fast before the test may decrease the amount of bacteria by diluting stomach contents or removing contents through digestion.
- Therapy with antibiotics such as tetracycline and aminoglycosides can weaken bacilli, causing false-negative culture results.
- The presence of saprophytic mycobacteria in gastric contents may cause false-positive acid-fast smears because these bacteria can't be microscopically distinguished from pathogenic mycobacteria.

Gastrin, serum

Gastrin is a polypeptide hormone produced and stored primarily by specialized G cells in the antrum of the stomach and, to a lesser degree, by the islets of Langerhans, in the pancreas. The main function of gastrin is to facilitate digestion of food by triggering gastric acid secretion in the parietal area of the stomach in response to food (especially proteins), vagal stimulation, or decreased stomach acidity. Secondarily, gastrin stimulates the release of pancreatic enzymes and the gastric enzyme pepsin, increases gastric and intestinal motility, and stimulates bile flow from the liver. Through a strong negative feedback control mechanism, acid in the gastric antrum inhibits gastrin release in response to all stimuli. However, abnormal secretion of gastrin can result from tumors (gastrinomas) and from pathologic disorders, especially achlorydria (absence of gastric acid) affecting the stomach, pancreas, and less commonly, the esophagus and the small bowel.

This radioimmunoassay, a quantitative analysis of gastrin levels, has significant diagnostic usefulness in patients suspected of having gastrinomas (Zollinger-Ellison syndrome). In doubtful situations, provocative testing may be necessary (see *Gastrin-stimulation tests,* page 290). However, gastrin estimation has limited value in persons with duodenal ulcer because the role of gastrin in peptic ulcers is unclear.

Purpose
- To confirm diagnosis of gastrinoma, the gastrin-secreting tumor in Zollinger-Ellison syndrome
- To aid differential diagnosis of gastric and duodenal ulcers and pernicious anemia

Patient preparation
Explain that this test helps determine the cause of GI symptoms. Instruct the patient to abstain from alcohol for at least 24 hours before the test and to fast for 12 hours before the test (water is permitted). Tell the patient that the test requires a blood sample.

Withhold all medications that may interfere with test results, especially anticholinergics, such as atropine and belladonna, or insulin. If these medications must be continued, note this on the laboratory slip.

Because stress can increase gastrin levels, the patient should be relaxed and recumbent for at least 30 minutes before the test.

Gastrin-stimulation tests

Because some patients with duodenal or gastric ulcers have normal fasting levels of gastrin, provocative testing is necessary to identify them: A protein-rich test meal serves this purpose. In a patient with duodenal or gastric ulcers, gastrin levels increase markedly after such a meal, whereas these levels rise only moderately in a healthy person.

Provocative testing is also necessary to distinguish a patient with duodenal or gastric ulcers from one suspected of having Zollinger-Ellison syndrome because both may show similar baseline gastrin levels. The most commonly used and effective provocative test is the secretion test, which requires an I.V. bolus infusion of 2 clinical units/kg of secretion. In patients with gastrinoma, gastrin levels rise, usually by more than 200 pg/ml within 10 minutes of infusion. In healthy patients, gastrin secretion levels do not change.

Another effective test involves I.V. infusion of calcium gluconate in a dosage of 5 mg/kg body weight over 3 hours. After the infusion, 10 ml of venous blood is drawn and sent to the laboratory. Gastrin levels double, rising to about 500 pg/ml, in a patient with Zollinger-Ellison syndrome; a patient with duodenal or gastric ulcers shows only a moderate rise or no change at all.

A third indication for provocative testing is an abnormally, but not strikingly, high fasting serum gastrin level. This is possible in both Zollinger-Ellison syndrome and in patients with pernicious anemia. To distinguish between the two, hydrochloric acid may be infused into the stomach through a nasogastric tube. Such infusion causes a sharp drop in gastrin levels in patients with pernicious anemia, but not in patients with Zollinger-Ellison syndrome.

Procedure Perform a venipuncture, and collect the sample in a 10- to 15-ml *red-top* tube.

Handle the sample gently to avoid hemolysis. To prevent destruction of serum gastrin by proteolytic enzymes, immediately send the sample to the laboratory to have the serum separated and frozen.

Values Serum gastrin levels are less than 200 pg/ml (ng/L).

Implications of results Strikingly high serum gastrin levels (over 1,000 pg/ml [ng/L]) confirm Zollinger-Ellison syndrome. (Levels as high as 450,000 pg/ml [ng/L] have been reported.)

Gastrin levels may be high in various conditions, but the concomitant findings of extremely low gastric juice pH and extremely high serum gastrin level indicate autonomous hormone secretion not governed by a negative feedback mechanism. Increased serum levels of gastrin may occur in a few patients with duodenal ulceration (less than 1%) and in patients with achlorhydria (with or without pernicious anemia) or with extensive stomach cancer (because of hyposecretion of gastric juices and hydrochloric acid).

Post-test care
- If a hematoma develops at the venipuncture site, applying warm soaks eases discomfort.
- The patient can resume a normal diet and discontinued medications.

Interfering factors
- Failure to observe restrictions of diet, medications, or physical activity may interfere with accurate determination of test results.
- Gastrin secretion is increased by amino acids (especially glycine), calcium carbonate, acetylcholine, calcium chloride, and ethanol; gastrin secretion is decreased by anticholinergics (atropine) or secretin (a strongly basic polypeptide).
- Insulin-induced hypoglycemia increases gastrin secretion.
- Hemolysis caused by excessive agitation of the sample may interfere with accurate determination of test results.

GI tract biopsy

Endoscopy allows direct visualization of the GI tract and any site that requires biopsy of tissue samples for histologic analysis. This relatively painless procedure helps detect, support diagnosis of, or monitor GI tract disorders. Its complications, notably hemorrhage, perforation, and aspiration, are rare.

Purpose
To detect, diagnose, and monitor GI tract disorders

Patient preparation
Careful patient preparation is vital. Describe the procedure and reassure the patient that he will be able to breathe with the endoscope in place. Tell him to fast for at least 8 hours before the procedure. (For lower GI biopsy, clean the bowel, as ordered.) Make sure the patient or a responsible family member has signed a consent form.

Just before the procedure, the patient should receive a sedative, as appropriate. The patient should be relaxed but not asleep because his cooperation promotes smooth passage of the endoscope. Spray the back of the patient's throat with a local anesthetic to suppress the gag reflex. To prevent aspiration and excessive bleeding, have suction equipment and bipolar cauterizing electrodes available.

Procedure
After the examiner passes the endoscope into the upper or lower GI tract and visualizes a lesion, node, or other abnormal area, he advances biopsy forceps through a channel in the endoscope until the forceps can be seen. Then he opens the forceps, positions them at the biopsy site, and closes them on the tissue. The closed forceps and tissue sample are removed from the endoscope, and the tissue is taken from the forceps. The specimen is placed in fixative. After the sample collection, the endoscope is removed. The tissue samples are sent to the laboratory immediately.

Findings
Normal GI tract tissue will contain single-layer columular epithelial cells.

Implications of results
Endoscopic biopsy of the GI tract can diagnose cancer, lymphoma, amyloidosis, candidiasis, and gastric ulcers; support diagnosis of Crohn's disease, chronic ulcerative colitis, gastritis, esophagitis, and melanosis coli in laxative abuse; and monitor progression of Barrett's esophagus, multiple gastric polyps, colon cancer and polyps, and chronic ulcerative colitis.

Post-test care
• The patient should be assisted into a comfortable position and allowed to rest before being moved to an appropriate recovery area for additional monitoring.
• Monitor vital signs and check for recovery from premedication.
• Monitor for and tell the patient to report immediately chest or abdominal pain, expectoration of blood, difficulty in breathing, or pain on swallowing.
• The patient should not be allowed to eat or drink until recovery from local anesthetic allows normal swallowing.

Interfering factor
Barium swallow within the preceding 48 hours may interfere with accurate test results.

Glomerular basement membrane antibody, serum

Antibodies specific for the glomerular basement membrane (GBM) and other renal components can bind to their specific antigens, causing an immune response that leads to various anti-GBM diseases, including glomerular nephritis and Goodpasture's syndrome (which may result in renal failure and death).

This renal immunofluorescence test reveals a linear deposition of immunoglobulin G along the basement membrane in Goodpasture's syndrome; in idiopathic membranes, GBM causes a granular pattern.

Purpose
To aid diagnosis of anti-GBM induced glomerular nephritis

Patient preparation
Explain the purpose of this test, and inform the patient that the test requires a blood sample.

Procedure
Perform a venipuncture and collect a blood sample. The test requires 4.0 ml of serum.

Findings
Normal test result is negative for anti-GBM antibodies.

Implications of results
The indirect immunofluorescence test detects anti-GBM antibodies in 87% of patients with anti-GBM–associated Goodpasture's syndrome, and in about 60% of patients with anti-GBM–associated glomerular nephritis.

Post-test care
If a hematoma develops at the venipuncture site, applying warm soaks eases discomfort.

Interfering factors
None

Glucagon, serum

Glucagon, a polypeptide hormone secreted by the alpha cells of the islets of Langerhans in the pancreas, acts primarily on the liver to promote glucose production and control glucose storage. Glucagon is secreted in response to hypoglycemia; secretion is inhibited by the other pancreatic hormones, insulin and somatostatin. Normally, the coordinated release of glucagon, insulin, and somatostatin ensures an adequate and constant fuel supply while maintaining blood glucose levels within relatively stable limits.

This test, a quantitative analysis of serum glucagon by radioimmunoassay, evaluates patients suspected of having glucagonoma (alpha-cell tumor) or hypoglycemia caused by idiopathic glucagon deficiency or pancreatic dysfunction. Glucagon is usually measured concomitantly with serum glucose and insulin, which influence glucagon secretion.

Purpose
To aid diagnosis of glucagonoma and hypoglycemia caused by chronic pancreatitis or idiopathic glucagon deficiency

Patient preparation
Explain that this test, which requires a blood sample, helps evaluate pancreatic function. Instruct the patient to fast for 10 to 12 hours before the test.

Withhold insulin, catecholamines, and other medications that could influence test results. If these drugs must be continued, note this on the laboratory slip. Because exercise and stress elevate serum glucagon levels, the patient should be relaxed and recumbent for 30 minutes before the test.

Procedure
Perform a venipuncture, and collect a blood sample in a chilled 10-ml *lavender-top* tube. Place the sample on ice and send it to the laboratory immediately. Handle the sample gently to prevent hemolysis.

Values
Fasting glucagon levels are normally 75 to 150 pg/ml (ng/L).

Implications of results
Markedly elevated fasting glucagon levels occur in glucagonoma; values may range from 900 to 7,800 pg/ml (ng/L). Elevated levels also occur in diabetes mellitus, acute pancreatitis, and pheochromocytoma.

Abnormally low glucagon levels are associated with idiopathic glucagon deficiency and hypoglycemia caused by chronic pancreatitis. Stimulation or suppression tests may be necessary to confirm diagnosis.

Post-test care
• If a hematoma develops at the venipuncture site, applying warm soaks eases discomfort.

- The patient can resume pretest diet and medications.

Interfering factors
- Prolonged fasting, undue stress, or use of catecholamines or insulin before the collection of blood samples may elevate glucagon levels.
- Failure to pack the sample in ice and send it to the laboratory immediately may affect test results.
- Hemolysis caused by excessive agitation of the sample may interfere with accurate determination of test results.

Glucose, fasting
Fasting blood sugar (FBS)

Commonly used to screen for disorders of glucose metabolism, primarily diabetes mellitus, the fasting plasma glucose test measures plasma glucose levels following an overnight fast.

In the fasting state, blood glucose levels drop, thereby stimulating release of the hormone glucagon. Glucagon then acts to raise plasma glucose by accelerating glycogenolysis, stimulating glyconeogenesis, and inhibiting glycogen synthesis. Normally, secretion of insulin checks this rise in glucose levels. In diabetes, however, absence or deficiency of insulin allows persistently high glucose levels.

Purpose
- To screen for diabetes mellitus and hypoglycemia
- To monitor drug or dietary therapy in patients with diabetes mellitus
- To aid determination of insulin requirements in patients with diabetes mellitus and in those who require parenteral or enteral nutritional support

Patient preparation
Explain that this test detects disorders of glucose metabolism and aids diagnosis of diabetes. Advise the patient to fast — taking only water — for 8 to 12 hours before the test. Tell him this test requires a blood sample.

Withhold drugs that affect test results. If the patient is known to have diabetes, blood should be drawn before administration of insulin or oral antidiabetic drugs.

➤ *Clinical alert:* Alert the patient to the symptoms of hypoglycemia — weakness, restlessness, nervousness, hunger, and sweating — and tell him to report such symptoms immediately.

Self-monitoring of blood glucose requires one large drop of blood from a fingertip and can be performed with a glucometer. For self-testing, teach the correct use of testing equipment and the method to obtain the blood sample.

Procedure

Perform a venipuncture, and collect the sample in a 5-ml *gray-top* tube.

Send the sample to the laboratory immediately because blood glucose levels decrease when the sample is left at room temperature. If transport is delayed, refrigerate the sample.

Specify on the laboratory slip the time of the patient's last pretest meal, the sample collection time, and the time the last pretest insulin or oral hypoglycemic dose (if applicable) was given.

Values

Normal range for fasting blood glucose varies according to the laboratory procedure. Generally, normal values after an 8- to 12-hour fast are as follows: fasting serum, 70 to 100 mg/dl (3.9 to 5.6 mmol/L); fasting whole blood, 60 to 100 mg/dl (3.3 to 5.6 mmol/L).

Implications of results

Fasting blood glucose levels of 140 mg/dl (7.8 mmol/L) or higher, obtained on two or more occasions, may be considered diagnostic of diabetes mellitus if other possible causes of hyperglycemia have been ruled out. Although increased fasting blood glucose levels most commonly indicate diabetes, such levels can also result from pancreatitis, recent acute illness (such as myocardial infarction), Cushing's syndrome, pituitary adenoma, pancreatitis, hyperthyroidism, and pheochromocytoma. Hyperglycemia may also stem from chronic hepatic disease, brain trauma, chronic illness, or chronic malnutrition, and is typical in eclampsia, anoxia, and seizure disorders.

Depressed glucose levels can result from hyperinsulinism (overdose of insulin is the most common cause), insulinoma, von Gierke's disease, functional or reactive hypoglycemia, hypothyroidism, adrenal insufficiency, congenital adrenal hyperplasia, hypopituitarism, islet cell carcinoma of the pancreas, hepatic necrosis, and glycogen storage disease.

Post-test care

- If a hematoma develops at the venipuncture site, applying warm soaks eases discomfort.
- Provide a balanced meal or a snack, especially if the patient is about to engage in a physical activity, such as driving a car.
- The patient may resume pretest diet and medications.

Interfering factors

- Drugs known to elevate plasma glucose levels are chlorthalidone, thiazide diuretics, furosemide, triamterene, oral contraceptives (estrogen-progestogen combination), benzodiazepines, phenytoin, phenothiazines, lithium, epinephrine, arginine, phenolphthalein, dextrothyroxine, diazoxide, large doses of nicotinic acid, corticosteroids, and recent I.V. glucose infusions. Ethacrynic acid may also cause hyperglycemia, but large doses can produce hypoglycemia in patients with uremia.
- Salicylates, antitubercular agents, sulfonylureas, sulfonamides, ethanol, clofibrate, and monoamine oxidase inhibitors can cause decreased blood glucose levels.
- Failure to observe dietary restrictions may elevate plasma glucose levels.
- Recent illness, infection, or pregnancy can elevate plasma glucose levels; strenuous exercise can depress them.
- Glycolysis resulting from failure to refrigerate the sample or to send it to the laboratory immediately can result in false-negative results, particularly in a patient with a disease that has an elevated white blood cell count, such as chronic leukemia.
- Administration of insulin or an oral antidiabetic drug within 8 hours of the sample collection may cause false-low values.

Glucose oxidase test

The glucose oxidase test — which involves the use of plastic-coated reagent strips (Chemstrip UG, Clinistix, Diastix, Kyotest UG) or Tes-Tape — is a specific, qualitative test for glycosuria. Although indicated in routine urinalysis, this test is now used less frequently to monitor urine glucose in patients with diabetes because of the availability of more precise techniques for blood glucose self-monitoring.

Purpose
- To detect glycosuria
- To monitor control of diabetes mellitus

Patient preparation
Explain to the patient that this test determines urine glucose concentration. Teach the newly diagnosed patient with diabetes how to perform a reagent strip test. Have the patient void; after 30 to 45 minutes, collect a second-voided specimen.

Instruct the patient not to drink water between voidings (the diluted urine will decrease the glucose concentration) or to contaminate the urine specimen with toilet tissue or stool.

If the patient is receiving levodopa, ascorbic acid, phenazopyridine, salicylates, peroxides, or hypochlorites, use Clinitest tablets instead.

Equipment
Specimen container, glucose test strips, reference color blocks
Note: Keep the test strip container tightly closed to prevent deterioration of strips by exposure to light or moisture. Store it in a cool place (under 86° F [30° C]) to avoid heat degradation. Don't use discolored or darkened Clinistix or Diastix or dark yellow or yellow-brown Tes-Tape.

Procedure
Collect a second-voided specimen.
Clinistix test: Dip the test area of the reagent strip into the specimen for 2 seconds. Remove excessive urine by tapping the strip against a clean surface or the side of the container, and begin timing. Hold the strip in the air, and "read" the color *exactly 10 seconds* after taking the strip out of the urine by comparing it with the reference color blocks on the label of the container. Record the results. Ignore color changes that develop after 10 seconds.
Diastix test: Dip the reagent strip into the specimen for 2 seconds. Remove excessive urine by tapping the strip against the container, and begin timing. Hold the strip in the air, and compare the color with the color chart *exactly 30 seconds* after taking the strip out of the urine. Record the results. Ignore color changes that develop after 30 seconds.
Tes-Tape: Withdraw about 1½" (3.8 cm) of the reagent tape from the dispenser; dip ¼" (0.6 cm) into the specimen for 2 seconds. Remove excessive urine by tapping the strip against the side of the container, and begin timing. Hold the tape in the air, and compare the color of the darkest part of the tape with the color chart *exactly 60 seconds* after taking

the strip out of the urine. If the tape indicates 0.5% or higher, wait an additional 60 seconds to make the final color comparison. Record the results.

Findings

Normally, glucose is not present in urine.

Implications of results

A positive test for glycosuria may occur in persons with normal blood glucose levels (for example, after a heavy meal or in persons with a low tubular reabsorption rate). However, glucosuria is usually abnormal and usually results from uncontrolled diabetes. The greater the concentration of glucose in the urine, the less controlled the diabetes. Glycosuria occurs in diabetes mellitus; adrenal and thyroid disorders; hepatic and central nervous system diseases; Fanconi's syndrome; other conditions involving low renal threshold, toxic renal tubular disease, heavy metal poisoning, glomerulonephritis, nephrosis, and pregnancy; with administration of large amounts of glucose, total parenteral nutrition, and such drugs as asparaginase, corticosteroids, carbamazepine, ammonium chloride, thiazide diuretics, dextrothyroxine, large doses of nicotinic acid, lithium carbonate; and with prolonged use of phenothiazines.

Post-test care

Provide written guidelines and a flow sheet so the patient can record the test results for home monitoring.

Interfering factors

• Dilute, stale urine or bacterial contamination of the specimen may interfere with the determination of test results.

• Reducing substances, such as levodopa, ascorbic acid, phenazopyridine, methyldopa, or salicylates, may cause false-negative results.

• Tetracyclines also produce false-negative test results.

• Using reagent strips after the expiration date or failure to keep the reagent strip container tightly closed or to record the reagent strip method used interferes with accurate determination of test results.

Glucose-6-phosphate dehydrogenase (G6PD)

Glucose-6-phosphate dehydrogenase (G6PD), an enzyme found in most body cells, is part of the pentose phosphate pathway (hexose monophosphate shunt) that metabolizes glucose. This test, which measures G6PD levels in red blood cells (RBCs), detects deficiency of this enzyme. Such deficiency is a hereditary, sex-linked condition carried on the female X chromosome (with clinical disease found mostly in males) that impairs the stability of the RBC membrane and makes RBCs susceptible to destruction by strong oxidizing agents. RBC enzyme levels normally decrease as the cells age, but G6PD deficiency accelerates this process, making older RBCs more prone to destruction than younger ones. In mild deficiency, young RBCs retain enough G6PD to ward off destruction; in severe deficiency, all RBCs fail to survive.

About 10% of all black males in the United States inherit mild G6PD deficiencies; certain peoples of Mediterranean origin inherit severe deficiencies. In some whites, consumption of fava beans may produce hemolytic episodes. Although deficiency of G6PD provides partial immunity to falciparum malaria, it precipitates an adverse reaction to antimalarials.

Purpose
- To detect hemolytic anemia caused by G6PD deficiency
- To aid differential diagnosis of hemolytic anemia

Patient preparation

Explain that this test, which requires a blood sample, detects inherited enzyme deficiency that may affect the life span of RBCs.

Check the patient's history, and report recent blood transfusion, or recent ingestion of aspirin, sulfonamides, phenacetin, nitrofurantoin, vitamin K derivatives, antimalarials (such as primaquine), or fava beans because these substances can provoke hemolysis in G6PD-deficient persons.

Procedure

Perform a venipuncture, and collect the sample in a 7-ml *lavender-top* tube.

Completely fill the collection tube, and invert it gently several times to adequately mix the sample and the anticoagulant. Handle the sample gently to prevent hemolysis.

Values
: RBC values of G6PD vary according to the method used. For example, with the fluorescent spot-screening method, values are simply reported as normal or abnormal; with the spectrophotometric kinetic method, test values are reported as units/gram (8.6 to 18.6 U/g in adults) of hemoglobin.

Implications of results
: The following screening tests can detect but not confirm G6PD deficiency: the incubated Heinz body test, dye reduction test of Motulsky, methemoglobin reduction (Brewer's) test, fluorescence of NADPH test, ascorbate cyanide test, or glutathione stability test.

Post-test care
: If a hematoma develops at the venipuncture site, applying warm soaks eases discomfort.

Interfering factors
: • Performing the test after a hemolytic episode or a blood transfusion can cause false-negative results.
: • Failure to use a collection tube containing the proper anticoagulant or to adequately mix the sample and anticoagulant may hinder accurate determination of test results.
: • Hemolysis caused by excessive agitation of the sample may affect the accuracy of test results.
: • The following substances decrease G6PD enzyme activity and precipitate hemolytic episodes: aspirin, sulfonamides, nitrofurantoin, vitamin K derivatives, primaquine, and fava beans.

Glucose tolerance test, oral

The oral glucose tolerance test, the sole method of evaluating borderline diabetes mellitus, measures carbohydrate metabolism after ingestion of a challenge dose of glucose. The body absorbs this dose rapidly, causing plasma glucose levels to rise and peak within 1 hour. The pancreas responds by secreting more insulin, causing glucose levels to return to normal after 2 to 3 hours. During this period, plasma glucose levels are monitored to assess insulin secretion and the body's ability to metabolize glucose. Occasionally, levels are monitored an additional 2 to 3 hours to aid diagnosis of hypoglycemia and malabsorption syndrome.

In a patient with non-insulin-dependent diabetes (Type II), fasting plasma glucose levels may be within normal range; however, insufficient secretion of insulin after ingestion of carbohydrates causes plasma glucose to rise sharply and return to normal slowly.

The oral glucose tolerance test is not used in patients with fasting plasma glucose values above 140 mg/100 ml (7.7 mmol/L) or postprandial plasma glucose above 200 mg/100 ml (11.1 mmol/L).

Purpose
- To confirm diabetes mellitus in selected patients
- To aid diagnosis of hypoglycemia and malabsorption syndrome

Patient preparation
Explain that this test evaluates glucose metabolism. Instruct the patient to maintain a high-carbohydrate diet for 3 days and then to fast for 10 to 16 hours before the test; to avoid smoking, coffee, alcohol; and to avoid strenuous exercise for 8 hours before and during the test. Tell the patient this test requires five blood samples. Suggest bringing a book or other quiet diversions to the test, because the procedure usually takes 3 hours but can last as long as 6 hours.

If possible, drugs that affect test results should be discontinued 3 days before. If these drugs must be continued, note this on the laboratory slip.

➤ *Clinical alert:* Alert the patient to the symptoms of hypoglycemia — weakness, restlessness, nervousness, hunger, and sweating — and tell him to report such symptoms immediately.

Procedure
Between 7 a.m. and 9 a.m., perform a venipuncture to obtain a fasting blood sample. Draw this sample into a 7-ml *gray-top* tube. (Collect a urine specimen at the same time if this is included as part of the test.) After collecting these samples, administer the test load of 75 g of oral glucose, and record the time of ingestion. Start the timing when the patient begins to drink the solution. Encourage the patient to drink the entire glucose solution within 5 minutes.

Draw blood samples 30 minutes, 1 hour, 2 hours, and 3 hours after giving the loading dose, using 7-ml *gray-top* tubes to collect them.

Tell the patient to lie down if he feels faint.

Send blood samples to the laboratory immediately or refrigerate them. Specify when the patient last ate and the blood sample collection times. If appropriate, record the time of the patient's last pretest insulin or oral antidiabetic drug dose.

Precautions   If the patient develops severe hypoglycemia, draw a blood sample, record the time on the laboratory slip, and discontinue the test. Have the patient drink a glass of orange juice, or administer glucose I.V. to reverse the reaction.

Values   Normal plasma glucose levels peak at 160 to 180 mg/100 ml (8.9 to 10.0 mmol/L) within 1 hour after administration of an oral glucose test dose and return to fasting levels or lower within 2 to 3 hours. Normal levels are less than 120 mg/dl (6.7 mmol/L).

Implications of results   If the 2-hour sample and at least one other sample between 0 and 2 hours after 75 g oral glucose shows a glucose level of 200 mg/dl (11.1 mmol/L) or greater, this test result confirms diabetes in a non-pregnant adult (see *Diagnostic criteria for diabetes mellitus, impaired glucose tolerance, and gestational diabetes,* page 304).

Increased glucose levels are associated with other serious conditions such as Cushing's disease, pheochromocytomas, central nervous system lesions, cirrhosis of the liver, myocardial or cerebral infarction, hyperthyroidism, pregnancy, and anxiety states.

Decreased levels occur in islet-cell adenoma, malabsorption syndrome, adrenocortical insufficiency (Addison's disease), hypothyroidism, or hypopituitarism.

Post-test care   • If a hematoma develops at the venipuncture site, applying warm soaks eases discomfort.
• Provide a balanced meal or a snack, but observe for hypoglycemic reaction.
• The patient may resume withheld medications.

Interfering factors   • Elevated plasma glucose levels may result from chlorthalidone, thiazide diuretics, furosemide, oral contraceptives (estrogen-progestogen combination), triamterene, benzodiazepines, lithium, phenytoin, phenothiazines, epinephrine, phenolphthalein, caffeine, arginine, dextrothyroxine, diazoxide, large doses of nicotinic acid, corticosteroids, and recent glucose I.V. infusions.
• Depressed glucose levels may be caused by ingestion of beta-adrenergic blockers, amphetamines, ethanol, clofibrate, insulin, oral anti-

Diagnostic criteria for diabetes mellitus, impaired glucose tolerance, and gestational diabetes

In nonpregnant adults

Diabetes mellitus: Diagnosis of diabetes mellitus in nonpregnant adults should be restricted to those who have *one* of the following:

- random plasma glucose level of 200 mg/dl (11.1 mmol/L) or greater *plus* classic signs and symptoms of diabetes mellitus, including polydipsia, polyuria, polyphagia, ketonuria, and weight loss
- fasting plasma glucose level of 140 mg/dl (7.8 mmol/L) or greater on at least two occasions
- fasting plasma glucose level less than 140 mg/dl *plus* sustained elevated plasma glucose levels during at least two oral glucose tolerance tests. The 2-hour glucose level and at least one other between 0 and 2 hours after a 75-g glucose dose should be 200 mg/dl or greater. Oral glucose tolerance testing is not necessary if the patient has a fasting plasma glucose level of 140 mg/dl or greater.

Impaired glucose tolerance: Diagnosis of impaired glucose tolerance in nonpregnant adults should be restricted to those who have *all* of the following:

- fasting plasma glucose level of less than 140 mg/dl
- two-hour oral glucose tolerance test plasma glucose level greater than 140 mg/dl
- intervening oral glucose tolerance test plasma glucose level of 200 mg/dl or greater.

In pregnant adults

Gestational diabetes: After an oral glucose load of 100 g, diagnosis of gestational diabetes may be made if two plasma glucose values equal or exceed:

Fasting	**1 hour**	**2 hours**	**3 hours**
105 mg/dl	190 mg/dl	165 mg/dl	145 mg/dl
(5.8 mmol/L)	(10.5 mmol/L)	(9.2 mmol/L)	(8.1 mmol/L)

In children

Diabetes mellitus: Diagnosis of diabetes mellitus in children should be restricted to those who have *one* of the following:

- random plasma glucose level of 200 mg/dl or greater *plus* classic signs and symptoms of diabetes mellitus, including polyuria, polydipsia, polyphagia, ketonuria, and rapid weight loss
- fasting plasma glucose level of 140 mg/dl or greater on at least two occasions *and* sustained, elevated plasma glucose levels during at least two oral glucose tolerance tests. Both the 2-hour plasma glucose level and at least one other between 0 and 2 hours after a glucose dose (1.75 g/kg ideal body weight, up to 75 g) should be 200 mg/dl or greater.

Impaired glucose tolerance: Diagnosis of impaired glucose in children should be restricted to those who have *both* of the following:

- fasting plasma glucose level less than 140 mg/dl
- two-hour oral glucose tolerance test plasma glucose level greater than 140 mg/dl.

diabetic drugs, and monoamine oxidase inhibitors.
- Failure to adhere to dietary and exercise restrictions may interfere with accurate determination of test results.
- Carbohydrate deprivation before the test can produce impaired tolerance (abnormal increase in plasma glucose, with a delayed decrease), because the pancreas is unaccustomed to responding to high-carbohydrate load.
- Persons over age 50 tend toward decreasing carbohydrate tolerance, which causes an increase in glucose levels, to upper limits of about 1 mg/100 ml (0.05 mmol/L) for every year over age 50.

Glucose, 2-hour postprandial, plasma

Two-hour postprandial blood sugar

The 2-hour postprandial plasma glucose test reflects metabolic response to a carbohydrate challenge; normally, blood glucose returns to the fasting level within 2 hours. This test, performed on a blood sample taken after a meal, is used to monitor therapy and to confirm diabetes in a patient with borderline fasting blood glucose levels.

Purpose
- To monitor drug or diet therapy in patients with diabetes mellitus
- To identify disorders associated with abnormal glucose metabolism

Patient preparation
Explain to the patient that this test evaluates glucose metabolism and helps detect diabetes. The patient should observe an overnight fast (allowing water only) followed by a high carbohydrate breakfast (including milk, orange juice, cereal with sugar, and toast). The patient should avoid smoking and strenuous exercise after the meal. Tell the patient this test requires a blood sample, which will be drawn 2 hours after the meal.

Procedure
Perform a venipuncture, and collect the sample in a 5-ml *gray-top* tube.

Send the sample to the laboratory immediately or refrigerate it.

Specify on the laboratory slip the time of the meal, the sample collection time, and the time the last pretest insulin or oral antidiabetic drug dose (if applicable) was given.

Values

Normal glucose values are less than 120 mg/dl (6.7 mmol/L).

Implications of results

Values above 140 mg/dl (7.8 mmol/L) are abnormal in adults under age 50; values above 160 mg/dl (8.9 mmol/L) are abnormal in persons over age 60.

High glucose levels may also occur with pancreatitis, uncontrolled diabetes mellitus, Cushing's syndrome, acromegaly, pheochromocytoma, and chronic hepatic disease.

Depressed glucose levels occur in hyperinsulinism, insulinoma, von Gierke's disease, functional or reactive hypoglycemia, hypothyroidism, adrenal insufficiency, congenital adrenal hyperplasia, hypopituitarism, islet-cell carcinoma of the pancreas, hepatic necrosis, and glycogen storage disease.

Post-test care

- If a hematoma develops at the venipuncture site, applying warm soaks eases discomfort.
- Patient may resume diet, normal activity, and medications that were discontinued.

Interfering factors

- Failure to follow dietary instructions may interfere with accurate test results.
- Smoking or drinking coffee during the 2 hours after the test meal may cause false-high values.
- Recent illness, infection, or pregnancy may raise glucose levels; strenuous exercise or stress may depress them.
- Drugs known to cause plasma glucose elevations are chlorthalidone, thiazide diuretics, furosemide, triamterene, oral contraceptives (estrogen-progestogen combination), benzodiazepines, phenytoin, phenothiazines, lithium, epinephrine, arginine, phenolphthalein, dextrothyroxine, diazoxide, large doses of nicotinic acid, corticosteroids, and recent I.V. glucose infusions. Ethacrynic acid may also cause hyperglycemia, but large doses can cause hypoglycemia in patients with uremia.
- Depressed glucose levels may result from the use of beta-adrenergic blockers, amphetamines, ethanol, clofibrate, insulin, oral antidiabetic drugs, and monoamine oxidase inhibitors.

- Glycolysis caused by failure to refrigerate the sample or to send it to the laboratory immediately can depress glucose levels.

Gonorrheal culture

A positive stained smear of genital exudate showing gram-negative diplococci can be confirmed by a gonorrhea culture in 90% of males with characteristic symptoms. Possible culture sites include the urethra (usual site in males), endocervix (usual site in females), anal canal, and oropharynx.

Gonorrhea, a still prevalent venereal disease, nearly exclusively results from sexual transmission of *Neisseria gonorrhoeae*. Its most common effect in females is a greenish yellow cervical discharge; but in many females, it produces no symptoms at all — a factor that contributes to the epidemic prevalence of this infection. In males, gonorrhea generally causes painful urination and a mucopurulent urethral discharge, symptoms of acute anterior urethritis.

Purpose   To confirm gonorrhea

Patient preparation   Describe the procedure, and explain that this test confirms gonorrhea. Instruct the female patient not to douche for 24 hours before the test. Tell the male patient that he should not void during the hour preceding the test. Warn him that males sometimes experience nausea, sweating, weakness, and fainting associated with discomfort when the cotton-tipped applicator or wire loop is introduced into the urethra.

Equipment   Sterile gloves, sterile cotton-tipped applicator, wire bacteriologic loop or thin urogenital alginate swabs (for male), vaginal speculum (for female), ring forceps, cotton balls

Procedure   *Endocervical culture:* The patient is placed in the lithotomy position, draped, and instructed to take deep breaths. A vaginal speculum, lubricated only with warm water, is inserted. Mucus is cleaned from the cervix, using cotton balls in ring forceps. Then a dry, sterile cotton-tipped applicator is inserted into the endocervical canal and rotated from side to side. The applicator is left in place for several seconds for optimum absorption of organisms.

Urethral culture: Place the patient in the supine position, and drape appropriately. Clean the urethral meatus with sterile gauze or a cotton sponge; then insert a thin urogenital alginate swab or a wire bacteriologic loop ⅜" to ¾" (1 to 2 cm) into the urethra, and rotate the swab or loop from side to side. Leave it in place for several seconds for optimum absorption of organisms. If permitted, the patient may milk the urethra, bringing urethral secretions to the meatus for collection on a cotton-tipped applicator.

Rectal culture: After obtaining an endocervical or urethral specimen (while the patient is still on the examination table), insert a sterile cotton-tipped applicator into the anal canal about 1" (2.5 cm), move the applicator from side to side, and leave it in place for several seconds for optimum absorption. If the applicator is contaminated with feces, discard it, and repeat the procedure with a clean applicator.

Throat culture: Position the patient with his head tilted back and his eyes closed. Check his throat for inflamed areas, using a tongue blade. Rub a sterile cotton-tipped applicator from side to side over the tonsillar areas, including any inflamed or purulent sites. Be careful not to touch the teeth, cheeks, or tongue with the applicator.

If laboratory facilities aren't readily available: Insert the applicator of test material into a Transgrow medium specimen bottle, making sure to uncap the bottle only just before insertion. Keep the bottle upright to minimize loss of carbon dioxide. With the cotton-tipped applicator, absorb the excess moisture within the bottle; then roll the applicator across the Transgrow medium. Discard the applicator, and place the lid on the bottle. Label the bottle appropriately.

After collecting the specimens, carefully dispose of gloves, applicators, and speculum, to prevent staff exposure to the organism.

Send the specimen to the laboratory immediately, or arrange for immediate transport of the Transgrow bottle because the specimen requires subculturing within 24 to 48 hours to obtain successful growths.

Precautions • Place the male patient in supine position to prevent falling if vasovagal syncope occurs during introduction of the cotton-tipped applicator or wire loop into the urethra. Observe for profound hypotension, bradycardia, pallor, and sweating.

- To prevent loss of urethral secretions, collect a urethral specimen at least 1 hour after the patient has voided.

Findings

Normally, no *N. gonorrhoeae* appears in the culture.

Implications of results

A positive culture confirms gonorrhea.

Post-test care

- Advise the patient to avoid intercourse and all sexual contact until test results are available. Explain that treatment usually begins after confirmation of positive culture, except in a patient with symptoms of gonorrhea or in a person who has had intercourse with someone known to have gonorrhea.
- Advise the patient that a repeat culture is required 1 week after completion of treatment to evaluate therapy.
- Inform the patient that positive culture findings must be reported to the local health department.
- Strongly recommend that the patient adhere to antibiotic regimen.

Interfering factors

- Improper collection technique may provide a nonrepresentative specimen or may contaminate the specimen.
- Fecal material may contaminate an anal culture.
- In males, voiding within 1 hour of specimen collection washes secretions out of the urethra, making fewer organisms available for culture.
- In females, douching within 24 hours of specimen collection washes out cervical secretions, making fewer organisms available for culture.

Granulocyte antibodies, serum

White blood cell antibodies

This test (formerly the leukoagglutinin test) detects granulocyte antibodies — antibodies that react with white blood cells (WBCs) and may cause a transfusion reaction. These antibodies usually develop after exposure to foreign WBCs through transfusions, pregnancies, or allografts.

If a blood recipient has these antibodies, a febrile nonhemolytic reaction may occur 1 to 4 hours after the start of whole blood, red blood cell, platelet, or granulocyte transfusion. (All these blood products contain some granulocytes, which react with the antibodies.) This nonhemolytic reaction (marked by fever and severe chills, sometimes with nausea, headache, and transient hypertension) must be distinguished from a true hemolytic reaction before further transfusion can proceed.

If a blood donor has these antibodies, the recipient may develop acute, noncardiogenic pulmonary edema after transfusion of the donor's blood. In this case, the donor's blood must be tested for granulocyte antibodies to determine if these have caused the recipient's reaction.

Purpose
- To detect granulocyte antibodies in blood recipients who develop transfusion reactions, thus differentiating between hemolytic and febrile nonhemolytic transfusion reactions
- To detect granulocyte antibodies in blood donors after transfusion of donor blood causes a reaction

Patient preparation
If a blood recipient is being tested, explain that this test helps determine the cause of the transfusion reaction. If a blood donor is being tested, explain that this test determines if his blood caused a transfusion reaction and predicts if he'll have a reaction to a transfusion in the future.

A pretransfusion blood sample taken from the blood bank's crossmatched sample is preferred for this test. If such a sample isn't available, tell the patient that the test requires a blood sample.

Note the recent administration of blood or dextran or testing with I.V. contrast media on the laboratory slip.

Procedure
If a pretransfusion sample isn't available from the blood bank, perform a venipuncture and collect a blood sample in a 10-ml *red-top* tube. (The laboratory will require 3 to 4 ml of serum for testing.) Label the sample with the patient's name, room number, and hospital or blood bank number. Include on the laboratory slip the patient's suspected diagnosis and any history of blood transfusions, pregnancies, and drug therapy.

Findings
Normally, test results are negative for agglutination because serum contains no antibodies.

Implications of
results

In a recipient's blood, a positive result indicates the presence of granulocyte antibodies, which identifies the recipient's transfusion reaction as a febrile nonhemolytic reaction to these antibodies.

In a donor's blood, a positive result indicates the presence of granulocyte antibodies, identifying the cause of a recipient's reaction as an acute, noncardiogenic pulmonary edema.

Post-test care

- If a hematoma develops at the venipuncture site, applying warm soaks eases discomfort.
- If a donor has a positive granulocyte antibody test, explain the meaning of this result to help prevent future transfusion reactions.

➤ *Clinical alert:* If a transfusion recipient has a positive granulocyte antibody test, continued transfusions require premedication with acetaminophen 1 to 2 hours before the transfusion, specially prepared leukocyte-poor blood, or both to prevent further reactions.

Interfering
factor

Previous administration of dextran or I.V. contrast media causes aggregation resembling agglutination.

Growth hormone, serum

Human growth hormone, somatotrophic hormone

Growth hormone (hGH), a protein secreted by acidophiles of the anterior pituitary gland, is the primary regulator of human growth. Unlike other pituitary hormones, hGH has no easily defined feedback mechanism or single target gland — it affects many body tissues. Like insulin, hGH promotes protein synthesis and stimulates amino acid uptake by cells.

In addition, hGH raises plasma glucose by inhibiting glucose uptake and utilization by cells, and increases free fatty acid concentrations by enhancing lipolysis. Secretion of hGH appears to be regulated by the hypothalamus by means of a growth hormone–releasing factor and a growth hormone release-inhibiting factor (somatostatin). Secretion of hGH is diurnal and varies with such factors as exercise, sleep, stress, and nutritional status. Hyposecretion or hypersecretion of this hormone may induce pathologic states (such as dwarfism or gigantism). Altered hGH levels are common in patients with pituitary dysfunction.

This test, a quantitative analysis of plasma hGH levels, is usually performed as part of an anterior pituitary stimulation or suppression test.

Purpose
- To aid differential diagnosis of dwarfism because retarded growth in children can result from pituitary or thyroid hypofunction
- To confirm diagnosis of acromegaly and gigantism
- To aid diagnosis of pituitary or hypothalamic tumors
- To help evaluate hGH therapy

Patient preparation
Explain to the patient or to the parents (if the patient is a child) that this test measures hormone levels and helps determine the cause of abnormal growth. Instruct the patient to fast and limit physical activity for 10 to 12 hours before the test. Tell the patient that the test requires a blood sample and another sample may have to be drawn the following day for comparison.

Withhold all medications that affect hGH levels, such as corticosteroids, as appropriate. If these medications must be continued, note this on the laboratory slip. The patient should be relaxed and recumbent for 30 minutes before the test because stress and physical activity elevate hGH levels.

Procedure
Between 6 a.m. and 8 a.m. on two consecutive days, draw at least 7 ml of venous blood into a 10-ml *red-top* collection tube.

Handle the sample gently to prevent hemolysis; send it to the laboratory immediately because hGH has a half-life of only 20 to 25 minutes.

Values
Normal hGH levels for males range from undetectable to 5 ng/ml (µg/L); for females, from undetectable to 10 ng/ml (µg/L). Higher values in females are due to estrogen effects. Children generally have higher hGH levels; nevertheless, they may range from undetectable to 16 ng/ml (µg/L).

Implications of results
Diagnostic use of hGH levels always requires growth hormone suppression or stimulation testing (see individual test entries). Increased hGH levels may indicate a pituitary or hypothalamic tumor (frequently an adenoma), which causes gigantism in children and acromegaly in adults and adolescents. Patients with diabetes mellitus sometimes

have elevated hGH levels without having acromegaly. Suppression testing is necessary to confirm the diagnosis.

Pituitary infarction, metastatic disease, or tumors may reduce hGH levels. Dwarfism may be caused by low hGH levels, although only 15% of all cases of growth failure are related to endocrine dysfunction. Confirmation of diagnosis requires stimulation testing with arginine or insulin.

Post-test care

- If a hematoma develops at the venipuncture site, applying warm soaks eases discomfort.
- The patient can resume discontinued diet and medications.

Interfering factors

- Failure to follow restrictions of diet, medications, or physical activity may alter test results.
- Arginine, levodopa, insulin (induced hypoglycemia), beta-blockers (propranolol), or estrogens raise hGH secretion.
- Phenothiazines (such as chlorpromazine) and corticosteroids reduce hGH secretion.
- Radioactive scan performed within 1 week before the test may affect results because plasma hGH levels are determined by radioimmunoassay.
- Hemolysis caused by excessive agitation of the sample may interfere with the accuracy of test results.

Growth hormone stimulation test

Arginine test

This test measures plasma growth hormone (hGH) levels after I.V. administration of arginine, an amino acid that normally stimulates hGH secretion, and is commonly used to identify pituitary gland dysfunction in infants and children with growth retardation and to confirm hGH deficiency. This test may be performed concomitantly with an insulin tolerance test or after administration of other hGH stimulants, such as glucagon, vasopressin, and levodopa.

Purpose

- To aid diagnosis of pituitary tumors
- To confirm hGH deficiency in infants and children with low baseline levels

Patient preparation	Explain that this test identifies hGH deficiency. Instruct the patient to fast, and explain that this test requires venous infusion of a drug and collection of several blood samples.
	Before the test, withhold all steroid medications. If these medications must be continued, record this on the laboratory slip.
Procedure	Between 6 a.m. and 8 a.m., draw 6 ml of venous blood (basal sample) into a 10- to 15-ml *red-top* collection tube. Start I.V. infusion of arginine (0.5 g/kg body weight to a maximum dose of 30 mg) in normal saline solution, and continue for 30 minutes. Use of an indwelling venous catheter avoids repeated venipunctures and minimizes stress and anxiety. Discontinue the I.V. infusion; then draw a total of four 6-ml samples at 30-minute intervals. Collect each sample in a 10- to 15-ml *red-top* tube, and label it appropriately.
	Draw each sample at the scheduled time, and specify the collection time on the laboratory slip. Send each sample to the laboratory immediately because hGH has a half-life of 20 to 25 minutes. Handle the samples gently to prevent hemolysis.
Values	Arginine should raise hGH levels to more than 10 ng/ml (µg/L) in males, 15 ng/ml (µg/L) in females, and 48 ng/ml (µg/L) in children. Such an increase may appear in the first sample drawn 30 minutes after arginine infusion is discontinued, or in the samples drawn 60 and 90 minutes afterward.
Implications of results	Elevated levels while fasting and during sleep help to rule out hGH deficiency. Failure of hGH levels to rise after arginine infusion indicates decreased anterior pituitary hGH reserve. In children, this deficiency causes dwarfism; in adults, it can indicate panhypopituitarism. When hGH levels fail to reach 10 ng/ml, retesting is required at the same time of day as the original test.
Post-test care	• If a hematoma develops at the venipuncture site, applying warm soaks eases discomfort.
	• The patient can resume discontinued diet and medications.
Interfering factors	• Failure to observe restrictions of diet, medications, and physical activity may affect test results.

- Radioactive scan performed within 1 week before the test may affect results.
- Hemolysis caused by excessive agitation of the sample may affect test results.

Growth hormone suppression test
Glucose loading

This test evaluates excessive baseline levels of growth hormone (hGH) from the anterior pituitary gland by measuring the secretory response to a loading dose of glucose. In a patient with excessive hGH levels, failure of suppression indicates anterior pituitary dysfunction and confirms diagnosis of acromegaly and gigantism.

Purpose
- To assess elevated baseline hGH levels
- To confirm diagnosis of gigantism in children and acromegaly in adults

Patient preparation
Explain that this test helps determine the cause of abnormal growth. Instruct the patient to fast and limit physical activity for 10 to 12 hours before the test. Tell the patient two blood samples will be drawn, and warn that nausea may occur after drinking the glucose solution and some discomfort may result from the needle punctures.

Before the test, withhold steroids; and if these or other medications must be continued, note it on the laboratory slip.

Because hGH levels rise after exercise or excitement, the patient should be relaxed and recumbent for 30 minutes before the test.

Procedure
Between 6 a.m. and 8 a.m., draw 6 ml of venous blood (basal sample) into a 10- to 15-ml *red-top* collection tube. Administer 100 g of glucose solution orally. To prevent nausea, advise the patient to drink the glucose slowly. After 1 hour, draw another 6 ml of venous blood into a second 10- to 15-ml *red-top* collection tube. Handle the samples gently to prevent hemolysis. Send each sample to the laboratory immediately because hGH has a half-life of only 20 to 25 minutes.

Values
Normally, glucose suppresses hGH to levels ranging from undetectable to 3 ng/ml (μg/L) in 30 min-

utes to 2 hours. In children, rebound stimulation may occur after 2 to 5 hours.

Implications of results
In a patient with active acromegaly, basal levels are elevated (75 ng/ml [µg/L]) and are not suppressed to less than 5 ng/ml (µg/L) during the test. Unchanged or rising hGH levels in response to glucose loading indicate hGH hypersecretion and may confirm suspected acromegaly or gigantism. This response may be verified by repeating the test after a 1-day rest.

Post-test care
• If a hematoma develops at the puncture sites, applying warm soaks eases discomfort.
• The patient can resume discontinued diet and medications.

Interfering factors
• Failure to observe restrictions of diet, medications, and physical activity may interfere with the accuracy of test results.
• Release of hGH may be impaired by corticosteroids and phenothiazines (chlorpromazine), and may be increased by arginine, levodopa, amphetamines, glucagon, niacin, or estrogens.
• Radioactive scan performed within 1 week before the test may affect results because hGH levels are determined by radioimmunoassay.
• Hemolysis caused by excessive agitation of the sample may interfere with the accuracy of test results.

H

Hallucinogens, urine

This qualitative medicolegal screening test detects hallucinogens in a random urine specimen. The analytic laboratory method used depends on the particular hallucinogen and may include chromatography, thin-layer chromatography, or enzyme-multiplied immunoassay technique (EMIT). At present, no routine method is available to measure hallucinogen levels in blood or urine.

The hallucinogens — lysergic acid diethylamide (LSD), phencyclidine (PCP), mescaline, dipropyltryptamine (DPT), diethyltryptamine (DET), dimethyltryptamine (DMT), and marijuana *(Cannabis sativa)* — are natural and synthetic drugs that distort perception, cause illusions, may produce euphoria or panic, or induce psychotic behavior. They can also induce elevated blood pressure and pulse rate, reflex hyperactivity, and mydriasis. Their metabolic effects vary. For example, LSD, which has a half-life of 3 hours, is metabolized by the liver and excreted in feces. Marijuana, which is rapidly metabolized, may produce lingering symptoms because some of its own metabolites are active hallucinogens.

Purpose
To detect presence of hallucinogens in the body for medicolegal purposes

Patient preparation
Explain that this test detects ingestion, inhalation, or parenteral administration of hallucinogens. Tell the patient that the test requires a urine specimen, and explain the proper collection technique.

Make sure that the patient or responsible member of the family has signed a consent form. Check the patient's recent medication history, noting the time and route of administration.

Procedure
Collect a random urine specimen. Send the specimen to the laboratory immediately or refrigerate it. For a medicolegal test, observe the appropriate precautions.

Findings
Normally, no hallucinogens are found in urine.

Implications of results	Because hallucinogens aren't used therapeutically, their presence in any amount confirms drug abuse.
Post-test care	Restrain the patient, if necessary, to protect him from self-imposed or sensory injury.
Interfering factor	Unknown interfering substances in normal urine may give false-positive LSD findings.

Haloperidol, serum

Haloperidol is a neuroleptic drug used to treat psychotic disorders, to control the tics and verbal utterances associated with Gilles de la Tourette's syndrome, and to manage severe hyperexcitability in children who do not respond to other treatment. Serum levels of haloperidol are measured by high-performance liquid chromatography (HPLC) with electrochemical detection.

Although its mechanism of action is not fully understood, haloperidol is thought to exert its effects by postsynaptic blockade of dopamine receptors in the central nervous system, thereby inhibiting dopamine-mediated effects. Haloperidol is converted by the liver to reduced haloperidol, its major metabolite, which has minimal pharmacologic activity. HPLC detects both. The elimination half-life ranges from 13 to 35 hours. Toxic symptoms include irreversible tardive dyskinesia, extrapyramidal effects, neuroleptic malignant syndrome, hypertension or hypotension, seizures, arrhythmias, hypothermia or hyperthermia, autonomic nervous system dysfunction, and deep, unarousable sleep and possible coma.

Purpose	• To determine the most effective drug dosage • To assess adverse reactions and changes associated with coadministered drugs • To assess patient compliance, particularly in patients who show a poor therapeutic response to haloperidol • To monitor haloperidol toxicity
Patient preparation	Explain the purpose of this test and inform the patient that the test requires a blood sample. For consistency, collect the serum sample at least 12 hours after the last dose (trough level). Also tell the patient that he need not restrict food or fluids.

Procedure Perform a venipuncture and obtain a blood sample. This test requires 3.0 ml of serum collected into a 7-ml *red-top* or *green-top* tube. Send the specimen refrigerated.

Values Therapeutic range of haloperidol normally is 5 to 15 ng/ml. However, during low-dose therapy, it ranges from 2 to 5 ng/ml; during high-dose therapy, from 10 to 40 ng/ml. Toxicity may occur at values greater than 50 ng/ml.

Implications of results Studies designed to demonstrate a relationship between serum haloperidol concentration and therapeutic response have given inconsistent results. For patients who respond to haloperidol, a serum concentration of at least 5 ng/ml appears to be necessary to ensure a positive response, and increasing the concentration beyond 15 to 20 ng/ml may result in no additional clinical improvement. Because of interindividual variations in haloperidol serum levels, the serum concentration should be interpreted in conjunction with the patient's clinical status.

Post-test care If a hematoma develops at the venipuncture site, applying warm soaks eases discomfort.

Interfering factors
- Monitoring serum concentration prior to the achievement of steady state (which should be determined after 1 week of therapy or any change in total dosage) may produce significantly underestimated values.
- Diphenhydramine may interfere with some HPLC methods used to measure haloperidol.

Ham test
Acidified serum lysis test

The Ham test is performed to determine the cause of undiagnosed hemolytic anemia, hemoglobinuria, and bone marrow aplasia. It helps establish a diagnosis of paroxysmal nocturnal hemoglobinuria (PNH), a rare hematologic disease.

The Ham test relies on the susceptibility of red blood cells (RBCs) to lysis: RBCs from patients with PNH are unusually susceptible to lysis by complement. To perform the test, washed RBCs are mixed with ABO-compatible normal serum and acid. After incubation at 98.6° F (37° C), the cells are examined for hemolysis. In the presence of acidified human serum, many PNH cells are lysed, whereas normal RBCs show no hemolysis.

Purpose To help establish a diagnosis of PNH

Patient preparation Explain that this test, which requires a blood sample, helps determine the cause of anemia or other hematologic diseases.

Procedure Because the blood sample must be defibrinated immediately, laboratory personnel must perform the venipuncture and collect the sample.

Findings Normally, RBCs undergo no hemolysis.

Implications of results Hemolysis of RBCs indicates PNH.

Post-test care If a hematoma develops at the venipuncture site, applying warm soaks eases discomfort.

Interfering factors
- Blood containing large numbers of spherocytes may produce false-positive results.
- Patients with congenital dyserythropoietic anemia or hereditary erythroblastic multinuclearity associated with a positive acidified serum will show false-positive results.

Haptoglobin, serum

Using radial immunodiffusion, this test measures serum levels of haptoglobin, an alpha$_2$-globulin, which binds free hemoglobin and prevents its accumulation in plasma, permitting clearance by reticuloendothelial cells and conserving body iron. Free hemoglobin released from intravascular cell destruction is quickly bound to haptoglobin; the resulting hemoglobin-haptoglobin complex prevents the renal excretion of plasma hemoglobin and is eventually removed from circulation by the liver. Thus, significant hemolysis is associated with lower concentration or absence of serum haptoglobin. After severe hemolysis, low haptoglobin levels may persist for 5 to 7 days until the liver can synthesize more of this glycoprotein.

Purpose
- To serve as an index of hemolysis
- To investigate hemolytic transfusion reactions
- To identify suspected ahaptoglobinemia
- To help establish proof of paternity, using genetic (phenotypic) variations in haptoglobin structure

Patient preparation
Explain the purpose of this test and inform the patient that the test requires a blood sample. Check the patient's medication history for drugs that may influence haptoglobin levels.

Procedure
Draw a venous blood sample into a 10- to 15-ml *red-top* tube. Handle the sample gently to prevent hemolysis.

Values
Normally, serum haptoglobin concentrations, measured in terms of the protein's hemoglobin-binding capacity, are 38 to 270 mg/dl (380 to 2,700 mg/L).

Implications of results
Markedly depressed serum haptoglobin levels are characteristic of acute and chronic hemolysis, severe hepatocellular disease, infectious mononucleosis, and transfusion reactions. Hepatocellular disease inhibits the synthesis of haptoglobin. In hemolytic transfusion reactions, haptoglobin levels begin falling after 6 to 8 hours and drop to 40% of pretransfusion levels after 24 hours.

➤ *Clinical alert:* If serum haptoglobin values are extremely low, watch for symptoms of hemolysis: chills, fever, back pain, flushing, distended neck veins, tachycardia, tachypnea, and hypotension.

Although haptoglobin is absent in 90% of neonates, in most of these infants, levels gradually rise to normal by age 4 months. In about 1% of the population — including 4% of blacks — haptoglobin is permanently absent; this disorder is known as congenital ahaptoglobinemia. It has no identified harmful consequences.

Strikingly elevated serum haptoglobin levels occur in diseases marked by chronic inflammatory reactions or tissue destruction, such as rheumatoid arthritis, chronic infections, and malignant neoplasms.

Post-test care
If a hematoma develops at the venipuncture site, applying warm soaks eases discomfort.

Interfering
factors

- Steroids and androgens can elevate haptoglobin levels and mask hemolysis in patients with inflammatory disease.
- Hemolysis caused by excessive agitation of the sample can interfere with accurate determination of test results.

Heinz bodies

Heinz bodies are particles of denatured hemoglobin that have precipitated out of the cytoplasm of red blood cells (RBCs), and that have collected in small masses and attached to the cell membranes. They form as a result of drug injury to RBCs, the presence of unstable hemoglobins, unbalanced globin chain synthesis caused by thalassemia, or a RBC enzyme deficiency (such as glucose-6-phosphate dehydrogenase deficiency). Although Heinz bodies are rapidly removed from RBCs in the spleen, they are a major factor in causing hemolytic anemias.

Using a whole blood sample, Heinz bodies can be detected by phase microscopy or with supravital stains, such as crystal violet, brilliant cresyl blue, or new methylene blue. However, when Heinz bodies do not form spontaneously, various oxidant drugs are added to the whole blood sample to induce their formation.

Purpose
To help detect causes of hemolytic anemia

Patient
preparation
Explain that this test, which requires a blood sample, helps determine the cause of anemia.

Review the patient's medication history for drugs that may interfere with accurate determination of test results. As appropriate, withhold antimalarials, furazolidone, nitrofurantoin, phenacetin, procarbazine, and sulfonamides. If these medications must be continued, note this on the laboratory slip.

Procedure
Perform a venipuncture, and collect the sample in a 7-ml *lavender-top* tube. Completely fill the sample collection tube, and invert it gently several times to adequately mix the sample and the anticoagulant.

Findings
Absence of Heinz bodies is the normal (negative) test result.

Implications of results	The presence of Heinz bodies — a positive test result — may indicate an inherited RBC enzyme deficiency, the presence of unstable hemoglobins, thalassemia, or drug-induced RBC injury. Heinz bodies may also be present after splenectomy.

Post-test care
- If a hematoma develops at the venipuncture site, applying warm soaks eases discomfort.
- The patient may resume withheld medications.

Interfering factors
- Antimalarials, furazolidone (in infants), nitrofurantoin, phenacetin, procarbazine, and sulfonamides can cause false-positive results.
- Failure to use the appropriate anticoagulant in the collection tube, to fill the collection tube completely, to adequately mix the sample and the anticoagulant, or to send the sample to the laboratory immediately may interfere with accurate test results.

Helicobacter pylori, serum

Campylobacter pylori, serum

This test detects antibodies for immunoglobulins G and A that are specific for *Helicobacter pylori,* which may be the leading cause of gastritis and peptic ulcer disease, and also may be the causative agent of duodenal ulcer. An association between *H. pylori* and gastric cancer may also exist.

Purpose
- To detect *H. pylori* infection
- To aid diagnosis of gastritis and peptic ulcer disease

Patient preparation
Explain to the patient that this test, which requires a blood sample, identifies the presence of *H. pylori* in the stomach.

Procedure
Perform a venipuncture and collect the sample in a *red-top* tube.

Findings
Normally, antibodies to *H. pylori* are not present.

Implications of results
Presence of *H. pylori* bacteria indicates a *H. pylori* infection.

Post-test care   If a hematoma develops at the venipuncture site, applying warm soaks eases discomfort.

Interfering factors
- Strain-to-strain antigenic variability in *H. pylori* may make the test less sensitive to the presence of the bacteria.
- Serologic tests have limited usefulness because they remain positive for months following antibiotic therapy.

Hematocrit (HCT)

Hematocrit (HCT) measures the percentage by volume of packed red blood cells (RBCs) in a whole blood sample; for example, a HCT level of 40% (0.40) means that a 100-ml sample contains 40 ml of packed RBCs. This packing is achieved by centrifugation of anticoagulated whole blood in a capillary tube, so that RBCs are tightly packed without hemolysis. The HCT level depends primarily on the number of RBCs, but is also influenced by the average size of the RBC. For example, conditions such as elevated concentrations of blood glucose and sodium, which cause swelling of erythrocytes may produce elevated HCT levels.

Test results may be used to calculate two erythrocyte indices: mean corpuscular volume and mean corpuscular hemoglobin concentration.

Purpose
- To aid diagnosis of abnormal states of hydration, polycythemia, and anemia
- To aid in calculating RBC indices
- To monitor fluid imbalance
- To monitor blood loss and evaluate blood replacement
- To conduct routine screening as part of the complete blood count

Patient preparation   Explain that this test detects anemia and other abnormal conditions of the blood. Inform the patient that the test requires a blood sample. Explain to the parents (and to the child, if appropriate) that a small amount of blood will be drawn from the finger or earlobe.

Procedure   Perform a finger stick, using a heparinized capillary tube with a red band on the anticoagulant end. Fill the capillary tube from the red-banded end to about two-thirds capacity, and seal this end with clay. Send the sample to the laboratory immediately.

Values

Typically, HCT values vary, depending on the patient's sex and age, type of sample, and the laboratory performing the test. Reference values range from 40% to 54% (0.40 to 0.54) for males, and 37% to 47% (0.37 to 0.47) for females.

Implications of results

Low HCT values may indicate anemia or hemodilution; high HCT values suggest polycythemia or hemoconcentration caused by blood loss.

Post-test care

If a hematoma develops at the venipuncture site, applying warm soaks eases discomfort.

Interfering factors

- Failure to use the proper anticoagulant in the collection tube and to fill it appropriately may interfere with accurate determination of test results.
- Hemolysis caused by excessive agitation of the sample may affect test results.
- Tourniquet constriction for longer than 1 minute causes hemoconcentration and typically raises the HCT level by 2.5% to 5% (0.02 to 0.05).
- Taking the blood sample from the same arm that is being used for I.V. infusion of fluids causes hemodilution.
- Failure to adequately mix the sample and anticoagulant may hinder accurate determination of test results.
- Excessive centrifugation of the sample results in hemolysis.

Hemoglobin, glycosylated
Total fasting hemoglobin, glycohemoglobin

The glycosylated hemoglobin (Hb) test is a diagnostic tool for monitoring diabetes therapy. The three minor hemoglobins measured in this test — A_{1a}, A_{1b}, and A_{1c} — are variants of Hb A formed by glycosylation, a chemical reaction in which glucose is chemically incorporated in Hb A. Because glycosylation occurs at a constant rate during the 120-day life span of an erythrocyte, glycosylated Hb levels reflect the average blood glucose level during the preceding 4 to 6 weeks, and therefore can be used for evaluating long-term effectiveness of diabetes therapy.

Because the goal of diabetes therapy is to establish and maintain near-normal carbohydrate metabolism to prevent sequelae, the glycosylated Hb test adds information supplied by blood or urine glucose tests. Measuring blood or urine glucose levels reflects glucose control only at the time of collection. Measuring glycosylated Hb requires only one venipuncture every 6 to 8 weeks and reflects diabetes control over several months.

Glycosylated Hb is usually measured by processing red cell hemolysates through a cation exchange chromatography column, to separate glycosylated hemoglobins from Hb A.

Purpose To monitor long-term control of diabetes mellitus

Patient preparation Explain that this test evaluates the effectiveness of diabetes therapy. Advise the patient that the test requires a blood sample. Instruct the patient to maintain his prescribed medication or diet regimen.

Procedure Perform a venipuncture, and collect the sample in a 5-ml *lavender-top* tube. Completely fill the collection tube, and invert it gently several times to mix the sample and anticoagulant adequately.

Values Glycosylated Hb values are reported as a percentage of the total Hb within an erythrocyte. Because Hb A_{1c} is present in a larger quantity than the other minor hemoglobins, it's the variant commonly measured. Normal values for Hb are usually 6% to 8% A_{1c} (0.06 to 0.08). Hb A_{1a} and Hb A_{1b} account for about 1.6% and 0.8% (0.016 and 0.008), respectively; Hb A_{1c} accounts for approximately 5% (0.05); and total glycosylated Hb accounts for 5.5% to 9% (0.055 to 0.09).

Implications of results As effective therapy brings diabetes under control, glycosylated Hb levels approach normal range.

Post-test care
• If a hematoma develops at the venipuncture site, applying warm soaks eases discomfort.
• The patient should be scheduled for appropriate follow-up testing in 6 to 8 weeks.

Interfering factor Failure to mix the sample and anticoagulant adequately may influence and interfere with accurate determination of test results.

Hemoglobin, total

This test, usually performed as part of a complete blood count, measures the grams of hemoglobin (Hb) found in a deciliter (100 ml) of whole blood. Hb concentration usually correlates closely with the red blood cell (RBC) count. In the laboratory, Hb is chemically converted to pigmented compounds and is measured by spectrophotometric or colorimetric technique.

Purpose
- To measure the severity of anemia or polycythemia and monitor response to therapy
- To supply figures for calculating mean corpuscular hemoglobin concentration

Patient preparation
Explain that this test helps determine if the patient has anemia or polycythemia or it assesses response to treatment. Inform the patient that the test requires a blood sample. Explain to the parents or to the child, if appropriate, that a small amount of blood will be drawn from the finger or earlobe.

Procedure
For adults and older children, perform a venipuncture, and collect the sample in a 7-ml *lavender-top* tube. For younger children and infants, collect capillary blood in a pipette. Completely fill the collection tube, and invert it gently several times to adequately mix the sample and the anticoagulant. Handle the sample gently to prevent hemolysis.

Values
Hb concentration varies, depending on the patient's age and sex and on the type of blood sample drawn. Except for infants, values for age groups listed in *Normal hemoglobin levels,* page 328, are based on venous blood samples.

Implications of results
Low Hb concentration may indicate anemia, recent hemorrhage, or fluid retention, causing hemodilution; an elevated Hb suggests hemoconcentration from polycythemia or dehydration.

Post-test care
If a hematoma develops at the venipuncture site, applying warm soaks eases discomfort.

Interfering factors
- Failure to use the proper anticoagulant in the collection tube or to adequately mix the sample and anticoagulant may interfere with the accuracy of test results.

Normal hemoglobin levels	
Age	**Hemoglobin level**
< 7 days	17 to 22 g/dl
1 week	15 to 20 g/dl
1 month	11 to 15 g/dl
Children	11 to 13 g/dl
Adult males	14 to 18 g/dl
Elderly males	12.4 to 14.9 g/dl
Adult females	12 to 16 g/dl
Elderly females	11.7 to 13.8 g/dl

- Hemolysis caused by excessive agitation of the sample may adversely affect the test results.
- Prolonged tourniquet constriction may cause hemoconcentration.
- Extremely high white blood cell counts, lipemia, or red blood cells that are resistant to lysis will falsely elevate Hb values.

Hemoglobin, unstable

Unstable hemoglobin (Hb) is a rare congenital red blood cell defect caused by amino acid substitution in the normally stable structure of Hb. These abnormal replacements produce a molecule that spontaneously denatures into clumps and aggregations called Heinz bodies, which separate from the red cell cytoplasm and accumulate at the cell membrane. Although Heinz bodies are usually efficiently removed by the spleen or liver, they may cause mild to severe hemolysis.

Unstable Hb is best detected by precipitation tests (heat stability or isopropanol solubility) performed in the laboratory. Although Hb electrophoresis and the Heinz body test may demonstrate certain unstable Hb, these tests don't always confirm their presence. Globin chain analysis identifies unstable Hb more reliably, but this procedure is time-consuming and technically complex and, therefore, is not performed routinely.

Purpose	To detect unstable Hb
Patient preparation	Explain that this test detects abnormal Hb in the blood. Inform the patient that the test requires a blood sample. Withhold antimalarials, furazolidone (from infants), nitrofurantoin, phenacetin, procarbazine, and sulfonamides before the test because these drugs may induce hemolysis. If these medications must be continued, note this on the laboratory slip.
Procedure	Perform a venipuncture, and collect the sample in a 7-ml *lavender-top* tube. Completely fill the collection tube, and invert it gently several times to mix the sample and the anticoagulant adequately. Don't shake the tube vigorously because hemolysis may result.
Findings	When no unstable Hb appears in the sample, the heat stability test is reported as negative; the isopropanol solubility test, as stable.
Implications of results	A positive heat stability or unstable solubility test, especially with hemolysis, strongly suggests the presence of unstable Hb.
Post-test care	• If a hematoma develops at the venipuncture site, applying warm soaks eases discomfort. • The patient may resume withheld medications.
Interfering factors	• Antimalarials, furazolidone (in infants), nitrofurantoin, phenacetin, procarbazine, and sulfonamides can induce Heinz body formation and result in a positive or unstable test. • High levels of Hb F may cause a false-positive isopropanol test. • Failure to use the proper anticoagulant in the collection tube, to fill the tube completely, or to mix the sample and the anticoagulant adequately may interfere with accurate determination of test results. • Hemolysis caused by excessive agitation of the sample or hemoconcentration caused by prolonged tourniquet constriction may influence test results.

Hemoglobin, urine

Free hemoglobin (Hb) in the urine — an abnormal finding — may occur in hemolytic anemias or in severe intravascular hemolysis resulting from a transfusion reaction. Hb consists of heme — an iron-protoporphyrin complex — and globin — a polypeptide. Hb combines with oxygen and carbon dioxide to allow red blood cells (RBCs) to transport these gases between the lungs and the tissues. Aging RBCs are constantly being destroyed by normal mechanisms within the reticuloendothelial system. However, when RBC destruction occurs within the circulation, as in intravascular hemolysis, free Hb enters the plasma and binds with haptoglobin, a plasma alpha$_2$-globulin. If the plasma level of Hb exceeds that of haptoglobin, the excess of unbound Hb is excreted in the urine (hemoglobinuria).

This test is based on the fact that heme proteins act like enzymes that catalyze oxidation of organic substances, such as guaiac or orthotoluidine. This reaction produces a blue coloration; the intensity of color varies with the amount of Hb present. Microscopic examination is required to identify intact RBCs in urine (hematuria), which can occur in the presence of unbound Hb.

Purpose
To aid diagnosis of hemolytic anemias or severe intravascular hemolysis from a transfusion reaction

Patient preparation
Explain that this test detects excessive RBC destruction. Inform the patient that the test requires a random urine specimen, and teach the proper collection technique. If the female patient is menstruating, reschedule the test because contamination of the specimen with menstrual blood alters test results.

Check the patient's medication history for drugs that may affect free Hb levels. Review your findings with the laboratory, and discontinue these medications before the test, as appropriate.

Procedure
Collect a random urine specimen. Send the specimen to the laboratory immediately.

Findings
Normally, Hb is not present in the urine.

Implications of results

Hemoglobinuria may result from severe intravascular hemolysis caused by a blood transfusion reaction, burns, or a crushing injury; from acquired hemolytic anemias caused by chemical or drug intoxication or malaria; or from the hemolytic anemia known as paroxysmal nocturnal hemoglobinuria. Hemoglobinuria may also result from congenital hemolytic anemias, as in hemoglobinopathies or enzyme defects, and, less commonly, is associated with cystitis, ureteral calculi, or urethritis.

Hemoglobinuria and hematuria occur in renal epithelial damage (as in acute glomerulonephritis or pyelonephritis), renal tumor, and tuberculosis.

Post-test care

The patient may resume discontinued medications.

Interfering factors

- Lysis of RBCs in stale or alkaline urine and contamination of the specimen with menstrual blood alter test results.
- Bacterial peroxidases in highly infected specimens can produce false-positive test results.
- Large doses of vitamin C or of medications that contain vitamin C as a preservative (such as certain antibiotics) can inhibit reagent activity, producing false-negative results. Nephrotoxic drugs (such as amphotericin B) or anticoagulants (such as warfarin) may cause a positive result for hemoglobinuria or hematuria.

Hemoglobin derivatives

This quantitative test measures the percentage of total hemoglobin (Hb) containing abnormal derivatives — primarily carboxyhemoglobin, sulfhemoglobin, and methemoglobin — after onset of signs of toxicity, such as cyanosis and anoxia. By changing the pH or adding a reducing substance and then analyzing the blood with a spectrophotometer, the specific form of Hb present can be determined, and thus the diagnosis can be confirmed.

When combined with certain chemicals or drugs, Hb is converted into compounds that are incapable of transporting oxygen. One such compound is carboxyhemoglobin, which results from the union of Hb and carbon monoxide. (Carbon monoxide's affinity for Hb is 210 times greater than that of oxygen.) The major effect of carbon monoxide toxicity is tissue hypoxia, because carboxyhemoglobin cannot carry oxygen and also because it prevents the release of oxygen from as yet unaffected Hb. Treatment with 100% oxygen or with 95% oxygen and 5% carbon dioxide can help to reverse carbon monoxide toxicity. The principal sources of carbon monoxide include tobacco smoke and exhaust from incomplete combustion of petroleum and natural gas fuels, such as that from gasoline and diesel motors, unvented natural gas heaters, and defective gas stoves.

Another compound, sulfhemoglobin, results from combining Hb with certain drugs, such as phenacetin or sulfonamides. Methemoglobin results from the oxidation of ferrous iron to the ferric form. Such oxidation usually results from chemicals and drugs — such as nitrates, nitrites, sulfonamides, aniline, chlorates, or phenacetin — or from primary methemoglobinemia. Sulfhemoglobin can't be removed by therapy and disappears only with the destruction of the affected red blood cells.

Purpose
- To rule out abnormal Hb derivatives as a cause of cyanosis or anoxia
- To monitor suspected overexposure to a substance causing cyanosis or anoxia, such as carbon monoxide

Patient preparation
Explain that this test helps determine if the Hb in the blood has the normal capacity to combine with oxygen. Inform the patient that the test requires a blood sample.

If the test is being performed for medicolegal purposes, make sure the patient or a responsible family member has signed a consent form. Check the patient's history for recent exposure to drugs and other potentially toxic substances.

Procedure
Perform a venipuncture, and collect the sample in a 4.5-ml *blue-top* tube for carboxyhemoglobin, or in a 7-ml *green-top* (heparinized) tube for sulfhemoglobin or methemoglobin. Seal the container to prevent air contamination, and send the sample to the laboratory immediately or refrigerate it. For a medicolegal test, observe appropriate precautions.

Values
Normally, carboxyhemoglobin concentration is 3% (0.03) of the total Hb (up to 15% [0.15] in tobacco smokers); methemoglobin concentration, less than 3% (0.03); and sulfhemoglobin concentration, undetectable.

Implications of
results

Levels depend on duration of exposure as well as concentration. Treatment of toxicity and exposure limitations depend on identification of various types of Hb and levels noted.

In acute carbon monoxide poisoning, symptoms occur when carboxyhemoglobin levels reach 20% (0.20); severe poisoning exists at 30% (0.30); fatal poisoning, at 50% (0.50) to 80% (0.80). Lower carboxyhemoglobin concentrations can produce serious symptoms in children and in persons with chronic carbon monoxide poisoning. Methemoglobin values of 10% (0.10) to 25% (0.25) produce cyanosis (but are tolerated); values of 35% (0.35) to 40% (0.40) produce exertional dyspnea and headache; values over 60% (0.60) produce lethargy and stupor; values over 70% (0.70), death. Sulfhemoglobin values of 10 g/dl (100 g/L) produce cyanosis but cause few or no toxic symptoms.

Post-test care

If a hematoma develops at the venipuncture site, applying warm soaks eases discomfort.

Interfering
factor

Air contamination of the sample may affect the accuracy of test results.

Hemoglobin electrophoresis

Hemoglobin (Hb) electrophoresis separates normal and certain abnormal hemoglobins. The electrophoresis apparatus consists of an anode (+) and a cathode (–), separated by a cellulose acetate membrane, on which different types of Hb migrate at different speeds when an electrical current is passed through the medium.

The laboratory may change the medium (from cellulose acetate to starch gel), or its pH (from 6.2 to 8.6), to clearly separate different types of Hb and to expand the range of this test beyond those routinely checked: A, A_2, S, C, and H.

Purpose

• To detect abnormal types of Hb and quantify their relative proportions
• To aid diagnosis of thalassemias

Patient
preparation

Explain that this test evaluates the types of Hb present in the blood. Inform the patient that the test will require a blood sample.

Check the patient's history for recent blood transfusion (within the past 4 months).

Procedure
: Perform a venipuncture, and collect the sample in a 7-ml *lavender-top* tube. Completely fill the collection tube, and invert it gently several times to mix the sample and anticoagulant adequately. Don't shake the tube vigorously because hemolysis may result.

Values
: The most common form of Hb found in normal adults is Hb A, which accounts for over 95% (0.95) of all hemoglobins; Hb A_2, 2% to 3% (0.02 to 0.03); and Hb F, less than 1% (0.01). In neonates, Hb F normally accounts for half the total. Hb S, H, or C are present only in hemoglobinopathies.

Implications of results
: Changes in the proportion of normal types of Hb may imply a hemolytic disease. The most common abnormality is increased Hb A_2, which is associated with α-thalassemia minor. Hb S is associated with sickle cell disease; Hb C, with hemoglobin C disease. More than 350 variants of Hb have been recognized.

Post-test care
: If a hematoma develops at the venipuncture site, applying ice, followed later by warm soaks, eases discomfort.

Interfering factors
:
- If the patient has received a blood transfusion within the past 4 months, this may invalidate test results.
- Failure to use the proper anticoagulant in the collection tube, to fill the tube completely, or to mix the sample and the anticoagulant adequately may interfere with accurate test results.
- Hemolysis caused by excessive agitation of the sample may interfere with accurate test results.

Hemoglobin S
Sickle cell test

Sickle cells are severely deformed red blood cells (RBCs). The sickling phenomenon results from a hemoglobinopathy — most commonly, the polymerization of hemoglobin (Hb) S, in the presence of low pH, low oxygen tension, elevated osmolarity, and elevated temperature, to form elongated structures (tactoids) that deform RBCs. Reversing these conditions depolymerizes Hb S and allows the RBCs to resume their normal shape. However, repeated sickling leads to permanent RBC deformity. Hb S is found almost exclusively in blacks; 0.2% of blacks born in the United States have sickle cell anemia.

Persons with sickle cell disease (who are homozygous for Hb S) usually show abundant spontaneously sickled RBCs on a peripheral blood smear. Persons with sickle cell trait (who are heterozygous for Hb S) or those who are doubly heterozygous for Hgb S and another abnormal hemoglobin may have normal RBCs that can be easily changed to sickled forms by lowering oxygen tension. This tendency to sickle can be identified by sealing a drop of blood between a glass slide and coverslip and adding a reducing agent, such as sodium metabisulfite. The RBCs can then be observed under a microscope and compared with a central slide containing blood and normal saline solution. The prevalence and rapidity of the sickling that follows are governed by the concentration of Hb S.

Although this test is useful as a rapid screening procedure, it may produce false-positive and false-negative results; consequently, a hemoglobin electrophoresis should be performed if the presence of Hb S is strongly suspected.

Purpose	To identify sickle cell disease and sickle cell trait

Patient preparation
Explain that this test, which requires a blood sample, helps detect sickle cell disease.

Check the patient's history for blood transfusion within the past 3 months.

Procedure
Perform a venipuncture, and collect the sample in a 7-ml *lavender-top* tube. Completely fill the collection tube, and invert it gently several times to adequately mix the sample and the anticoagulant. Don't shake the tube vigorously because hemolysis may result.

Findings
Results of this test are reported as positive or negative. A normal, or negative, test suggests the absence of Hb S.

Implications of results
A positive test may indicate the presence of sickle cells, but hemoglobin electrophoresis is needed to distinguish between homozygous and heterozygous forms. Rarely, other abnormal types of Hb may cause sickling of RBCs in the absence of Hb S.

Post-test care   If a hematoma develops at the venipuncture site, applying warm soaks eases discomfort.

Interfering factors
- Hb concentration under 10% (0.10), elevated Hb F levels in infants under age 6 months, and blood transfusion within the past 3 months may produce false-negative test results.
- Failure to use the proper anticoagulant in the collection tube, to completely fill the tube, or to adequately mix the sample and the anticoagulant may interfere with accurate determination of test results.
- Hemolysis caused by excessive agitation of the sample may affect test results.

Hemosiderin, urine

This test measures the urine level of hemosiderin, a colloidal iron oxide and one of the two forms of storage iron deposited in body tissue. When iron storage mechanisms fail to manage iron overload, excess iron may escape to cells unaccustomed to high iron concentrations and may produce toxic effects. Particularly vulnerable to such toxicity are the liver, myocardium, bone marrow, pancreas, kidneys, and skin, which tend to develop tissue damage known as hemochromatosis. This disorder may occur in a rare hereditary form known as primary hemochromatosis and in exogenous forms. Elevated tissue storage of iron without associated tissue damage is called hemosiderosis and is often confused with hemochromatosis.

Purpose   To aid diagnosis of hemochromatosis

Patient preparation   Explain that this test helps determine if the body is accumulating excessive amounts of iron. Inform the patient that no restrictions are necessary before the test and that the test requires a urine specimen.

Procedure   Collect a random urine specimen of approximately 30 ml. Use a plastic urine container, securely seal the container, and send the specimen to the laboratory immediately.

Findings   Normally, hemosiderin is not found in urine.

Implications of results	The presence of hemosiderin, appearing as yellow-brown granules in urinary sediment, indicates hemochromatosis; liver or bone marrow biopsy is necessary for confirmation of primary hemochromatosis. Hemosiderin may also suggest pernicious anemia, chronic hemolytic anemia, multiple blood transfusions, and paroxysmal nocturnal hemoglobinuria, the result of excessive iron injections or dietary intake of iron.
Post-test care	None
Interfering factor	Failure to send the specimen to the laboratory immediately may interfere with accurate determination of test results.

Heparin monitoring, plasma

Heparin functions as an anticoagulant by forming a complex with plasma antithrombin (AT, formerly known as antithrombin-III). In the presence of heparin, plasma AT inactivates coagulation factors IIa, Xa, IXa, and XIa. Several coagulation tests, including activated partial thromboplastin time (APTT), prothrombin time (PT), and thrombin clotting time assay, can be affected by the presence of heparin in samples. Tests used to monitor standard heparin therapy include the APTT, protamine titration assays, and anti-Xa based assays. Low molecular weight heparins function primarily by inhibiting factor Xa and can be monitored only by anti-Xa assays. The PT is less sensitive to heparin than the APTT.

Most laboratories monitor heparin treatment with the APTT test, comparing the patient's results with the values obtained from plasmas containing therapeutic heparin concentrations. Because of variability in commercial reagents, each laboratory should determine what the therapeutic range is for their APTT test.

Protamine sulfate neutralizes heparin and can be used in a thrombin clot time assay to confirm the presence of heparin in a sample (shortened clotting time with protamine). Additionally, titration of the heparin with protamine can be used to determine the concentration of heparin in plasma. Anti-Xa based assays can also be used to determine plasma heparin levels and are the test of choice for monitoring patients with heparin resistance and for monitoring therapeutic anticoagulation with low molecular weight heparins. These tests are performed by incubating the patient's plasma (the source of heparin) with Xa, followed by measurement of residual Xa activity.

Failure to reach therapeutic heparin levels on the first day of heparin therapy is associated with a higher risk for rethrombosis.

Purpose To monitor therapeutic heparin levels

Patient preparation Explain to the patient that this test is necessary to determine the appropriate heparin dosage and if blood clotting time is too long. Inform the patient that a blood sample is required. Note the use of heparin or warfarin on the laboratory slip.

Procedure Perform a venipuncture, and collect the sample in a 7-ml *blue-top* tube. To prevent hemolysis, avoid excessive probing of the venipuncture site and handle the sample gently. Completely fill the collection tube, invert it gently several times, and send it to the laboratory immediately or place it on ice.

Values Heparin levels of 0.2 to 0.4 units/ml (protamine titration or anti-Xa activity) are considered therapeutic. For most laboratories and APTT reagents, this corresponds to an APTT of 1.5 to 2.8 times the mean value of normal controls.

Implications of results
- Subtherapeutic heparin levels are associated with recurrent thrombosis. Excessively high heparin levels may predispose the patient to bleeding.
- Heparin resistance may occur in patients with high levels of heparin-binding proteins. These patients should be monitored by measuring anti-Xa heparin levels.

Post-test care If a hematoma develops at the venipuncture site, applying warm soaks eases discomfort.

Interfering factors
- Hemolysis or poor venipuncture technique can interfere with test results.
- Failure to mix the sample and anticoagulant properly or to send the sample to the laboratory promptly may alter test results.

- Avoid collection of samples from heparinized infusion lines. This can result in falsely elevated heparin levels. If it is unavoidable and several blood samples must be drawn, the sample from the heparinized line should be drawn last to allow the line to be flushed out.
- Heparin monitoring by APTT is sensitive to other factors that influence the APTT result. Baseline testing before initiating anticoagulation is important. Other assays for heparin levels are less sensitive to these influences.

Hepatitis A antibody (anti-HAV, IgM), serum

Hepatitis A, also known as infectious hepatitis, is transmitted by feces, saliva, and contaminated food and water. The hepatitis A virus (HAV) is fairly common — approximately 50% of U.S. citizens become infected by the time they reach adulthood, most of them experiencing minimal or no symptoms at all. This type of hepatitis does not lead to chronic hepatitis, cirrhosis, or liver cancer. Patients with HAV are usually not hospitalized, and the risk to caregivers is low. HAV does not have a carrier state and provides lifelong immunity after the acute infection is resolved.

Purpose
To aid differential diagnosis of viral hepatitis

Patient preparation
Explain that this test helps to identify HAV, which causes hepatitis A. Inform the patient that the test requires a blood sample.

Procedure
Perform a venipuncture, and collect the blood sample in a 7-ml *red-top* tube. This test requires 2.0 ml of serum. Freeze the sample and send it to the laboratory.

Findings
Normal serum is negative for immunoglobulin M (IgM) antibodies to HAV.

Implications of results
The presence of IgM antibodies to HAV indicates acute hepatitis A infection. IgM antibodies develop within 1 week of onset of symptoms, peak in 3 months, and disappear after 6 months. The presence of immunoglobulin G antibodies to HAV signifies an old infection and is usually not clinically rel-

evant, but does not rule out acute hepatitis B or non-A, non-B hepatitis.

Post-test care If a hematoma develops at the venipuncture site, applying warm soaks eases discomfort.

Interfering factors None

Hepatitis B surface antigen
Hepatitis-associated antigen, Australia antigen

Hepatitis B surface antigen (HBsAg) is the earliest and most reliable serologic marker of viral hepatitis infection. It appears in the sera of patients with hepatitis B virus (HBV) —formerly called serum hepatitis or long-incubation hepatitis—as early as 14 days after exposure and persists during acute illness. It can be detected by radioimmunoassay or, less commonly, by reverse passive hemagglutination during the extended incubation period and usually during the first 3 weeks of acute infection or if the patient is a carrier.

Because transmission of hepatitis is one of the gravest complications associated with blood transfusion, all donors must be screened for HBV before their blood is stored. This screening, required by the Food and Drug Administration's Center for Biologics, has helped reduce the incidence of hepatitis. However, this test does not screen for hepatitis A, hepatitis C, or non-A, non-B viruses.

Purpose
- To screen blood donors for HBV
- To screen persons at high risk for contracting HBV (such as hemodialysis nurses)
- To aid differential diagnosis of viral hepatitis

Patient preparation Explain that this test, which requires a blood sample, helps identify a type of viral hepatitis. If the patient is giving blood, explain the donation procedure.

Procedure Perform a venipuncture, and collect the sample in a 7-ml *red-top* tube.

Findings Normal serum is negative for HBsAg.

Implications of results
: Presence of HBsAg in a patient with hepatitis confirms hepatitis B. In chronic carriers and persons with chronic active hepatitis, HBsAg may be present in serum several months after onset of acute infection. HBsAg may also occur in more than 5% of patients with certain diseases other than hepatitis, such as hemophilia, Hodgkin's disease, and leukemia. If the antigen is found in donor blood, this blood must be discarded because it carries a 40% to 70% risk of transmitting hepatitis. However, blood samples that test positive should be retested for HBsAg because inaccurate results do occur.

Post-test care
: Notify the blood donor if test results are positive for the antigen. Report confirmed viral hepatitis to public health authorities. This is a reportable disease in most states.

Interfering factors
: None

Hepatitis C antibody (anti-HCV), serum

Hepatitis C virus (HCV) causes more than 90% of non-A, non-B hepatitis cases, and more than 80% of community-acquired non-A, non-B hepatitis cases are attributed to HCV infection. Causes include I.V. drug use and abuse, transfusions, dialysis, and needle sticks. The application of the test for HCV has decreased the incidence of post-transfusion hepatitis.

Purpose
: • To detect HCV specific antibodies
  • To aid differential diagnosis of viral hepatitis
  • To screen blood units for transfusion safety

Patient preparation
: Explain that this test is used to identify anti-HCV and to reduce risk of HCV during transfusions. Inform the patient that a blood sample is required. If the patient is giving blood, explain the donation procedure.

Procedure
: Perform a venipuncture, and collect the sample in a *red-top* tube. This test requires 0.5 ml of serum. Freeze the sample and send it to the laboratory.

Findings
: Normal serum is negative for anti-HCV.

Implications of results	The presence of anti-HCV in a patient with acute hepatitis confirms hepatitis C (post-transfusion non-A, non B).
Post-test care	Notify the blood donor if test results are positive for HCV. In most states, you must report confirmed hepatitis to public health authorities.
Interfering factors	None

Hepatitis D antibody (anti-HDV), serum

Hepatitis D virus (HDV), also known as delta hepatitis, occurs only when the patient is already infected with the hepatitis B virus (HBV), either during its acute phase or as a chronic carrier. HDV needs HBV for its replication. HDV is extremely cytopathic for the liver cells it infects, and patients with HDV and HBV have a greater incidence of fulminant hepatitis than patients with HBV alone because HBV is not cytopathic. Clinically, HDV cannot be distinguished from other types of hepatitis. HDV frequently leads to chronic active hepatitis and death but presently is not a reportable disease in most states.

Purpose	To aid differential diagnosis of chronic, recurrent, and acute viral hepatitis
Patient preparation	Explain that this test, which requires a blood sample, helps to identify HDV. If the patient is giving blood, explain the donation procedure. Schedule radioisotope tests after this test.
Procedure	Perform a venipuncture, and collect a 2-ml sample of blood in a 7-ml *red-top* tube. This test requires 2.0 ml of serum. Freeze the sample and send it to the laboratory.
Findings	Normal serum is negative for anti-HDV.
Implications of results	Presence of anti-HDV in patients with HBV indicates infection with HDV.

Post-test care   Notify the blood donor if test results are positive for the antigen.

Interfering   Patients with lipemia or high-titer rheumatoid fac-
factors   tor may have false-positive results.

Hepatitis profile, prenatal

Pregnant patients with acute or chronic hepatitis B virus (HBV) infection have a high potential to pass the disease to their infants through blood transmission during delivery. Neonates infected at birth are at slight risk for acute fulminant hepatitis, which may prove fatal, and at great risk later for chronic hepatitis with all of its associated complications.

Various tests are used to screen pregnant patients for the presence of HBV infection. Routine prenatal screening typically includes hepatitis B surface antigen (HBsAg), hepatitis B e antigen (HBeAg), and Hepatitis B e antibody (anti-HBe). Further investigation may include two other tests. HBV-deoxyribonucleic acid (DNA), which detects the presence of infectious HBV particles in serum, is the most sensitive and accurate test for determining ongoing viral replication and infection. Hepatitis B core antibody (anti-HBc immunoglobulin M [IgM]) can help distinguish between acute and chronic HBV infections.

Purpose   To screen pregnant patients at risk for HBV

Patient   Explain that this test helps detect the presence of
preparation   HBV so that appropriate measures can be taken to protect the neonate at delivery. Inform the patient that the test requires a blood sample.

Procedure   Perform a venipuncture, and collect the sample in a 5-ml *red-top* tube. Send the sample to the laboratory immediately, or refrigerate it if testing is delayed.

Precautions   Because the patient is considered at risk for infection, follow infection prevention techniques throughout the sample collection procedure. Wash your hands thoroughly before and after patient contact, discard used needles and syringes immediately after use in appropriate containers, and handle blood samples with care during collection and transportation to the laboratory. Immediately report any needle sticks or other exposure to the patient's blood.

Findings   No HBsAg, HBeAg, anti-HBe, HBV-DNA, or anti-HBc IgM is normally found in serum.

Implications of results

Positive results for HBsAg indicate active HBV infection. In acute infection HBsAg usually disappears within 1 to 3 months; persistence longer than 6 months may point to chronic hepatitis or a chronic carrier state.

Positive results for HBeAg indicates a highly infectious state; persistence for more than 10 weeks suggests progression to possible chronic hepatitis and carrier state. Anti-HBe indicates decreasing infectivity. Association with anti-HBc without HBsAg and anti-HBs confirms recent acute infection.

Positive results for HBV-DNA indicates the presence of viral DNA in the serum. This is the most accurate assessment of viral replication and infection.

The earliest specific antibody to anti-HBc is IgM. In the anti-HBc IgM test, positive results typically indicate current acute HBV infection and can differentiate acute from chronic HBV. However, anti-HBs and anti-HBcs can persist in a patient's serum for years.

Because mothers with HBV infection usually pass the disease to their infants — 90% of infants born to HBsAg- and HBcAg-positive mothers develop HBV infection — prompt treatment is necessary to protect the infant after birth. One effective treatment involves administration of hepatitis B immune globulin, followed by immunization with HBV vaccine. This provides the infant with both short- and long-term protection against infection. Because the infant will remain at risk for HBV infection throughout childhood, active immunization is required.

Post-test care   If a hematoma develops at the venipuncture site, applying warm soaks eases discomfort.

Interfering factors

• Heparin may impair normal clotting, yielding false-positive results. For this reason, clearly label any sample drawn from a patient receiving heparin therapy so that the laboratory can treat the sample with thrombin or protamine sulfate to ensure complete clotting.

- Although the evidence is still inconclusive, hepatitis B vaccine may yield a false-positive result.

Hereditary angioneurotic edema test

A common genetic abnormality associated with complement, hereditary angioneurotic edema is characterized by episodes of acute edema in subcutaneous tissue, the GI tract, or the upper respiratory tract. Acute respiratory involvement may be life-threatening. The disorder, inherited as an autosomal dominant trait, can result from a low concentration of C1 esterase inhibitor or from the presence of an abnormal, nonfunctional inhibitor protein; either condition disrupts normal regulation of the classical complement pathway, causing excessive breakdown of C4 and C2 and generation of a kininlike fragment of C2.

In this test, designed to confirm diagnosis of hereditary angioneurotic edema, the concentration of C1 esterase inhibitor is determined through a nephelometric assay, in which a specific antiserum is reacted with the patient's serum sample, with the resultant turbidity compared with a known standard. The assay for C1 esterase inhibitor, the second part of the test, detects the presence of abnormal inhibitor protein. In this assay, patient serum is activated with aggregated human immunoglobulin, then monitored in a radial immunodiffusion plate.

However, most laboratories make a tentative diagnosis of hereditary angioneurotic edema with the far simpler C4 assay, and hereditary angioneurotic edema is then confirmed by a C1 esterase inhibitor assay.

Purpose To confirm diagnosis of hereditary angioneurotic edema

Patient preparation Explain that this test panel can confirm whether symptoms are caused by hereditary angioneurotic edema. Inform the patient that fasting is required for at least 12 hours before the test and that the test requires a blood sample.

Procedure Perform a venipuncture, and collect the sample in a 7-ml *red-top* tube. Send the sample to the laboratory immediately. Serum must be separated from the clot and tested within 8 hours of sample collection, or the sample must be frozen at –94° F (–70° C) until testing can be completed.

Values   Normal serum concentration of C1 esterase inhibitor ranges from 8 to 24 mg/dl. For the assay, absence of reaction indicates presence of a normal functional inhibitor protein; reaction indicates abnormal inhibitor protein.

Implications of results   None

Post-test care   If a hematoma develops at the venipuncture site, applying warm soaks eases discomfort.

Interfering factor   Improper sample handling or a delay in testing can cause false-low readings for C4 and C1 esterase inhibitor.

Herpes simplex antibodies, serum

Herpes simplex virus (HSV), a member of the herpesvirus group, causes diseases of varying severity, including oral-pharyngeal infection, gingivostomatitis, genital lesions, keratitis or conjunctivitis, generalized dermal lesions, and pneumonia. Severe involvement is associated with intrauterine or neonatal infections and encephalitis; such infections are most severe in immunosuppressed patients. Of the two closely related antigenic types, type 1 usually causes infections above the waistline; type 2 infections predominantly involve the external genitalia.

Primary contact with this virus occurs in early childhood as acute stomatitis or, more commonly, as an inapparent infection. The virus then exists in a latent form that can be reactivated by ultraviolet light, stress, or immunocompromised conditions. Generally, the prevalence of antibodies to HSV in adults is over 50%; indeed, a majority of adults have been infected with HSV by age 20. Sensitive assays, such as indirect immunofluorescence or enzyme immunoassay (but not complement fixation) are used to demonstrate immunoglobulin M (IgM) class antibodies to HSV or to detect a fourfold or greater increase in immunoglobulin G (IgG) class antibodies between acute- and convalescent-phase sera.

Purpose

To confirm systemic infections caused by HSV

Patient preparation

Explain the purpose of this test and inform the patient that the test will require a blood sample.

Procedure

Perform a venipuncture to collect 5 ml of sterile blood in a tube. Allow the blood to clot for at least 1 hour at room temperature. Handle the sample gently to prevent hemolysis. Transfer the serum to a sterile tube or vial and send it to the laboratory promptly. If transfer must be delayed for 1 or 2 days, store the serum at 39.2° F (4° C) or; if longer, store at –4° F (–20° C) to avoid microbial contamination.

Findings

Patients who experience primary infections with HSV will develop both IgM and IgG class antibodies. Reportedly, over 50% of adults have IgG class antibodies to HSV because of prior infection. Reactivated infections caused by HSV can be recognized serologically only by an increase in IgG class antibodies between acute- and convalescent-phase sera.

Implications of results

HSV infections can be ruled out in patients whose sera show no detectable antibodies to the virus. The presence of IgM or a fourfold or greater increase in IgG antibodies indicates active HSV infection. However, because HSV antibodies are prevalent in the adult population, other procedures, such as direct examination of tissue specimens by an immunofluorescent antibody test, enzyme immunoassay for viral antigens, or culturing, are warranted to make a diagnosis.

Post-test care

If a hematoma develops at the venipuncture site, applying warm soaks eases discomfort.

Interfering factor

Patients with preexisting HSV who are infected with the varicella-zoster virus may have elevated HSV titers caused by cross-reactivity. In such cases, direct examination of tissue specimens by immunofluorescent antibody or enzyme immunoassay for viral antigens or by culturing are needed to make a definitive diagnosis.

Herpes simplex virus culture

Herpes simplex virus (HSV), a herpesvirus, produces a wide spectrum of clinical manifestations, including keratitis, gingivostomatitis, encephalitis, and oftentimes disseminated diseases in immunocompromised individuals. Of the six members of the herpesvirus group (Epstein-Barr virus, cytomegalovirus [CMV], varicella-zoster virus [VZV], human herpesvirus-6, and the two closely related serotypes of HSV — type 1 and type 2 [HSV-1 and HSV-2]) only CMV, VZV, and HSV replicate in the standard cell cultures used in diagnostic laboratories. Of these herpesviruses, HSV replicates most rapidly in cell cultures; approximately 50% of the strains can be detected by characteristic cytopathic effect (CPE) within 24 hours after the laboratory receives the specimen. An additional 5 to 7 days are required to detect the remaining HSV strains. These strains are present in low titers in specimens and thus require a few days in culture to replicate and produce detectable CPE. Alternatively, early antigens of HSV can be detected by monoclonal antibodies in shell vial cell cultures within 16 hours after receipt of the specimen with the same sensitivity and specificity as standard tube cell cultures and detection of the virus by CPE.

Purpose

To confirm diagnosis of HSV infection by culturing the virus from specimens

Patient preparation

Explain that this test will be performed to detect infection by HSV. Specimens should be collected from suspected lesions during the prodromal and acute stages of clinical infection to ensure the best chance of recovering a virus in cell cultures.

Procedure

Collect a specimen for culture into the appropriate collection device as listed below —
Throat, skin, eye, genital area: microbiological transport swab
Body fluids or other respiratory specimens (washings, lavage): sterile screw-capped jar.

Specimens should be transported to the laboratory as soon as possible after collection. If the anticipated time between collection and inoculation of cell cultures is more than 2 to 3 hours, the specimen should be transported at 39.2° F (4° C). Do not freeze the specimen or allow it to dry.

Findings	HSV is rarely recovered from immunocompetent patients who show no overt signs of disease. However, like other herpesviruses, HSV can be shed from immunosuppressed patients intermittently in the absence of apparent disease. For epidemiologic purposes, HSV detected by CPE in standard tube cell cultures must be confirmed and identified by transfer of infected cells to slides with subsequent immunologic serotyping as HSV-1 or HSV-2. In the shell vial assay, this step occurs as part of the initial detection of the virus.
Implications of results	HSV detected in specimens taken from dermal lesions, the eye, cerebrospinal fluid, or tissue are highly significant. Specimens from the upper respiratory tract may be associated with intermittent shedding of the virus, particularly in an immunocompromised patient.
Post-test care	None
Interfering factor	Administration of antiviral drugs before collection of the specimen may interfere with detection of the virus.

Heterophile agglutination tests

Heterophile agglutination tests detect and identify two immunoglobulin antibodies in human serum that agglutinate sheep and horse red cells. The heterophile antibody, also known as the Paul-Bunnell antibody, is the hallmark of the Epstein-Barr virus (EBV) found in the sera of patients with infectious mononucleosis (see Epstein-Barr Virus Antibodies and Infectious Mononucleosis Screening Test). Another antibody, the Forssman antibody, present in some normal serum as well as in conditions such as serum sickness, also agglutinates with sheep red cells, thus rendering test results inconclusive for infectious mononucleosis.

If the Paul-Bunnell test establishes a presumptive titer, the Davidsohn differential absorption test can then be used to distinguish between EBV antibodies and Forssman antibodies.

The B lymphocytes that are infected with EBV produce a variety of antibodies, including the diagnostic heterophile antibody and antibodies against

EBV. Associated antigens include viral capsid antigen, early antigen, and nuclear antigen.

Purpose To aid differential diagnosis of infectious mononucleosis

Patient preparation Explain that this test helps detect infectious mononucleosis. Tell the patient that the test requires a blood sample.

Procedure Perform a venipuncture, and collect the sample in a 7-ml *red-top* tube.

Values Normally, the titer is less than 1:56 but may be higher in elderly patients. Some laboratories refer to a normal titer as "negative" or as having "no reaction."

Implications of results Although heterophile antibodies are present in the sera of approximately 80% of patients with infectious mononucleosis 1 month after onset, a positive finding — a titer higher than 1:56 — does not confirm this disorder; for example, a high titer can result from systemic lupus erythematosus, syphilis, cryoglobulinemia, or the presence of antibodies to nonsyphilitic treponemata (yaws, pinta, bejel).

A gradual increase in titer to about 1:224 during week 3 or 4, followed by a gradual decrease during weeks 4 to 8, proves most conclusive for infectious mononucleosis. However, a negative titer doesn't always rule out this disorder; occasionally, the titer becomes reactive 2 weeks later. Therefore, if symptoms persist, the test should be repeated in 2 weeks.

Confirmation of infectious mononucleosis depends on heterophile agglutination tests and hematologic tests that show absolute lymphocytosis, with 10% to 30% or more atypical lymphocytes.

Post-test care
- If the titer is positive and infectious mononucleosis is confirmed, instruct the patient in the treatment plan. If the titer is positive but infectious mononucleosis isn't confirmed, or if the titer is negative but symptoms persist, explain that additional testing will be necessary in a few days or weeks to confirm diagnosis and plan effective treatment.
- If a hematoma develops at the venipuncture site, applying warm soaks eases discomfort.

Interfering
factors

- If treatment for mononucleosis begins before development of heterophile antibodies, the titer is usually negative.
- Patients addicted to opiates may have high titers. False-positive titers may occur in patients with opiate addiction, serum sickness, leukemia, hepatitis, or pancreatic cancer.

Hexosaminidase A and B, serum

This fluorometric test measures the hexosaminidase A and B content of serum samples drawn by venipuncture or collected from a neonate's umbilical cord or of amniotic fluid obtained by amniocentesis.

Hexosaminidase is a group of enzymes necessary for the metabolism of gangliosides — watersoluble glycolipids found primarily in brain tissue. Deficiency of hexosaminidase A (one of the two hexosaminidase isoenzymes) causes Tay-Sachs disease. In this autosomal recessive disorder, G_{M2} ganglioside accumulates in brain tissue, causing progressive destruction and demyelination of central nervous system cells and usually death by age 3. This disorder most commonly affects persons of Ashkenazic Jewish ancestry. Sandhoff's disease, which results from total hexosaminidase deficiency (both A and B), is an uncommon, virulent variant that produces more rapid deterioration and is not prevalent in any ethnic group.

Hexosaminidase deficiency can also be identified by testing ? culture of skin fibroblasts. However, because this procedure is costly and technically complex, analysis of blood or of amniotic fluid is the prevalent method. A reference center for congenital diseases should be consulted for the best current screening method and the preferred specimen it requires.

Purpose

- To confirm or rule out Tay-Sachs disease in neonates
- To screen for Tay-Sachs carriers
- To establish prenatal diagnosis of hexosaminidase A deficiency

Patient
preparation

When testing an adult, explain that this test identifies a carrier of Tay-Sachs disease. Emphasize the test's importance to an Ashkenazic Jewish couple who plan to have children, and explain that they both must carry the defective gene to transmit Tay-Sachs disease to their offspring. Tell the patient the test requires a blood sample.

When testing a neonate, explain to the parents that this test detects Tay-Sachs disease. Tell them the test requires a blood sample.

Inform the patient or parents that no pretest restrictions of food or fluid are necessary. If the test is being performed prenatally, advise the patient of preparations for amniocentesis.

Procedure

Perform a venipuncture or collect a sample of cord blood. Collect the sample in a 7-ml *red-top* tube. Handle the collection tube gently to prevent hemolysis.

When testing a neonate, check with the laboratory concerning its preferred method and site for collecting serum samples.

Values

Total serum levels of hexosaminidase range from 5 to 12.9 U/L, with hexosaminidase A accounting for 55% to 76% of the total.

Implications of results

Absence of hexosaminidase A indicates Tay-Sachs disease (total hexosaminidase levels can be normal).

Absence of hexosaminidase A and hexosaminidase B (the other isoenzyme) indicates Sandhoff's disease.

Post-test care

- If both parents are carriers for Tay-Sachs disease, refer them for genetic counseling. Be sure to stress the importance of having amniocentesis performed as early as possible during pregnancy.
- If only one partner is a carrier, reassure the couple that there's no risk of their offspring inheriting the disease, since both parents must be carriers to transmit Tay-Sachs disease.
- If a hematoma develops at the venipuncture site, applying warm soaks eases discomfort.

Interfering factor

Hemolysis caused by excessive agitation of the sample may interfere with accurate determination of test results.

HIV antibody, serum enzyme immunoassay

This enzyme immunoassay is a screening test designed to detect the presence of antibodies directed to human immunodeficiency virus (HIV) antigens (see HIV Antibody, Western Blot Assay, the test that confirms the presence of HIV antibodies). Because this test is highly sensitive, it is routinely used to test all donated blood for transfusion and is also used to help diagnose HIV infection. The antibody is produced in response to exposure to the virus, usually within 6 to 8 weeks after that exposure, but, occasionally, a more prolonged "window" period exists between exposure and development of antibody.

Purpose
- To aid in diagnosis of HIV infection
- To detect exposure to HIV

Patient preparation
Be sure to inform patients or blood donors that their blood will be tested for the antibody to HIV. In certain states, reporting a positive test to the state health authorities is mandatory so that epidemiologic studies can be done and probable contacts can be alerted and counseled. Explain that the test requires a blood sample, but requires no dietary or other restrictions before the test.

Procedure
Perform a venipuncture and collect a blood sample in a 7-ml test tube without anticoagulant. Let the sample stand at room temperature to allow clotting to occur, and then send it to the laboratory.

Findings
Normal individuals will test negative, but in populations with an extremely low prevalence of HIV infection, a high percentage of false-positive test results may occur.

Implications of results
A positive test may not indicate exposure to HIV; the test's specificity has been found to be as low as 30%. Because false-positive results are possible, this immunoassay test must always be confirmed by another test method, such as the Western blot, before major decisions regarding the patient's lifestyle, health care, or precautions are taken.

Post-test care
- If the test is confirmed by another method, then the patient and the patient's sexual partner must

have counseling regarding prevention of spread of the virus. The patient's previous sexual partners may also require evaluation and counseling.
- If a hematoma develops at the venipuncture site, applying warm soaks eases discomfort.

Interfering factor

Occasionally, false-positive test results may occur in patients with autoimmune diseases such as systemic lupus erythematosus or patients with antibodies to human leukocyte antigens. Improved test methods may reduce the likelihood of false positives.

HIV antibody, Western blot assay

This test is based upon the principle that antibodies to human immunodeficiency virus (HIV) particles can be detected in an immunoblotting test that separates HIV antigens by their molecular weight. Thus, antibodies can be identified as reacting with specific antigens of particular molecular weights, which are known as bands.

Purpose

To confirm the presence of antibodies to HIV in persons who have reacted with a positive enzyme immunoassay for HIV antibodies

Patient preparation

It is extremely important that patients or blood donors be fully aware that they will be tested for the antibody and, in certain states, the patient's written consent must be obtained. It is also mandatory in certain states that a positive test be reported to the state health authorities so that epidemiologic studies can be done and probable contacts can be alerted and counseled. Inform the patient that the test requires a blood sample, but requires no dietary or other restrictions before the test.

Procedure

Perform a venipuncture and collect one sample in a 7-ml tube without anticoagulant. Let the sample stand at room temperature to allow clotting to occur, and then send it to the laboratory.

Findings

The normal test result is negative for antibodies to HIV.

Implications of results	A positive test confirms that the patient has antibodies to HIV. As in the enzyme immunoassay, a positive test result does not mean that the patient now has acquired immunodeficiency syndrome (AIDS) but that it is likely to develop within about 10 years; however, the length of time between infection and the development of clinical AIDS varies greatly.
Post-test care	• Patients who have a positive test result should receive expert counseling and medical attention to plan and carry out the most effective preventive therapy and treatment for AIDS and its various complications. The patient's contacts who may have been exposed to the virus through sexual activity or needle sharing also should be tested and counseled appropriately. • If a hematoma develops at the venipuncture site, applying warm soaks eases discomfort.
Interfering factor	Various antibodies to a variety of antigens may occasionally result in bands that do not correspond exactly to those required for a positive diagnosis of HIV. The causes of many of these indeterminate test results are not known at this time. Because of its grave implications for the patient's life and future, interpretation of Western blot tests for HIV requires the greatest possible care.

Homovanillic acid, urine

This test is a quantitative analysis of urine levels of homovanillic acid (HVA), one of three major catecholamines and a metabolite of dopamine. Synthesized primarily in the brain, dopamine is a precursor to epinephrine and norepinephrine, the other principal catecholamines. The liver breaks down most dopamine into HVA for eventual excretion; a minimal amount of dopamine is excreted in the urine.

Using two-dimensional chromatography, urine HVA levels are usually measured simultaneously with the major catecholamines and other catecholamine metabolites —metanephrine, normetanephrine, and vanillylmandelic acid. The principal indication for this test is suspected neuroblastoma or ganglioneuroma, which usually affects young children and adolescents.

Purpose
- To aid diagnosis of neuroblastoma and ganglioneuroma
- To rule out pheochromocytoma

Patient preparation

Explain that this test assesses secretion of certain hormones. Inform the patient that restriction of food or fluids is not required before the test, but that stressful situations and excessive physical exercise should be avoided during the collection period. Tell the patient the test requires collection of a 24-hour urine specimen, and teach the proper collection technique.

Check the patient's history for medications that may affect test results. As ordered, withhold these drugs before the test.

Procedure

To keep the specimen at a pH of 2.0 to 4.0, collect a 24-hour urine specimen in a bottle containing a preservative. Refrigerate the specimen or keep it on ice during the collection period. When the collection is completed, send the specimen to the laboratory immediately.

Values

Normally, the urine HVA value for adults is less than 8 mg/day (40 mmol/day). The range of normal urine HVA (mcg/mg creatinine) values in children varies with age:

Age (years)	HVA µg/ mg creatinine	HVA µmol/ mmol creatinine
0 to 1	1.2 to 35	0.7 to 21
1 to 2	4 to 23	2.4 to 14
2 to 5	0.5 to 13.5	0.3 to 8
5 to 10	0.5 to 9	0.3 to 5.4
10 to 15	0.25 to 12	0.2 to 7.2
15 to 17	0.5 to 2	0.3 to 1.2

Implications of results

Elevated urine HVA levels suggest neuroblastoma, a malignant soft-tissue tumor that develops in infants and young children, or ganglioneuroma, a tumor of the sympathetic nervous system that develops in older children and adolescents and rarely metastasizes. HVA levels don't usually rise in patients with pheochromocytoma because this tumor secretes mainly epinephrine, which metabolizes primarily into vanillylmandelic acid. Thus, abnormally high urine HVA levels generally rule out pheochromocytoma.

Post-test care   The patient may resume withheld medications and normal activity.

Interfering factors

- Monoamine oxidase inhibitors decrease urine HVA levels by inhibiting dopamine metabolism. Aspirin, methocarbamol, and levodopa may raise or lower HVA levels.
- Failure to observe drug restrictions, to collect all urine during the test period, or to store the specimen properly may interfere with test results.
- Excessive physical exercise or emotional stress during the collection period may increase HVA levels.

Human chorionic gonadotropin (hCG), serum

Human chorionic gonadotropin (hCG) is a glycoprotein hormone produced by the trophoblastic cells of the placenta. If conception occurs, a specific assay for hCG — commonly called the beta-subunit assay — may detect this hormone in the blood 9 days after ovulation. This interval coincides with the implantation of the fertilized ovum into the uterine wall. With progesterone, hCG maintains the corpus luteum during early pregnancy.

Production of hCG increases steadily during the first trimester, peaking around the 10th week of gestation. Levels then fall to less than 10% of first trimester peak levels during the remainder of the pregnancy. At approximately 2 weeks after delivery, the hormone may no longer be detectable.

This serum radioimmunoassay, a quantitative analysis of the hCG beta-subunit level, is slightly more sensitive (and far more costly) than modern urine pregnancy tests.

Purpose

- To detect early pregnancy
- To determine adequacy of hormonal production in high-risk pregnancies (for example, habitual spontaneous abortion)
- To aid diagnosis of trophoblastic tumors, such as hydatidiform moles or choriocarcinoma, and especially to monitor for tumor recurrence after completion of successful therapy
- To monitor induction of ovulation and conception

Patient preparation	Explain the purpose of this test. Inform the patient that restriction of food or fluids before the test is not required and that the test requires a blood sample. Perform radioisotope scans after collection.
Procedure	Perform a venipuncture, and collect the sample in a 7-ml *red-top* tube. Handle the sample gently to prevent hemolysis, and send it to the laboratory immediately.
Values	Normal values for hCG are less than 3 mIU/ml (U/L). During pregnancy, hCG levels vary and depend partially on the number of days after the last normal menstrual period.
Implications of results	Elevated hCG beta-subunit levels indicate pregnancy; significantly higher concentrations are present in a multiple pregnancy. Increased levels may also suggest hydatidiform mole, trophoblastic neoplasms of the placenta, or nontrophoblastic carcinomas that secrete hCG (including gastric, pancreatic, and ovarian adenocarcinomas). Low hCG beta-subunit levels can occur in ectopic pregnancy or pregnancy of less than 9 days. Beta-subunit levels cannot differentiate between pregnancy and tumor recurrence because these levels are high in both conditions.
Post-test care	If a hematoma develops at the venipuncture site, applying warm soaks eases discomfort.
Interfering factors	• Heparin anticoagulants or EDTA depresses plasma hCG levels and may interfere with accurate determination of test results. Check with the laboratory about whether the test should be performed on plasma or serum. • Hemolysis caused by excessive agitation of the sample may affect test results. • Radioisotope scans will also affect test results.

Human chorionic gonadotropin (hCG), urine
Pregnancy test

As a qualitative analysis of urine levels of human chorionic gonadotropin (hCG), this test can detect pregnancy as early as 10 days after a missed menstrual period. Quantitative measurements can evaluate suspected hydatidiform mole or hCG-secreting tumors. After conception occurs, placental trophoblastic cells start to produce hCG, a glycoprotein, which prevents degeneration of the corpus luteum at the end of the normal menstrual cycle. The corpus luteum then secretes large quantities of progesterone and estrogen, promoting early development of the endometrium, placenta, and fetus. During the first trimester, hCG levels rise steadily and rapidly, peaking around the 10th week of gestation, subsequently tapering off to less than 10% of peak levels.

The most common method of evaluating hCG in urine is hemagglutination inhibition. This laboratory procedure, based on an antigen-antibody reaction, can provide both qualitative and quantitative information. The qualitative urine test is easier and less costly than the serum hCG test (beta-subunit assay), and thus is used more frequently to detect pregnancy. The earliest possible determination of pregnancy (as early as 7 days after conception) can be achieved only through the serum hCG test.

Purpose	• To detect and confirm pregnancy • To aid diagnosis of hydatidiform mole or hCG-secreting tumors
Patient preparation	Explain to the patient the purpose of this test. Inform her that she needn't restrict food or fluids before the test, and that the test requires a first-voided morning specimen or a 24-hour urine collection, depending on whether the test is qualitative or quantitative. Check the patient's recent medication history for use of drugs that may affect hCG levels.
Procedure	For verification of pregnancy (qualitative analysis), collect a first-voided morning specimen. If this is not possible, collect a random specimen. For quantitative analysis of hCG, collect a 24-hour urine specimen. Refrigerate the 24-hour specimen or keep it on ice during the collection period. Specify the date of the patient's last menstrual period on the laboratory slip.
Values	In qualitative analysis, test results are positive when agglutination fails to occur, thus indicating pregnancy. In quantitative analysis, urine hCG levels in the first trimester of a normal pregnancy may be as

high as 500,000 IU/day; in the second trimester, they range from 10,000 to 25,000 IU/day; and in the third trimester, from 5,000 to 15,000 IU/day. After delivery, hCG levels decline rapidly and within a few days are undetectable.

Measurable hCG shouldn't be found in the urine of males or nonpregnant females.

Implications of results

During pregnancy, elevated urine hCG levels may indicate multiple pregnancy or erythroblastosis fetalis; depressed urine hCG levels may indicate threatened abortion or ectopic pregnancy. Measurable levels of hCG in males and nonpregnant females may indicate choriocarcinoma, ovarian or testicular tumors, melanoma, multiple myeloma, or gastric, hepatic, pancreatic, or breast cancer.

Post-test care

The patient may resume discontinued medications.

Interfering factors

- Gross proteinuria (in excess of 1 g/day), hematuria, or an elevated erythrocyte sedimentation rate may produce false-positive results, depending on the laboratory method used.
- Early pregnancy, ectopic pregnancy, or threatened spontaneous abortion may produce false-negative test results.
- Phenothiazines may cause false-negative or false-positive test results.
- Contamination of the specimen with tap water or soap may produce false-positive test results.

Human chorionic somatomammotropin

Human placental lactogen (hPL)

A polypeptide hormone secreted by placental syncytial trophoblasts, human placental lactogen (hPL) displays lactogenic and somatotropic (growth hormone) properties in the pregnant patient. In combination with prolactin, hPL prepares the breasts for lactation. It also promotes lipolysis, liberating free fatty acids to provide energy for maternal metabolism and fetal nutrition. By exerting an anti-insulin effect, hPL causes the pancreas to secrete more insulin in response to rising blood sugar levels, thus facilitating protein synthesis and mobilization essential to fetal growth. Secretion is autonomous, beginning about the 5th week of gestation and declining rapidly after delivery. According to some evidence, this hormone may not be essential for a successful pregnancy.

This radioimmunoassay measures plasma hPL levels, which are roughly proportional to placental mass, as evidenced by higher levels in a multiple pregnancy. Such assays may be required in high-risk pregnancies (patients with diabetes mellitus, hypertension, or toxemia) or in suspected placental tissue dysfunction. Because values vary widely during the last half of pregnancy, serial determinations over several days provide the most reliable test results. This test, when combined with measurement of estriol levels, is a reliable indicator of placental function as well as fetal well-being. This test may also be useful as a tumor marker in certain malignant states, such as ectopic tumors that secrete hPL.

Purpose
- To assess placental function
- To aid diagnosis of hydatidiform mole and choriocarcinoma (human chorionic gonadotropin levels are more diagnostic in these conditions)
- To aid diagnosis and monitor treatment of ectopic nontrophoblastic tumors that secrete hPL

Patient preparation
Explain the purpose of this test and tell the patient that the test requires a blood sample. Inform the pregnant patient that this test may be repeated during her pregnancy.

Procedure
Perform a venipuncture, and collect the sample in a 7-ml *red-top* tube. Handle the sample gently to prevent hemolysis, and send it to the laboratory promptly.

Values
For pregnant females, values are as follows:

Weeks of gestation	Normal hPL levels
25 to 27	4.6 µg/ml (mg/L)
28 to 31	2.4 to 6.1 µg/ml (mg/L)
32 to 35	3.7 to 7.7 µg/ml (mg/L)
36 to term	5 to 8.6 µg/ml (mg/L)

At term, females with diabetes mellitus may have mean levels of 9 to 11 µg/ml (mg/L).

Normal levels for nonpregnant females are less than 0.5 µg/ml (mg/L); normal levels for males, less than 0.5 µg/ml (mg/L).

Implications of results

For reliable interpretation, hPL levels must be correlated with gestational age; for example, after 30 weeks' gestation, levels below 4 µg/ml (mg/L) may indicate placental dysfunction. Subnormal concentrations of hPL are also associated with trophoblastic neoplastic disease, such as hydatidiform mole or choriocarcinoma. Low hPL concentrations are also characteristically associated with postmaturity syndrome, retardation of intrauterine growth, and toxemia of pregnancy. However, low hPL concentrations don't confirm fetal distress, although declining concentrations may help differentiate incomplete spontaneous abortion from threatened spontaneous abortion.

Conversely, hPL concentrations over 4 µg/ml after 30 weeks' gestation don't guarantee fetal well-being because elevated levels have been reported after fetal death. An hPL value above 6 µg/ml after 30 weeks' gestation may suggest an unusually large placenta, commonly occurring in patients with diabetes mellitus, multiple pregnancy, or Rh isoimmunization. Nevertheless, this test has limited use in predicting fetal death in a patient with diabetes or in managing Rh isoimmunization during pregnancy.

Abnormal concentrations of hPL have been found in the sera of patients with various malignant diseases, including bronchogenic cancer, hepatoma, lymphoma, and pheochromocytoma. In these patients, hPL levels are used as tumor markers for evaluation of chemotherapy, for monitoring tumor growth and recurrence, and for detection of residual tissue after excision.

Post-test care

If a hematoma develops at the venipuncture site, applying warm soaks eases discomfort.

Interfering factor

Hemolysis caused by excessive agitation of the sample may interfere with accurate determination of test results.

Human leukocyte antigen (HLA) typing

Human leukocyte antigens (HLA) are molecules on the surface of cells that present to processed antigens so that they can be recognized by T cells. These molecules are of two main classes: class I and class II. Class I molecules are expressed on nearly all cells and bind antigens made within these cells, including fragments of viral proteins and normal cellular proteins. $CD8^+$ T cells recognize antigens bound to class I molecules and, if the cells are infected, kill them. Class II molecules are only expressed on macrophages, B cells, and activated T cells. Foreign antigens (from bacteria, fungi, or parasites) are taken up by these cells, processed, and presented to $CD4^+$ T cells by class II molecules. $CD4^+$ T cells regulate how B cells produce immunoglobulin.

Matching for these antigens is important in organ transplantation and also in the selection of the most appropriate platelet donors for patients who are refractory to random platelets. Some HLA antigens are associated with certain diseases, for example, HLA-B27 with ankylosing spondylitis or HLA-DR2 with narcolepsy. Occasionally a test may be ordered for and restricted to the detection of one specific HLA antigen (for example, HLA-B27).

Purpose
- To identify the closest match between donor and recipient for the purpose of organ transplantation
- To identify a marker for a particular disease
- To aid interpretation in cases of disputed parentage

Patient preparation
Explain the purpose of this test and inform the patient that the test requires a blood sample. Advise the patient that no dietary or other restrictions are necessary before the test.

Procedure
Perform a venipuncture and collect 15 ml of blood in tubes containing acid-citrate-dextrose solution B. Mix the tubes well. Label them appropriately and send them to the laboratory immediately. Do not refrigerate or freeze the samples.

Findings
Results will be expressed to indicate the numerical designation of the antigens found. Each person can

have two antigens detected at each of the loci indicated above.

HLA typing results between the potential donor and recipient may be found to have various degrees of matching. This correlates with the ability to transplant bone marrow and with the long-term graft results of kidney and, perhaps, liver, heart, or pancreas transplantations.

HLA class I antigen matching for platelets correlates with the function and life span of the transfusion platelets in a patient who is refractory to treatment.

Comparison of results in a mother, child, and putative father may rule out or indicate a high probability of paternity.

Post-test care

If a hematoma develops at the venipuncture site, applying warm soaks eases discomfort.

Interfering factors

None

Hydroxybutyric dehydrogenase (HBD)
Alpha-hydroxybutyric dehydrogenase

Hydroxybutyric dehydrogenase (HBD) is one of five isoenzymes of lactate dehydrogenase (LD), known as LD_1. Measurement of serum HBD is sometimes used as a substitute for LD isoenzyme fractionation because this analysis is easier to perform and less costly than LD electrophoresis. Because HBD levels remain elevated for 18 days after myocardial infarction (MI) when other cardiac enzymes have returned to normal, this test is used to aid diagnosis of MI.

Although HBD concentration predominately reflects LD_1 and LD_2 activity, it may also show LD_5 activity, if enough of this isoenzyme is present (as it is in some forms of hepatic disease). Therefore, this test isn't consistently reliable in distinguishing between myocardial and hepatic cellular damage.

Purpose

• To aid diagnosis of MI when LD isoenzyme assay is unavailable
• To monitor cardiac isoenzyme activity when LD_1 level is elevated

- To detect MI after other enzyme levels drop to normal (HBD remains elevated longer)
- To support diagnosis of conditions associated with elevated HBD levels (leukemia, lymphomas, melanomas, muscular dystrophy, nephrotic syndrome, and hemolytic and megaloblastic anemias)
- To aid in differentiating between cardiac and hepatic cellular damage when total LD is elevated (LD-HBD ratio is commonly used)

Patient preparation

Explain that this test evaluates the function of the heart or liver. Inform the patient that no restriction of food or fluids is required before the test and that the test requires a blood sample. Tell the patient suspected of having an MI that the test will be repeated on subsequent mornings to monitor his progress.

Procedure

Perform a venipuncture, and collect the sample in a 7-ml *red-top* tube. For patients with MI, draw blood at the same time each morning.

Handle the collection tube gently to prevent hemolysis, because red blood cells contain LD_1. Because HBD activity is unstable at room temperature, send the sample to the laboratory immediately or refrigerate it at 32° to 39.2° F (0° to 4° C).

Values

Serum HBD values range from 114 to 290 U/L. Ratio of serum LD to HBD normally varies from 1.2 to 1.6:1.

Implications of results

In patients with MI, HBD levels peak 72 hours after onset of chest pain and remain elevated for 2 weeks. The LD-HBD ratio is decreased because of greater activity of LD_1 and LD_2, as reflected in HBD levels; total LD rises less markedly. HBD levels are also raised by hemolytic or megaloblastic anemia, muscular dystrophy, and moderate-to-severe acute hepato-cellular damage. Acute hepatitis increases the LD-HBD ratio, because HBD levels are less sensitive to hepatocellular damage than LD levels, which increase moderately.

Post-test care

If a hematoma develops at the venipuncture site, applying warm soaks eases discomfort.

Interfering factors
- Failure to draw the sample on schedule, thereby missing peak levels, may interfere with accurate determination of values.
- Failure to send the sample to the laboratory promptly or to refrigerate the sample may influence test results.
- Hemolysis of the blood sample may raise serum HBD levels.
- Surgery or cardioversion can elevate serum HBD levels.

17-Hydroxycorticosteroids, urine

This test measures urine levels of 17-hydroxycorticosteroids (17-OHCS) — metabolites of the hormones that regulate glyconeogenesis. More than 80% of all urinary 17-OHCS are metabolites of cortisol, the primary adrenocortical steroid. Test findings thus reflect cortisol secretion and, indirectly, adrenocortical function. Because cortisol secretion varies diurnally and in response to stress and many other factors, urine 17-OHCS levels are most accurately determined from a 24-hour urine specimen. Spectrophotofluorometry is used to measure 17-OHCS levels. Levels of plasma cortisol, urine free cortisol, and urine 17-ketosteroids may be measured, and adrenocorticotropic hormone (ACTH) stimulation and suppression testing performed to confirm results of this test.

Purpose
To assess adrenocortical function

Patient preparation
Explain that this test evaluates function of the adrenal glands. Inform the patient that restriction of food or fluids is not required, but that he should avoid excessive physical exercise and stressful situations during the testing period. Tell the patient this test requires collection of a 24-hour urine specimen, and teach the proper collection technique.

Check the patient's medication history for drugs that may affect 17-OHCS levels. As ordered, restrict these medications before the test.

Procedure
To prevent deterioration of the specimen, collect a 24-hour urine specimen in a bottle containing a preservative. Refrigerate the specimen or place it on ice during the collection period.

Values   Normally, urine 17-OHCS values range from 4.5 to
12 mg/day (12 to 23 μmol/day) in males, and from
2.5 to 10 mg/day (7 to 27 μmol/day) in females.
Children ages 8 to 12 normally excrete less than 4.5
mg/day (12 μmol/day); younger children excrete
less than 1.5 mg/day (4 μmol/day). Levels normally increase slightly during the first trimester of
pregnancy. Patients who are obese or extremely
muscular may excrete slightly higher amounts of
17-OHCS, because of increased cortisol catabolism.

Implications of   Elevated urine 17-OHCS levels may indicate Cush-
results   ing's syndrome, adrenal carcinoma or adenoma, or
pituitary tumor. Increased levels may also occur in
patients with virilism, hyperthyroidism, and severe
hypertension. Extreme stress induced by conditions such as acute pancreatitis and eclampsia, can
also cause urine 17-OHCS levels to increase.
    Low urine 17-OHCS levels may indicate Addi-
son's disease, hypopituitarism, or myxedema.

Post-test care   The patient may resume restricted activity and
medications.

Interfering   • Drugs that may elevate urine 17-OHCS levels
factors   include meprobamate, phenothiazines, spirono-
             lactone, ascorbic acid, chloral hydrate, glutethi-
             mide, chlordiazepoxide, penicillin G, hydroxyzine,
             quinidine, quinine, the iodides, and methena-
             mine.
           • Drugs that may suppress urine 17-OHCS levels
             include hydralazine, phenytoin, thiazide diuret-
             ics, ethinamate, nalidixic acid, and reserpine.
           • Failure to follow drug restrictions, to collect all
             urine during the test period, or to store the spec-
             imen properly may interfere with test results.

5-Hydroxyindoleacetic acid (5-HIAA), urine

This quantitative analysis of urine levels of 5-
hydroxyindoleacetic acid (5-HIAA) is used primarily to screen for carcinoid tumors (argentaffinomas). Urine 5-HIAA levels reflect plasma
concentrations of serotonin (5-hydroxytryptam-
ine). This powerful vasopressor is produced by
argentaffin cells, primarily in the intestinal mucosa,

and is metabolized through oxidative deamination into 5-HIAA. Carcinoid tumors, found generally in the intestine or appendix, secrete an excessive amount of serotonin, which is reflected by high 5-HIAA levels. This test measures 5-HIAA levels by the colorimetric technique and is most accurately performed with a 24-hour urine specimen, which can detect small or intermittently secreting carcinoid tumors.

Purpose

To aid diagnosis of carcinoid tumors (argentaffinomas)

Patient preparation

Explain the purpose of this test. Instruct the patient to avoid foods containing serotonin, such as bananas, plums, pineapples, avocados, eggplant, tomatoes, or walnuts, for 4 days before the test. Tell the patient this test requires collection of a 24-hour urine specimen, and teach the proper collection technique.

Check the patient's medication history for recent use of drugs that may affect test results. As ordered, withhold these drugs before the test.

Procedure

To keep the specimen at a pH of 2.0 to 4.0, collect a 24-hour urine specimen in a bottle containing a preservative. Refrigerate the specimen or keep it on ice during the collection period. When the collection is completed, send the specimen to the laboratory immediately.

Values

Normally, urine 5-HIAA values are less than 6 mg/day (30 mmol/day).

Implications of results

Marked elevation of urine 5-HIAA levels, possibly as high as 200 to 600 mg/day (1,000 to 3,000 mmol/day), indicates a carcinoid tumor. However, because these tumors vary in their capacity to store and secrete serotonin, some patients with carcinoid syndrome (metastatic carcinoid tumors) may not show elevated levels. Repeated testing is often necessary.

Post-test care

The patient may resume restricted medications and a normal diet.

Interfering factors

• Melphalan, reserpine, and fluorouracil raise urine 5-HIAA levels. Ethanol, tricyclic antidepressants, monoamine oxidase inhibitors, methyldopa, and isoniazid characteristically suppress 5-HIAA levels.

- Methenamine compounds, phenothiazines, salicylates, guaifenesin, methocarbamol, and acetaminophen may raise or lower 5-HIAA levels.
- Failure to observe drug and dietary restrictions, to collect all urine during the test period, or to store the specimen properly may interfere with accurate determination of test results.
- Severe GI disturbance or diarrhea may interfere with accurate determination of test results.

Hydroxyproline, urine

The test measures total urine levels of hydroxyproline, an amino acid found mainly in collagen (a component of skin and bone). Urine hydroxyproline levels are a good index of bone matrix turnover because levels increase when collagen breaks down during bone resorption. Bone matrix turnover and hydroxyproline levels normally rise in children during periods of rapid skeletal growth. However, they also rise in disorders that increase bone resorption, such as Paget's disease, metastatic bone tumors, and certain endocrine disorders. This test helps diagnose these disorders, but it's more commonly used to monitor response to drug therapy in conditions marked by rapid bone resorption.

Hydroxyproline levels are most often determined colorimetrically on a timed urine sample; they may also be determined by ion-exchange or gas-liquid chromatography. A collagen-restricted diet is essential for this test because hydroxyproline levels reflect collagen intake. Free hydroxyproline, a small component of total hydroxyproline and a sensitive indicator of dietary collagen intake, may be measured to validate results.

Purpose	• To monitor treatment for disorders characterized by bone resorption, primarily Paget's disease • To aid diagnosis of disorders characterized by bone resorption
Patient preparation	Explain that this test helps monitor treatment or detect an amino acid disorder related to bone formation. Tell the patient to avoid meat, fish, poultry, jelly, or any food containing gelatin for 24 hours be-

fore and during the test. Inform the patient that this test requires a 2-hour or 24-hour urine specimen, as appropriate, and teach the proper collection technique.

Note the patient's age and sex on the laboratory slip. Check the patient's medication history for drugs that may alter test results. Restrict such drugs, as appropriate.

Procedure
Collect a 2-hour or 24-hour urine specimen, as ordered, in a container that has a preservative that prevents degradation of hydroxyproline. Refrigerate the specimen or keep it on ice during the collection period, and send it to the laboratory immediately.

Values
Normal values for adults are 14 to 45 mg/day (110 to 350 μmol/day). For a 2-hour specimen, normal values are 0.4 to 5 mg (3 to 40 μmol/day) for males and 0.4 to 2.9 mg (3 to 20 μmol/day) for females. Normal values for children are much higher and peak between ages 11 and 18. Values also rise during the third trimester of pregnancy, reflecting fetal skeletal growth.

Implications of results
Hydroxyproline levels should decrease slowly during therapy for bone resorption disorders. Elevated levels may indicate bone disease, metastatic bone tumors, or endocrine disorders that stimulate hormonal secretion.

Post-test care
The patient may resume withheld foods and medications.

Interfering factors
• Ascorbic acid, vitamin D, aspirin, glucocorticoids, calcitonin (used to treat Paget's disease), and plicamycin can decrease urine hydroxyproline levels.
• Failure to observe appropriate restrictions, to collect all urine during the test period, or to store the specimen correctly may alter test results.
• Psoriasis and burns can promote collagen turnover, elevating urine hydroxyproline levels.

Hypothyroidism, congenital screening test

This test measures serum thyroxine (T_4) levels in the neonate to detect congenital hypothyroidism. Characterized by absence or low levels of T_4, congenital hypothyroidism affects roughly 1 in 5,000 neonates, occurring in girls three times more often than in boys. This disorder can result from thyroid dysgenesis or hypoplasia, congenital goiter, or maternal use of thyroid inhibitors during pregnancy. If untreated, congenital hypothyroidism can lead to irreversible brain damage by age 3 months. Because clinical signs are few, this disorder typically went undetected until cretinism became apparent or death followed respiratory distress. Recently, however, radioimmunoassays for T_4 and thyroid-stimulating hormone (TSH) have been used effectively to screen neonates for congenital hypothyroidism. This test is now mandatory in some states.

Purpose To screen neonates for congenital hypothyroidism

Patient preparation Explain to the parents that although hypothyroidism is uncommon in infants, this screening test detects the disorder early enough to begin therapy before irreversible brain damage occurs. Tell the parents that the test will be performed before the infant is discharged from the hospital and again 4 to 6 weeks later. Emphasize the importance of the screening and the need for following the test protocol.

Because false-positive findings can result from variations in the test procedure or from a congenital thyroxine-binding globulin (TBG) defect, inform the parents that a second test may be necessary.

Equipment Alcohol or povidone-iodine sponges, sterile lancet, specially marked filter paper, $2'' \times 2''$ sterile gauze pads, small adhesive bandage strip, labels

Procedure After assembling the necessary equipment and washing your hands thoroughly, wipe the neonate's heel with an alcohol or a povidone-iodine sponge. Then dry it thoroughly with a gauze pad.

Perform a heelstick. Squeezing the heel gently, fill the circles on the filter paper with blood. Make sure the blood saturates the paper. Apply gentle pressure with a gauze pad to ensure hemostasis at the puncture site. When the filter paper is dry, label it appropriately and send it to the laboratory.

Values
Immediately after birth, neonatal T_4 levels are considerably higher than normal adult levels. By the end of the first week, however, T_4 values decrease markedly:

Age (days)	Total T_4 level	
	(μg/dl)	(nmol/L)
1 to 3	10.1 to 20.9	130 to 280
7 to 14	9.8 to 16.6	125 to 215
15 to 28	8.2 to 16.6	110 to 215
30 to 120	7.1 to 15.0	100 to 195

Implications of results
Low serum T_4 levels in the neonate require TSH testing for confirmation of the diagnosis. Decreased T_4 levels accompanied by elevated TSH readings (more than 25 mIU/liter) indicate primary congenital hypothyroidism (thyroid gland dysfunction). If both T_4 and TSH levels are depressed, secondary congenital hypothyroidism (resulting from pituitary or hypothalamic dysfunction) should be suspected. If T_4 levels are subnormal in the presence of normal TSH readings, further testing is required.

Serum TBG levels must be analyzed to identify infants with low total T_4 resulting from congenital defects in TBG. This low T_4-normal TSH pattern also occurs in a transient form of congenital hypothyroidism, which may accompany prematurity or prenatal hypoxia.

A complete thyroid workup — including serum T_3, TBG, and free T_4 levels — is necessary for unequivocal diagnosis of congenital hypothyroidism before treatment begins.

Post-test care
• Heelsticks heal readily and require no special care.
• If results of the screening test suggest congenital hypothyroidism, tell the parents additional testing will be required to confirm the disorder.
• If diagnosis is confirmed, inform the parents that replacement therapy can restore normal thyroid gland function. Emphasize that such therapy is lifelong and that dosage will increase until adult requirement is reached.

- If the sample is not processed in the hospital laboratory, be sure parents are notified when test results are available.

Interfering factors

Failure to allow the filter paper to dry completely or to follow special directions for obtaining the sample may interfere with determination of accurate results.

I-J

Imipramine and desipramine, serum

Imipramine and desipramine are tricyclic antidepressants (TCAs) used to treat endogenous depression. Imipramine is also used to treat childhood enuresis. These drugs, which inhibit the reuptake of the neurotransmitters norepinephrine and serotonin at the synaptic cleft, are thought to potentiate synaptic transmission in the central nervous system (CNS). Because imipramine is metabolized to desipramine, both drugs are present in serum after the administration of imipramine. Reverse conversion does not occur; therefore, after the administration of desipramine, only this drug is present in serum.

Monitoring the serum levels of TCAs has proved useful because evaluation of depressive symptoms is subjective, while clinical studies have reported a superior response rate in patients whose serum levels were kept within a defined therapeutic range. Unlike nortriptyline, imipramine and desipramine have less evidence for a "therapeutic window" (see Amitriptyline and Nortriptyline, Serum). Nevertheless, patients with serum levels below the therapeutic threshold tend to show poorer clinical response rates than those with levels within the therapeutic range. In serious overdose, cardiac and CNS toxicities may predominate.

Imipramine and desipramine are most commonly measured in serum by enzyme immunoassay or high-performance liquid chromatography.

Purpose
- To monitor and maintain drug dosage at therapeutic levels
- To assess patient compliance
- To help assess toxicity after overdose

Patient preparation
Explain the purpose of this test, and inform the patient that the test requires a blood sample, but does not require fasting before the test.

When a patient begins therapy with either imipramine or desipramine, at least 7 days are required to achieve a steady state serum level. Monitoring serum levels before the attainment of steady state is not recommended because the results are uninterpretable. Similarly, any change in the total daily dose requires at least 7 days to establish a new steady state. For patients at steady state on single daily doses, samples should be collected between 10 and 14 hours after the last dose. For patients on a divided daily dose, samples should be collected 4 to 6 hours after the last dose.

Procedure
Perform a venipuncture, and collect a blood sample into a 7-ml *red-top* tube. (Collection tubes containing a gel separator should not be used.) Serum should be separated from the clot within 1 hour. Handle the sample gently to prevent hemolysis because these drugs are concentrated in erythrocytes. Heparinized plasma is also suitable.

Imipramine and desipramine are stable in serum or plasma for at least 5 days at room temperature and for longer periods when refrigerated at 39.2° F (4° C).

Values
For patients treated with imipramine, the therapeutic range for the *total* of imipramine plus desipramine is 125 to 275 ng/ml (0.45 to 1.35 μmol/L). For patients treated with desipramine, the therapeutic range is 75 to 225 ng/ml (0.45 to 1.35 μmol/L).

Total tricyclic levels less than 450 ng/ml (1.6 μmol/L) are often associated with toxicity; levels less than 1,000 ng/ml (3.6 μmol/L) are usually associated with severe toxicity.

Implications of results
Serum levels below the therapeutic range are associated with an increased probability of poor therapeutic response. Patients with steady state levels within the therapeutic range who have not responded after 3 or 4 weeks of therapy may require treatment with a different antidepressant.

Post-test care
If a hematoma develops at the venipuncture site, applying warm soaks may ease discomfort.

Interfering factor
Hemolysis of the sample may cause false-high serum levels.

Immune complex assays, serum

Circulating immune complex

Immune complexes are combinations of antigens and antibodies that can activate the complement cascade. In the blood, soluble, circulating immune complexes may cause severe damage, usually in the renal glomeruli, the aorta, and other large blood vessels. When they are produced faster than they can be cleared by the lymphoreticular system, they can cause severe inflammatory disorders. Immune complexes are commonly present in autoimmune disorders such as systemic lupus erythematosus (SLE), postinfectious syndromes, serum sickness, drug sensitivity, and rheumatoid arthritis.

Various methods are currently used to detect circulating complexes of various sizes and properties. Physical methods include ultracentrifugation and gel filtration, cryoprecipitation, and nephelometry. Reactions with rheumatoid factor or complement include precipitin reactions, inhibition of agglutination of immunoglobulin G-coated latex particles, C1q binding, radio assay, and conglutinin binding. Interactions with cell receptors include the platelet aggregation test, inhibitions of phagocytosis, and the Raji cell assay.

The most common methods for diluting circulatory immune complexes include assays that detect C1q binding and methods that detect C3 activation, such as the Raji cell assay. Other test methods may be appropriate, using C1 or the rheumatoid factor (RF). More than one test may be required to achieve accurate results.

Purpose
- To demonstrate circulating immune complexes in serum
- To monitor response to therapy
- To estimate severity of disease

Patient preparation
Explain that these tests help evaluate immune system function, that the test may be repeated to monitor the response to therapy, and that the test requires a blood sample.

If the patient is scheduled for C1q assays, check the patient's history for recent heparin therapy, which may affect test results. Report such therapy to the laboratory.

Procedure   Perform a venipuncture, and collect the sample in a 7-ml *red-top* tube.

Send the sample to the laboratory immediately to prevent deterioration of immune complexes.

Findings   Normally, immune complexes are not detectable in serum.

Implications of results   The presence of detectable immune complexes in serum has etiologic importance in many autoimmune diseases, such as SLE and rheumatoid arthritis. However, for a definitive diagnosis, the presence of these complexes must be considered with the results of other studies. For example, in SLE, immune complexes are associated with high titers of antinuclear antibodies and circulating antinative deoxyribonucleic acid (DNA) antibodies.

Because of their filtering function, renal glomeruli seem most vulnerable to immune complex deposition, although blood vessel walls and choroid plexuses (vascular folds in the ventricles of the brain) can be affected. A renal biopsy to detect immune complexes can provide conclusive evidence for immune complex (Type III) glomerulonephritis, differentiating it from other types of glomerulonephritis.

Post-test care   If a hematoma develops at the venipuncture site, applying warm soaks may ease discomfort.

Interfering factors   • Failure to send the serum sample to the laboratory immediately may alter test results because complement deteriorates rapidly at room temperature.
• The presence of cryoglobulins in the patient's serum can interfere with accurate determination of test results.
• Inability to standardize RF inhibition tests and platelet aggregation assays can interfere with accurate determination of test results.

Immunoglobulin G (IgG) subclass measurement

Immunoglobulin G are antibodies that are generally made against bacteria, viruses, and toxins, and are the predominant antibodies in the secondary antibody response. Minor variations in the heavy chains establishes the four IgG subclasses. Measurement of the four subclasses of human immunoglobulin IgG — IgG$_1$, IgG$_2$, IgG$_3$, and IgG$_4$ — is recommended in patients with unexplained recurrent sinopulmonary or ear infections. Reportedly, deficiency of IgG$_2$ or IgG$_3$ is an immune deficiency that allows recurring infections by *Streptococcus pneumoniae* and *Haemophilus influenzae*. Increased IgG$_4$ has been found in atopic allergy. One of two methods is used: radial immunodiffusion for most samples, or enzyme-linked immunosorbent assay for very low-level samples.

Purpose
- To aid diagnosis of immunoglobulin deficiencies
- To aid diagnosis in children with recurring infections

Patient preparation
Explain that this test helps detect abnormally low levels of proteins, which are needed to combat infections, and that the test requires a blood sample.

Procedure
Perform a venipuncture, and collect the blood sample in a 3 -ml *red-top* tube. Send the specimen to the laboratory immediately, or freeze it at –4° F (–20° C) if prolonged storage is necessary.

Values
For a range of normal values by age, see *Normal levels of IgG subclass proteins*.

Implications of results
Diminished levels of all IgG subclasses are associated with several primary immunodeficiencies, including hypogammaglobulinemia, ataxia-telangiectasia, and Wiskott-Aldrich syndrome.

IgG$_2$ and IgG$_4$ deficiency may occur in certain patients with IgA deficiency. Isolated IgA deficiency is common and often asymptomatic; concomitant IgG$_2$ and IgG$_4$ deficiency may predispose to recurrent sinopulmonary infection.

In children, both isolated and combined deficiencies of IgG$_2$, IgG$_3$, and IgG$_4$ can produce recurrent sinopulmonary infections and otitis media. Such children show impaired antibody response to *H. influenzae* type B and *S. pneumoniae* despite normal total IgG levels.

Post-test care
If a hematoma develops at the venipuncture site, applying warm soaks may ease discomfort.

Normal levels of IgG subclass proteins (mg/dl)

Age	IgG$_1$	IgG$_2$	IgG$_3$	IgG$_4$
Fetus (cord blood)	435 to 1,084	143 to 453	27 to 146	1 to 47
1 to 7 days	381 to 937	117 to 382	21 to 115	1 to 44
8 to 14 days	327 to 790	92 to 310	16 to 85	1 to 40
3 to 4 weeks	218 to 496	40 to 167	4 to 23	1 to 33
2 months	194 to 480	35 to 164	4 to 36	1 to 30
3 months	167 to 447	28 to 157	4 to 52	1 to 24
4 months	143 to 394	23 to 147	4 to 65	1 to 14
5 months	158 to 392	24 to 132	6 to 68	1 to 13
6 months	175 to 390	24 to 115	8 to 72	1 to 11
7 months	190 to 388	25 to 100	10 to 75	1 to 10
8 months	200 to 417	26 to 123	10 to 76	1 to 16
9 months	211 to 450	26 to 149	10 to 77	1 to 22
10 to 12 months	241 to 543	28 to 221	10 to 80	1 to 39
13 to 20 months	281 to 692	30 to 343	10 to 88	1 to 68
21 months to 2 years	310 to 729	46 to 387	10 to 96	1 to 77
3 years	348 to 773	72 to 441	10 to 105	1 to 87
4 years	370 to 804	88 to 455	11 to 108	1 to 97
5 years	375 to 835	94 to 468	12 to 111	1 to 106
6 years	380 to 866	100 to 481	14 to 115	1 to 115
7 years	385 to 896	105 to 494	16 to 118	1 to 124
8 years	390 to 927	111 to 507	18 to 122	1 to 133
9 years	395 to 958	117 to 520	19 to 125	1 to 142
10 years	400 to 989	123 to 534	21 to 129	1 to 151
11 years	405 to 1,020	128 to 547	23 to 132	1 to 160
12 years	410 to 1,051	134 to 560	25 to 136	1 to 169
13 years	415 to 1,081	140 to 573	27 to 139	1 to 178
14 years	419 to 1,102	145 to 582	28 to 141	1 to 184
> 15 years	423 to 1,112	149 to 586	29 to 142	1 to 187

None

Immunoglobulins G, A, and M

Immunoglobulins are serum antibodies that are produced by plasma cells of the B lymphocytes and are the major component of the humoral response to antigen stimulation. They are classified into five groups — immunoglobulin G (IgG), IgA, IgM, IgD, and IgE — that are normally present in serum in predictable percentages. In normal serum, IgG comprises about 80% of serum immunoglobulins and includes the warm-temperature type; IgA, about 15% of the total; IgM, 5% to 7% and includes ABO blood group isoagglutinins; IgD and allergen-specific IgE comprise less than 2%. (See *Major immunoglobulins.*) Deviations from normal immunoglobulin percentages are characteristic in many immune disorders — cancer, hepatic disorders, rheumatoid arthritis, and systemic lupus erythematosus, for example. Infection and inflammation may also cause immunoglobulin percentages to increase.

Immunoelectrophoresis identifies IgG, IgA, and IgM in a serum sample; the level of each is measured by radial immunodiffusion or nephelometry. Some laboratories detect immunoglobulin by indirect immunofluorescence and radioimmunoassay.

Purpose

- To diagnose paraproteinemias, such as multiple myeloma and Waldenström's macroglobulinemia
- To diagnose some B-cell malignant diseases
- To detect immunodeficiencies that are associated with abnormally low immunoglobulin levels
- To detect hypogammaglobulinemia and hypergammaglobulinemia, as well as nonimmunologic diseases, such as cirrhosis and hepatitis, that are associated with abnormally high immunoglobulin levels
- To assess the effectiveness of chemotherapy or radiation therapy

Patient preparation

Explain that this test measures antibody levels or evaluates the effectiveness of treatment, and that the test requires a blood sample. Instruct the patient to restrict food and fluids, except for water, for 12 to 14 hours before the test.

Major immunoglobulins

IgG has antibody activity against viruses, some bacteria, fungi, and toxins. It occurs as a secondary response after IgM and is the only immunoglobulin that crosses the placenta.

IgA protects the mucous membranes in the respiratory and GI tracts against invasion by microorganisms and activates the complement system. It includes antitoxins, antibacterial agglutinins, antinuclear antibodies, and allergic reagins. IgA exists in its secretory form in colostrum, saliva, tears, and in GI and bronchial secretions.

IgM is the first antibody to appear after antigenic stimulation. It produces antibody against rheumatoid factors and gram-negative organisms, forms the ABO blood group, and activates the complement system.

IgD is present in serum and umbilical cord blood. Its function is unknown. However, increased values are reported in chronic infections, connective tissue disorders, certain lever diseases, and IgD myeloma. Decreased values occur in hereditary and acquired deficiency syndromes.

IgE is present in serum and interstitial fluid. It has antibody activity for hypersensitivity reactions. Increased values occur in atopic skin diseases (eczema), parasitic infestations, hay fever, asthma, anaphylactic shock, and IgE myeloma.

Check the patient's medication history for drugs that may affect test results. If these medications must be continued, note this on the laboratory slip.

Procedure   Perform a venipuncture, and collect the sample in a 7-ml *red-top* tube. Send the sample to the laboratory immediately to prevent deterioration of immunoglobulins.

Values   Using nephelometry, serum immunoglobulin levels for adults range as follows —
IgG: 700 to 1,500 mg/dl (7.00 to 15.00 g/L)
IgA: 60 to 400 mg/dl (0.60 to 4.00 g/L)
IgM: 60 to 300 mg/dl (0.60 to 3.00 g/L).

These values are age-dependent. (See *Normal immunoglobulin values in children,* page 382.)

Implications of results   *Serum immunoglobulin levels in various disorders,* page 383, shows IgG, IgA, and IgM levels in various disorders. In congenital and acquired hypogammaglobulinemias, myelomas, and macroglobulinemia, the findings confirm the diagnosis. In hepatic and

Normal immunoglobulin values in children				
Age	**Values (mg/dl)**			
	IgG	**IgA**	**IgM (males)**	**IgM (females)**
2 to 4 months	141 to 930	5 to 64	14 to 142	16 to 125
5 to 8 months	250 to 1,190	10 to 87	24 to 167	50 to 163
9 to 14 months	320 to 1,250	17 to 94	30 to 212	29 to 216
15 to 23 months	470 to 1,600	22 to 178	35 to 189	44 to 240
2 to 3 years	400 to 1,620	7 to 192	41 to 168	33 to 196
3.5 to 4.5 years	620 to 1,510	42 to 238	31 to 272	37 to 425
5 to 6 years	630 to 1,530	44 to 334	38 to 197	30 to 248
7 to 8 years	620 to 1,660	42 to 285	24 to 225	35 to 282
9 to 10 years	770 to 1,560	46 to 435	35 to 208	43 to 348

autoimmune diseases, leukemias, and lymphomas, such findings are less important but can support the diagnosis based on other tests, such as biopsies and white blood cell differential, and on physical examination.

Post-test care
- Advise the patient with abnormally low immunoglobulin levels (especially of IgG or IgM) to protect himself against bacterial infection. When caring for such a patient, watch for signs of infection, such as fever, chills, rash, or skin ulcers.
- Instruct the patient with abnormally high immunoglobulin levels and symptoms of monoclonal gammopathies to report bone pain and tenderness. Such a patient has numerous antibody-producing malignant plasma cells in bone marrow, which hamper production of other blood components. When caring for such a patient, watch for signs of hypercalcemia, renal failure, and spontaneous pathologic fractures.
- If a hematoma develops at the venipuncture site, applying warm soaks eases discomfort.
- The patient may resume a normal diet and withheld medications.

Serum immunoglobin levels in various disorders

Disorder	IgG	IgA	IgM
Immunoglobulin (Ig) disorders			
Lymphoid aplasia	D	D	D
Agammaglobulinemia	D	D	D
Type 1 dysgammaglobulinemia (selective IgG, and IgA deficiency)	D	D	N or I
Type II dysgammaglobulinemia (absent IgA and IgM)	N	D	D
IgA globulinemia	N	D	N
Ataxia-telangiectasia	N	D	N
Multiple myeloma, macroglobulin-emia, lymphomas			
Heavy chain disease (Franklin's disease)	D	D	D
IgG myeloma	I	D	D
IgA myeloma	D	I	D
Macroglobulinemia	D	D	I
Acute lymphocytic leukemia	N	D	N
Chronic lymphocytic leukemia	D	D	D
Acute myelocytic leukemia	N	N	N
Chronic myelocytic leukemia	N	D	N
Hodgkin's disease	N	N	N
Hepatic disorders			
Hepatitis	I	I	I
Laënnec's cirrhosis	I	I	N
Biliary cirrhosis	N	N	I
Hepatoma	N	N	D
Other disorders			
Rheumatoid arthritis	I	I	I
Systemic lupus erythematosus	I	I	I
Nephrotic syndrome	D	D	N
Trypanosomiasis	N	N	I
Pulmonary tuberculosis	I	N	N

Key: N = Normal; I = Increased; D = Decreased

Interfering factors

- Failure to send the blood sample to the laboratory promptly may interfere with the accuracy of test results because of deterioration of the immunoglobulins.
- Radiation therapy or chemotherapy — for example, with methotrexate — may reduce immunoglobulin levels, because of these treatments' suppressive effects on bone marrow.
- Various drugs can affect test results. Aminophenazone, anticonvulsants, asparaginase, hydralazine, hydantoin derivatives, oral contraceptives, and phenylbutazone may raise all immunoglobulin levels. Methotrexate and severe

hypersensitivity to bacille Calmette-Guérin vaccine may lower all levels. Dextrans, phenytoin, and high doses of methylprednisolone lower IgG and IgA levels; dextrans and methylprednisolone lower IgM levels. Methadone raises IgG levels; alcoholism raises IgA levels; narcotics addiction may raise IgM levels.

Infectious mononucleosis screening test

The infectious mononucleosis screening test, commonly known as the monospot test, evaluates serum for heterophile antibodies. These antibodies appear in the serum within 6 to 10 days of contracting infectious mononucleosis. Titers will usually be highest within 2 to 3 weeks of illness. Antibody levels typically persist for 4 to 8 weeks, but may persist for up to a year. The antibody level activity doesn't relate to the degree of lymphocytosis or disease severity. See Epstein-Barr Virus Antibodies and Heterophile Agglutination Tests.

Purpose
: To diagnose infectious mononucleosis

Patient preparation
: Explain the purpose of this test, and tell the patient that the test requires a blood sample.

Procedure
: Perform a venipuncture, and collect a blood sample in a *red-top* tube.

Findings
: Normal serum is negative for heterophile antibodies.

Implications of results
: Correlating test results with clinical findings is essential because both false-positive and false-negative results have been reported. Approximately 10% of adults with infectious mononucleosis don't produce heterophile antibodies. The presence of Epstein-Barr virus antibodies is pertinent in these cases. In children, failure to develop these antibodies occurs more frequently. False-positive results (less than 2%) have been reported with the following diseases: acute lymphocytic leukemia, Burkitt's lymphoma, cytomegalovirus, Hodgkin's disease, infectious hepatitis, lymphoma, malaria, pancreatic cancer, rheumatoid arthritis, and rubella.

Post-test care	If a hematoma develops at the venipuncture site, applying warm soaks eases discomfort.

Interfering factors	None

Insulin, serum

This radioimmunoassay is a quantitative analysis of serum insulin levels, which are always measured concomitantly with glucose levels because glucose is the primary stimulus for insulin release from pancreatic islet cells. It helps evaluate patients suspected of having hyperinsulinemia caused by pancreatic tumor or islet cell hyperplasia.

Insulin, a hormone secreted by beta cells of the islets of Langerhans, regulates the metabolism and transport or mobilization of carbohydrates, amino acids, and lipids. Stimulated by increased plasma levels of glucose, insulin secretion reaches peak levels after meals, when metabolism and food storage are greatest. An insufficient level of insulin or resistance to its effects is the primary abnormality in diabetes mellitus.

Purpose

- To aid diagnosis of hypoglycemia resulting from tumor or hyperplasia of pancreatic islet cells, glucocorticoid deficiency, or severe hepatic disease
- To aid diagnosis of diabetes mellitus and insulin-resistant states

Patient preparation

Explain that this test, which requires a blood sample, helps evaluate pancreatic function. Instruct the patient to fast for 10 to 12 hours before the test. (Questionable results may make it necessary to repeat the test or, frequently, to perform a simultaneous glucose tolerance test.)

As ordered, withhold corticotropin, steroids (including oral contraceptives), thyroid supplements, epinephrine, or other medications that may influence test results. If these medications must be continued, note this on the laboratory slip. The patient should be relaxed and recumbent for 30 minutes before the test because agitation and stress may affect insulin levels.

Procedure

Perform a venipuncture, and collect one sample for insulin level in a 7-ml *red-top* tube; collect another sample for glucose in a *gray-top* tube. Handle the sample gently to prevent hemolysis. Pack the sample for insulin in ice, and send it, along with the glucose sample, to the laboratory immediately.

➤ *Clinical alert:* In the patient with a suspected insulinoma, there is always a risk of severe hypoglycemia. Keep dextrose 50% I.V. available to combat possible hypoglycemia. The most diagnostically useful insulin levels in such patients are those collected during a hypoglycemic episode.

Values

Serum insulin levels normally range from undetectable to 25 µU/ml (0 to 180 pmol/L).

Implications of results

Insulin levels are interpreted in light of the prevailing glucose concentration. A normal insulin level may be inappropriate for the glucose results. High insulin and low glucose levels after a significant fast or during a hypoglycemic episode suggest an insulinoma. Prolonged fasting or stimulation testing may be required to confirm the diagnosis. In insulin-resistant diabetic states (non-insulin-dependent diabetes mellitus), insulin levels are elevated; in non-insulin-resistant diabetes (insulin-dependent diabetes mellitus), they are low.

Post-test care

- If a hematoma develops at the venipuncture site, applying warm soaks eases discomfort.
- The patient may resume discontinued diet and medications.

Interfering factors

- Failure to observe diet and activity restrictions may affect test results.
- Use of corticotropin, steroids (including oral contraceptives), thyroid hormones, or epinephrine increases insulin requirements by exerting a hyperglycemic effect, thereby raising serum insulin levels.
- Use of insulin by non-insulin-dependent patients suppresses endogenous insulin secretion, lowering levels.
- In patients with insulin-dependent diabetes mellitus, high levels of insulin antibodies may interfere with the test.
- Failure to pack the insulin sample in ice and send it to the laboratory promptly, or hemolysis caused by excessive agitation of the sample may hinder accurate determination of test results.

Insulin antibodies, serum

Using radioimmunoassay, this test detects insulin antibodies in the blood of patients who receive insulin for treatment of diabetes mellitus. Most insulin preparations are derived from beef and pork pancreases and contain insulin-related peptides, which are the major immunogenic components in insulin. Immunoglobulin G antibodies that form in response to these peptides form a complex with subsequent insulin injections and neutralize the insulin, thereby impairing its glucose-regulating action.

Purpose
- To identify insulin resistance in patients who require excessive dosage of insulin
- To confirm factitious hypoglycemia
- To identify the cause of allergic reactions to insulin and to help determine the most appropriate preparation for treatment of diabetes

Patient preparation
Explain the purpose of this test, and tell the patient that the test requires a blood sample.

Procedure
Perform a venipuncture, and obtain a blood sample of at least 2 ml. Send it to the laboratory promptly.

Values
Normally, this test detects no insulin antibodies or detects less than 3% binding of labeled beef and pork insulin.

Implications of results
Detection of insulin antibodies confirms their formation as the cause of insulin resistance and suggests the need for alternate therapy to control hyperglycemia. Detection of insulin antibodies may also confirm factitious hypoglycemia, an unusual condition that results from insulin injection, rather than insulinoma or chronic pancreatitis.

Post-test care
If a hematoma develops at the venipuncture site, applying warm soaks eases discomfort.

Interfering factors
None

Intrinsic factor blocking antibody, serum

Intrinsic factor (IF) is formed in gastric parietal cells and secreted into the gastric lumen, where it binds to exogenous vitamin B_{12}. The IF-B_{12} complex facilitates absorption of B_{12}. In patients with pernicious anemia, failure of the gastric mucosa to form IF is associated with gastric mucosal atrophy. Because the sera of patients with pernicious anemia commonly show antibodies to IF, IF antibody detection is of diagnostic value.

Serum antibodies to IF include type I, the blocking antibody, and type II, the binding antibody. The blocking antibody inhibits uptake of vitamin B_{12} at its binding site of IF. The radioimmunoassay test for IF blocking antibody is positive in the sera of approximately half of all patients with pernicious anemia; the test is rarely positive in patients with other conditions.

Purpose   To aid diagnosis of pernicious anemia

Patient preparation   Explain the purpose of this test, and inform the patient that the test requires a blood sample.

Procedure   Perform a venipuncture to collect 5 ml of sterile blood in a *red-top* tube. Allow the blood to clot for at least 1 hour at room temperature. Avoid excessive agitation of the sample to prevent hemolysis. Transfer the serum to a sterile tube or vial, and send it frozen to the laboratory.

Values   A normal test result is negative for IF blocking antibody. The test is positive in 50% of patients with pernicious anemia.

Implications of results   A positive test result strongly supports a diagnosis of pernicious anemia and is useful in patients with low serum concentrations of vitamin B_{12}. However, the negative test alone does not rule out pernicious anemia because about half of patients with pernicious anemia test negative for this antibody.

Post-test care   If a hematoma develops at the venipuncture site, applying warm soaks eases discomfort.

Interfering
factor

Recent exposure to a radioisotope, and treatment with methotrexate or other folic acid antagonists interferes with accurate determination of test results.

Inulin clearance

Inulin, a polysaccharide of fructose obtained from dahlias and artichokes, is metabolically inert within the body. When injected I.V., inulin is almost entirely filtered by the glomeruli and is not reabsorbed by the tubules. Inulin clearance is therefore practically an exact measure of the glomerular filtration rate (GFR).

Despite its sensitivity and low incidence of side effects, the inulin clearance test is time-consuming, complex, and uncomfortable for the patient, and thus is infrequently performed. Less accurate tests, such as urea and creatinine clearance, are used instead. Iothalamate iodine 125 (^{125} I) can be substituted for inulin in a similar test procedure. Because the iodine content is negligible, ^{125} I can be given to patients with iodine hypersensitivity but is contraindicated during pregnancy, lactation, and periods of growth.

Purpose

To measure GFR

Patient
preparation

Explain that this test evaluates kidney function. Instruct the patient to fast for 4 hours before the test, to abstain from exercise the morning of the test, and to drink 1 liter of water 1 hour before the test. Encourage liquids during the test to maintain adequate urine flow. Tell the patient that the test will require five blood samples and five urine specimens, and that he will receive an I.V. infusion of inulin. Advise him that he may feel bloated or have the urge to void during urine collection, and that a catheter will be in place for 2 hours.

Equipment

25 ml of 10% inulin and 500 ml of 1.5% inulin, five 10-ml *green-top* (heparinized) tubes, equipment for venipuncture, equipment for indwelling urinary catheterization, clamp, five urine specimen containers, I.V. pump, I.V. solution (250 ml of dextrose 5% in water), I.V. tubing with a Y-port

Procedure

Perform a venipuncture, and collect 10 ml of blood in a *green-top* (heparinized) tube to be used as a control sample. Then, the patient should have a urinary catheter inserted. Make sure the bladder is empty, and save the urine for a baseline specimen. If the patient has a catheter in place before the test, the drainage bag should be emptied and the catheter clamped for 1 hour before a baseline specimen is taken.

Infuse the recommended priming dose of 25 ml of 10% inulin by I.V. bolus over 4 minutes. Allow 30 minutes for distribution. (*Note:* Use the solution for I.V. bolus within 1 hour of preparation. Before administration, shake the ampule, and warm it in boiling water to dissolve all crystals. Then, cool to body temperature.) Then, using an I.V. pump, infuse the maintenance solution of 500 ml of 1.5% inulin at a constant rate of 4 ml/minute. Tell the patient not to exert pressure on the arm with the I.V. site or to touch the control, and to promptly report if he feels a burning sensation.

Collect a urine specimen 30 minutes after starting the I.V. line, and three additional specimens at 20-minute intervals thereafter. Clamp the catheter between collections.

Draw a blood sample at the midpoint of each 20-minute period and at the end of the test. Handle blood samples gently to prevent hemolysis, and send specimens to the laboratory immediately after each collection. If more than 10 minutes will elapse before transport, refrigerate the urine specimen.

Record the inulin dosage on the laboratory slip. Properly label each specimen, and include the collection time.

Precautions   Inulin clearance should be used cautiously in patients with cardiac disease because increased fluid intake may cause congestive heart failure.

Values   Inulin clearance is normally 1.5 to 2.2 ml/second for age 21 and older; 1.4 to 2.1 ml/second, ages 11 to 20; and 1.4 to 2.0 ml/second, birth to age 10. Clearance may decrease as much as 45% after age 70.

Implications of results   Depressed clearance is characteristic in congestive heart failure, decreased renal blood flow, acute tubular necrosis, acute and chronic glomerulonephritis, advanced chronic bilateral pyelonephritis, nephrosclerosis, advanced bilateral renal lesions, bilateral ureteral obstruction, and dehydration.

Post-test care
- If a hematoma develops at the venipuncture site, applying warm soaks eases discomfort. If phlebitis develops at the I.V. site, elevate the patient's arm and apply warm soaks.
- Be sure the patient voids within 8 to 10 hours after the catheter is removed.
- The patient may resume restricted diet and activity.

Interfering factors
- Failure to infuse inulin at a constant rate, collect blood and urine specimens at the proper intervals, or adhere to dietary and exercise restrictions may prevent accurate test results.
- Hemolysis caused by excessive agitation of the blood samples may influence test results.

Iron, serum, and total iron-binding capacity

Iron is essential to the formation and function of hemoglobin, as well as many other heme and non-heme compounds. After iron is absorbed by the intestine, it is distributed to various body compartments for synthesis, storage, and transport. Iron in the plasma is almost all bound to a glycoprotein called transferrin.

Serum iron assay measures the amount of iron bound to transferrin; total iron-binding capacity (TIBC) measures the amount of iron that would appear in plasma if all the transferrin were saturated with iron. The percentage of saturation is obtained by dividing the serum iron result by the TIBC, which reveals the amount of saturated transferrin. Normally, transferrin is about 30% saturated.

Serum iron and TIBC are of greater diagnostic usefulness when performed with the serum ferritin assay. Bone marrow or liver biopsy, and iron absorption or excretion studies may yield more information.

Purpose
- To estimate total iron storage
- To aid diagnosis of hemochromatosis
- To help distinguish between iron deficiency anemia and anemia of chronic disease
- To aid evaluation of nutritional status

Patient preparation

Explain to the patient that this test, which requires a blood sample, evaluates the body's capacity to store iron.

Review the patient's medication history for drugs that may interfere with accurate determination of test results. Withhold chloramphenicol, iron supplements, and oral contraceptives, as appropriate. If such medications must be continued, note this on the laboratory slip.

Procedure

Perform a venipuncture, and collect the sample in a 7-ml *red-top* tube. Handle the sample gently to prevent hemolysis, and send it to the laboratory immediately.

Values

Normal serum iron and TIBC values are as follows:

Serum iron mcg/dl (µmol/L)	TIBC mcg/dl (µmol/L)	Saturation
Males:		
70 to 150 (12 to 27)	300 to 400 (54 to 72)	20% to 50%
Females:		
80 to 150 (14 to 27)	350 to 450 (54 to 81)	20% to 50%

Implications of results

In iron deficiency, serum iron levels drop and TIBC increases to decrease the saturation. In cases of chronic inflammation (such as in rheumatoid arthritis), serum iron may be low in the presence of adequate body stores, but TIBC may be unchanged or may drop to preserve normal saturation. A normal serum iron in the absence of iron supplements excludes iron deficiency. A low serum iron may be seen in iron deficiency or in inflammatory states; it is here that serum ferritin is helpful.

Iron overload may not alter serum levels until relatively late, but in general, serum iron increases and TIBC remains the same to increase the saturation.

Post-test care

• If a hematoma develops at the venipuncture site, applying warm soaks eases discomfort.
• The patient may resume withheld medications.

Interfering factors

• Chloramphenicol and oral contraceptives can cause false-positive test results. Iron supplements can cause false-positive serum iron values but false-negative TIBC.

- Hemolysis caused by excessive agitation of the sample, or failure to send the sample to the laboratory immediately may interfere with accurate determination of test results.

Isopropanol and methanol, serum

This toxicity determination, through gas chromatography, quantitatively measures serum isopropanol or methanol levels in patients suspected of ingesting these alcohols. Toxic symptoms produced by ingestion of isopropanol include gastritis, confusion, central nervous system depression, respiratory arrest, and coma; symptoms of methanol toxicity include nausea, vomiting, diarrhea, stupor, convulsions, respiratory arrest, blindness, metabolic acidosis, and coma, and may occur 8 to 36 hours after methanol ingestion. Ingestion of isopropanol or methanol can be fatal.

After ethanol, isopropanol and methanol are the most common volatile liquids. Isopropanol (rubbing alcohol) — used as a disinfectant, a liniment, and an industrial solvent — is more toxic than ethanol. Methanol — used as an industrial solvent and in bootleg liquor — is less inebriating but more toxic than ethanol, because it's partially oxidized to formaldehyde in the body.

Purpose
To confirm the cause and extent of intoxication suspected from the history or after onset of symptoms

Patient preparation
Explain that this test determines whether the blood contains a toxic level of isopropanol or methanol, and that the test requires a blood sample.

If the test is being performed for medicolegal purposes, make sure the patient or a responsible member of his family has signed a consent form. Check the patient's recent medication history, including the names and dosage schedules of any drugs the patient has used, and the amount and time of isopropanol or methanol ingestion.

Procedure
Clean the venipuncture site with benzalkonium chloride (aqueous 1:75 dilution) or povidone-iodine solution. Perform a venipuncture, and collect the sample in a 7-ml *red-top* tube.

Don't clean the venipuncture site with alcohol or tincture of iodine. This contaminates the specimen and interferes with test results.

Send the sample to the laboratory immediately or refrigerate it. For a medicolegal test, observe appropriate precautions.

Values

The presence of any concentration of isopropanol or methanol in serum is abnormal and potentially toxic. The lethal level of isopropanol is 150 mg/dl (25 mmol/L); the lethal level of methanol is 80 mg/dl (25 mmol/L).

Implications of results

Confirmation of serum levels of isopropanol or methanol guides treatment of toxicity.

Isopropanol is twice as toxic as ethanol. Methanol toxicity is likely to cause blindness in the presence of metabolic acidosis.

Post-test care

If a hematoma develops at the venipuncture site, applying warm soaks eases discomfort.

Interfering factor

Use of alcohol or tincture of iodine at the venipuncture site causes false-high levels.

K

Ketone test, urine

Ketone bodies, which result from the metabolism of fatty acid and fat, consist predominately of acetoacetic acid, acetone, and beta-hydroxybutyric acid. Excessive amounts of ketones are formed when altered carbohydrate metabolism causes fat to become the predominant body fuel. Ketonuria is generally associated with diabetes.

In this routine, semiquantitative screening test, the action of urine on a commercially prepared product (Acetest tablet, Chemstrip K, Ketostix, or Kyotest UK) measures the urine level of ketone bodies. Each product measures a specific ketone body. For example, Acetest measures acetone, while Ketostix measures acetoacetic acid. Urine determinations reflect serum concentration.

Purpose
- To screen for ketonuria
- To detect diabetic ketoacidosis and carbohydrate deprivation
- To distinguish between a diabetic and a nondiabetic coma
- To monitor control of diabetes mellitus, ketogenic weight reduction, and treatment of diabetic ketoacidosis

Patient preparation
Explain that the purpose of this test is to evaluate fat metabolism. If the patient has newly diagnosed diabetes, teach the patient how to perform the test. Instruct the patient to void; then give him a drink of water. About 30 minutes later, ask him to give a second-voided specimen.

If the patient is taking levodopa or phenazopyridine, or has recently received sulfobromophthalein, Acetest tablets must be used, because reagent strips will give inaccurate results.

Procedure
Collect a second-voided midstream specimen, and use one of the following procedures.

Acetest: Lay the tablet on a piece of white paper, and place one drop of urine on the tablet. After 30 seconds, compare the tablet color (white, lavender, or purple) with the color chart.

Ketostix: Dip the reagent stick into the specimen and remove it immediately. After 15 seconds, compare the stick color (buff or purple) with the color chart. Record the results as negative, small, moderate, or large amounts of ketones.

Kyotest UK: Dip the reagent strip into the freshly voided urine specimen for no longer than 1 second, or hold the test strip directly in the urine stream. Tap the edge of the strip against the container or a clean, dry surface to remove excess urine. When using the tape, the end held in the fingers should be kept dry. Observe for color change, usually a deepening shade of blue, which develops in 60 seconds. Compare with color chart on the container or instruction sheet. Ignore color changes that occur after 3 minutes.

Note: The specimen must be tested within 60 minutes after it is obtained, or it must be refrigerated. Allow refrigerated specimens to return to room temperature before testing. Don't use tablets or strips that have become discolored or darkened.

Findings

Normally, no ketones are present in urine.

Implications of results

Ketosis and ketonuria exist when carbohydrate intake is limited, fat metabolism is increased, or the diet has a high fat content. In patients with diabetes mellitus, ketones in the urine indicate that the diabetes is not adequately controlled and changes to the diet or medications are necessary as soon as possible. In nondiabetic patients, ketonuria suggests reduced carbohydrate metabolism and increased fat metabolism.

Post-test care

If the test will be performed at home, provide written guidelines and a flow sheet to help the patient record results.

Interfering factors

- Failure to keep the reagent container tightly closed to prevent absorption of light or moisture, or bacterial contamination of the specimen causes false-negative results.
- Levodopa, phenazopyridine, and sulfobromophthalein produce false-positive test results when Ketostix is used.
- Carbohydrate-free and high-fat and high-protein diets cause ketonuria.

17-Ketosteroid fractionation, urine

This test uses column chromatography or gas–liquid chromatography to quantitate urine levels of the following metabolites from the adrenal cortices and from the testes: androsterone, dehydroepiandrosterone, delta-5-pregnenetriol, etiocholanolone, 11-hydroxyandrosterone, 11-hydroxyetiocholanolone, 11-ketoandrosterone, 11-ketoetiocholanolone, 11-ketopregnanetriol, pregnanediol, and pregnanetriol. Androsterone, etiocholanolone, and dehydroepiandrosterone are the three major metabolites of androgens in the urine.

Purpose
- To evaluate adrenal and gonadal abnormalities
- To differentiate diagnosis of adrenal hyperplasia and carcinoma
- To aid diagnosis of arrhenoblastoma or Stein-Leventhal syndrome

Patient Preparation
Explain the purpose of this test. Inform the patient that the test requires 24-hour urine collection, and teach the proper collection technique. Emphasize the importance of collecting all urine specimens.

Procedure
Obtain a plastic container with acetic acid or hydrochloric acid as a preservative. Label the container with the patient's name, test, and date. Include the time the collection was started and the time it was completed. Send the specimen to the laboratory when the test is completed. If unable to sent the specimen to the laboratory immediately, keep it refrigerated.

Values
Normal values vary depending on the laboratory performing the test. They are often reported by age and sex. (See *17-Ketosteroid fractionation normal test values,* page 398.)

Implications of results
Elevated urine levels can result from adrenal hyperplasia and carcinoma. In females, elevated levels may indicate ovarian dysfunction such as Stein-Leventhal syndrome (polycystic ovarian disease) or arrhenoblastoma (a rare ovarian tumor).

Post-test care
If the test will be performed at home, provide written guidelines and a flow sheet to help the patient record results.

17-Ketosteroid fractionation normal test values

| | Adults | | Children ages 10 to 15 years | |
	Males	Females	Males	Females
Androsterone (mg/24 hours)	0.9 to 6.1	0 to 3.1	0.2 to 2.0	0.5 to 2.5
Dehydroepiandrosterone (mg/24 hours)	0 to 3.1	0 to 1.5	< 0.4	< 0.4
Delta-5-pregnenetriol (mg/24 hours)	0 to 0.4	0 to 0.4	< 0.3	< 0.3
Etiocholanolone (mg/24 hours)	0.9 to 5.2	0.1 to 3.5	0.1 to 1.6	0.7 to 3.1
11-Hydroxyandrosterone (mg/24 hours)	0.2 to 1.6	0 to 1.1	0.1 to 1.1	0.2 to 1.0
11-Hydroxyetiochol-anolone (mg/24 hours)	0.1 to 0.9	0.1 to 0.8	< 0.3	0.1 to 0.5
11-Ketoandrosterone (mg/24 hours)	0 to 0.5	0 to 0.3	< 0.1	< 0.1
11-Ketoetiocholanolone (mg/24 hours)	0 to 1.6	0 to 1.0	< 0.3	0.1 to 0.5
11-Ketopregnanetriol (mg/24 hours)	0 to 0.5	0 to 0.5	< 0.3	< 0.2
Pregnanediol (mg/24 hours)	0 to 1.9	0 to 4.5	0.1 to 1.2	0.1 to 0.7
Pregnanetriol (mg/24 hours)	0.2 to 2.0	0 to 1.4	0.2 to 0.6	0.1 to 0.6

Adapted with permission from *Mayo Medical Laboratories 1994 Test Catalog.* Rochester, Minn.: Mayo Medical Laboratories, 1994.

Interfering factors   An incomplete collection invalidates the results.

17-Ketosteroids, urine

This test uses the spectrophotofluorometric technique to measure urine levels of 17-ketosteroids (17-KS). Steroids and steroid metabolites characterized by a ketone group on carbon 17 in the steroid nucleus, 17-KS originate primarily in the adrenal glands but also in the testes, which produce one third of 17-KS in males, and in the ovaries, which produce a minimal amount of 17-KS in females. Although not all 17-KS are androgens, they cause androgenic effects. For example, excessive secretion of 17-KS may result in hirsutism and may increase clitoral or phallic size; in utero, elevated 17-KS levels may cause a female fetus to develop a male urogenital tract. Because 17-KS do not include all the androgens (testosterone, for example, the most potent androgen, is not a 17-KS), these levels provide only a rough estimate of androgenic activity. To provide information about androgen secretion, plasma testosterone levels may be measured concurrently; 17-KS fractionation may also be appropriate.

Purpose	• To aid diagnosis of adrenal and gonadal dysfunction
	• To aid diagnosis of adrenogenital syndrome (congenital adrenal hyperplasia)

Patient preparation

Explain that this test evaluates hormonal balance. Tell the patient that the test requires 24-hour urine collection, and teach the proper collection technique. The patient should avoid excessive physical exercise and stressful situations during the collection period.

If the female patient is menstruating, the urine collection may have to be postponed because blood in the specimen interferes with test findings.

Check the patient's medication history for drugs that may affect test results. Review findings with the laboratory, then restrict such drugs.

Procedure

Collect a 24-hour urine specimen in a bottle containing a preservative to keep the specimen at a pH of 4.0 to 4.5. Refrigerate the specimen or place it on ice during the collection period. When the collection is completed, send the specimen to the laboratory immediately.

Values

Normally, urine 17-KS values range from 6 to 21 mg/day (20 to 75 μmol/day) in males, and from 4 to 17 mg/day (15 to 60 μmol/day) in females. Children between ages 11 and 14 excrete 2 to 7 mg/day (5 to 25 μmol/day); younger children and infants excrete 0 to 3 mg/day (0 to 10 μmol/day).

Implications of results

Elevated urine 17-KS levels may result from adrenal hyperplasia, carcinoma or adenoma, or adrenogenital syndrome. In females, elevated levels may also indicate ovarian dysfunction — such as polycystic ovarian disease (Stein-Leventhal syndrome) — or lutein cell tumor of the ovary or androgenic arrhenoblastoma. In males, elevated 17-KS may indicate interstitial cell tumor of the testis. Characteristically, 17-KS levels also rise during pregnancy, severe stress, chronic illness, or debilitating disease.

Depressed urine 17-KS levels may result from Addison's disease, panhypopituitarism, eunuchoidism, or castration, and may occur in cretinism, myxedema, and nephrosis.

Post-test care The patient may resume restricted activity and medications.

Interfering factors
- Meprobamate, phenothiazines, spironolactone, and oleandomycin may elevate urine 17-KS levels. Estrogens, penicillin, ethacrynic acid, and phenytoin may suppress 17-KS levels. Nalidixic acid and quinine may elevate or suppress 17-KS levels.
- Failure to observe drug restrictions, to collect all urine, or to store the specimen properly may interfere with test results.

Lactate dehydrogenase (LD)

Lactate dehydrogenase (LD) is an enzyme that catalyzes the reversible conversion of tissue pyruvic acid into lactic acid. Because LD is present in almost all body tissues, cellular damage causes an elevation of total serum LD, thus limiting the diagnostic usefulness of LD. However, five tissue-specific isoenzymes can be identified and measured, using heat inactivation or electrophoresis: two of these isoenzymes, LD_1 and LD_2, appear primarily in the heart, red blood cells, and kidneys; LD_3, primarily in the lungs, white blood cells, and platelets; and LD_4 and LD_5, in the liver and the skeletal muscles.

The specificity of LD isoenzymes and their distribution pattern is useful in diagnosing hepatic, pulmonary, and erythrocytic damage. But its widest clinical application (with other cardiac enzyme tests) is in diagnosing acute myocardial infarction (MI). LD isoenzyme assay is also useful when creatine kinase (CK) hasn't been measured within 24 hours of an acute MI. The myocardial LD level rises later than CK (12 to 48 hours after infarction begins), peaks in 2 to 5 days, and drops to normal in 7 to 10 days, if tissue necrosis doesn't persist.

Purpose
- To aid differential diagnosis of MI, pulmonary infarction, anemias, and hepatic disease
- To support CK isoenzyme test results in diagnosing MI, or to provide diagnosis when CK-MB samples are drawn too late to display elevation
- To monitor patient response to some forms of chemotherapy

Patient preparation
Explain the purpose of this test, and mention that the test requires a blood sample. Tell the patient suspected of having an MI that the test will be repeated on the next two mornings to monitor progressive changes.

Procedure
Perform a venipuncture, and collect the sample in a 7-ml *red-top* tube. Draw the samples on schedule to avoid missing peak levels, and mark the collection time on the laboratory slip.

Handle the sample gently to prevent artifact blood sample hemolysis because red blood cells contain LD_1. Send the sample to the laboratory immediately or, if transport is delayed, keep the sample at room temperature. Changes in temperature reportedly inactivate LD_5, thus altering isoenzyme patterns.

Values   Total LD levels, which will vary with the method used and are higher in children, normally range from 94 to 257 U/L. Normal distribution is as follows —

LD_1: 17.5% to 28.3% of total
LD_2: 30.4% to 36.4% of total
LD_3: 19.2% to 24.8% of total
LD_4: 9.6% to 15.6% of total
LD_5: 5.5% to 12.7% of total

Implications of results   Because many common diseases cause elevations in total LD levels, isoenzyme electrophoresis is usually necessary for diagnosis. In some disorders, total LD may be within normal limits, but abnormal proportions of each enzyme indicate specific organ tissue damage. For instance, in acute MI, the concentration of LD_1 is greater than LD_2 within 12 to 48 hours after the onset of symptoms. This reversal of normal isoenzyme patterns is typical of myocardial damage and is referred to as flipped LD.

Post-test care   If a hematoma develops at the venipuncture site, applying warm soaks eases discomfort.

Interfering factors
- Hemolysis caused by excessive agitation of the sample may affect accurate determination of LD levels.
- For diagnosis of acute MI, failure to draw the sample on schedule may interfere with test results.
- Failure to send the sample to the laboratory immediately may influence determination of LD isoenzyme patterns.
- Recent surgery or pregnancy can cause elevated LD levels. Prosthetic heart valves may also increase LD levels, from chronic hemolysis.

Lactic acid and pyruvic acid

Lactic acid, present in blood as lactate ion, is derived primarily from muscle cells and erythrocytes.

It is an intermediate product of carbohydrate metabolism and is normally metabolized by the liver. Blood lactate concentration depends on the rate of production and on the rate of metabolism; lactate levels may rise significantly during exercise.

Lactate is the reduction product of pyruvate, a by-product of carbohydrate metabolism. Together these two compounds exist in an equilibrium that is regulated by oxygen supply. When oxygen levels are deficient, the equilibrium shifts toward increased lactate. When the hepatic system fails to metabolize lactate sufficiently or when excess pyruvate converts to lactate because of tissue hypoxia and circulatory collapse, lactic acidosis (lactate levels exceeding 2 mmol/L, with a pH below 7.37) may result. Measurement of blood lactate levels by enzymatic methods, using lactic dehydrogenase, is recommended for all patients with an unexplained anion gap.

Although arterial or venous blood can be used for lactate analysis, a venous sample is more convenient to obtain. However, unless the patient rests for 1 hour before the test, venous blood may yield higher values than arterial blood. Comparison of pyruvate and lactate levels reliably mirrors tissue oxidation, but measurement of pyruvate is technically difficult and infrequently performed.

Purpose
• To assess tissue oxidation
• To help determine the cause of lactic acidosis

Patient preparation
Explain that this test evaluates the oxygen level in tissues and that the test requires a blood sample. The patient should fast overnight and should rest for at least 1 hour before the test.

Procedure
Perform a venipuncture, and collect the sample in a 5-ml *gray-top* tube. Because venostasis will raise blood lactate levels, tell the patient that he must not clench his fist during the venipuncture.

Because lactate and pyruvate are extremely unstable, place the sample container in an ice-filled cup, and send it to the laboratory immediately.

Values
Blood lactate values range from 0.93 to 1.65 mmol/L; pyruvate levels, from 0.08 to 0.16 mmol/L. Normally, the lactate-pyruvate ratio is less than 10:1.

Implications of
results

Elevated blood lactate levels associated with hypoxia may result from strenuous muscle exercise, shock, hemorrhage, septicemia, myocardial infarction, pulmonary embolism, and cardiac arrest. When no reason for diminished tissue perfusion is apparent, increased lactate levels may result from systemic disorders — such as uncontrolled diabetes mellitus, leukemias and lymphomas, hepatic disease, and renal failure — and from enzymatic defects — such as von Gierke's disease (glycogen storage disease) and fructose 1,6-diphosphatase deficiency.

Lactic acidosis can follow ingestion of large doses of acetaminophen and ethanol, and I.V. infusion of epinephrine, glucagon, fructose, and sorbitol.

Post-test care

- If a hematoma develops at the venipuncture site, applying warm soaks eases discomfort.
- The patient may resume a normal diet.

Interfering
factors

- Failure to adhere to restrictions of diet and activity may interfere with accurate determination of test results.
- Failure to pack the sample in ice and to transport it to the laboratory immediately may elevate blood lactate levels.

Lactose tolerance test, oral

This test measures plasma glucose levels after ingestion of a challenge dose of lactose. It also is used to screen for lactose intolerance caused by lactase deficiency.

Lactose, a disaccharide, is found in milk and other dairy products. The intestinal enzyme lactase splits lactase into the monosaccharides glucose and galactose, for absorption by the intestinal epithelium. Absence or deficiency of lactase causes undigested lactose to remain in the intestinal lumen, producing such symptoms as abdominal cramps and watery diarrhea. True congenital lactase deficiency is rare. Usually, lactose intolerance is acquired, as lactase levels generally fall with age.

Purpose

To detect lactose intolerance

Patient
preparation

Explain the purpose of this test, and instruct the patient to fast and to avoid strenuous activity for 8 hours before the test. Tell the patient that the test requires four blood samples and may require a stool sample. Withhold drugs that may affect plasma glucose levels. If these drugs must be continued, note this on the laboratory slip.

Procedure After the patient has fasted for 8 hours, perform a venipuncture and collect a blood sample in a 7-ml *gray-top* tube. Then, administer the test load of lactose — for an adult, 50 g of lactose dissolved in 400 ml water; for a child, 50 g/m² of body surface area. Record the time of ingestion.

Draw a blood sample 30, 60, and 120 minutes after giving the loading dose, using 7-ml *gray-top* tubes. If a stool specimen is required, collect it 5 hours after giving the loading dose.

Send blood and stool specimens to the laboratory immediately, or refrigerate them if transport is delayed. Specify the time of collection on the laboratory slips.

Precautions Monitor for symptoms of lactose intolerance — abdominal cramps, nausea, bloating, flatulence, and watery diarrhea — caused by the loading dose.

Values Normally, plasma glucose levels exceed 160 mg/dl (8.9 mmol/L) within 15 to 60 minutes after ingestion of the lactose loading dose. Stool specimen analysis shows normal pH (7.0 to 8.0) and low glucose content (less than 1+ on a glucose-indicating dipstick).

Implications of results A rise in plasma glucose of less than 20 mg/dl (1.1 mmol/L) indicates lactose intolerance, as does stool acidity (pH of 5.5 or less) and high glucose content (greater than 1+ on the dipstick). Accompanying signs and symptoms provoked by the test also suggest but do not confirm it because such symptoms may develop in patients with normal lactase activity after receiving a loading dose of lactose. Measurement of breath hydrogen after oral lactose or a small-bowel biopsy with lactase assay may be performed to confirm the diagnosis.

Post-test care • If a hematoma develops at the venipuncture site, applying warm soaks eases discomfort.
• The patient may resume restricted diet, activity, and medications.

Interfering
factors

- Drugs that affect plasma glucose levels — such as thiazide diuretics, oral contraceptives, benzodiazepines, propranolol, and insulin — may alter test results.
- Delayed emptying of stomach contents can cause depressed glucose levels.
- Failure to follow diet and exercise restrictions may alter test results.
- Glycolysis may cause false-negative results.

Lead, blood

Lead, which serves no known biochemical function, should normally be undetectable in biological tissues and fluids. Because lead is ubiquitous in the environment (air, water, food, soil, paint), most individuals do have detectable levels of blood lead. In adults, these low levels are not considered harmful. However, acute or chronic exposure to significant amounts of environmental lead produces elevated lead levels and toxicity. Characteristic symptoms of such toxicity may include neurologic abnormalities (ataxia, irritability, inability to concentrate, sleep disturbances); GI abnormalities (nausea, vomiting, anorexia, constipation or diarrhea), neuromuscular abnormalities (fatigue, weakness); and hematologic (anemia), and renal abnormalities. Reportedly, infants and children are particularly sensitive to lead toxicity. Lead exposure is linked to deficits in intellectual development and other neurobehavioral dysfunction.

Lead can be found in all tissues, but 90% eventually accumulates in bone. However, an elevated blood lead level, if the analysis is performed accurately, is considered the best indicator of exposure to lead. Blood lead is usually assayed by atomic absorption spectroscopy.

Purpose

- To screen possible lead exposure in high-risk individuals (children in urban environments, industrial workers), and anyone manifesting signs and symptoms that suggest lead toxicity
- To periodically monitor persons with elevated blood levels of lead to determine if exposure is ongoing

Patient
preparation

Explain the purpose of this test and inform the patient that the test requires a blood sample.

Procedure   Perform a venipuncture, and collect a blood sample. The test requires 2 ml of whole blood in EDTA. For reliable results, the sample must be collected with a lead-free needle and syringe and transported to the laboratory in a lead-free container. Otherwise, environmental contamination of the sample may yield falsely elevated results. Laboratories performing high-quality metal analysis usually provide the appropriate supplies with instructions for their use.

Values   For adults, normal blood lead levels are less than 20 mcg/dl (1 μmol/L); levels greater than 30 mcg/dl (1.5 μmol/L) are considered elevated. For children, levels greater than 25 mcg/dl (1.25 μmol/L) are considered elevated.

Implications of results
- The Occupational Safety and Health Administration has set 30 mcg/dl (1.5 μmol/L) as a threshold for industrial exposure. Any worker equaling or exceeding that level must be removed from the workplace, with pay, until the blood level drops below 30 mcg/dl (1.5 μmol/L).
- An expert advisory committee for the Centers for Disease Control has defined lead poisoning in children as a blood level of 25 mcg/dl (1.25 μmol/L) with a free erythrocyte protoporphyrin level of 35 mcg/dl (1.75 μmol/L) even in children without overt symptoms. Studies investigating the association between blood lead levels and neurobehavioral deficits in children have not identified a threshold level below which immunity to such deficits occurs. Apparently, even blood lead levels as low as 10 mcg/dl (0.5 μmol/L) may be potentially deleterious during critical developmental periods.

➤ *Clinical alert:* Persons with elevated blood lead levels as defined above must be separated from the source of lead exposure immediately. Periodic monitoring of blood levels should continue until the level returns to normal to confirm cessation of exposure. If the blood lead level exceeds 80 mcg/dl (4.0 μmol/L), toxic symptoms are usually evident and may require chelation therapy with edetate calcium disodium to accelerate renal excretion of lead.

Post-test care   If a hematoma develops at the venipuncture site, applying warm soaks eases discomfort.

<table>
<tr><td>Interfering
factor</td><td>Handling the sample with equipment that is not lead-free can yield spurious test results.</td></tr>
</table>

Legionella pneumophila, culture

Legionella organisms are tiny gram-negative rods that require special media for culture. Most are associated with respiratory tract infection — most commonly an influenza-like illness or an atypical pneumonia — that is most likely to develop in persons who are immunocompromised or have decreased resistance to infection. *Legionella* can be cultured from a sputum specimen, but the organism yield is much better from transtracheal aspiration, bronchial washings, or pleural fluid. (For additional information on the detection of *Legionella,* see *Legionella pneumophila smear* and *Legionella pneumophila antibody, serum.*)

Purpose	To detect *Legionella* infection in persons with respiratory tract illness
Patient preparation	Explain the purpose of this test, and inform the patient about the site and method of collecting the test specimen.
Procedure	A specimen of respiratory tract material (pleural fluid, sputum, bronchial washings, transtracheal aspirate, or lung tissue) is collected into a sterile container and transported according to specific instructions from the testing laboratory.

Legionella pneumophila, smear

The direct fluorescent antibody test detects *Legionella pneumophila* in fresh or fixed lung tissue, or smears of respiratory tract fluids. This test is used in association with culture and histopathologic staining.

A smear prepared from the specimen is fixed on a slide and covered with antigen-specific fluorescein-labeled globulin. The resulting antigen-antibody complex fluoresces under ultraviolet light, revealing *Legionella* organisms as fluorescent yellow-green rods.

| ***Legionella pneumophila* antibody, serum** |

The *Legionella* indirect fluorescent antibody (IFA) test is used to detect *Legionella pneumophila* antibodies in serum. This test must be used in association with isolation of the organism from a specimen. More than 39 species with 54 serogroups have been identified.

Serologic confirmation of recent infection with *Legionella* shows a fourfold rise in titer between the acute and convalescent phase (3 to 6 weeks after onset of fever) of the illness. In the *Legionella* IFA test, the titer must rise to 1:128 to be considered positive. A titer of 1:256 is evidence of previous *Legionella* infection.

Findings A normal test result is negative for *Legionella* organisms.

Implications of results Positive culture results confirm respiratory infection with *Legionella* organisms.

Post-test care None

Interfering factors
- Failure to follow specific instructions for collection and transport of the specimen may cause failure to recover the organism.
- Antibiotics may interfere with culture or smear results.

Leucine aminopeptidase
Amino acid arylamidase

Leucine aminopeptidase (LAP) is a proteolytic enzyme found in all body tissues but concentrated in several isoenzyme forms in the liver, pancreas, and small intestine. Its metabolic function in the body is to hydrolyze the peptide bonds of alpha-amino acids involved in cellular energy production. LAP levels tend to parallel those of alkaline phosphatase in hepatic disease and normal pregnancy; but unlike alkaline phosphatase, LAP remains normal in skeletal disease. Despite its relative hepatobiliary specificity, this test — which measures serum LAP levels — isn't commonly performed. In the past, it has been used to diagnose pancreatic cancer but has proven unreliable for this purpose. Recent research suggests that LAP isoenzyme determination may be beneficial in evaluating neonatal jaundice.

Purpose
- To aid in differentiating hepatic disease from skeletal disease when LAP is elevated from an unknown cause
- To help distinguish between congenital biliary atresia and neonatal hepatitis

Patient preparation

Explain that this test helps assess liver function. Advise the patient whether restriction of food or fluids is required (this varies with individual laboratory procedure). Tell the patient that the test requires a blood sample.

Determine if the patient is taking estrogen or progesterone because these drugs elevate LAP levels.

Procedure

Perform a venipuncture, and collect the sample in a 7-ml *red-top* tube.

Precautions

Handle the sample gently to prevent hemolysis, because LAP is contained in serum.

Values

LAP levels typically range from 12 to 33 U/L (with higher values in males) but depend on the test method.

Implications of results

Because alkaline phosphatase rises in both skeletal and hepatic diseases and LAP rises only in the latter, normal LAP with elevated alkaline phosphatase suggests skeletal disease. High LAP levels occur with obstructive jaundice resulting from intrahepatic cholestasis (such as liver metastases) and extrahepatic diseases, such as common bile duct calculus or cancer of the head of the pancreas. Slight elevations occur when hepatocellular damage doesn't cause biliary obstruction, and in hepatitis, cirrhosis, and pancreatitis. However, LAP levels may rise before alkaline phosphatase levels in persons without jaundice. In infants with jaundice, high total LAP (more than 500 U/L) and two zones of electrophoretic activity suggest biliary atresia. Neonatal hepatitis causes milder LAP elevation (less than 500 U/L), and only a single isoenzyme is detected by fractionation.

Post-test care

If a hematoma develops at the venipuncture site, applying warm soaks eases discomfort.

Interfering factors

- Estrogens, progesterone, pregnancy, and oral contraceptives can cause elevated LAP levels.
- Hemolysis caused by excessive agitation of the sample may hinder accurate determination of test results.

Leukocyte alkaline phosphatase stain

Levels of leukocyte alkaline phosphatase (LAP), an enzyme found in neutrophils, may be altered by infection, stress, chronic inflammatory diseases, Hodgkin's disease, and hematologic disorders. Most of these conditions elevate LAP levels; only a few, notably chronic myelogenous leukemia (CML), depress them.

Purpose

To differentiate CML from other disorders that raise the white blood cell count

Patient preparation

Explain the purpose of this test and tell the patient that the test requires a blood sample.

Procedure

Obtain a blood sample by venipuncture or finger stick. The venous blood sample is collected in a 7-ml *green-top* tube and transported immediately to the laboratory, where a blood smear is prepared; the peripheral blood sample is smeared on a 3″ × 1″ glass slide and fixed in cold formalin-methanol. The blood smear is then stained to show the amount of LAP present in the cytoplasm of the neutrophils.

Values

One hundred neutrophils are counted and assessed; each is assigned a score of 0 to 4, according to the degree of LAP staining. Normal values for LAP range from 40 to 100, depending on the laboratory's standards.

Implications of results

Depressed LAP values typically indicate CML; however, low values may also occur in paroxysmal nocturnal hemoglobinuria, aplastic anemia, and infectious mononucleosis. Elevated values may indicate Hodgkin's disease, polycythemia vera, or a neutrophilic leukemoid reaction — a response to such conditions as infection, chronic inflammation, or pregnancy.

After a diagnosis of CML, the LAP stain may also be used to help detect onset of the blastic phase of the disease, when LAP levels typically rise. However, LAP levels also increase toward normal in response to therapy; consequently, test results must be correlated with the patient's condition.

Post-test care If a hematoma develops at the venipuncture site, applying warm soaks eases discomfort.

Interfering factors None

Lipase, serum

Lipase is produced in the pancreas and secreted into the duodenum, where it converts triglycerides and other fats into fatty acids and glycerol. Destruction of pancreatic cells, which occurs in acute pancreatitis, releases large amounts of lipase into the blood.

Typically, this test measures serum lipase levels by the kinetic turbidimetric technique; it's most useful in diagnosing acute pancreatitis when performed with a serum or urine amylase test. Other methods that use synthetic substrates are also common. Test methods using synthetic substrates are also common.

Purpose To aid diagnosis of acute pancreatitis

Patient preparation Explain that this test, which requires a blood sample, evaluates pancreatic function. Instruct the patient to fast the night before the test.

Withhold cholinergics, codeine, meperidine, and morphine. If such medications must be continued, note this on the laboratory slip.

Procedure Perform a venipuncture, and collect the sample in a 7-ml *red-top* tube. Handle the collection tube gently to prevent hemolysis.

Values Serum levels by a typical method range from 32 to 80 U/L. Serum levels by a method using synthetic substrates range from 56 to 239 U/L.

Implications of results High lipase levels suggest acute pancreatitis or pancreatic duct obstruction. After an attack of acute pancreatitis, levels frequently remain elevated up to 14 days. Lipase levels may also rise in pancreatic injury not caused by acute pancreatitis, such as perforated peptic ulcer with chemical pancreatitis caused by gastric juices, and in patients with high intestinal obstruction, pancreatic cancer, or renal disease with impaired excretion.

Post-test care
- If a hematoma develops at the venipuncture site, applying warm soaks eases discomfort.
- The patient may resume discontinued medications.

Interfering factors
- Cholinergics, codeine, meperidine, and morphine cause spasm of the sphincter of Oddi, producing false-positive results.
- Hemolysis caused by excessive agitation of the sample may interfere with accurate determination of lipase values.

Lipids, fecal

Lipids excreted in feces include monoglycerides, diglycerides, triglycerides, phospholipids, glycolipids, soaps (fatty acids and fatty acid salts), sterols, and cholesterol esters. These lipids are derived from intestinal bacterial cells and epithelial cells, unabsorbed dietary lipids, and GI secretions. Normally, dietary lipids emulsified by bile are almost completely absorbed in the small intestine, provided biliary and pancreatic secretions are adequate. However, excessive excretion of fecal lipids — steatorrhea — occurs in various malabsorption syndromes. Both qualitative and quantitative tests can detect excessive excretion of lipids in patients with signs of malabsorption: weight loss, abdominal distention, and scaly skin. In the qualitative test, a specimen from a random stool is stained with Sudan III dye and examined microscopically for evidence of malabsorption — undigested muscle fibers and various fats. In the quantitative test, the entire 72-hour specimen is dried and weighed; the lipids therein are extracted with a solvent, evaporated, and weighed. Only the quantitative test can confirm steatorrhea.

Purpose
To confirm steatorrhea

Patient preparation
Explain that this test evaluates digestion of fats. Instruct him to abstain from alcohol and to maintain a high-fat diet (100 g/day) for 3 days before the test

and during the collection period. Tell him the test requires a 72-hour stool collection.

Withhold drugs that may affect test results. If these medications must be continued, note this on the laboratory slip.

Teach the patient how to collect a timed stool specimen, and provide him with the necessary equipment. Tell the patient to avoid contaminating the stool specimen with urine or toilet tissue.

Procedure   Collect a 72-hour stool specimen. Don't use a waxed collection container because wax may become incorporated in the stool and interfere with accurate testing. Refrigerate the collection container between defecations, and keep it tightly covered.

Values   Fecal lipids normally comprise less than 20% of excreted solids, with excretion of less than 7 g/day (24 mmol/day).

Implications of results   Both digestive and absorptive disorders cause steatorrhea. Digestive disorders may affect the production and release of pancreatic lipase or bile; absorptive disorders may affect the integrity of the intestine. In pancreatic insufficiency, impaired lipid digestion may result from insufficient production of lipase. Pancreatic resection, cystic fibrosis, chronic pancreatitis, or ductal obstruction by stone or tumor may prevent the normal release or action of lipase. In impaired hepatic function, faulty lipid digestion may result from inadequate production of bile salts. Biliary obstruction, which may accompany gallbladder disease, may prevent the normal release of bile salts into the duodenum. Extensive small bowel resection or bypass may also interrupt normal enterohepatic circulation of bile salts.

Diseases of the intestinal mucosa affect normal absorption of lipids; regional ileitis and atrophy caused by malnutrition cause gross structural changes in the intestinal wall, whereas celiac disease and tropical sprue produce mucosal abnormalities. Scleroderma, radiation enteritis, fistulas, intestinal tuberculosis, small intestine diverticula, and altered intestinal flora may also cause steatorrhea. Whipple's disease and lymphomas cause lymphatic obstruction that may inhibit fat absorption.

Post-test care   The patient may resume a normal diet and restricted medications.

Interfering
factors

- The following substances may produce inaccurate test results by inhibiting absorption or affecting chemical digestion: azathioprine, bisacodyl, cholestyramine, kanamycin, neomycin, colchicine, aluminum hydroxide, calcium carbonate, alcohol, potassium chloride, and mineral oil.
- Failure to observe pretest instructions pertaining to diet and ingestion of alcohol, use of a waxed collection container, contamination of the sample, and incomplete stool specimen collection (total weight less than 300 g) interfere with accurate testing.

Lipoprotein-cholesterol fractionation

Lipoprotein fractionation tests isolate and measure the cholesterol in serum bound to low-density lipoproteins (LDLs) and high-density lipoproteins (HDLs). HDL is selectively precipitated and its cholesterol measured. LDL is calculated using HDL cholesterol, total cholesterol, and total triglyceride. The cholesterol in LDL and HDL fractions is significant because the Framingham Heart Study has shown that the cholesterol in HDL ("good" cholesterol) is inversely related to the incidence of coronary artery disease (CAD) — the higher the HDL level, the lower the incidence of CAD; conversely, the higher the LDL level ("bad" cholesterol), the higher the incidence of CAD.

Purpose

To assess the risk of CAD

Patient
preparation

Explain that this test, which requires a blood sample, helps determine the risk of CAD. Instruct the patient to maintain a normal diet for 2 weeks before the test, to abstain from alcohol for 24 hours before the test, and to fast and avoid exercise for 12 to 14 hours before the test. As ordered, withhold thyroid hormones, oral contraceptives, and antilipemics, which alter test results.

Procedure

Perform a venipuncture, and collect the sample in a 7-ml *red-top* tube. Send the sample to the laboratory immediately because spontaneous redistribution of cholesterol occurs among lipoproteins. If the sample can't be transported immediately, it should be refrigerated but not frozen.

Values

Because normal cholesterol values vary according to age, sex, geographic region, and ethnic group, check the laboratory for normal values. Normal HDL-cholesterol levels range from 29 to 77 mg/100 ml (0.8 to 2.0 mmol/L) and normal LDL-cholesterol levels range from 62 to 185 mg/100 ml (1.6 to 4.7 mmol/L).

Implications of results

High LDL levels increase the risk of CAD. Elevated HDL levels generally reflect a healthy state but can also indicate chronic hepatitis, early-stage primary biliary cirrhosis, or alcohol consumption. Rarely, a sharp rise (to as high as 100 mg/dl) in a second type of HDL (alpha$_2$-HDL) may signal CAD. Although cholesterol fractionation provides valuable information about the risk of heart disease, other sources of such risk — diabetes mellitus, hypertension, cigarette smoking — are at least as important.

Post-test care

- If a hematoma develops at the venipuncture site, applying warm soaks eases discomfort.
- The patient may resume restricted diet and medications.

Interfering factors

- Values are lowered by antilipemic medications, such as clofibrate, cholestyramine, colestipol, dextrothyroxine, niacin, probucol, and gemfibrozil.
- Oral contraceptives, disulfiram, alcohol, miconazole, and high doses of phenothiazines may increase values.
- Estrogens usually increase but may decrease values.
- Failure to send the sample to the laboratory immediately may allow spontaneous redistribution of the lipoproteins and alter test results.
- Collecting the sample in a heparinized tube may produce false elevation of values through activation of the enzyme lipase, which, in turn, causes the release of fatty acids from triglycerides.
- Presence of bilirubin, hemoglobin, salicylates, iodine, vitamins A and D, or some other substances may affect accurate determination of values. Some procedures (for example, Abell-Kendall) are less susceptible to interference than others.
- Concurrent illness, especially if accompanied by fever, recent surgery, or myocardial infarction, may interfere with accurate test results.

Lipoprotein phenotyping

In lipoprotein phenotyping, ultracentrifugation and electrophoresis of a blood sample determine lipoprotein levels, chylomicrons, very-low-density lipoproteins (VLDLs), low-density lipoproteins (LDLs), and high-density lipoproteins (HDLs).

For transportation through the blood, most lipids must combine with water-soluble proteins (apoproteins) to form lipoproteins. Several types of lipoproteins normally exist in the body, but in certain familial disorders, the blood levels of these types change. Classification of patients by the pattern of their lipoprotein levels identifies hyperlipoproteinemias and hypolipoproteinemias.

Purpose
To determine classification of hyperlipoproteinemia or hypolipoproteinemia

Patient preparation
Explain that this test, which requires a blood sample, helps determine how the body metabolizes fats. Instruct the patient to abstain from alcohol for 24 hours before the test, to have a low-fat meal the night before the test, and to fast after midnight the night before the test.

Check the patient's medication history for use of heparin. Withhold antilipemics, such as cholestyramine, about 2 weeks before the test.

Notify the laboratory if the patient is hospitalized for any other condition that might significantly alter lipoprotein metabolism, such as diabetes mellitus, nephrosis, or hypothyroidism.

Procedure
Perform a venipuncture, and collect the sample in a 7-ml *lavender-top* tube. Fill the collection tube completely, and invert it gently several times to mix the sample and the anticoagulant. Handle the sample gently to prevent hemolysis, which can alter test results.

When drawing multiple samples, collect the sample for lipoprotein phenotyping first, because venous obstruction for more than 2 minutes can affect test results.

Findings
The types of hyperlipoproteinemias or hypolipoproteinemias are identified by their characteristic electrophoretic patterns. The laboratory reports the type of lipoproteinemia present. (See *Familial hyperlipoproteinemias,* pages 418 and 419, for patterns in the six types of hyperlipoproteinemias.)

Familial hyperlipoproteinemias

Type	Causes and incidence	Clinical signs	Laboratory findings
I	Deficient lipoprotein lipase, resulting in increase chylomicrons	Eruptive xanthomas Lipemia	Increased chylomicron, total cholesterol, and triglyceride levels
	May be induced by alcoholism, hyper-insulinemic states, pregnancy	Abdominal pain	Normal or slightly increased very-low-density lipoprotein (VLDL) level
	Incidence: rare		Normal or decreased low-density lipoprotein (LDL) and high-density lipoprotein (HDL) levels
			Cholesterol-triglyceride ratio under 0.2
IIa	Deficient LDL-cell receptor, resulting in increased LDL and excessive cholesterol synthesis	Premature coronary artery disease (CAD) Arcus cornea Xanthelasma	Increased LDL level Normal VLDL level Cholesterol-triglyceride ratio over 2.0
	May be induced by hypothyroidism	Tendinous and tuberous xanthomas	
	Incidence: common		
IIb	Unknown cause resulting in increased cholesterol synthesis	Premature CAD Obesity	Increased LDL, VLDL, total cholesterol, and triglyceride levels
	May be induced by dysgammaglobulinemia, hypothyroidism, uncontrolled diabetes mellitus, and nephrotic syndrome	Possible xanthelasmas	
	Incidence: common		
III	Unknown cause, result-ing in deficient VLDL-to-LDL conversion	Premature CAD Arcus cornea	Increased total cholesterol, VLDL, and triglyceride levels
	May be induced by hypothyroidism, uncontrolled diabetes mellitus, and paraproteinemia	Eruptive tuberous xanthomas	Normal or decreased LDL level Cholesterol-triglyceride ratio of VLDL over 0.4
	Incidence: rare		Broad beta band ob-served on electrophoresis

Familial hyperlipoproteinemias *(continued)*

Type	Causes and incidence	Clinical signs	Laboratory findings
IV	Unknown cause, resulting in decreased levels of lipoprotein lipase May be induced by uncontrolled diabetes mellitus, alcoholism, pregnancy, steroid or estrogen therapy, dysgammaglobulinemia, and hyperthyroidism Incidence: common	Possible premature CAD Obesity Hypertension Peripheral neuropathy	Increased VLDL and triglyceride levels Normal LDL levels Cholesterol-triglyceride ratio of VLDL under 0.25
V	Unknown cause, resulting in defective triglyceride clearance May be induced by alcoholism, dysgammaglobulinemia, uncontrolled diabetes mellitus, nephrotic syndrome, pancreatitis, and steroid therapy Incidence: rare	Premature CAD Abdominal pain Lipemia retinalis Eruptive xanthomas Hepatosplenomegaly	Increased VLDL, total cholesterol, and triglyceride levels Chylomicrons present Cholesterol-triglyceride ratio under 0.6

Implications of results

Familial lipoprotein disorders are classified as either hyperlipoproteinemias or hypolipoproteinemias.

The hyperlipoproteinemias break down into six types — I, IIa, IIb, III, IV, and V. Types IIa, IIb, and IV are relatively common. The hypolipoproteinemias are rare and include hypobetalipoproteinemia, abetalipoproteinemia (Bassen-Kornzweig's syndrome), and alpha-lipoprotein deficiency (Tangier disease).

Although research into the apolipoproteins and their genetic variants in assessing cardiac risk in hyperproteinemia continues, the mainstay of diagnosis and monitoring of therapy is an assay of total cholesterol, HDL-cholesterol, and triglyceride. Apolipoprotein B, estimated by immunoassay, has a place in type IV hyperlipidemia in refining the information obtainable from calculated LDL-cholesterol. Apoprotein E genotyping by polyacrylamide isoelectric focusing has relevance in identifying the

E2/E2 genotype that characterizes type III hyperlipidemia.

In familial combined hyperlipidemia, the most common form of hyperlipidemia, the patient has a family history of early onset coronary heart disease associated with elevation of both cholesterol and triglycerides, and a phenotype corresponding to type IIa, IIb, or IV hyperlipidemia. There is also increased production of apolipoprotein B by the liver.

Post-test care
- If a hematoma develops at the venipuncture site, applying warm soaks eases discomfort.
- The patient may resume a normal diet and restricted medications.

Interfering factors
- Hemolysis caused by excessive agitation of the sample may interfere with accurate test results.
- Failure to observe diet and alcohol restrictions, or recent use of antilipemics, which lower lipid levels, may interfere with accurate determination of values.
- Administration of heparin (which activates the enzyme lipase, producing fatty acids from triglycerides) or collection of the sample in a heparinized tube may falsely elevate values.

Lithium, serum

Lithium carbonate, which is used to treat bipolar affective disorders, has a narrow therapeutic index. It produces toxic effects at levels only slightly above those required to achieve a satisfactory therapeutic response. Such toxicity most commonly produces GI symptoms (nausea, vomiting, diarrhea), but may also cause cardiac, central nervous system, renal, and thyroid toxicities as well. Because lithium is chemically related to sodium and substitutes for sodium in certain physiological processes, changes in sodium metabolism can affect lithium levels. For example, patients on salt-restricted diets can show significantly increased serum lithium levels and concomitant toxicity resulting from increased tubular reabsorption even though their lithium dosage is unchanged.

For these reasons, lithium therapy requires careful monitoring of serum lithium levels. During initial therapy, serum levels are typically monitored once or twice weekly until the desired therapeutic level is achieved and maintained. Thereafter, blood levels are commonly monitored at 2- to 3- month intervals or whenever toxicity or suboptimal response is suspected. Because of the potential for toxicity, periodic monitoring also includes electrolyte levels, electrocardiograms, and thyroid tests (thyroxin, triiodothyronine uptake, thyroid-stimulating hormone) and renal (blood urea nitrogen, creatinine) function. Lithium is assayed by flame photometry, atomic absorption spectroscopy, or by ion selective electrode.

Purpose
- To verify appropriate lithium dosage for maintaining therapeutic serum levels
- To detect or confirm lithium toxicity
- To assess patient compliance

Patient preparation
Explain the purpose of this test, and inform the patient that the test requires a blood sample.

Procedure
Perform a venipuncture and collect a blood sample. This test requires 1 ml of serum. In most patients, serum lithium levels reach steady state in approximately 5 days. Unless toxicity is suspected, testing serum levels before steady state is achieved is not recommended because such testing yields results that are difficult to interpret. At steady state, blood samples should be collected 10 to 14 hours after the last dose.

Values
Therapeutic range of lithium is 0.8 to 1.2 mEq/L (mmol/L).

Implications of results
Because of individual variation, some patients develop signs of toxicity at serum levels within the therapeutic range; others may show no overt toxicity at much higher levels. In fact, some require levels between 1.2 and 2.0 mEq/L (mmol/L) to achieve optimum response. Consequently, the serum level should be used as a guide and must be interpreted in light of clinical presentation. Levels greater than 2.0 mEq/L (mmol/L) are associated with toxicity in most patients, and levels greater than 3.0 mEq/L (mmol/L) may cause fatal toxicity.

Post-test care
If a hematoma develops at the venipuncture site, applying warm soaks eases discomfort.

None

Liver biopsy, percutaneous

Percutaneous biopsy of the liver is the needle aspiration of a core of tissue for histologic analysis. This procedure is performed under a local or general anesthetic. Such analysis can identify hepatic disorders after ultrasonography, computed tomography, and radionuclide studies have failed to detect them. Because many patients with hepatic disorders have clotting defects, testing for hemostasis should precede liver biopsy.

Purpose

To diagnose hepatic parenchymal disease, malignant disease, and granulomatous infections

Patient
preparation

Explain that this test helps diagnose liver disorders. Describe the procedure, and answer any questions the patient has about the test. Instruct the patient to restrict food and fluids for 4 to 8 hours before the test.

Make sure that the patient or an appropriate family member has signed a consent form. Check the patient's history for hypersensitivity to the local anesthetic. Make sure prothrombin time and platelet count tests have been performed and that the results are recorded on the patient's chart.

Just before the biopsy, tell the patient to void. Inform the patient that he will receive a local anesthetic but may experience pain similar to that of a punch in his right shoulder, as the biopsy needle passes the phrenic nerve.

Procedure

For aspiration biopsy using the Menghini needle, the patient is placed in a supine position, with his right hand under his head. Instruct the patient to maintain this position and remain as still as possible during the procedure. The liver is palpated, the biopsy site is selected and marked, and the anesthetic is then injected. The needle flange is set to control the depth of penetration, and 2 ml of sterile normal saline solution are drawn into the syringe. The syringe is attached to the biopsy needle, and the needle is introduced into the subcutaneous tissue, through the right eighth or ninth intercostal space, between the anterior and posterior axillary lines. One milliliter of normal saline solution is injected to clear the needle and the plunger, then the plunger is drawn back to the 4-ml mark to create negative pressure. At this point in the procedure, the patient is asked to take a deep breath, exhale, and hold his breath at the end of expiration to prevent any movement of the chest wall. As the patient holds his breath, the biopsy needle is quickly inserted into the liver and withdrawn in 1 second. After the needle is withdrawn, the patient can resume breathing normally. The tissue specimen is then placed in a properly labeled specimen cup containing 10% formalin solution. This is done by releasing negative pressure while the point of the needle is in the formalin solution. Again, 1 ml of normal saline solution is injected to clear the needle of the tissue specimen. Apply pressure to the biopsy site to halt bleeding. Send the specimen to the laboratory immediately.

Precautions
Percutaneous liver biopsy is contraindicated in a patient with a platelet count below 100,000; prothrombin time longer than 15 seconds; empyema of the lungs, pleurae, peritoneum, biliary tract, or liver; vascular tumor; hepatic angiomas; hydatid cyst; or tense ascites. If extrahepatic obstruction is suspected, ultrasonography or subcutaneous transhepatic cholangiography should rule out this condition before the biopsy is considered.

Findings
The normal liver consists of sheets of hepatocytes supported by a reticulin framework.

Implications of results
Hepatic tissue may show diffuse disease, such as cirrhosis or hepatitis, or granulomatous infections, such as tuberculosis. Primary malignant tumors include hepatocellular carcinoma, cholangiocellular carcinoma, and angiosarcoma, but hepatic metastases are more common.

Nonmalignant findings with a known focal lesion require further studies — laparotomy, or laparoscopy with biopsy, for example.

Post-test care
• Position the patient on the right side for 2 hours, with a small pillow or sandbag under the costal margin to provide extra pressure. Advise bed rest for 24 hours.
• The patient may resume a normal diet.

- The patient may experience pain, which may persist for several hours after the test, and may require analgesic medication.
- Check the patient's vital signs every 15 minutes for 1 hour, then every 30 minutes for 4 hours, and every 4 hours thereafter for 24 hours. Throughout, observe carefully for signs of shock.

➤ *Clinical alert:* Watch for bleeding or signs of bile peritonitis — tenderness and rigidity around the biopsy site. Be alert for symptoms of pneumothorax: rising respiration rate, depressed breath sounds, dyspnea, persistent shoulder pain, and pleuritic chest pain.

Interfering factor

Failure to obtain a representative specimen, to place the specimen in the proper preservative, or to transport the specimen immediately to the laboratory may interfere with accurate determination of test results.

Lung biopsy

In a biopsy of the lung, a specimen of pulmonary tissue is excised by closed or open technique for histologic examination. Closed technique, performed under local anesthetic, includes both needle and transbronchial biopsies; open technique, performed under general anesthetic in the operating room, includes both limited and standard thoracotomies. Needle biopsy is appropriate when the lesion is readily accessible, or when it originates in the lung parenchyma, is confined to it, or is affixed to the chest wall; it provides a much smaller specimen than the open technique. Transbronchial biopsy, the removal of multiple tissue specimens through a fiber-optic bronchoscope, is appropriate for diffuse infiltrative pulmonary disease, tumors, or when severe debilitation contraindicates open biopsy. Open biopsy is appropriate for the study of a well-circumscribed lesion that may require resection.

Generally, a biopsy of the lung is recommended after chest X-ray, computed tomography scan, and bronchoscopy have failed to identify the cause of diffuse parenchymal pulmonary disease or of a pulmonary lesion. Complications of lung biopsy may include bleeding, infection, and pneumothorax.

Purpose To confirm diagnosis of diffuse parenchymal pulmonary disease and pulmonary lesions

Patient preparation Explain that this test assesses the condition of the lungs. Describe the procedure and answer any questions. Instruct the patient to fast after midnight before the procedure. (Sometimes the patient is permitted to have clear liquids the morning of the test.)

Tell the patient that a chest X-ray and blood studies (prothrombin time, activated partial thromboplastin time, and platelet count) will be performed before the biopsy.

Make sure that the patient or an appropriate family member has signed a consent form. Check the patient's history for hypersensitivity to the local anesthetic. A mild sedative may be administered 30 minutes before the biopsy to help the patient relax. The patient will receive a local anesthetic but may experience a sharp, transient pain when the biopsy needle touches the lung.

Procedure After the biopsy site is selected, lead markers are placed on the patient's skin, and X-rays are ordered to verify their correct placement. The patient is placed in a sitting position, with arms folded on a table in front, and is instructed to maintain this position, remaining as still as possible, and to refrain from coughing. The skin over the biopsy site is prepared, and the area is draped. With a 25G needle, the local anesthetic is injected just above the lower rib to prevent damage to the intercostal nerves and vessels. Using a 22G needle, the examiner anesthetizes the intercostal muscles and parietal pleura, makes a small incision (2 to 3 mm) with a scalpel, and introduces the biopsy needle through the incision, chest wall, and pleura, into the tumor or the pulmonary tissue.

If the intercostal space at the incision site is wide, the needle is inserted at a 90-degree angle; if the ribs overlap and the intercostal space is narrow, at a 45-degree angle. When the needle is in the tumor or pulmonary tissue, the specimen is obtained and the needle is withdrawn. The specimen is divided immediately: the tissue for histology is placed in a properly labeled bottle containing 10% neutral buffered formaldehyde solution; the tissue for microbiology is placed in a sterile container.

Pressure is exerted on the biopsy site to stop the bleeding, and then a small bandage is applied.

Precautions

A needle biopsy is contraindicated in patients with a lesion that has separated from the chest wall or is accompanied by emphysematous bullae, cysts, or gross emphysema, and in patients with coagulopathy, hypoxia, pulmonary hypertension, or cardiac disease with cor pulmonale.

During biopsy, observe carefully for signs of respiratory distress — shortness of breath, elevated pulse, and cyanosis (late sign). Because coughing or movement during biopsy can cause tearing of the lung by the biopsy needle, keep the patient calm and still during the procedure.

Findings

Normal pulmonary tissue shows uniform texture of the alveolar ducts, alveolar walls, bronchioles, and small vessels.

Implications of results

Histologic examination of a pulmonary tissue specimen can reveal squamous cell or oat cell carcinoma, and adenocarcinoma. Such examination supplements the results of microbiologic cultures, deep-cough sputum specimens, chest X-rays, bronchoscopy, and the patient's physical history, in confirming cancer or parenchymal pulmonary disease.

Post-test care

• Check vital signs every 15 minutes for 1 hour, every hour for 4 hours, then every 4 hours. Watch for bleeding, shortness of breath, elevated pulse, diminished breath sounds on the biopsy side, and, eventually, cyanosis. Make sure the chest X-ray is repeated immediately after the biopsy is completed.
• The patient may resume a normal diet.

Interfering factor

Failure to obtain a representative tissue specimen or to store the specimens for histology and microbiology in the appropriate containers may interfere with accurate determination of test results.

Lupus erythematosus (LE) cell preparation

Lupus erythematosus (LE) cell preparation is an in vitro procedure used in the diagnosis of systemic lupus erythematosus (SLE). This test is less sensitive and reliable than the antinuclear antibody (ANA) or the anti-deoxyribonucleic acid (DNA) antibody test, which have largely replaced it. However, it may be used because it requires minimal equipment and reagents.

In this test, a blood sample is mixed with laboratory-treated nucleoprotein (the antigen). If the sample contains ANA, the ANA reacts with the nucleoprotein, causing swelling and rupture. Phagocytes from the serum then engulf the extruded nuclei, forming LE cells, which are then detected by microscopic examination of the sample.

Purpose
- To aid diagnosis of SLE
- To monitor treatment of SLE (about 60% of successfully treated patients fail to show LE cells after 4 to 6 weeks of therapy)

Patient preparation
Explain that this test helps detect antibodies to tissue. Inform the patient that the test requires a blood sample and may be repeated to monitor response to therapy.

Check the patient's medication history for drugs, such as isoniazid, hydralazine, and procainamide, that may affect test results. If such drugs must be continued, note this on the laboratory slip.

Procedure
Perform a venipuncture, and collect the sample in a 7-ml *red-top* tube. Handle the sample gently to prevent hemolysis.

Findings
Normally, no LE cells are present.

Implications of results
The presence of at least two LE cells may indicate SLE. Although these cells occur primarily in SLE, they may also form in chronic active hepatitis, rheumatoid arthritis, scleroderma, and drug reactions. Also, up to 25% of patients with SLE demonstrate no LE cells. Apart from supportive clinical signs, definitive diagnosis of SLE may necessitate a confirming ANA or anti-DNA test. The ANA test detects autoantibodies in the sera of many SLE patients with negative LE cell tests. Anti-DNA antibodies appear in two-thirds of all SLE patients but are rare in other conditions; the presence of such antibodies is strong evidence of SLE.

Post-test care
- Because many patients with SLE have compromised immune systems, keep a clean, dry ban-

dage over the venipuncture site for at least 24 hours, and check for infection.
- If a hematoma develops at the venipuncture site, applying warm soaks eases discomfort.
- If test results indicate SLE, tell the patient that further diagnostic tests may be required.

Interfering factors
- Hemolysis caused by excessive agitation of the sample may interfere with accurate determination of test results.
- Certain drugs — most commonly isoniazid, hydralazine, and procainamide — can produce a syndrome resembling SLE. Other such drugs include para-aminosalicylic acid, chlorpromazine, clofibrate, phenytoin, griseofulvin, ethosuximide, methyldopa, oral contraceptives, gold salts, penicillin, propylthiouracil, phenylbutazone, methysergide, streptomycin, sulfonamides, tetracyclines, mephenytoin, quinidine, primidone, reserpine, and trimethadione.

Luteinizing hormone (LH), plasma

Interstitial-cell-stimulating hormone

This test, usually ordered for anovulation and infertility studies and performed most often on females, is a quantitative analysis of plasma luteinizing hormone (LH) levels. For accurate diagnosis, results must be evaluated in light of findings obtained from related hormone tests (follicle-stimulating hormone [FSH], estrogen, and testosterone, for example). LH is a glycoprotein secreted by basophilic cells of the anterior pituitary gland. In females, cyclic LH secretion (with FSH) causes ovulation and transforms the ovarian follicle into the corpus luteum, which, in turn, secretes progesterone. In males, continuous LH secretion stimulates the interstitial (Leydig) cells of the testes to release testosterone, which stimulates and maintains spermatogenesis (with FSH).

Purpose
- To detect ovulation
- To assess male or female infertility
- To evaluate amenorrhea
- To monitor therapy designed to induce ovulation
- To aid evaluation of children with endocrine problems associated with precocious puberty

Patient preparation	Explain that this test helps evaluate secretion of female hormones. Tell the patient that the test requires a blood sample.

Withhold drugs, such as steroids (including estrogens or progesterone), that may interfere with plasma LH levels for 48 hours before the test. If these medications must be continued, note this on the laboratory slip.

Procedure Perform a venipuncture, and collect the sample in a 7-ml *red-top* tube. Handle the sample gently to prevent hemolysis.

If the patient is a female, indicate the date of her last menstrual cycle or indicate menopause on the laboratory slip.

Values Normal values may have a wide range —
Children: 4 to 20 mIU/ml (IU/L)
Adult males: 5 to 20 mIU/ml (IU/L)
Adult females: Values vary, depending on the phase of the menstrual cycle — follicular phase: 5 to 15 mIU/ml (IU/L); midcycle (ovulation): 30 to 60 mIU/ml (IU/L); luteal phase: 5 to 15 mIU/ml (IU/L)
Postmenopausal females: 50 to 100 mIU/ml (IU/L)

Implications of results In females, absence of a midcycle peak in LH secretion may indicate anovulation. Decreased or low-normal levels may indicate hypogonadotropism; these findings are commonly associated with amenorrhea. High LH levels may indicate congenital absence of ovaries or ovarian failure associated with Stein-Leventhal syndrome (polycystic ovary syndrome), Turner's syndrome (ovarian dysgenesis), menopause, or early-stage acromegaly. Infertility can result from either primary or secondary gonadal dysfunction.

In males, low values may indicate secondary gonadal dysfunction (of hypothalamic or pituitary origin); high values may indicate testicular failure (primary hypogonadism) or destruction or congenital absence of testes.

Post-test care • If a hematoma develops at the venipuncture site, applying warm soaks eases discomfort.
• The patient may resume discontinued medications.

Interfering factors

- Failure to observe restrictions of medications may interfere with accurate determination of test results. Steroids (including estrogens, progesterone, and testosterone) may decrease plasma LH levels.
- Radioactive scan performed within 1 week before the test may influence test results because plasma LH levels are determined by radioimmunoassay.
- Hemolysis caused by excessive agitation of the sample may interfere with accurate determination of test results.

Lyme disease serology

Lyme disease is a multisystem disorder characterized by dermatologic, neurologic, cardiac, and rheumatic manifestations in various stages. Epidemiologic and serologic studies implicate the tickborne spirochete, *Borrelia burgdorferi,* as the causative agent. Serologic tests, both indirect immunofluorescent and enzyme-linked immunosorbent assays, measure antibody response to this spirochete and indicate current infection or past exposure. These assays identify 50% of patients with early-stage Lyme disease; essentially 100% of patients with later complications of carditis, neuritis, and arthritis; and 100% of patients in remission.

In an indirect immunofluorescent assay, *B. burgdorferi* is grown in culture, fixed to a microscope slide, and incubated with a human serum sample. A fluorescein-labeled antiglobulin is then introduced into the antigen-antibody complex. Any human antibody that binds to the spirochete is detected by viewing (under an ultraviolet microscope) the fluorescent antiglobulin that attaches to it.

Purpose

To confirm diagnosis of infection with *B. burgdorferi*

Patient preparation

Explain that this test helps determine whether his symptoms are caused by Lyme disease. Tell the patient that the test requires a blood sample.

Procedure

Perform a venipuncture, and collect the sample in a 7-ml *red-top* tube. Handle the specimen carefully to prevent hemolysis.

Findings   Normal serum values are nonreactive. Positive results may be confirmed by additional testing.

Implications of results   A positive Lyme serology can help confirm diagnosis but is not definitive. Other treponemal diseases and high rheumatoid factor titers can cause false-positive results. Patients with other treponemal diseases demonstrate considerable cross-reactivity, and, although rheumatoid factor isn't normally associated with Lyme disease, up to 20% of patients with high rheumatoid factor titers may have positive Lyme disease reactions.

Post-test care   If a hematoma develops at the venipuncture site, applying warm soaks eases discomfort.

Interfering factors
- Analysis of serum with high lipid levels may cause inaccurate test results and requires repetition of the test after a period of restricted fat intake.
- Hemolysis caused by excessive agitation of the sample can interfere with accurate determination of test results.

Lymph node biopsy

Lymph node biopsy is the surgical excision of an active lymph node or the needle aspiration of a nodal specimen for histologic examination. Both techniques usually employ a local anesthetic and sample the superficial nodes in the cervical, supraclavicular, axillary, or inguinal region. Excision is the preferred technique, because it provides a larger specimen.

Lymph nodes swell from their usually flat, bean shape during infection but return to normal size as infection clears. When nodal enlargement is prolonged and is accompanied by backache, leg edema, breathing and swallowing difficulties, and later, weight loss, weakness, severe itching, fever, night sweats, cough, hemoptysis, or hoarseness, biopsy is indicated. Generalized or localized lymph node enlargement is typical of diseases such as chronic lymphatic leukemia, Hodgkin's disease, infectious mononucleosis, and rheumatoid arthritis.

Complete blood count, liver function studies, liver and spleen scans, and X-rays should precede this test.

Purpose
- To determine the cause of lymph node enlargement
- To distinguish between benign and malignant lymph node tumors
- To stage metastatic carcinoma

Patient preparation

Explain that this test allows microscopic study of lymph node tissue. Describe the procedure and answer any questions. For excisional biopsy, the patient must restrict food from midnight and to drink only clear liquids on the morning of the test (if general anesthetic is needed for deeper nodes, he must also restrict fluids). For needle biopsy, the patient needn't restrict food or fluids.

Make sure that the patient or a responsible family member has signed a consent form. Check the patient's history for hypersensitivity to the anesthetic.

If the patient will receive a local anesthetic, explain that he may experience discomfort during injection. Just before the biopsy, record baseline vital signs.

Procedure

Excisional biopsy: Prepare the skin over the biopsy site; drape the area for privacy. The anesthetic is then administered. The examiner makes an incision, removes an entire node, and places it in a properly labeled bottle containing normal saline solution. Then the wound is sutured, and a sterile dressing is applied.

Needle biopsy: After preparing the biopsy site and administering a local anesthetic, the examiner grasps the node between his thumb and forefinger, inserts the needle directly into the node, and obtains a small core specimen. The needle is then removed, and the specimen is placed in a properly labeled bottle containing normal saline solution. Pressure is exerted on the biopsy site to control bleeding, and an adhesive bandage is applied.

Storing the tissue specimen in normal saline solution instead of in 10% formaldehyde solution allows part of the specimen to be used for cytologic impression smears, which are studied along with the biopsy specimen.

Findings

The normal lymph node is encapsulated by collagenous connective tissue and is divided into smaller lobes by tissue strands called trabeculae. It has an outer cortex, composed of lymphoid cells and nodules or follicles containing lymphocytes, and an inner medulla, composed of reticular phagocytic cells that collect and drain fluid.

Implications of results

Histologic examination of the tissue specimen distinguishes between malignant and nonmalignant causes of lymph node enlargement. Lymphatic malignancy accounts for up to 5% of all cancers and is slightly more prevalent in males than in females. Hodgkin's disease, a lymphoma affecting the entire lymph system, is the leading cancer affecting adolescents and young adults. Lymph node malignancy may also result from metastasizing carcinoma.

When histologic results aren't clear or nodular material isn't involved, mediastinoscopy or laparotomy can provide another nodal specimen. Occasionally, lymphangiography can furnish additional diagnostic information.

Post-test care

- Check vital signs, and watch for bleeding, tenderness, and redness at the biopsy site.
- Patient may resume his usual diet.

Interfering factors

- Improper specimen storage or failure to obtain a representative tissue specimen may alter test results.
- Inability to differentiate nodal pathology may interfere with accurate determination of test results.

Lymphocyte marker assay

T- and B-cell surface markers, T- and B-lymphocyte subset assay

Lymphocytes are divided into two major functionally distinct groups: T cells, which are thymus derived; and B cells, which are bone marrow derived. T lymphocytes arise in the thymus gland and migrate to peripheral organs (lymph nodes, spleen, and blood) during embryonic development. They function as regulators of B-cell responses. B cells are thymic-independent immunoglobulin-producing cells that develop in bone marrow. They function as specific antigen receptors by using endogenous immunoglubulins that evolve on their surface membrane.

T- and B-cell assays are commonly performed and have contributed greatly to clinical understanding of immunodeficiency, autoimmune disorders, tumor immunity, and infectious disease. Such assays can be performed by microscopy or flow cytometry with specific antibodies linked to fluorescent dyes. These tests are most commonly performed on cells from peripheral blood, but can also be performed on tissue sections or cells from bone marrow or other organs. Results of tests for T- and B-cell markers should be expressed as the absolute number of cells per microliter (μliter) of whole blood. Results that report a percentage of cells carrying a specific marker are subject to misinterpretation because such a result could represent a relative increase in one cell group or a decrease in another.

In 1983, the First International Workshop on Human Leukocyte Differentiation Antigens established new nomenclature for cellular types and subtypes. They defined a series of "clusters of differentiation" (CD types) that define cellular antigens. A second workshop in 1984 refined and expanded this nomenclature (see *Cell types and nomenclature,* pages 435 and 436). CD nomenclature is rapidly replacing older antibody designations (such as OKT 4 and Leu 3).

Purpose	• To evaluate immune function by identifying specific cells involved in immune response
	• To aid diagnosis of lymphocytic leukemia, lymphoma, and acquired immunodeficiency syndrome (AIDS)
	• To aid diagnosis and treatment of chronic infections, hepatitis, and autoimmune disorders

Patient preparation   Explain the purpose of this test, and inform the patient that the test requires a blood sample.

Procedure   Perform a venipuncture, and collect a whole blood sample. Do not refrigerate or freeze the sample. Send it to the laboratory promptly.

Values   Normal values of T and B surface markers are as follows—
Percentage B cells (CD19): 5% to 20%
Percentage T cells (CD3): 53% to 88%
Percentage Helper T cells (CD4): 32% to 61%
Percentage Suppressor/cytotoxic T cells (CD8): 18% to 42%
Percentage natural killer cells (CD16): 4% to 32%
Lymphocyte counts: 0.66 to 4.60 thousand/μliter

Cell types and nomenclature

Cell type	CD designation	Antibody designation	Comments
Cortical thymocytes	CD1	Leu 6 OKT 6 T6	Early T cell antigen also occur on Langerhans cells, associated with B_2-microglobulin not present on peripheral T cells.
T cells, natural killer cells	CD2	Leu 5b OKT 11 T11	Pan-T cell antigen sheep red blood cell receptor on T cells. To differentiate lymphoproliferative disorders of T-cell origin, such as T-cell lymphocytic leukemia and lymphoblastic lymphoma, from those of non-T-cell origin.
Mature T cells	CD3	Leu 4 OKT 3 T3	Also present on T-cell acute lymphocytic leukemia and cutaneous T-cell lymphoma; part of T-antigen receptor complex.
Helper T cells	CD4	Leu 3a OKT 4 T4	Receptor for major histocompatibility complex class II module. Used to identify and characterize the proportion of T-helper cells in autoimmune or immunoregulatory disorders; to detect immunodeficiency disorders, such as acquired immunodeficiency syndrome; to differentiate T-cell acute lymphoblastic leukemia from T-cell lymphomas and other lymphoproliferative disorders.
Pan-T and pan-B cell subpopulation	CD5	Leu 1 OKT 1 T1	Used to identify B-cell lymphoproliferative disorders, such as B-cell chronic lymphocytic leukemia.
Mature T- and B-cell subpopulation	CD6	T12	Malignant T cells
Pan-T cell, thymocytes	CD7	Leu 9 3A1	T-cell leukemias
Suppressor/cytotoxic T cells	CD8, CD11a, CD11b, CD11c, CD16, CD56	Leu 2a OKT 8 T8	Receptor for major histocompatibility complex class I molecule. Used to identify suppressor/cytotoxic T cells in autoimmune and immunoregulatory disorders and to characterize lymphoproliferative disorders.
B cells	CD19	Leu 12 B4	None

(continued)

Cell types and nomenclature *(continued)*

Cell type	CD designation	Antibody designation	Comments
B cells	CD20	Leu 16 B1	Used to differentiate lymphoproliferative disorders of B-cell origin, such as B-cell chronic lymphocytic leukemia, from those of T-cell origin.
Mature B cells	CD21	B2	C3d receptor
CALLA(common acute lymphocytic leukemia antigen) marker	CD10	Not known	Used to identify bone marrow regeneration; to identify non-T-cell acute lymphocytic leukemia.
Lymphocyte subset panel	CD4, CD5, CD7, CD8, and CD4:CD8 ratio	Not known	Used to evaluate immunodeficiencies; to identify immunoregulation associated with autoimmune disorders, to characterize lymphoid malignancies.
Lymphocytic leukemia marker panel	CD2, CD7, CD10, CD20	Leu 5b, Leu 9, B1, BA-1, CALLA	Used to characterize lymphocytic leukemias as T, B, non-T, or non-B, regardless of the stage of differentiation of the malignant cells.

B-cell count CD19): 99 to 426 cells/µliter
T-cell count (CD3): 812 to 2,318 cells/µliter
Helper T cell count (CD4): 589 to 1,505 cells/µliter
Suppressor/cytotoxic T cell count (CD8): 325 to 997 cells/µliter
Natural killer cell count (CD16): 78 to 602 cells/µliter
CD4-CD8 ratio: ≥ 1.0.

Implications of results

B cells are decreased in transient hypogammaglobulinemia of infancy, X-linked hypogammaglobulinemia, selective deficiency of IgG, IgA, IgM, lymphomas, nephrotic syndrome, and multiple myeloma.

T cells are decreased in DeGeorge's syndrome, Nezelof's syndrome, Hodgkin's or other malignant disease, and acute viral infection.

Both B and T cells are decreased in autosomal or sex-linked recessive immunodeficiency, Wiskott-Aldrich's syndrome; decrease of B and T cells may also result from radiation, and aging. T cells increase in Graves' disease; B cells increase in active lupus erythematosus and chronic lymphocytic leukemia.

Decreased lymphocyte totals usually follow immunosuppressant and cytotoxic drug therapy.

In patients with AIDS, the CD_4-CD_8 ratio decreases (less than 1) because of loss of helper T lymphocytes.

Post-test care If a hematoma develops at the venipuncture site, applying warm soaks eases discomfort.

Interfering factors None

Lymphocyte transformation tests

Transformation tests evaluate lymphocyte competency without injection of antigens into the patient's skin. These in vitro tests eliminate the risk of adverse effects but can still accurately assess the ability of lymphocytes to proliferate and to recognize and respond to antigens.

The mitogen assay, performed using nonspecific plant lectins, evaluates the mitotic response of T and B lymphocytes to a foreign antigen. The mitogens phytohemagglutinin (PHA) and concanavalin A stimulate T lymphocytes preferentially, whereas pokeweed primarily stimulates B lymphocytes, and T lymphocytes to a lesser extent. In the mitogen assay, a purified culture of lymphocytes from the patient's blood is incubated with a nonspecific mitogen for 72 hours — the interval during which the greatest effect on deoxyribonucleic acid (DNA) synthesis usually occurs. The culture is then pulse-labeled with tritiated thymidine, which is incorporated in the newly formed DNA of dividing cells. The uptake of radioactive thymidine can be measured by a liquid scintillation spectrophotometer in counts per minute (cpm), which parallels the rate of mitosis. Lymphocyte responsiveness, or the extent of mitosis, is then reported as a stimulation index, determined by dividing the cpm of the stimulated culture by the cpm of a control culture. The antigen assay uses specific antigens, such as purified protein derivative, *Candida,* mumps, tetanus toxoid, and streptokinase, to stimulate lymphocyte transformation. After incubation of 4½ to 7 days, transformation is measured by the same method used in the mitogen assay.

The mixed lymphocyte culture (MLC) assay tests the response of lymphocytes to histocompatibility antigens (HLA) determined by the D locus of the 6th chromosome. The MLC assay is useful in matching transplant recipients and donors and in testing immunocompetence. In this assay, lymphocytes from a recipient and potential donor are cultured together for 5 days to test compatibility. Recipient and potential donor lymphocytes (if viable and unaltered) will recognize any genetic differences and undergo transformation (grow and divide), demonstrating incompatibility. In the one-way MLC, one group of lymphocytes is pretreated with radiation or mitomycin C so that it can't divide but can still stimulate the other group of lymphocytes. Lymphocyte transformation is identified by an increased incorporation of radioactive thymidine labeling and reported as the stimulation index. After the culture is labeled with radioactive thymidine, the MLC stimulation index is then determined.

Purpose
- To assess and monitor genetic and acquired immunodeficiency states
- To provide histocompatibility typing of both tissue transplant recipients and donors

Patient preparation
Explain that this test evaluates lymphocyte function, which is the keystone of the immune system. If needed, inform the patient that the test monitors response to therapy. For histocompatibility typing, explain that this test helps determine the best match for a transplant. Tell the patient that the test requires a blood sample. If a radioisotope scan is scheduled, be sure the serum sample for this test is drawn first.

Procedure
Perform a venipuncture. If the patient is an adult, collect the sample in a 7-ml *green-top* (heparinized) tube; for a child, use a 5-ml *green-top* tube.

Precautions
Completely fill the collection tube, and invert it gently several times to mix the sample and anticoagulant. Send the sample to the laboratory immediately.

Findings
In the mitogen assay, the normal stimulation index exceeds 10; in the antigen assay, the normal stimulation index exceeds 3. In the MLC assay, unresponsiveness indicates histocompatibility for the D locus antigens.

Implications of
results
In the mitogen and antigen assays, a low stimulation index or unresponsiveness indicates a depressed or defective immune system. Serial testing can be performed to monitor the effectiveness of therapy in a patient with an immunodeficiency disease.

In the MLC test, the stimulation index is a measure of compatibility. A high index indicates poor compatibility. Conversely, a low stimulation index indicates good compatibility.

Post-test care
• Because many of these patients may have a compromised immune system, take special care to keep the venipuncture site clean and dry.
• If a hematoma develops at the venipuncture site, applying warm soaks eases discomfort.

Interfering
factors
• Pregnancy or the use of oral contraceptives depresses lymphocyte response to PHA and thus causes a low stimulation index.
• Chemotherapy may hinder accurate determination of test results unless pretherapy baseline values are available for comparison.
• A radioisotope scan performed within 1 week before test, and failure to send the sample to the laboratory immediately can affect accuracy of test results.

Lysozyme, urine
Muramidase

Lysozyme, a low-molecular weight enzyme, is present in mucus, saliva, tears, skin secretions, and various internal body cells and fluids. This enzyme splits, or lyses, the cell walls of gram-positive bacteria and, with complement and other blood factors, acts to destroy them. Lysozyme seems to be synthesized in granulocytes and monocytes, and it first appears in serum after destruction of such cells. When serum lysozyme levels exceed three times normal, the enzyme appears in the urine. However, because renal tissue also contains lysozyme, renal injury alone can cause measurable excretion of this enzyme.

This test measures urine lysozyme levels turbidimetrically. Serum lysozyme determinations, using the same method, confirm the results of urine testing.

Purpose To aid diagnosis of acute monocytic or granulocytic leukemia, and to monitor the progression of these diseases

Patient preparation Explain that this test evaluates the immune system. Tell the patient that the test requires collection of a 24-hour urine specimen, and teach the correct procedure for collecting the specimen. Tell the patient to avoid contaminating the urine specimen with toilet tissue or stool.

If the female patient is menstruating, the test may have to be rescheduled.

Procedure Collect a 24-hour urine specimen. Cover and refrigerate the specimen throughout the collection period. If the patient has an indwelling urinary catheter in place, keep the collection bag on ice. Send the specimens to the laboratory immediately when the test is completed.

Values Normally, urine lysozyme values range from 0 to 1.4 µg/ml (0.097 µmol/L).

Implications of results Urine levels rise markedly after acute onset or relapse of monocytic or myelomonocytic leukemia, and rise moderately after acute onset or relapse of granulocytic (myeloid) leukemia. Urine lysozyme levels remain normal or decrease in lymphocytic leukemia, and remain normal in myeloblastic and myelocytic leukemias.

Post-test care None

Interfering factors
- The presence of bacteria in the specimen decreases urine lysozyme levels; blood or saliva in the specimen increases lysozyme levels.
- Failure to collect all urine during the test period may interfere with accurate test results.

Magnesium, serum

This test, a quantitative analysis, measures serum levels of magnesium, the most abundant intracellular cation after potassium. Vital to neuromuscular function, this often overlooked electrolyte helps regulate intracellular metabolism, activates many essential enzymes, and affects the metabolism of nucleic acids and proteins. Magnesium also helps transport sodium and potassium across cell membranes and, through its effect on the secretion of parathyroid hormone, influences intracellular calcium levels. Most magnesium is found in bone and in intracellular fluid; a small amount is found in extracellular fluid. Magnesium is absorbed by the small intestine and is excreted in the urine and feces.

Purpose
- To evaluate electrolyte status
- To assess neuromuscular or renal function

Patient preparation
Explain that this test, which requires a blood sample, determines the magnesium content of the blood. Instruct the patient to avoid using magnesium salts (such as milk of magnesia or Epsom salt) for at least 3 days before the test, but not to restrict food or fluids.

Procedure
Perform a venipuncture, and collect the sample in a 10- to 15-ml *red-top* tube. Handle the sample gently to prevent hemolysis. *Note:* The prevention of hemolysis is especially important with this test because 75% of the blood's magnesium is located in red blood cells.

Values
Normally, serum magnesium levels range from 1.8 to 2.4 mg/dl (atomic absorption) or from 0.7 to 1.2 mmol/L.

Implications of results
Elevated serum magnesium levels (hypermagnesemia) most commonly occur in renal failure, when the kidneys excrete inadequate amounts of magnesium. Adrenal insufficiency (Addison's disease) can also elevate serum magnesium.

➤ *Clinical alert:* In suspected or confirmed hypermagnesemia, observe the patient for lethargy; flushing; diaphoresis; decreased blood pressure; slow, weak pulse rate; diminished deep tendon reflexes; muscle weakness; and slow, shallow respirations.

Suppressed serum magnesium levels (hypomagnesemia) most commonly result from chronic alcoholism. Other causes include malabsorption syndrome, diarrhea, faulty absorption following bowel resection, prolonged bowel or gastric aspiration, acute pancreatitis, primary aldosteronism, severe burns, hypercalcemic conditions (including hyperparathyroidism), and certain diuretic therapies.

➤ *Clinical alert:* In hypomagnesemia, watch for leg and foot cramps, hyperactive deep tendon reflexes, cardiac arrhythmias, muscle weakness, seizures, twitching, tetany, and tremors.

Post-test care
If a hematoma develops at the venipuncture site, applying warm soaks eases discomfort.

Interfering factors
- Excessive use of antacids or cathartics or excessive infusion of magnesium sulfate raises magnesium levels.
- Prolonged I.V. infusions that do not contain magnesium suppress magnesium levels. Excessive use of diuretics, including thiazides and ethacrynic acid, decreases levels by increasing magnesium excretion in the urine.
- I.V. administration of calcium gluconate may falsely decrease serum magnesium levels if measured by the Titan yellow method.
- Hemolysis caused by excessive agitation of the sample causes falsely elevated serum magnesium levels.

Magnesium, urine

This test — which measures the urine level of magnesium, an important cation absorbed in the intestinal tract and excreted in the urine — is especially useful because magnesium deficiency is detectable in urine before it changes serum magnesium levels. Measurement of urine magnesium is becoming more important to rule out magnesium deficiency as the cause of neurologic symptoms and to help evaluate glomerular function in suspected renal disease.

Magnesium is found primarily in the bones and in intracellular fluid; a small amount is present in extracellular fluid. This element activates many enzyme systems, helps transport sodium and potassium across cell membranes, affects nucleic acid and protein metabolism, and influences intracellular calcium levels through its effect on secretion of parathyroid hormone. Magnesium deficiency usually results from poor absorption typically related to increased absorption of calcium; magnesium absorption increases as dietary intake of calcium decreases.

Purpose
- To rule out magnesium deficiency in patients with symptoms of central nervous system irritation
- To detect excessive urinary excretion of magnesium
- To help evaluate glomerular function in renal disease

Patient preparation
Explain that this test, which determines urine magnesium levels, requires a 24-hour urine specimen.

If the patient is receiving magnesium-containing antacids, diuretics (for example, ethacrynic acid and spironolactone), or aldosterone, note this on the laboratory slip.

Procedure
Collect a 24-hour urine specimen in a plastic container. Make sure hydrochloric acid has been added as a preservative. Tell the patient to be careful not to contaminate the urine specimen with toilet tissue or stool.

Values
Normal urinary magnesium levels are 7.3 to 12.2 mg/dl (3 to 5 mmol/day), although values differ between laboratories.

Implications of results
Low urine magnesium levels may result from malabsorption, acute or chronic diarrhea, diabetic acidosis, dehydration, pancreatitis, advanced renal failure, primary aldosteronism, or decreased dietary intake of magnesium.

Elevated urine magnesium levels may result from early chronic renal disease, adrenocortical insufficiency (Addison's disease), chronic alcoholism, or long-term ingestion of magnesium-containing antacids.

Post-test care   None

Interfering   • Failure to collect all urine during the test period
factors   may interfere with accurate determination of test
              results.
              • Ethacrynic acid, thiazide diuretics, aldosterone,
              or excessive amounts of magnesium-containing
              antacids increase urine magnesium levels.
              • Spironolactone decreases urine magnesium lev-
              els.
              • Acidosis, hypercalcemia, and hypophosphatemia
              inhibit the reabsorption of magnesium.

Manganese, serum

This test, an analysis by atomic absorption spectroscopy, measures serum levels of manganese, a
trace element. Manganese is found throughout the
body but is concentrated in the pituitary, the pineal,
and lactating mammary glands, as well as in the
liver and bones. Although the function of this element is only partially understood, manganese is
known to activate several enzymes — including
cholinesterase and arginase — that are essential to
metabolism. Arginase, for example, is necessary
for the formation of urea during protein catabolism.

Because of poor intestinal absorption, the body
retains only a fraction of the manganese supplied by
foods such as unrefined cereals, green leafy vegetables, and nuts. Industrial workers exposed to potentially dangerous levels of manganese may require
testing for toxicity. Such toxicity can follow inhalation of manganese dust or fumes — a constant hazard in the steel and dry-cell battery industries — or
ingestion of contaminated water.

Purpose   • To detect manganese exposure and toxicity
           • To monitor manganese therapy in total nutrition
           therapy

Patient   Explain that this test, which requires a blood sam-
preparation ple, determines the manganese level in the blood.
            Check the patient's history for use of medica-
            tions that may influence serum manganese levels.

Procedure   Perform a venipuncture, and collect the sample in
            a metal-free collection tube. Laboratories will sup-
            ply a special kit for this test on request. Handle the

sample gently to prevent hemolysis, and send it to the laboratory immediately.

Values
: Normally, serum manganese values range from 0.43 to 0.76 ng/ml (7.8 to 13.8 nmol/L).

Implications of results
: Significantly elevated serum levels indicate manganese toxicity, which requires prompt medical attention because it can lead to central nervous system deterioration. Depressed serum manganese levels may indicate deficient dietary intake, although such deficiency has not been linked to disease.

Post-test care
: If a hematoma develops at the venipuncture site, applying warm soaks eases discomfort.

Interfering factors
: • High dietary intake of calcium and phosphorus can interfere with intestinal absorption of manganese and subsequently decrease serum levels.
: • Serum manganese levels are influenced by estrogen, which increases levels, and by glucocorticoids, which alter its distribution in the body.
: • Hemolysis caused by excessive agitation of the sample may alter test results.
: • Failure to use a metal-free collection tube interferes with accurate determination of test results.
: • Be careful when evaluating toxicity because serum levels of manganese may have returned to normal while neurologic damage continues to exist.
: • Keep in mind that manganese levels are lower in patients receiving hemodialysis.

Melanin, urine

This relatively rare test measures urine levels of melanin, the brown-black pigment that colors the skin, hair, and eyes. An end product of tyrosine metabolism, melanin is normally elaborated by specialized cells called melanocytes. Cutaneous melanomas — malignant tumors that produce excessive amounts of melanin — develop most often around the head and neck but may also originate in mucous membranes (as in the rectum), the retinas, or the central nervous system, where melanocytes appear. Patients with these tumors may excrete melanin precursors — melanogens — in their urine. If the urine is left standing, exposure to air converts the melanogens to melanin in about 24 hours.

Thormählen's test uses sodium nitroprusside to detect melanogens or melanin in urine, based on characteristic color changes. More specific tests for melanin, such as chromatography, isolate and measure the pigment.

Purpose	To aid diagnosis of malignant melanomas
Patient preparation	Explain the purpose of this test. Inform the patient that the test requires a random urine specimen, and teach the correct collection technique.
Procedure	Collect a random urine specimen. Send the specimen to the laboratory immediately.
Findings	Normally, urine does not contain melanogens or melanin.
Implications of results	In the presence of a visible skin tumor, large quantities of melanin or melanogens in urine indicate metastasis. Because malignant melanomas may also develop in internal organs, large quantities of melanin or melanogens in a urine specimen, in the absence of a visible skin tumor, indicate an internal melanoma.
Post-test care	None
Interfering factor	Failure to send the urine specimen to the laboratory immediately may interfere with accurate test results.

Multiple sclerosis (MS) screening panel

The variable progression of multiple sclerosis (MS), with its periodic exacerbations and remissions, often makes early diagnosis difficult. This test panel, consisting of two tests performed on cerebrospinal fluid (CSF) samples, helps screen patients for MS and also for certain other demyelinating diseases. Certain abnormalities in CSF — increased total protein (which occurs primarily from increased immunoglobulin G [IgG] synthesis) and detectable IgG proteins that appear as oligoclonal bands on electrophoresis — point to

MS or possibly other demyelinating disease. The first test in the screening panel, the CSF-IgG index test, detects IgG synthesis in the central nervous system. The index is determined by calculating and then comparing the ratio of IgG to albumin in both CSF and serum samples. A CSF ratio greater than the serum ratio suggests IgG synthesis in central nervous system tissue. The second test in the panel, the oligoclonal band test, uses electrophoresis to inspect and compare the immunoglobulin region of both CSF and serum samples.

Purpose
To aid diagnosis of MS

Patient preparation
Explain the purpose of this test, and inform the patient that the test will require samples of blood and CSF. Warn the patient to expect transient discomfort during the injection of local anesthetic and insertion of the spinal needle during CSF collection. Tell the patient that headache may occur during lumbar puncture, but that cooperation during the test will minimize this and other possible adverse effects. Make sure that the patient or a responsible family member has signed a consent form. The anxious patient may require a mild sedative before the procedure.

Procedure
Perform a venipuncture, and collect the blood samples in 7-ml *red-top* tubes. Then, within 2 hours of blood sample collection, a lumbar puncture should be performed and at least 3 ml of CSF collected in a sterile tube that contains no additives.

Record the CSF collection time on the test form. Send properly labeled samples to the laboratory immediately. *Note:* Never freeze CSF samples.

Precautions
During the lumbar puncture, observe the patient closely for signs of adverse reactions, such as elevated pulse rate, pallor, or clammy skin.

Values
Normal IgG values in CSF include the following —
CSF IgG: ≤8.4 mg/dl
CSF albumin: ≤26.0 mg/dl
Serum IgG: 640 to 1,430 mg/dl
Serum albumin: 2,584 to 4,792 mg/dl
CSF-IgG index: ≤0.77
CSF IgG-albumin ratio: 0.15 to 0.38
Serum IgG-albumin ratio: 0.15 to 0.41.

Normal oligoclonal banding is 0 to 1 band in both serum and CSF.

Implications of results

Greater than normal IgG ratios are consistent with MS, as well as with other demyelinating diseases such as neurosyphilis, acute inflammatory polyradiculopathy, and subacute sclerosing panencephalitis.

Multiple oligoclonal bands present in CSF but not in serum are consistent with MS but also may occur in other diseases, including neurosyphilis, subacute sclerosing panencephalitis, cryptococcal meningitis, idiopathic polyneuritis, and chronic rubella panencephalitis.

Post-test care

- The patient should remain supine for at least 8 hours after lumbar puncture.
- Encourage the patient to increase fluid intake.
- Monitor vital signs and neurologic status frequently.
- If a hematoma develops at the venipuncture site, applying warm soaks eases discomfort.

Interfering factor

Improper handling of blood or CSF samples or excessive delay before CSF testing may cause falsenegative results for oligoclonal banding.

Myasthenia gravis test panel

Most patients with myasthenia gravis (MG) have detectable levels of various antibodies to acetylcholine receptors (AChR) and sometimes to other components of skeletal muscle. This four-test panel aids diagnosis of MG by determining serum levels of these antibodies.

The first test in the panel, the AChR-binding antibody test, detects antibodies directed at several different sites on solubilized AChR protein. In addition to confirming the diagnosis of MG, this test is also used to screen for subclinical MG in patients with thymoma (a usually benign tumor associated with MG) who show no overt signs of MG.

The second test, the AChR-modulating antibody test, detects antibodies with the potential to cause muscle weakness (which bind to AChR sites on the surface of intact muscle membranes). This test is particularly useful as a second-line test after a negative AChR-binding antibody test, which may occur in patients with recent, mild, or ocular-restricted MG symptoms.

The AChR-blocking antibody test, a third-line test for MG, detects antibodies that bind near the AChR neurotransmitter binding site. Results are positive in over 50% of patients with MG.

The striational antibody test detects antibodies that bind to the contractile elements of skeletal muscle. These antibodies are often associated with thymoma; positive results occur in about 80% of patients with thymoma related to MG and in 24% of those with thymoma unrelated to MG.

Purpose
- To confirm diagnosis of acquired (autoimmune) MG
- To determine the baseline level of specific autoantibodies
- To aid diagnosis of thymoma

Patient preparation
Explain that this test panel helps determine the presence and severity of myasthenia gravis. Tell the patient that the test requires a blood sample.

Procedure
Perform a venipuncture, and collect the sample in a 10-ml *red-top* tube. Send the sample to the laboratory immediately, or refrigerate the sample. If prolonged storage is necessary, freeze the sample at –4° F (–20° C).

Values and implications of results
See *Myasthenia gravis test panel: Values and implications of results,* page 450, for a discussion of test outcomes.

Post-test care
If a hematoma develops at the venipuncture site, applying warm soaks eases discomfort.

Interfering factors
- Immunosuppressant drug therapy may cause false-negative results.
- False-positive results for AChR-binding antibodies may occur in patients with amyotrophic lateral sclerosis, especially if they have received treatment with snake venom.
- Muscle relaxants used during general anesthesia may cause false-positive results in tests for AChR-modulating and AChR-blocking antibodies in serum obtained perioperatively.
- Anticoagulants and preservatives may interfere with results for AChR-modulating antibodies.

	Myasthenia gravis test panel: Values and implications of results	
Test	**Normal values**	**Implications**
Acetylcholine receptor (AChR)-binding antibodies	≤ 0.03 nmol/l	Positive in 86% of myasthenia gravis (MG) patients (71% with ocular MG). Titers are generally low in patients with ocular MG (0.4 to 1.0 nmol/L).
AChR-modulating antibodies	0% to 20% loss of AChR	Positive in 86% of MG patients (in 72% with ocular MG). Percentage of AChR loss is usually high in patients with thymoma or generalized MG.
AChR-blocking antibodies	0% to 25% blockade of AChR	Positive in 52% of MG patients (in 30% with ocular MG). The prevalence and percentage of AChR blockade are higher in generalized MG.
Striational antibodies	Negative	Positive in 30% of patients with adult MG. Incidence increases with age (rare in patients under age 20). Positive in 55% in patients over age 60, positive in 80% of patients with MG and thymoma, and in 24% of patients with thymoma without MG.

- D-penicillamine can stimulate production of AChR and striational antibodies and can induce MG.

Myelin basic protein

Composed of various lipids and proteins, myelin acts as the brain's electrical insulator, allowing conduction of electrical impulses. Destruction of myelin, or demyelination, occurs in several neurologic disorders — most commonly in multiple sclerosis (MS).

Demyelination releases various components of myelin into the cerebrospinal fluid (CSF). The most specific of these components, myelin basic protein, can be quantified by radioimmunoassay to evaluate demyelination.

Elevated levels of myelin basic protein also have been found in encephalopathies, central nervous system (CNS) infarction, hemorrhage, and trauma. As a result, definitive diagnosis of demyelinating disease requires further testing, such as electrophoretic detection of oligoclonal banding in serum and CSF, and quantitative studies of CSF immuno-globulin levels.

This test is most useful as a measurement of active demyelination rather than as a diagnostic test for any specific disease. When performed periodically, it can help track the progress of disease by marking periods of increased and decreased demyelination.

Purpose   To detect and evaluate active demyelination within the CNS

Patient preparation   Explain that this test helps determine the underlying cause of neurologic symptoms and that the test requires a specimen of CSF, taken through a lumbar puncture. Warn the patient that the test may cause headache and discomfort at the puncture site, but that these effects are transient. Before the procedure, make sure that the patient or a responsible family member has signed a consent form.

Procedure   A lumbar puncture is performed and at least 3 ml of CSF is collected in a sterile tube that contains no additives.

Record the CSF collection time on the laboratory slip, and send the properly labeled specimen to the laboratory immediately. If prolonged storage is necessary, refrigerate or freeze the specimen.

Precautions   During lumbar puncture, observe the patient closely for signs of adverse reactions, such as elevated pulse rate, pallor, or clammy skin.

Values   Normal CSF values of myelin basic protein are less than 4 ng/ml (μg/L).

Implications of results   Usually, values below 4 ng/ml (μg/L) are associated with the absence of active demyelination or a state of disease remission. Values between 4 and 8 ng/ml (μg/L) are considered weakly positive and indicate either chronic disease with slowly progressive demyelination or the recovery phase of an acute exacerbation. Levels of 9 ng/ml (μg/L) or greater are strongly positive and indicate active demyelination.

Post-test care   • The patient should remain supine for at least 8 hours after lumbar puncture and increase his fluid intake.

- Monitor vital signs and neurologic status frequently.
- Monitor for any redness, swelling, or continued leakage of CSF from the lumbar puncture site.

Interfering factors   None

Myoglobin, serum

Using radioimmunoassay, this test measures serum levels of myoglobin, an oxygen-binding muscle protein similar to hemoglobin. Myoglobin binds, stores, and transports oxygen to the muscle cells' mitochondria, where oxygen generates energy by converting glucose into carbon dioxide and water. Myoglobin is normally found in skeletal and cardiac muscle, but is released into the blood after muscle damage caused by trauma, ischemia or inflammation. However, because myoglobin levels don't indicate the site of injury, they're commonly used to confirm other studies, such as total creatine kinase (CK) or the myocardial-specific isoenzyme, CK-MB. In myocardial infarction (MI), serum myoglobin levels peak in approximately 4 to 8 hours after onset of pain.

Purpose
- To estimate damage caused by MI or skeletal muscle injury
- To predict exacerbation of polymyositis, a degenerative muscle disease

Patient preparation   Explain that this test, which requires a blood sample, helps determine the severity of muscle damage.

Procedure   Perform a venipuncture, and collect the sample in a 10 *red-top* tube.

Collect a blood sample 4 to 8 hours after the onset of an acute MI, when myoglobin levels peak. *Note:* Don't collect a blood sample from a patient who has recently had an episode of angina or has undergone cardioversion.

Values   Normal serum myoglobin levels range from 30 to 90 ng/ml (µg/L).

Implications of results	Elevated serum myoglobin levels help estimate the severity of damage after MI or skeletal muscle injury. In a patient with polymyositis, elevated levels may signal exacerbation of the disease. However, elevated myoglobin levels are also associated with dermatomyositis, systemic lupus erythematosus, cold injury (hypothermia), shock, or severe renal failure. Because test results are nonspecific, elevated serum levels must be correlated with the patient's signs and symptoms.

Post-test care	If a hematoma develops at the venipuncture site, applying warm soaks eases discomfort.

Interfering factors	• Recent cardioversion or an anginal episode may increase myoglobin levels.
	• Performing this test immediately after onset of an acute MI produces misleading results, because myoglobin levels don't start to increase for at least 2 hours.
	• Testing 12 hours or later after onset of MI can produce misleading results. By 12 hours after onset, serum levels may already have returned to normal range.
	• Radioactive scan performed within 1 week before the test may affect results.

Myoglobin, urine

This test detects the presence in urine of myoglobin, a red pigment found in cardiac and skeletal muscle. Myoglobin probably serves as a reservoir of oxygen, facilitating its movement within muscle. When muscle cells are extensively damaged, as by disease, cold injury, or severe crushing trauma, myoglobin is released into the blood, quickly cleared by renal glomerular filtration, and eliminated in the urine (myoglobinuria). Myoglobin appears in the urine as early as 3 hours after myocardial infarction (MI). Because of the marked structural similarities of urine myoglobin and urine hemoglobin, they are not satisfactorily differentiated by qualitative assays. Specific antibodies to myoglobin that do not react with hemoglobin enable myoglobin to be identified unequivocally by immunoassay.

Purpose	• To aid diagnosis of muscular disease
	• To detect extensive infarction of muscle tissue

- To assess the extent of muscular damage from crushing trauma

Patient preparation Explain that this test detects a red pigment found in muscle cells and helps evaluate muscle injury or disease. Inform the patient that the test requires a random urine specimen, and teach the correct technique for collecting the specimen.

Procedure Collect a random urine specimen, and send it to the laboratory immediately.

Findings Normally, myoglobin does not appear in the urine.

Implications of results Myoglobinuria occurs in acute or chronic muscular disease, alcoholic polymyopathy, familial myoglobinuria, and extensive MI. Myoglobinuria also results from severe trauma to the skeletal muscles (as in a crushing injury, extreme hypothermia, or severe burns). Transient myoglobinuria ("march" myoglobinuria) may follow severe or prolonged exertion in predisposed subjects. This form of myoglobinuria disappears after a period of rest. Myoglobinuria has also been reported in patients with diabetic acidosis, hypokalemia, systemic infection with fever, and barbiturate toxicity.

Post-test care None

Interfering factors
- Extremely dilute urine can reduce test sensitivity.
- Because myoglobin is excreted through the kidneys, renal function also influences test results.

N

Nasopharyngeal culture

This test evaluates nasopharyngeal secretions for the presence of pathogenic organisms. Direct microscopic inspection of a gram-stained smear of the specimen provides preliminary identification of organisms that may guide clinical management, and determines the need for additional testing. Streaking a culture plate with nasopharyngeal secretions and allowing any organisms present to grow permit isolation and identification of pathogens. Cultured pathogens may then require sensitivity testing to determine appropriate antibiotic therapy. Nasopharyngeal cultures are often useful for identifying *Bordetella pertussis* and *Neisseria meningitidis*, especially in very young, elderly, or debilitated patients.

A nasopharyngeal culture can also be used to isolate viruses, especially to identify carriers of influenza virus A and B. However, the laboratory procedure required for such testing is complex, time consuming, and costly and therefore is performed infrequently.

Purpose
- To identify pathogens causing upper respiratory tract symptoms
- To detect carriers of infectious organisms such as *N. meningitidis* and *B. pertussis*

Patient preparation
Describe the procedure, and explain that this test isolates the cause of nasopharyngeal infection and allows identification of the organism and testing for antibiotic sensitivity. Tell the patient that secretions will be obtained from the back of the nose and the throat, using a cotton-tipped applicator. Warn that he may experience slight discomfort and may gag, but reassure him that obtaining the specimen takes only a few seconds.

Equipment
Penlight; sterile, flexible wire cotton-tipped applicator; small, sterile, open-ended heat-resistant glass tube or sterile nasal speculum; tongue blade; culture tube; transport medium (broth)

Procedure
Ask the patient to cough before you begin collection of the specimen. Then, position the patient with his head tilted back. Using a penlight and a tongue blade, inspect the nasopharyngeal area. Next, gently pass the cotton-tipped applicator through the nostril and into the nasopharynx, keeping it near the septum and floor of the nose.

Make sure that the applicator doesn't touch the sides of the patient's nostril or his tongue to prevent any contamination of the specimen. Rotate the applicator quickly, and remove it. Or place the glass tube in the patient's nostril, and carefully pass the applicator through the tube into the nasopharynx. Rotate the applicator for 5 seconds, and then place it in the culture tube with transport medium. Remove the glass tube.

Label the specimen appropriately, including the date and time of collection, and the origin of the material. Note recent antibiotic therapy or chemotherapy on the laboratory slip. Indicate the suspected organism. Also inform the laboratory if certain organisms, such as *Corynebacterium diphtheriae* and *B. pertussis,* are suspected because they require special growth media.

If the specimen is being collected for isolation of a virus, check with the laboratory for the recommended collection techniques. Refrigerate or freeze a viral specimen according to the laboratory's procedure.

Findings
The presence or absence of normal flora or absence of a pathogen is usually reported. Flora commonly found in the nasopharynx include nonhemolytic streptococci, alpha-hemolytic streptococci, *Neisseria* (except *N. gonorrhoeae*), coagulase-negative staphylococci such as *Staphylococcus epidermidis,* and, occasionally, the coagulase-positive *S. aureus.*

Implications of results
Pathogens include group A, and occasionally groups B, C, and G, beta-hemolytic streptococci; *B. pertussis*; *C. diphtheriae*; and *S. aureus.*

Post-test care
None

Interfering factors
• Recent antibiotic therapy decreases bacterial growth.
• Improper collection technique may contaminate the specimen.

- Failure to place the specimen in transport medium allows the specimen to dry out and the bacteria to deteriorate.
- Failure to send the specimen to the laboratory immediately after collection permits proliferation of organisms.
- Failure to keep a viral specimen cold allows the viruses to deteriorate.

5'-Nucleotidase

The enzyme 5'-nucleotidase (5'NT) is a phosphomonoesterase formed almost entirely in the hepatobiliary tissues. Unlike alkaline phosphatase, an enzyme that is nonspecific, this enzyme hydrolyzes nucleoside 5'-phosphate groups only. Although serum 5'NT, alkaline phosphatase, and leucine aminopeptidase (LAP) levels rise in hepatic metastasis, hepatocarcinoma, and biliary tract obstruction, only 5'NT remains normal in skeletal disease and pregnancy, and so is more specific for hepatic dysfunction than alkaline phosphatase or LAP.

This test, which measures serum 5'NT levels, is used most often to determine whether alkaline phosphatase elevation originates from skeletal or hepatic disease.

Purpose
- To distinguish between hepatobiliary and skeletal disease when the source of elevated alkaline phosphatase levels is uncertain
- To help differentiate biliary obstruction from acute hepatocellular damage
- To detect hepatic metastasis in the absence of jaundice

Patient preparation
Explain that this test, which requires a blood sample, helps evaluate liver function.

Procedure
Perform a venipuncture, and collect the sample in a 7-ml *red-top* tube. Handle the sample gently to prevent hemolysis because red blood cells contain this enzyme.

Values
Serum 5'NT values for adults range from 2 to 17 U/L. Values for children may be lower.

Implications of results
Highest 5'NT elevations occur in common bile duct obstruction by calculi or tumors in diseases that

cause severe intrahepatic cholestasis, such as neoplastic infiltrations of the liver. Slight-to-moderate increases may reflect acute hepatocellular damage or active cirrhosis. Simultaneous elevation of 5′NT and alkaline phosphatase confirms biliary disease as the cause of elevated alkaline phosphatase. Normal levels support a diagnosis of bone disease as the cause of elevated alkaline phosphatase levels.

Post-test care   If a hematoma develops at the venipuncture site, applying warm soaks eases discomfort.

Interfering factors

- Hemolysis of the sample may interfere with accurate determination of serum levels.
- Ingestion of cholestatic drugs, such as phenothiazines, morphine, meperidine, and codeine, elevates 5′NT levels.

Opiates, urine

These tests, performed using thin-layer chromatography or enzyme-multiplied immunoassay technique, detect the presence of opiates in patients with acute drug toxicities or adverse drug reactions, and help determine drug dependence and progress of detoxification. Testing for opiates is usually qualitative, but quantitative testing for confirmation can also be performed on morphine, codeine, meperidine, methadone, and propoxyphene. Although urine is the preferred specimen for detecting opiates, gastric contents may also be analyzed.

Used primarily as central nervous system depressants for relieving pain, opiates, which include morphine, heroin, hydromorphone, codeine, meperi-dine, methadone, propoxyphene, and oxycodone, are absorbed slowly from the GI tract, with peak effects occurring approximately 1 hour after ingestion. Opiates are detoxified by the liver and eliminated in the urine within 48 hours of administration, with 90% excreted in 24 hours.

Purpose
- To determine the cause of acute drug toxicity or adverse drug reaction suspected from history
- To help monitor drug dependence or the progress of detoxification
- To detect the presence of opiates for medicolegal purposes

Patient preparation
Explain that this test determines the presence of opiate drugs in the urine. For a monitoring test, inform the patient that restriction of food or fluids is not required. For methadone testing, tell the patient that a 24-hour urine specimen is required, and teach the proper collection technique; for all other tests to detect the presence of narcotic analgesics, random urine specimens are used.

For a medicolegal test, make sure that the patient or responsible family member has signed a consent form. Record the patient's recent medication history, including dosage schedule and route of administration.

Procedure   Instruct the patient to collect a 24-hour urine specimen to measure methadone levels or a random
urine specimen for other drugs in this group.

Send the specimen to the laboratory immediately, or refrigerate the specimen during the collection period.

For a medicolegal test, observe proper precautions.

Values   Tests for heroin and oxycodone are qualitative.
Most other tests are also reported qualitatively.

Some opiates can be measured quantitatively.
Toxic concentrations of these drugs follow —
Morphine: > 0.005 mg/dl (0.2 μmol/L)
Codeine: > 0.005 mg/dl (0.2 μmol/L)
Hydromorphone: > 0.1 mg/dl (5 μmol/L)
Meperidine: > 0.5 mg/dl (20 μmol/L)
Methadone: > 0.2 mg/dl (10 μmol/L)
Propoxyphene: > 0.5 mg/dl (20 μmol/L).

Implications of   Detoxification is based on urine levels. Detection of
results   opiates may have medicolegal implications.

Post-test care   None

Interfering   Delayed transport may produce false-negative test
factor   results in a urine specimen analyzed by thin-layer
chromatography.

Osmotic fragility

Osmotic fragility measures resistance to hemolysis
of red blood cells (RBCs), or erythrocytes, when
exposed to a series of increasingly dilute saline solutions. The test is based on osmosis — movement
of water across a membrane from a less concentrated solution to a more concentrated one, in a natural
tendency to correct the imbalance.

RBCs suspended in an isotonic saline solution —
one with the same salt concentration (osmotic pressure) as normal plasma (0.85 g/dl) — keep their
shape. If RBCs are added to a hypotonic (less concentrated) solution, they take up water until they
burst; if added to a hypertonic solution, they shrink.

The degree of hypotonicity needed to produce
hemolysis varies inversely with the osmotic fragility of RBCs; the closer saline tonicity is to normal
physiologic values when hemolysis occurs, the
more fragile the cells. Normal RBCs can swell sig-

nificantly before exceeding their membrane capacity; but spherocytes and RBCs with damaged membranes burst in solutions that are only slightly more dilute than normal saline. In certain other diseases, such as sickle cell disease and thalassemia, RBCs are strongly resistant to damage by hypotonic solutions. In some cases, RBCs do not hemolyze immediately, and their incubation in solution for 24 hours improves test sensitivity.

This test offers quantitative confirmation of RBC morphology and should supplement the stained cell examination.

Purpose

- To aid diagnosis of hereditary spherocytosis
- To confirm morphologic RBC abnormalities

Patient preparation

Explain that this test, which requires a blood sample, helps identify the cause of anemia.

Procedure

Because this is not a routine test, notify the laboratory before drawing the sample.

Perform a venipuncture, and collect the sample in a 7-ml *green-top* (heparinized) tube, or secure a special heparinized tube for collecting defibrinated blood.

Completely fill the tube, and invert it gently several times to mix the sample and anticoagulant adequately. Handle the sample gently to prevent hemolysis.

Findings

Osmotic fragility values are reported as the percent of the solution at which the RBCs swell and rupture. Normal RBCs will rupture in solutions of 0.30% to 0.45% saline. RBC rupture in solutions of over 50% saline indicates increased fragility. Resistance to rupture in solutions below 30% saline indicates decreased fragility.

Implications of results

Low osmotic fragility (increased resistance to hemolysis) is characteristic of thalassemia, iron deficiency anemia, sickle cell anemia, and other RBC disorders in which codocytes (target cells) and leptocytes are found. Low osmotic fragility also occurs in patients with liver disease, polycythemia vera, and obstructive jaundice as well as after splenectomy.

High osmotic fragility (decreased resistance to hemolysis) is characteristic in patients with hereditary spherocytosis, in spherocytosis associated with autoimmune hemolytic anemia, severe burns, chemical poisoning, and in hemolytic disease of the newborn (erythroblastosis fetalis). Increased fragility is also associated with conditions involving mechanical trauma to RBCs (such as prosthetic heart valves or disseminated intravascular coagulation), transfusion with incompatible blood, and certain enzyme deficiencies.

Post-test care   If a hematoma develops at the venipuncture site, applying warm soaks eases discomfort.

Interfering factors   The following factors may affect the accurate determination of test results:

- failure to use the proper anticoagulant in the collection tube, to fill the tube completely, or to mix the sample and anticoagulant adequately
- hemolysis caused by excessive agitation of the sample
- presence of hemolytic organisms in the sample
- severe anemia, or other conditions in which fewer red cells are available for testing.

Ova and parasites (O&P), sputum

This test evaluates a sputum specimen for parasites. Such infection is rare in the United States but may result from exposure to *Entamoeba histolytica, Ascaris lumbricoides, Echinococcus granulosus, Strongyloides stercoralis, Paragonimus westermani,* or *Necator americanus.* The specimen is obtained by expectoration or by tracheal suctioning.

Purpose   To identify pulmonary parasites

Patient preparation   Explain that this test helps identify parasitic pulmonary infection. Tell the patient that the test requires a sputum specimen or, if necessary, tracheal suctioning. Explain that an early morning collection is preferred because secretions accumulate overnight.

For expectoration, encourage fluid intake the night before collection, to help sputum production. Teach the patient how to expectorate by taking three deep breaths and forcing a deep cough. Before tracheal suctioning, warn the patient to expect some discomfort from the catheter.

Equipment *For expectoration:* Sterile, disposable, impermeable container with screw cap or tight-fitting cap; nebulizer; intermittent positive-pressure breathing (IPPB) ventilator; 10% sodium chloride, acetylcysteine, or sterile or distilled water aerosols, to induce cough

For tracheal suctioning: size 16 or 18 French suction catheter, sterile gloves, sterile specimen container or sputum trap, sterile normal saline solution

Procedure *Expectoration:* Instruct the patient to breathe deeply a few times and then to cough deeply and expectorate into the container. If cough is nonproductive, use chest physiotherapy, heated aerosol spray (nebulization), or IPPB with prescribed aerosol to induce sputum, as appropriate. Close the container securely, and clean the outside of it. Dispose of equipment properly; take proper precautions in sending the specimen to the laboratory.

Tracheal suctioning: Administer oxygen before and after the procedure, if necessary. Attach a sputum trap to the suction catheter. While wearing sterile gloves, lubricate the tip of the catheter, and pass the catheter through the patient's nostril, without suction. (The patient will cough when the catheter passes into the larynx.) Advance the catheter into the trachea. To obtain the specimen, apply suction for no longer than 15 seconds. Stop suctioning, and gently remove the catheter. Discard the catheter and glove in a proper receptacle. Then, detach the sputum trap from the suction apparatus and cap the opening.

Label all specimens carefully. Send the specimen to the laboratory immediately, or place it in preservative.

Precautions • Tracheal suctioning is contraindicated in patients with esophageal varices or cardiac disease.
• In a patient with asthma or chronic bronchitis, watch for aggravated bronchospasm with use of more than 10% concentration of sodium chloride or acetylcysteine in an aerosol.
• During tracheal suctioning, suction for only 5 to 10 seconds at a time. *Never* suction longer than 15 seconds. If the patient becomes hypoxic or cyanotic, remove the catheter immediately, and administer oxygen.

Findings — Normally, no parasites or ova are present in sputum.

Implications of results — The parasite identified indicates the type of pulmonary infection and the presence of adult-stage intestinal infection as follows —

E. histolytica trophozoites: pulmonary amebiasis
A. lumbricoides larvae and adults: pneumonitis
E. granulosus cysts of larval stage: hydatid disease
S. stercoralis larvae: strongyloidiasis
P. westermani ova: paragonimiasis
N. americanus larvae: hookworm disease.

Post-test care
- Provide good mouth care.
- After suctioning, offer water; monitor vital signs every hour until stable.

Interfering factors
- Recent therapy with anthelmintics or amebicides may alter test results.
- Improper collection may produce a nonrepresentative specimen.

Ova and parasites (O&P), stool

Examination of a stool specimen can detect several types of intestinal parasites. Some of these parasites are nonpathogenic; others cause intestinal disease. In the United States, the most common parasites include the protozoa *Dientamoeba fragilis, Entamoeba histolytica* and *Giardia lamblia;* the roundworms *Ascaris lumbricoides* and *Necator americanus* (commonly called hookworm); and the tapeworms *Diphyllobothrium latum, Taenia saginata,* and, rarely, *T. solium.*

Purpose — To diagnose intestinal parasitic infection and disease

Patient preparation — Explain that this test detects intestinal parasitic infection. The patient should avoid treatments with castor or mineral oil, bismuth, magnesium or antidiarrheal compounds, barium enemas, and antibiotics for 7 to 10 days before the test. Tell the patient that the test requires three stool specimens — one every other day or every third day.

If the patient has diarrhea, record recent dietary and travel history. Check and record the patient's medication history for use of antiparasitic agents.

Equipment   Waterproof specimen container with a preservative and a tight-fitting lid, bedpan (if necessary), tongue blade, gloves

Procedure   Collect a stool specimen directly into the container. If the patient is bedridden, collect the specimen into a clean, dry bedpan; then, using a tongue blade, transfer it into a properly labeled container. Note on the laboratory slip the date and time of collection, specimen consistency, any recent or current antibiotic therapy, and any pertinent travel or dietary history. Also note any unusual parasites that may need to be identified.

Do not contaminate the stool specimen with urine, which can destroy trophozoites. Don't collect stool from a toilet bowl because water is toxic to trophozoites and may contain organisms that interfere with test results.

Place the specimen in the preservative and mix well. If the entire stool can't be sent to the laboratory, include macroscopic worms or worm segments, and bloody and mucoid portions of the specimen.

Observe aseptic precautions when handling the specimen, disposing of equipment, sealing the container, and transporting it.

Special requests for unusual parasites need to be indicated on the laboratory slip.

Findings   Normally, no parasites or ova appear in stool.

Implications of   The presence of *E. histolytica* confirms amebiasis;
results   *G. lamblia,* giardiasis. If amebiasis is suspected but stool examinations are negative, specimen collection after a saline cathartic using buffered sodium biphosphate or during sigmoidoscopy may be necessary. If giardiasis is suspected but stool examinations are negative, examination of duodenal contents may be necessary.

Eosinophilia may also indicate parasitic infection. Helminths may migrate from the intestinal tract, producing pathologic changes in other parts of the body. For example, the roundworm *Ascaris* may perforate the bowel wall, causing peritonitis, or may migrate to the lungs, causing pneumonitis. Hookworms can cause hypochromic microcytic anemia secondary to bloodsucking and hemorrhage, especially in patients with iron-deficient diets. The tapeworm *D. latum* may cause megaloblastic anemia by removing vitamin B_{12}.

Post-test care The patient may resume discontinued medications.

Interfering factors

- Improper collection technique or the presence of urine may cause false-negative results.
- Collection of too few specimens may cause failure to detect the organism.
- Exposure of the specimen to excessive heat or cold can destroy parasites.
- Failure to observe pretest restrictions of castor or mineral oil, bismuth, magnesium or antidiarrheal compounds, barium enemas, or antibiotics may interfere with microscopic analysis or reduce the number of parasites.

Oxalate, urine

This test measures urine levels of oxalate, a salt of oxalic acid. Oxalate is an end product of metabolism and is excreted almost exclusively in the urine. Most important, the test detects hyperoxaluria, a disorder in which oxalate accumulates in the soft and connective tissue, especially in the kidneys and bladder, causing chronic inflammation and fibrosis. Calcium oxalate deposits are the most common cause of renal calculi, which may produce kidney damage.

Purpose

- To detect primary hyperoxaluria in patients with malabsorption
- To rule out hyperoxaluria in renal insufficiency

Patient preparation Explain the purpose of this test. Tell the patient that the test requires a 24-hour urine specimen, and teach the appropriate collection method. The patient should restrict intake of vitamin C for 24 hours before the collection of urine begins.

Procedure Collect a 24-hour urine specimen in a light-protected plastic container with hydrochloric acid. The patient should not urinate directly into the 24-hour specimen container and should not contaminate the urine specimen with toilet tissue or stool.

Values	Urine oxalate levels 10 to 41 mg/day (0.11 to 0.46 µmol/day) are considered normal.
Implications of results	Hyperoxaluria results from excessive metabolic production of oxalate or increased oxalate intake. Levels as high as 100 to 400 mg/day (1,000 to 4,000 µmol/day) can occur.

Implications of results — Hyperoxaluria results from excessive metabolic production of oxalate or increased oxalate intake. Levels as high as 100 to 400 mg/day (1,000 to 4,000 µmol/day) can occur.

Primary hyperoxaluria, a rare inborn metabolic disorder, causes excessive production and urinary excretion of oxalate. Characteristically, in this type of hyperoxaluria, elevated urine oxalate levels precede elevated serum levels.

Secondary hyperoxaluria can result from pancreatic insufficiency, diabetes mellitus, cirrhosis, pyridoxine deficiency, Crohn's disease, ileal resection, ingestion of antifreeze (ethylene glycol) or stain remover, or a reaction to a methoxyflurane anesthetic.

Post-test care — None

Interfering factors

- Failure to collect all urine during the test period may interfere with accurate determination of the test results.
- Improper storage of the specimen during the collection period may interfere with accurate test results.
- Ingestion of vitamin C will alter the test results because it increases urine oxalate levels.
- A high intake of animal protein, beans, beets, calcium, chocolate, cocoa, gelatin, pepper, purines, rhubarb, spinach, strawberries, tea, and tomatoes may cause hyperoxaluria.

P

Papanicolaou (Pap) test

The Papanicolaou (Pap) test, a cytologic test, is widely known for its use in early detection of cervical cancer. For this test, secretions are scraped from the patient's cervix and spread onto a slide. After the slide is immersed in a fixative, it is sent to the laboratory for cytologic analysis. This test relies on the ready exfoliation of malignant cells from the cervix. Although cervical scrapings are the most common test specimen, this test also permits cytologic evaluation of the vaginal pool, prostatic secretions, urine, gastric secretions, cavity fluids, bronchial aspirations, sputum, and solid tumor cells obtained by fine needle aspiration. It also shows cell maturity, metabolic activity, and morphology variations.

The American Cancer Society recommends a Pap test every year for women who are sexually active or those who are age 18 or older (or less frequently, as ordered, if three consecutive annual Pap tests are normal). Annual tests (or at intervals dictated by the patient's physician) are advisable for women over age 40, for those in a high-risk category, and for those who have had a positive test. If a Pap test is positive or suggests malignancy, cervical biopsy can confirm diagnosis.

Purpose	• To detect malignant cells • To detect inflammatory tissue changes • To assess response to chemotherapy and radiation therapy • To detect viral, fungal, and, occasionally, parasitic invasion
Patient preparation	Explain to the patient that the test allows the study of cervical cells. Stress its importance as an aid for detection of cancer at a stage when the disease is often asymptomatic and still curable. The test should not be scheduled during the menstrual period: the best time is midcycle. Instruct the patient not to douche or insert vaginal medications for 24 hours before the test because doing so can wash away cellular deposits and change the vaginal pH. Tell her the test requires that the cervix be scraped.

Obtain an accurate patient history that includes answers to the following questions: When did you last have a Pap test? Have you ever had an abnormal Pap test? When was your last menstrual period? Are your periods regular? How many days do they last? Is bleeding heavy or light? Have you taken or are you currently taking hormones or oral contraceptives? Do you use an intrauterine device? Do you have any vaginal discharge, pain, or itching? What, if any, gynecologic disorders have occurred in your family? Have you ever had gynecologic surgery, chemotherapy, or radiation therapy? If so, what kind? Note any pertinent patient history on the laboratory slip. If the patient is anxious, be supportive and tell her that test results should be available within a few days.

Just before the test, the patient should empty her bladder.

Equipment   Drape; vaginal speculum; collection device, such as a Pap stick (wooden spatula), cotton-tipped applicator, or clean, dry glass pipette with rubber bulb; normal saline solution; glass microscopic slides; fixative (commercial spray or 95% ethyl alcohol solution in a jar) for slides

Procedure   After instructing the patient to disrobe from the waist down and to drape herself, ask her to lie on the examining table and to place her heels in the stirrups. (She may be more comfortable if she keeps her shoes on.) Tell her to slide her buttocks to the edge of the table. Adjust the drape to minimize exposure.

To avoid startling the patient, tell her when the examination will begin. First, an unlubricated speculum is inserted into the vagina. To make insertion easier, the speculum may be moistened with saline or warm water.

After locating the cervix, the examiner will collect secretions from the cervix and material from the endocervical canal with a saline-moistened cotton-tipped applicator or wooden spatula. Then the specimen is spread onto the slide, according to laboratory recommendation, and the slide is immediately immersed in or sprayed with a fixative. Alternatively, posterior vaginal pool secretions and pancervical material may be collected and smeared onto a single slide, which must be fixed immediately according to laboratory instructions.

Be sure the cervical specimen is aspirated and scraped from the cervix. Aspiration of the posterior fornix of the vagina can supplement a cervical specimen but should not replace it. If vaginal or vulval lesions are present, scrapings taken directly from the lesion are preferred. For an elderly patient whose uterus is involuted or atrophied, use a small pipette, if necessary, to aspirate cells from the squamocolumnar junction and the cervical canal. Preserve the slides immediately.

Label the specimen appropriately, including the date; the patient's name, age, and date of her last menstrual period; and the secretion collection site and method.

Findings Normally, no malignant cells or abnormalities are present.

Implications of results Usually, malignant cells have relatively large nuclei and only small amounts of cytoplasm. They show abnormal nuclear chromatin patterns and marked variation in size, shape, and staining properties, and may have prominent nucleoli.

A Pap smear may be graded in different ways, so check your laboratory's reporting format. The following is the traditional classification method —

Class I: normal pattern; absence of atypical or abnormal cells

Class II: benign abnormality; atypical, but nonmalignant, cells present

Class III: atypical cells consistent with dysplasia

Class IV: suggestive of, but inconclusive for, malignant cells

Class V: conclusive for malignant cells.

In current practice, however, many clinicians prefer to classify Pap test results according to the following descriptive terminology —

Normal

Metaplasia

Inflammation

Minimal atypia: koilocytosis

Mild dysplasia: cervical intraepithelial neoplasia (CIN I)

Moderate dysplasia: CIN II

Severe dysplasia: carcinoma in situ (CIN III)

Invasive carcinoma.

To confirm a suggestive or positive cytology report, the test may be repeated or followed by a cervical biopsy.

Post-test care
- If cervical bleeding occurs, supply the patient with a sanitary napkin.
- Tell the patient when to return for her next Pap test.

Interfering factors
- Delay in fixing a specimen allows the cells to dry, destroys the effectiveness of the nuclear stain, and makes cytologic interpretation difficult.
- Use of lubricating gel on the speculum can alter the specimen.
- Douching within 24 hours before a Pap test can wash away cellular deposits.
- Exclusive use of a specimen collected from the vaginal fornix may yield false-negative test results.
- Collecting the specimen during menstruation may interfere with accurate determination of test results.

Parathyroid hormone (PTH), serum

Parathormone

Parathyroid hormone (PTH), a polypeptide secreted by the parathyroid glands, regulates plasma concentration of calcium and phosphorus. Normally, PTH release is regulated by a negative feedback mechanism involving serum calcium. Normal or elevated circulating ionized calcium inhibits PTH release; a decrease in calcium ions stimulates PTH release. The overall effect of PTH is to raise plasma levels of calcium while lowering phosphorus levels by stimulating osteoclasts and osteocytes to mobilize both calcium and phosphorus from bone, by acting on renal tubular cells to promote calcium reabsorption and phosphorus excretion (phosphaturia), and (with biologically active vitamin D [1,25-dihydroxycholecalciferol]) by promoting intestinal absorption of calcium.

Circulating PTH exists in three distinct molecular forms: the intact PTH molecule, which originates in the parathyroids, and two smaller circulating forms — N-terminal fragments and C-terminal fragments — that are cleaved from the intact molecule by the kidneys, liver, and, to a lesser extent for the C-fragment, the parathyroids. Currently, radioimmunoassays are available to detect intact PTH, and the N- and C-terminal fragments. The assays for intact PTH are accurate, widely available, and clinically useful; however, the C-terminal assays show falsely high values in patients with renal disease, and have limited value. An inappropriate excess or deficiency of PTH has clinical and diagnostic consequences directly related to the effects of PTH on bone and on the renal tubules, and to its interaction with ionized calcium and biologically active vitamin D. Consequently, measuring serum calcium, phosphorus, and creatine levels with serum PTH is useful in identifying states of pathologic parathyroid function. Suppression or stimulation tests may be of confirming value.

Purpose

To aid the differential diagnosis of parathyroid disorders

Patient preparation

Explain that this test helps evaluate parathyroid function. Instruct the patient to observe an overnight fast because food may affect PTH levels and interfere with the test results. Tell the patient that this test requires a blood sample.

Procedure

Draw 3 ml venous blood into two separate 7-ml *red-top* tubes. Handle the sample gently to prevent hemolysis. Send it to the laboratory immediately so that the serum can be separated and frozen for assay.

Values

Normal serum PTH levels vary, depending on the laboratory, and must be interpreted in association with serum calcium levels. Typical values are as follows —
PTH: 20 to 70 μliterEq/ml
N-terminal fraction: 236 to 630 pg/ml
C-terminal fraction: 410 to 1,760 pg/ml.

Implications of results

Measured concomitantly with serum calcium levels, abnormally elevated PTH values may indicate primary, secondary, or tertiary hyperparathyroidism.

High PTH levels with high to normal calcium levels occur in patients with primary hyperparathyroidism resulting from parathyroid adenoma (or rarely carcinoma) or parathyroid hyperplasia. High PTH levels with low calcium levels (a normal response to low calcium levels) occur in secondary hyperparathyroidism possibly associated with chronic renal disease, severe vitamin D deficiency, calcium malabsorption, or pregnancy and lactation.

High PTH levels with high-to-normal calcium levels occur in tertiary hyperparathyroidism associated with progressive secondary hyperparathyroidism in which autonomous parathyroid function has developed.

Low PTH with low calcium levels indicate hypoparathyroidism usually resulting from accidental removal of the parathyroid glands during surgery, occasionally associated with autoimmune disease, and occasionally idiopathic. Low PTH levels with high calcium levels may indicate malignant tumors such as squamous cell carcinoma of the lung; and renal, pancreatic, or ovarian cancers in which high calcium levels are caused by secretion of a parathormone-like hormone that does not cross-react with PTH assay.

Post-test care   If a hematoma develops at the venipuncture site, applying warm soaks eases discomfort.

Interfering factors
- Failure to observe an overnight fast may interfere with the accurate determination of test results.
- Ingestion of milk may cause false-low PTH levels.
- Elevated blood lipids interfere with accurate test results.
- Hemolysis caused by excessive agitation of the sample may interfere with accurate test results.

Peritoneal fluid analysis

Accumulation of fluid in the peritoneal space — ascites — can be caused by conditions such as hepatic, renal, or cardiovascular disorders; inflammation; infection; or neoplasm.

Peritoneal fluid analysis includes examination of gross appearance, red blood cell (RBC) and white blood cell (WBC) counts, cytologic studies, microbiological studies for bacteria and fungi, and determinations of protein, glucose, amylase, ammonia, alkaline phosphatase, creatinine, and carcinoembryonic antigen (CEA) levels.

This test assesses a sample of peritoneal fluid obtained by paracentesis, a procedure requiring a local anesthetic that entails inserting a trocar and cannula through the abdominal wall. If the sample of fluid is being removed for therapeutic purposes, the trocar can be connected to a drainage system. If only a small amount of fluid is being removed for diagnostic purposes, an 18G needle can be substituted for the trocar and cannula. In a four-quadrant tap, fluid is aspirated from each quadrant of the abdomen to verify abdominal trauma and confirm the need for surgery.

Complications associated with this test include shock and hypovolemia, perforation of abdominal organs, hemorrhage, and hepatic coma.

Purpose
- To determine the cause of ascites
- To detect abdominal trauma
- To detect perforation of the bladder as indicated by increased levels of ammonia, creatinine, and urea
- To detect bacterial peritonitis
- To detect peritoneal effusion caused by pancreatitis, pancreatic trauma, or GI perforation or necrosis

Patient preparation
Describe the procedure and explain the purpose of the test. Inform the patient that restriction of food or fluids is not required before the test, that the test requires a peritoneal fluid specimen, that blood may be drawn for analysis, and that a local anesthetic will be given to minimize discomfort. Inform the patient with severe ascites that the procedure will relieve discomfort and ease breathing.

Provide psychological support to decrease anxiety, and assure the patient that complications are rare.

Make sure the patient or responsible family member has signed a consent form. Record baseline vital signs and weight for comparison with posttest readings; abdominal girth measurements may also be ordered.

Just before the test, tell the patient to void. This helps prevent accidental bladder injury during needle insertion.

Procedure
The patient is positioned seated, with feet flat on the floor and back well supported, or in high Fowler's position.

The puncture site is then shaved, the skin prepared, and the area draped. A local anesthetic is injected, and the needle or trocar and cannula are usually inserted 1″ to 2″ (2.5 to 5 cm) below the umbilicus. However, insertion may also be through the flank, the iliac fossa, the border of the rectus, or at each quadrant of the abdomen. If a trocar and cannula are used, a small incision is made to facilitate insertion. When the needle pierces the peritoneum, it "gives" with a popping sound. The trocar is removed, and fluid is aspirated with a 50-ml syringe. Specimens of peritoneal or ascitic fluid are placed in appropriate containers, labeled, and sent promptly to the laboratory. If the patient has received antibiotic therapy, note this on the laboratory slip. Avoid contamination of specimens, which alters their bacterial content.

Additional fluid may then be aspirated (no more than 1,500 ml). After aspiration, the trocar or needle is removed, and a pressure dressing is applied.

Precautions
- Peritoneal fluid analysis should be used cautiously in patients who are pregnant and in those with bleeding tendencies or unstable vital signs.
- Check vital signs every 15 minutes during the procedure. Watch for deviations from baseline findings. Observe for dizziness, pallor, perspiration, and increased anxiety.
- If rapid fluid aspiration induces hypovolemia and shock, reduce the vertical distance between the trocar and the collection bag, to slow the drainage rate. If necessary, stop drainage by turning the stopcock off or by clamping the tubing.

Values
See *Peritoneal fluid analysis,* page 476, for normal contents of peritoneal fluid.

Implications of results
Milk-colored peritoneal fluid may result from chyle escaping from a thoracic duct that is damaged or blocked by carcinoma, lymphoma, tuberculosis, parasitic infection, adhesion, or hepatic cirrhosis; a pseudochylous condition may result from the presence of WBCs or tumor cells. Differential diagnosis of true chylous ascites depends on the presence of elevated triglyceride levels (greater than or equal to 400 mg/dl [4.5 mmol/L]) and microscopic fat globules.

Cloudy or turbid fluid may indicate peritonitis caused by primary bacterial infection, ruptured bowel (after trauma), pancreatitis, strangulated or infarcted intestine, or appendicitis.

Bloody fluid may result from a benign or malignant tumor, hemorrhagic pancreatitis, or a traumatic tap; however, if the fluid fails to clear on continued aspiration, traumatic tap isn't the cause.

Peritoneal fluid analysis	
Element	**Normal value or finding**
Gross appearance	Sterile, odorless, clear to pale yellow color; scant amount (< 50 ml)
Red blood cells	None
White blood cells	< 300/μliter
Protein	0.3 to 4.1 g/dl (albumin, 50% to 70%; globulin, 30% to 45%; fibrinogen, 0.3% to 4.5%)
Glucose	70 to 100 mg/dl
Amylase	138 to 404 amylase units/liter
Ammonia	< 50 μg/dl
Alkaline phosphatase	Male over age 18: 90 to 239 units/liter Female under age 45: 76 to 196 units/liter Female over age 45: 87 to 250 units/liter
Lactate dehydrogenase	Equal to serum level
Cytology	No malignant cells present
Bacteria	None
Fungi	None
Carcinoembryonic antigen	< 2.5 mg/ml

Bile-stained green fluid may indicate a ruptured gallbladder, acute pancreatitis, perforated intestine or duodenal ulcer.

RBC count greater than 100/μliter (0.1×10^9/L) indicates neoplasm or tuberculosis; a count greater than 100,000/μliter (100×10^9/L) indicates intra-abdominal trauma.

WBC count greater than 300/μliter (0.3×10^9/L), with more than 25% neutrophils, occurs in 90% of patients with spontaneous bacterial peritonitis and in 50% of those with cirrhosis. A high percentage of lymphocytes suggests tuberculous peritonitis or chylous ascites. Numerous mesothelial cells indicate tuberculous peritonitis.

Protein levels rise above 3 g/dl (30 g/L) in malignant disease and above 4 g/dl (40 g/L) in tuberculosis.

Glucose levels fall below 60 mg/dl (3.3 mmol/L) in 30% to 50% of patients with tuberculous peritonitis and peritoneal carcinomatosis.

Amylase levels rise in about 90% of patients with pancreatic trauma, pancreatic pseudocyst, or acute pancreatitis, and may also rise in intestinal necrosis or strangulation.

Alkaline phosphatase levels rise to more than twice the normal serum levels in about 90% of patients with ruptured or strangulated small intestine.

Ammonia levels also exceed twice the normal serum levels in ruptured or strangulated large and small intestines, and in ruptured ulcer or appendix.

Creatine levels in peritoneal fluid aid in the differential diagnosis of peritoneal effusion from urinary extravasation; the presence of creatine is indicative of a ruptured urinary bladder, which causes urinary extravasation.

Protein ascitic fluid-serum ratio of 0.5 or greater, a lactate dehydrogenase (LD) ascitic fluid-serum ratio over 0.6, and an ascitic fluid LD level over 400 mU/ml (U/L) suggest malignant, tuberculous, or pancreatic ascites. Any two of these findings indicates a nonhepatic cause; absence of all three usually suggests uncomplicated hepatic disease.

Albumin gradient between ascitic fluid and serum greater than 1 g/dl (10 g/L) indicates chronic hepatic disease; a lesser value suggests malignancy.

Cytologic examination of peritoneal fluid accurately detects malignant cells.

Microbiological examination can reveal coliforms, anaerobes, and enterococci, which can enter the peritoneum from a ruptured organ, or from infections accompanying appendicitis, pancreatitis, tuberculosis, or ovarian disease. Gram-positive cocci often indicate primary peritonitis; gram-negative organisms, secondary peritonitis. The presence of fungi may indicate histoplasmosis, candidiasis, or coccidioidomycosis.

Elevated CEA levels are associated with abdominal malignancy.

Post-test care
- Apply a gauze dressing to the puncture site. Make sure it's thick enough to absorb all drainage. Check the dressing frequently, whenever you check vital signs; reinforce or apply a pressure dressing, if needed.
- Monitor vital signs until stable. If the patient's recovery is poor, check vital signs every 15 minutes. Weigh the patient and measure abdominal

girth; compare these with baseline measurements.

- Allow the patient to rest and, if possible, withhold treatment or procedures that may cause undue stress.
- Monitor urine output for at least 24 hours, and watch for hematuria, which may indicate bladder trauma.
- Watch for signs of hemorrhage and shock or for increasing pain and abdominal tenderness. These may indicate a perforated intestine or, depending on the site of the tap, puncture of the inferior epigastric artery, hematoma of the anterior cecal wall, or rupture of the iliac vein or bladder.
- Observe the patient with severe hepatic disease for signs of hepatic coma, which may result from the loss of sodium and potassium that accompanies hypovolemia. Watch for mental changes, such as drowsiness and stupor. Such a patient is also prone to uremia, infection, hemorrhage, and protein depletion.
- Administer I.V. infusions and albumin as ordered. Check the laboratory report for serum electrolytes (especially sodium) and protein levels.

➤ *Clinical alert:* If a large amount of fluid was aspirated, watch for signs of vascular collapse (color change, elevated pulse rate and respiration rates, decreased blood pressure and central venous pressure, mental changes, and dizziness). Administer fluids orally if the patient is alert and can tolerate them.

Interfering factors
- Failure to send the specimen to the laboratory immediately or unsterile collection technique interferes with accurate testing.
- Injury to underlying structures during paracentesis may contaminate the sample with bile, blood, urine, or feces.

Phenobarbital, serum

Phenobarbital is an anticonvulsant drug used principally to manage generalized tonic-clonic (grand mal) seizures as well as simple and complex partial seizures. It is the drug of choice for treating febrile seizures and is also used to control neonatal seizures. Phenobarbital can be administered alone or in conjunction with other antiepileptic drugs such as phenytoin or valproic acid.

This quantitative test measures serum phenobarbital levels and is used to monitor efficacy of therapy, compliance with therapy, or suspected toxicity.

Purpose
- To determine if drug dosage is appropriate for optimizing therapeutic efficacy and minimizing adverse effects
- To assess patient compliance, particularly in patients who show poor therapeutic response
- To assess suspected toxicity

Patient preparation
Two to three weeks of phenobarbital therapy are required to achieve a steady-state serum concentration, before which serum monitoring is not recommended. Explain that this test helps determine the optimum drug dosage. Inform the patient that he needn't restrict food or fluids before the test and that the test requires a blood sample. Also check the patient's recent medication history, noting dosage and route of administration.

Procedure
Perform a venipuncture, and collect the sample in a *red-top* tube. A minimum serum volume of 0.5 ml is required for analysis.

Values
The therapeutic level for adults ranges from 20 to 40 µg/ml; in children, 15 to 30 µg/ml. In most patients, the frequency of adverse effects increases if serum levels exceed 40 µg/ml. Levels above 55 µg/ml are usually considered toxic, and adverse effects are usually severe with levels above 60 µg/ml. These effects become potentially life-threatening when levels exceed 100 µg/ml.

Implications of results
In patients showing a positive response to phenobarbital, seizures are usually controlled when the serum concentration is maintained in the therapeutic range. However, serum concentration is only one factor in patient management and should always be interpreted in conjunction with the patient's clinical status.

Post-test care
If a hematoma develops at the venipuncture site, applying warm soaks eases discomfort.

Interfering factors

- Patients who develop hepatic disease may experience an increase in serum concentration requiring a compensatory decrease in dosage.
- Although renal excretion contributes to drug clearance, serum concentration is relatively unaffected by changes in renal function.
- Coadministration of valproic acid, phenytoin, cimetidine, or chloramphenicol inhibits phenobarbital's metabolic clearance. A reduction in phenobarbital dosage by 30% to 50% may be required to avoid toxicity when valproic acid is being concomitantly administered.

Phenothiazines, serum

This screening test uses gas-liquid chromatography or fluorometry to measure serum phenothiazine levels in patients exhibiting symptoms of toxicity after treatment with phenothiazines. This group of drugs (including chlorpromazine, prochlorperazine, thioridazine, and trifluoperazine) is widely used to manage acute and chronic psychoses; to control nausea and vomiting; to augment the effects of anesthetics, analgesics, and sedatives; and to relieve acute symptoms during withdrawal from addicting drugs, including alcohol. Well absorbed from the GI tract, these drugs are rapidly distributed to all body tissues. After conversion by the liver, their metabolites are excreted in urine, bile, and feces.

Purpose

- To check for phenothiazine toxicity suspected from history or after onset of clinical symptoms
- To monitor patient compliance with therapy
- To determine the presence of phenothiazines for medicolegal purposes

Patient preparation

Explain the purpose of the test, and tell the patient the test requires a blood sample.

If the test is being performed for medicolegal purposes, make sure that the patient or a responsible family member has signed a consent form. Check and record the patient's medication history.

Procedure

Perform a venipuncture, and collect the sample in a 7-ml *red-top* tube. Send the sample to the laboratory immediately or refrigerate it.

In serial testing, maintain a constant time span between drug administration and sample collection. For a medicolegal test, observe the proper precautions.

Values
Therapeutic levels of prochlorperazine, chlorpromazine, and trifluoperazine are less than 0.5 mcg/ml (950 nmol/L); toxic levels exceed 1.0 mcg/ml (1,900 nmol/L). Therapeutic levels of thioridazine are less than 1.25 mcg/ml (1.1 μmol/L); toxic levels exceed 10 mcg/ml (1.9 μmol/L).

Implications of results
Serial serum levels of phenothiazines guide adjustment of therapeutic dosage. Identification of toxic levels guides treatment of toxicity.

Post-test care
If a hematoma develops at the venipuncture site, applying warm soaks eases discomfort.

Interfering factor
Antacids, anticholinergics, and barbiturates decrease serum phenothiazine levels.

Phenylalanine screening, serum

Guthrie screening test

This test is a screening method used to detect elevated serum phenylalanine, an indication of possible phenylketonuria (PKU). Phenylalanine is a naturally occurring amino acid essential to growth and nitrogen balance. At birth, an infant with PKU usually has normal phenylalanine levels, but after milk or formula feeding begins (both contain phenylalanine), levels gradually rise because of a deficiency of the liver enzyme that converts phenylalanine to tyrosine. The serum phenylalanine screening test detects abnormal phenylalanine levels based on the growth rate of a mutant form of *Bacillus subtilis,* an organism that needs phenylalanine to thrive. To ensure accurate results, the test must be performed after 3 full days (preferably 4 days) of milk or formula feeding.

Purpose
To screen infants for PKU

Patient preparation
Explain to the parents that the test is a routine screening measure for possible PKU and is a required test in many states. Tell them the test requires a blood sample, and that a small amount of blood will be drawn from the infant's heel.

Procedure
Perform a heelstick, and collect three drops of blood — one in each circle — on the filter paper.

Note the infant's name, birth date, and date of the first milk or formula feeding on the laboratory slip, and send the sample to the laboratory immediately.

Values
In the laboratory, the sample is mixed with a culture medium containing a special phenylalanine–dependent strain of *B. subtilis* and a phenylalanine antagonist. A negative test indicates normal phenylalanine levels (less than 2 mg/dl [120 mmol/L]) and no appreciable danger of PKU.

Implications of results
Growth of *B. subtilis* on the filter paper indicates that serum phenylalanine levels are high enough to overcome the antagonist. An abnormal finding, or positive test, suggests the *possibility* of PKU. Diagnosis requires precise serum phenylalanine measurement and urine testing. A positive test may also result from hepatic disease, galactosemia, or delayed development of certain enzyme systems.

Post-test care
Reassure the parents of a child who may have PKU that although this disease occurs in 1 in 10,000 children, early detection and continuous treatment with a low-phenylalanine diet can prevent permanent mental retardation.

Interfering factor
Performing the test before the infant has received at least 3 full days of milk or formula feeding yields a false-negative finding.

Phenytoin, serum

Phenytoin (Dilantin) is an anticonvulsant drug used in the prophylactic management of partial and generalized tonic-clonic (grand mal) seizures and to treat patients in status epilepticus. It is frequently administered with other anticonvulsant drugs.

One test method uses the enzyme-multiplied immunoassay technique to measure serum levels of phenytoin, and is used to monitor patients for efficacy, compliance, or suspected toxicity. Another test method, the apoenzyme reactive immunoassay, is rapid, accurate, and is being increasingly used in outpatient testing.

Purpose
- To determine if drug dosage is appropriate for optimal therapeutic effects while minimizing adverse effects
- To assess patient compliance, particularly in patients who show a poor therapeutic response
- To assess suspected toxicity

Patient preparation
After a patient begins phenytoin therapy, 7 to 10 days are required to achieve a steady-state serum concentration, before which monitoring serum concentrations is not recommended. Explain that this test helps determine the optimum drug dosage. Inform the patient that he needn't restrict food or fluids before the test and that the test requires a blood sample. Also check the patient's recent medication history, noting dosage and route of administration.

Procedure
Perform a venipuncture and collect the sample in a *red-top* tube. A minimum serum volume of 0.5 ml is required for analysis.

Values
The therapeutic level for most patients ranges from 10 to 20 μg/ml. Levels of 25 μg/ml are usually considered toxic.

Implications of results
Most patients show a favorable response when serum levels are maintained within the therapeutic range. However, some patients may respond well at dosages below 10 μg/ml, whereas others may require concentrations in excess of 20 μg/ml to achieve an adequate response. Serum levels above 25 μg/ml may be associated with nystagmus, ataxia, and diplopia. Levels above 30 μg/ml usually cause drowsiness and lethargy. Extreme lethargy and coma occur at concentrations above 50 μg/ml.

A transition from linear to nonlinear elimination kinetics can occur at serum levels within or slightly above the upper limit of the therapeutic range. In such cases, small increases in administered dose can result in significant and unpredictable elevations in serum levels with concomitant increased risk of toxicity.

Post-test care
If a hematoma develops at the venipuncture site, applying warm soaks eases discomfort.

Interfering
factors

- Coadministration of enzyme inducers such as phenobarbital or carbamazepine can reduce serum phenytoin levels.
- Coadministration of enzyme inhibitors, such as cimetidine, erythromycin, or propoxyphene, can increase serum phenytoin levels.
- In uremic patients, metabolic products can displace phenytoin from its albumin binding sites, resulting in increased hepatic extraction of phenytoin and a decrease in total serum phenytoin concentration. However, the free phenytoin concentration may remain unchanged (the therapeutic range for free phenytoin ranges from 1 to 2 µg/ml).
- Coadministration of valproic acid can result in displacement of phenytoin from its albumin binding sites, resulting in a decrease in total serum phenytoin concentration. Measurement of free phenytoin concentration may be indicated to determine if a change in phenytoin dosage is required.
- Coadministration of disulfiram can increase phenytoin metabolism, lower phenytoin levels, and cause seizures.

Phosphates, serum

This test measures serum levels of phosphates, the dominant cellular anions. Phosphates help store and utilize body energy and help regulate calcium levels, carbohydrate and lipid metabolism, and acid-base balance. Phosphates are essential to bone formation; about 85% of the body's phosphates are found in bone. The intestine absorbs a considerable amount of phosphates from dietary sources, but adequate levels of vitamin D are necessary for their absorption. The kidneys excrete phosphates and serve as a regulatory mechanism. Because calcium and phosphate interact in a reciprocal relationship, urine excretion of phosphates increases or decreases in inverse proportion to serum calcium levels. Abnormal concentrations of phosphates result more often from improper excretion than from abnormal ingestion or absorption from dietary sources.

Purpose

- To aid diagnosis of renal disorders and acid-base imbalance

- To detect endocrine, skeletal, and calcium disorders

Patient preparation   Explain the purpose of the test. Inform the patient that restriction of food or fluids is not required before the test and that this test requires a blood sample. Check the patient's medication history for recent therapy with drugs that may alter phosphate levels.

Procedure   Perform a venipuncture, and collect the sample in a 10- to 15-ml *red-top* tube. Handle the sample gently to prevent hemolysis.

Values   Normally, serum phosphate levels range from 2.5 to 4.5 mg/dl (0.80 to 1.40 mmol/L) or from 1.8 to 2.6 mEq/liter. Children have higher serum phosphate levels than adults. Phosphate levels can rise as high as 7 mg/dl (2.25 mmol/L) during periods of increased bone growth.

Implications of results   Because serum phosphate values alone are of limited use diagnostically (only a few rare conditions directly affect phosphate metabolism), they should be interpreted in light of serum calcium results.

Depressed phosphate levels (hypophosphatemia) may result from malnutrition, malabsorption syndromes, hyperparathyroidism, renal tubular acidosis, or treatment of diabetic acidosis. In children, hypophosphatemia can suppress normal growth.

Elevated levels (hyperphosphatemia) may result from skeletal disease, healing fractures, hypoparathyroidism, acromegaly, diabetic acidosis, and renal failure. Hyperphosphatemia is rarely clinically significant; however, if prolonged, it can alter bone metabolism by causing abnormal calcium phosphate deposits.

Post-test care   If a hematoma develops at the venipuncture site, applying warm soaks eases discomfort.

Interfering factors
- Excessive vitamin D intake, phosphate administration, and drug therapy with anabolic steroids and androgens may elevate serum phosphorus levels.
- Improper handling of the sample, resulting in hemolysis, causes false-high serum phosphate levels.

- Suppressed phosphate levels may result from excessive phosphate excretion caused by prolonged vomiting and diarrhea, vitamin D deficiency (which interferes with phosphate absorption), prolonged I.V. infusion of dextrose 5% in water, ingestion of phosphate-binding antacids, and drug therapy with acetazolamide, insulin, and epinephrine.

Plasma thrombin time
Thrombin clotting time

The thrombin time test measures how quickly a clot forms when a standard amount of bovine thrombin is added to a platelet-poor plasma sample from the patient and to a normal plasma control sample. After thrombin is added, the clotting time for each sample is compared and recorded. Because thrombin rapidly converts fibrinogen to a fibrin clot, this test allows a quick but imprecise estimation of plasma fibrinogen levels, which are a function of clotting time.

Purpose
- To detect fibrinogen deficiency or defect
- To aid diagnosis of disseminated intravascular coagulation (DIC) and hepatic disease
- To monitor the effectiveness of treatment with heparin, streptokinase, or urokinase

Patient preparation
Explain that this test helps evaluate blood clotting. Inform the patient that restriction of food or fluids is not required before the test and that the test requires a blood sample.

Procedure
Perform a venipuncture, and collect the sample in a 7-ml *blue-top* tube. Fill the collection tube, invert it gently several times, and send it to the laboratory immediately or place it on ice.

To prevent hemolysis, avoid excessive probing during venipuncture.

Values
Normal thrombin times range from 10 to 15 seconds. Test results are usually reported with a normal control value.

Implications of results
A thrombin time greater than 1.3 times the control may indicate effective heparin therapy, hepatic disease, DIC, hypofibrinogenemia, or fibrinogenemia.

A repeat testing after protamine treatment (to neutralize heparin) will exclude heparin as a causative factor.

Patients with unexplained prolonged thrombin times require quantitation of fibrinogen levels; in suspected DIC, the test for fibrin split products is also necessary. Paraproteins, such as those present in myeloma, may also interfere with thrombin times.

Post-test care   If a hematoma develops at the venipuncture site, applying warm soaks eases discomfort.

Interfering factors
- Hemolysis caused by excessive probing during venipuncture or excessive agitation of the sample may alter test results.
- Failure to use the proper anticoagulant in the collection tube, to mix the sample and the anticoagulant adequately, to send the sample to the laboratory immediately, or to place it on ice may interfere with the accurate determination of test results.
- Sample collection from heparinized lines can also cause falsely prolonged results.
- Administration of heparin may prolong clotting time.

Plasminogen, plasma

Plasminogen, the precursor molecule of plasmin, is measured to assess fibrinolysis. During fibrinolysis, plasmin dissolves fibrin clots to prevent excessive coagulation and the resultant impairment of blood flow. Plasmin doesn't circulate in active form, so it can't be measured directly. However, its circulating precursor, plasminogen, *can* be measured to evaluate fibrinolysis.

This test assesses plasminogen levels by adding streptokinase, a plasminogen activator, to a plasma sample. Streptokinase converts plasminogen to active plasmin; the plasmin is then measured using a chromogenic substrate.

Purpose
- To assess fibrinolysis
- To detect congenital and acquired fibrinolytic disorders

Patient preparation   Explain that this test evaluates blood clotting. Inform the patient that restriction of food or fluids is not required before the test and that the test requires a blood sample. Check the patient's history for use of streptokinase or other medications that may cause inaccurate test results. If these drugs must be continued, note this on the laboratory slip.

Procedure   Perform a venipuncture and collect the sample in a 7-ml *blue-top* tube.

Collect the sample as quickly as possible to prevent stasis, which can slow blood flow, causing coagulation and plasminogen activation.

Immediately after collection, invert the tube gently several times; then send the sample to the laboratory. If testing is delayed, plasma must be separated and frozen at –94°F (–70°C).

Precautions   To prevent hemolysis, avoid excessive probing during venipuncture.

Values   Normal plasminogen levels are 65% or greater (expressed as a percentage of normal), or 2.7 to 4.5 μU/ml (U/L; expressed as activity units).

Implications of   Diminished plasminogen levels can result from disresults   seminated intravascular coagulation and liver diseases. Inherited plasminogen deficiencies are rare.

Post-test care   • If a hematoma develops at the venipuncture site, applying warm soaks eases discomfort.
• The patient may resume restricted medications.

Interfering   • Failure to use the proper specimen tube, to mix
factors   the sample and citrate adequately, to send the sample immediately, or to have it separated and frozen may alter results.
• Hemolysis from excessive probing during venipuncture or excessive agitation of the sample may alter results.
• Prolonged tourniquet use before venipuncture may cause stasis, resulting in false-low plasminogen levels.
• Oral contraceptives may slightly increase plasminogen levels. Thrombolytic drugs, such as streptokinase or urokinase, may decrease levels.

Platelet aggregation

After vascular injury, platelets gather at the injury site and form an aggregate — or plug — that helps maintain hemostasis and promotes healing. The platelet aggregation test, an in vitro procedure, measures the rate at which the platelets in a sample of citrated platelet-rich plasma form a clump after the addition of an aggregating reagent (adenosine diphosphate, epinephrine, thrombin, collagen, or ristocetin). Because evenly suspended platelets are more turbid, the greater the aggregation and platelet clumping, the less turbid the sample. A spectrophotometer measures changes in turbidity and prints a graphic record of the results. This test is used for detecting von Willebrand's disease and inherited platelet defects such as Glanzmann's thrombasthenia, Bernard-Soulier's syndrome, and storage pool disorders.

Purpose
- To assess platelet aggregation
- To detect von Willebrand's disease or other congenital platelet bleeding disorders

Patient preparation
Explain that this test evaluates blood clotting and that the test requires a blood sample. Instruct the patient to fast or maintain a nonfat diet for 8 hours before the test because lipemia can affect test findings.

As appropriate, withhold aspirin and aspirin-containing compounds for 14 days, and phenylbutazone, sulfinpyrazone, phenothiazines, antihistamines, nonsteroidal anti-inflammatory drugs (NSAIDs), and tricyclic antidepressants (TCAs) for 48 hours before the test. If these medications must be continued, note this on the laboratory slip. Because the list of medications known to alter the results of this test is long and growing, the patient should be as free of drugs as possible before the test.

Procedure
Perform a venipuncture, and collect the sample in a 7-ml siliconized tube containing sodium citrate.

Completely fill the collection tube, and invert it gently several times to mix the sample and the anticoagulant adequately. Handle the sample gently to prevent hemolysis, and keep it between 71.6° F (22° C) and 98.6° F (37° C) to prevent aggregation.

Precautions   If a coagulation defect is suspected, avoid excessive probing at the venipuncture site; don't leave the tourniquet on too long (it causes bruising); and apply pressure to the venipuncture site for 5 minutes, or until the bleeding stops.

Findings   Results are compared with normal aggregation controls, and the presence and percentage of aggregation with each agonist (an aggregation inducer) is then reported. Collagen, adenosine diphosphate (ADP), arachidonic acid, and ristocetin are the most commonly used agonists.

Implications of results   Absent aggregation with all agonists except ristocetin is found in Glanzmann's thrombasthenia. Absent ristocetin agglutination is seen in Bernard-Soulier's syndrome (giant platelets) and in severe von Willebrand's disease. Hypersensitivity to ristocetin is seen in some forms of von Willebrand's disease. Abnormal responses to ADP, collagen, and arachidonic acid are seen in a variety of platelet defects.

Post-test care   • If a hematoma develops at the venipuncture site, applying warm soaks eases discomfort.
• The patient may resume diet and withheld medications.

Interfering factors   • Hemolysis caused by excessive agitation of the sample or by trauma at the venipuncture site may interfere with accurate determination of test results.
• Failure to use the proper anticoagulant or to mix the sample and anticoagulant adequately may alter test results.
• Drugs, especially NSAIDs, are the most common cause of abnormal results. Failure to observe dietary and medication restrictions also may impair accurate determination of test results. Platelet aggregation is inhibited by aspirin and aspirin compounds, dipyridamole, caffeine, aminophylline, phenylbutazone, sulfinpyrazone, phenothiazines, antihistamines, anti-inflammatory drugs, and TCAs.

Platelet count

Platelets, or thrombocytes, are the smallest formed elements in the blood. They are vital to the formation of the hemostatic plug in vascular injury and promote coagulation by supplying phospholipids to the intrinsic thromboplastin pathway. The platelet count is one of the most important screening tests of platelet function. Accurate counts are vital for monitoring chemotherapy, radiation therapy, or severe thrombocytosis and thrombocytopenia. A platelet count that falls below 50,000 can cause spontaneous bleeding; when it drops below 5,000, fatal central nervous system bleeding or massive GI hemorrhage is possible.

Properly prepared and stained peripheral blood films provide a reliable estimate of platelet number if the sample shows at least one platelet for every 10 to 20 red blood cells visible in an oil-immersion field. Most laboratories use automated cell counters. Nevertheless, results from such automated systems should always be checked against a visual estimate from a stained blood film.

Purpose	• To evaluate platelet production • To assess effects of chemotherapy or radiation therapy on platelet production • To aid diagnosis of thrombocytopenia and thrombocytosis • To confirm visual estimate of platelet number and morphology from a stained blood film
Patient preparation	Explain that this test evaluates blood clotting. Inform the patient that restriction of food or fluids is not required before the test and that the test requires a blood sample. Check the patient's history for use of medications that may affect test results. Notify the laboratory if such drugs have been used.
Procedure	Perform a venipuncture, and collect the sample in a 7-ml *lavender-top* tube. Completely fill the collection tube, and invert it gently several times to mix the sample and the anticoagulant adequately. To prevent hemolysis, avoid excessive probing at the venipuncture site.
Values	Normal platelet counts range from 150,000 to 400,000/mm³ (150 to 400 × 10⁹/L).
Implications of results	Low platelet counts can be caused by abnormal platelet production (vitamin B_{12} or folate deficiency, chemotherapy, leukemia, aplastic anemia, bone

marrow infiltration); accelerated platelet destruction (disseminated intravascular coagulation, sepsis, autoimmune thrombocytopenia, and heparin-, quinine-, or quinidine-induced thrombocytopenia); or increased sequestration of platelets in the spleen (hypersplenism). Drug-induced thrombocytopenia should always be considered in a patient with thrombocytopenia.

An increased platelet count (thrombocytosis), can result from hemorrhage; infectious disorders; malignant disease; iron deficiency anemia; recent surgery, pregnancy, or splenectomy; and inflammatory disorders, such as collagen vascular disease. In such cases, the platelet count returns to normal after the patient recovers from the primary disorder. However, the count remains elevated in primary thrombocytosis, myelofibrosis with myeloid metaplasia, polycythemia vera, and chronic myelogenous leukemia.

When the platelet count is abnormal, diagnosis usually requires further investigation.

Post-test care
If a hematoma develops at the venipuncture site, applying warm soaks eases discomfort.

Interfering factors
- Failure to use the proper anticoagulant or to mix the sample and anticoagulant promptly and adequately may interfere with the accurate determination of test results.
- Hemolysis caused by excessive agitation of the sample or by excessive probing at the venipuncture site may alter test results.
- Some patients have EDTA-dependent antibodies that cause platelets to clump when collected. Suspect this pseudothrombocytopenia when platelet clumps are observed on the blood film.
- Platelet counts normally increase at high altitudes, with persistent cold temperature, and during strenuous exercise and excitement; the platelet count decreases just before menstruation.

Platelet survival

The platelet survival test measures the rate at which platelets are destroyed and renewed in the peripheral circulation. Platelets labeled with radioactive indium (^{111}In) are injected into the bloodstream. For 7 days, labeled platelets remaining in the circulation are counted in serial samples of peripheral blood and are plotted to obtain a platelet survival curve. Findings are easily reproducible and closely express the life span of circulating platelets. This test provides important information for diagnosis of idiopathic thrombocytopenic purpura, a disorder marked by a shortened platelet life span.

This test should not be performed on pregnant women.

Purpose	• To monitor the effects of drugs known to alter platelet survival
	• To evaluate known or suspected disorders associated with destruction of platelets
	• To aid diagnosis of idiopathic thrombocytopenic purpura
	• To assess platelet survival and life span

Patient preparation   Explain that this test helps evaluate clotting and that the test requires a series of blood samples. A laboratory technologist will perform three or four venipunctures on the 1st day of the test and one venipuncture daily for the next 8 to 10 days.

Advise the patient that the test involves injection of a small, harmless dose of radioactive material.

Also note any previous history of transfusion or pregnancies on the laboratory slip.

Procedure   Three or four venipunctures are performed on the 1st day, and the samples collected in 7-ml *lavender-top* tubes. The first venipuncture is performed to obtain platelets for tagging with ^{111}In (donor platelets from a blood bag may be used instead). The labeled platelets are injected into the bloodstream. Then, two samples are drawn: one at 30 minutes and another after 2 hours after the platelet injection.

A venipuncture is performed daily for the next 7 days, and the blood samples are collected in 7-ml *lavender-top* tubes.

Precautions   If the patient has a suspected coagulation defect, avoid excessive probing during venipuncture; don't leave the tourniquet on too long (it will cause bruising); and be sure to apply pressure to the venipuncture site for 5 minutes, or until the bleeding stops.

Findings   Normally, half the radiolabeled platelets disappear from the circulation in 130 to 150 hours.

Implications of results
Diminished platelet survival time — which may be as brief as 1 to 4 hours — occurs in disorders with accelerated destruction, such as idiopathic (auto-immune) thrombocytopenic purpura. Normal survival with reduced recovery suggests splenic sequestration; normal survival is also seen in individuals with autosomal dominant thrombocytopenia. Imaging of the site of platelet destruction in ^{111}In platelet survival studies may be valuable in predicting the patient's response to splenectomy and in identifying accessory spleens after splenectomy.

Post-test care
If a hematoma develops at the venipuncture site, applying warm soaks eases discomfort.

Interfering factor
Presence of antiplatelet antibodies from previous transfusions or pregnancies may interfere with accurate test results by shortening platelet survival time.

Pleural biopsy

Pleural biopsy is the removal of pleural tissue by needle biopsy or open biopsy for histologic examination. Pleural needle biopsy requires a local anesthetic. It generally follows thoracentesis — aspiration of pleural fluid — that is performed when the etiology of the effusion is unknown, but it can be performed separately.

Open (surgical) pleural biopsy, performed in the absence of pleural effusion, permits direct visualization of the pleura and the underlying lung.

Purpose
- To differentiate between nonmalignant and malignant disease
- To diagnose viral, fungal, parasitic, and collagen vascular disease of the pleura

Patient preparation
Describe the procedure and answer the patient's questions. Explain that this test permits microscopic examination of pleural tissue. Inform the patient that blood studies will precede the biopsy, that chest X-rays will be taken before and after the biopsy, and that an anesthetic will be given to minimize pain.

Make sure that the patient or an appropriate family member has signed a consent form. Check the patient's history for hypersensitivity to the local anesthetic. Just before the procedure, record vital signs.

Procedure

The patient is seated on the side of the bed, with feet resting on a stool and arms supported by the overbed table or upper body. The patient should hold this position and remain still during the procedure. After the skin is prepared, a local anesthetic is administered.

Vim-Silverman needle biopsy: The needle is inserted through the appropriate intercostal space into the biopsy site, with the outer tip distal to the pleura and the central portion pushed in deeper and held in place. The outer case is inserted about ⅜″ (1 cm), the entire assembly rotated 360 degrees, and the needle and tissue specimen are withdrawn.

Cope's needle biopsy: The trocar is introduced through the appropriate intercostal space into the biopsy site. The sharp obturator is then removed and a hooked stylet is inserted through the trocar. The opened notch is directed against the pleura, along the intercostal space, and is slowly withdrawn. While the outer tube is held stationary, the inner tube is twisted to cut off the tissue specimen, and the assembly is withdrawn.

The specimen is immediately put in 10% neutral buffered formaldehyde solution in a labeled specimen bottle and sent to the laboratory immediately.

Clean the skin around the biopsy site, and apply an adhesive bandage.

Precautions

Pleural biopsy is contraindicated in patients with severe bleeding disorders.

Findings

The normal pleura consists primarily of mesothelial cells, flattened in a uniform layer. Layers of areolar connective tissue — containing blood vessels, nerves, and lymphatics — lie below.

Implications of results

Histologic examination of the tissue specimen can reveal malignant disease; tuberculosis; or viral, fungal, parasitic, or collagen vascular disease. Primary neoplasms of the pleura are generally fibrous and epithelial.

Post-test care

• Check vital signs every 15 minutes for 1 hour, then every hour for 4 hours or until stable. The chest X-ray should be repeated immediately after the biopsy.

- Observe the patient for signs of respiratory distress (shortness of breath), shoulder pain, and complications, such as pneumothorax (immediate) and pneumonia (delayed).

Interfering factor Failure to use the proper fixative or obtain adequate specimens may alter results.

Pleural fluid analysis
Thoracentesis

The pleura, a two-layer membrane covering the lungs and lining the thoracic cavity, maintains a small amount of lubricating fluid between its layers to minimize friction during respiration. Increased fluid in this space — the result of diseases such as cancer, tuberculosis, or blood or lymphatic disorders — can cause respiratory difficulty.

In pleural fluid aspiration (thoracentesis), the thoracic wall is punctured to obtain a specimen of pleural fluid for analysis or to relieve pulmonary compression and resultant respiratory distress. The specimen is examined for color, consistency, glucose and protein content, cellular composition, and the enzymes lactate dehydrogenase (LD) and amylase; it's also examined cytologically for malignant cells and cultured for pathogens. Preceding thoracentesis with physical examination and chest radiograph or ultrasound study, to locate the fluid, lessens the risk of puncturing the lung, liver, or spleen.

Purpose To provide a fluid specimen to determine the cause and nature of pleural effusion

Patient preparation Explain the purpose of the test and describe the procedure. Inform the patient that restriction of food or fluids is not required before the test, and that chest radiography or ultrasonography may precede the test. Check the patient's history for hypersensitivity to local anesthetics. Warn the patient that a stinging sensation will occur on injection of the anesthetic as well as some pressure during withdrawal of the fluid. To minimize the risk of injury to the lung, advise the patient not to cough, breathe deeply, or move during the test.

Equipment

Sterile collection bottles, sterile gloves, adhesive tape, sterile thoracentesis tray (a prepackaged, disposable tray) with the following: 70% alcohol or povidone-iodine solution, drapes, local anesthetic (usually 1% lidocaine), 5-ml sterile syringe for local anesthetic, 25G needle, 50-ml syringe for removing fluid, 17G aspiration needle, sterile specimen bottle or tube, three-way stopcock or sterile tubing to prevent air from entering the pleural cavity, small sterile dressing

Procedure

Record the patient's baseline vital signs. Shave the area around the needle insertion site, if necessary. Position the patient properly to widen the intercostal spaces and to allow easier access to the pleural cavity; make sure the patient is well-supported and comfortable. Preferably, seat the patient at the edge of the bed, with a chair or stool supporting the feet and the head and arms resting on a padded overbed table. Position a patient who can't sit up on the unaffected side, with the arm on the affected side elevated above the head. Remind the patient not to cough, breathe deeply, or move suddenly during the procedure.

Use strict aseptic techniques throughout. After the patient is properly positioned, the area is disinfected and draped, and a local anesthetic is injected into the subcutaneous tissue. The thoracentesis needle is inserted above the rib to avoid lacerating the intercostal vessels. When the needle reaches the pocket of fluid, the 50-ml syringe and the stopcock are attached, and the clamps on the tubing are opened to aspirate fluid into the container. During aspiration, check the patient for signs of respiratory distress, such as weakness, dyspnea, pallor, cyanosis, changes in heart rate, tachypnea, diaphoresis, blood-tinged frothy mucus, and hypotension.

After the needle is withdrawn, apply slight pressure and a small adhesive bandage to the puncture site.

Add a small amount (about 0.5 ml) of sterile heparin to the container to prevent coagulation of the fluid.

Label the specimen with the patient's name; record the date and time of the test as well as the amount, color, and character of the fluid (clear, frothy, purulent, bloody) on the laboratory slip. Also note the patient's temperature and antibiotic therapy, if applicable. Send the specimen to the laboratory immediately. Note any signs of distress the

Characteristics of pulmonary transudate and exudate

Characteristic	Transudate	Exudate
Appearance	Clear	Cloudy, turbid
Specific gravity	< 1.016	> 1.016
Clot (fibrinogen)	Absent	Present
Protein	< 3 g/dl	> 3 g/dl
White blood cells	Few lymphocytes	Many; may be purulent
Red blood cells	Few	Variable
Glucose	Equal to serum level	May be less than serum level
Lactate dehydrogenase	Low	High

patient exhibited during the procedure. Document the exact location where fluid was removed; this information may aid diagnosis.

Precautions Thoracentesis is contraindicated in patients who have histories of bleeding disorders.

Findings Normally, the pleural cavity maintains negative pressure and contains less than 20 ml of serous fluid. (See *Characteristics of pulmonary transudate and exudate*.)

Implications of results Pleural effusion results from the abnormal formation or reabsorption of pleural fluid. Certain characteristics classify pleural fluid as either a transudate (a low-protein fluid that has leaked from normal blood vessels) or an exudate (a protein-rich fluid that has leaked from blood vessels with increased permeability). Pleural fluid may contain blood (hemothorax), chyle (chylothorax), or pus and necrotic tissue. Blood-tinged fluid may indicate a traumatic tap; if so, the fluid should clear as aspiration progresses.

Transudative effusion generally results from diminished colloidal pressure, increased negative pressure within the pleural cavity, ascites, systemic and pulmonary venous hypertension, congestive heart failure, hepatic cirrhosis, and nephritis.

Exudative effusion results from disorders that increase pleural capillary permeability (possibly with changes in hydrostatic or colloid osmotic pressures), lymphatic drainage interference, infections, pulmonary infarctions, and neoplasms. Exudative effusion associated with depressed glucose levels, elevated LD, rheumatoid arthritis cells, and negative smears, cultures, and cytologic examination may indicate pleurisy associated with rheumatoid arthritis.

The most common pathogens that appear in culture studies of pleural fluid include *Mycobacterium tuberculosis, Staphylococcus aureus, Streptococcus pneumoniae* and other streptococci, *Haemophilus influenzae,* and in the case of a ruptured pulmonary abscess, anaerobes, such as bacteroides. Generally, cultures are positive during the early stages of infection; however, antibiotic therapy may produce a negative culture despite a positive Gram stain and grossly purulent fluid. Empyema may result from complications of pneumonia, pulmonary abscess, perforation of the esophagus, or penetration from mediastinitis. A high percentage of neutrophils suggests septic inflammation; predominating lymphocytes suggest tuberculosis or fungal or viral effusions.

Serosanguineous fluid may indicate pleural extension of a malignant tumor. Elevated LD in a nonpurulent, nonhemolyzed, nonbloody effusion may also suggest malignancy. Pleural fluid glucose levels that are 30 to 40 mg/dl (1.6 to 2.2 mmol/L) less than blood glucose levels may indicate malignant disease, bacterial infection, nonseptic inflammation, or metastases. Increased amylase levels occur with pleural effusions associated with pancreatitis, lung cancer, or esophageal perforation.

Post-test care
- Reposition the patient comfortably on the affected side or as appropriate. Tell the patient to remain on this side for at least 1 hour to seal the puncture site. Elevate the head of the bed to facilitate breathing.
- Monitor vital signs every 30 minutes for 2 hours, then every 4 hours until they are stable.
- Tell the patient to call for assistance immediately if he experiences difficulty breathing.
- Watch for signs of pneumothorax, tension pneumothorax, fluid reaccumulation and, if a large amount of fluid was withdrawn, pulmonary edema or cardiac distress caused by mediastinal

---

| **Recognizing complications of thoracentesis** |

Identify the following possible complications of thoracentesis by watching for their characteristic signs and symptoms:

- *pneumothorax:* apprehension, increased restlessness, cyanosis, sudden breathlessness, tachycardia, chest pain.
- *tension pneumothorax:* dyspnea, chest pain, tachycardia, hypotension, absent or diminished breath sounds on the affected side.
- *fluid reaccumulation:* increasing and persistent cough, respiratory distress, hemoptysis.
- *mediastinal shift:* labored breathing, cardiac arrhythmias, cardiac distress, pulmonary edema (pink frothy sputum, paradoxical pulse).

---

shift (see *Recognizing complications of thoracentesis* for more information). After the test, a radiograph is usually ordered to detect these complications before clinical symptoms appear.
- Check the puncture site for any fluid leakage. A large amount of leakage is abnormal.

Interfering factors
- Failure to use aseptic technique may contaminate the specimen.
- Antibiotic therapy before aspiration of fluid for culture may decrease the number of bacteria, making isolation of the infecting organism difficult.
- Failure to send the specimen to the laboratory immediately or to add heparin to the container may alter test results.

Polymerase chain reaction

The polymerase chain reaction (PCR), a new molecular technique, was first developed to diagnose sickle cell anemia prenatally. The PCR technique allows small deoxyribonucleic acid (DNA) particles to be duplicated millions of times for several hours, making it easier to identify a specific gene. Beside diagnosing diseases prenatally, this method can also detect and diagnose cancer and infectious diseases.

Purpose	• Prenatal detection of diseases, including cystic fibrosis, hemophilia, muscular dystrophy, and sickle cell anemia
	• Detection of cancers, including lymphoma and chronic myelogenous leukemia
	• Detection of infectious agents, such as the *Borrelia burgdorferi* spirochete that causes Lyme disease, and viruses, such as human immunodeficiency virus (HIV)

Patient preparation Explain the purpose of the test. Inform the patient that a blood sample, biopsy, or other specimens such as cerebrospinal fluid (CSF) or sputum will be required. Also, mention any precautions or restrictions as needed.

Procedure The specimen needed for the PCR assay depends on the type of analysis required. For instance, prenatal diagnosis requires amniotic fluid or chorionic villus biopsy. HIV detection requires a whole blood sample whereas CSF, discharge from wounds, serum biopsies, and sputum are necessary to detect infectious agents. Spinal or synovial fluid are required to detect *B. burgdorferi*, for example, and cancer diagnosis requires solid tissue biopsy.

Findings Normal tissue or the absence of infectious agents indicates a negative test result.

Implications of results The presence of DNA for a specific organism or cellular tissue indicates active disease.

Post-test care If a hematoma develops at the venipuncture site, applying warm soaks eases discomfort.

Interfering factor Because heparin inhibits the *B. burgdorferi* assay, it should not be used as a preservative.

Porphyrins, urine

This test is a quantitative analysis of urine porphyrins (most notably, uroporphyrins and coproporphyrins) and their precursors (porphyrinogens and porphobilinogen [PBG]). Porphyrins are compounds formed from delta-aminolevulinic acid that are produced during the formation of hemoglobin. They are normally excreted in urine in insignificant amounts. Elevated urine levels of porphyrins or porphyrinogens, therefore, reflect impaired heme biosynthesis. Such impairment may result from inherited enzyme deficiencies (congenital porphyrias) or from defects caused by disorders such as hemolytic anemias and hepatic disease (acquired porphyrias). Lead poisoning is the most common cause of acquired porphyria.

Determination of the specific porphyrins and porphyrinogens found in a urine specimen can help identify the impaired metabolic step in heme biosynthesis. Occasionally, a preliminary qualitative screening is performed on a random specimen; a positive finding on the screening test must be confirmed by the quantitative analysis of a 24-hour specimen. For correct diagnosis of a specific porphyria, urine porphyrin levels should be correlated with plasma and fecal porphyrin levels.

Purpose
- To detect excessive excretion of porphyrins
- To detect suspected lead poisoning as indicated by elevated excretion of porphyrins and PBG
- To aid diagnosis of congenital or acquired porphyrias
- To aid diagnosis of hepatic disease

Patient preparation
Explain the purpose of the test, and inform the patient that the test requires a 24-hour urine specimen. Teach the patient the collection technique. Tell the patient to avoid contaminating the specimen with toilet tissue or feces.

Check the patient's history for current pregnancy, menstruation, or drug use; such conditions may interfere with accurate determination of test results.

Procedure
Obtain a 24-hour urine specimen and send it to the laboratory in a light-protected container with preservative. If a preservative is not used, the specimen must be refrigerated until the collection is complete. Record the exact times the collection began and ended on the specimen container.

If a light-resistant container isn't available, protect the specimen from light exposure. If an indwelling urinary catheter is in place, put the collection bag in a dark plastic bag.

Refrigerate the specimen or keep it on ice during the collection period. Then send it to the laboratory immediately.

Values — Normal porphyrin and precursor values for urine fall in these ranges —

Uroporphyrins: in females, from 1 to 22 mcg/day (1 to 26 nmol/day); in males, from undetectable to 42 mcg/day (0 to 50 nmol/day)

Coproporphyrins: in females, from 1 to 57 mcg/day (1 to 86 nmol/day); in males, from undetectable to 96 mcg/day (0 to 146 nmol/day)

PBG: in both sexes, up to 1.5 mg/day (6.6 mmol/day).

Implications of results — In patients with porphyrias, the urine contains elevated levels of porphyrins and PBG. Elevated levels of porphyrins are also associated with cirrhosis, infectious hepatitis, Hodgkin's disease, central nervous system disorders, heavy metal toxicity, and carbon tetrachloride or benzene toxicity. *Urine porphyrin levels in porphyria,* page 504, shows typical findings for uroporphyrins, coproporphyrins, and PBG in porphyria. Because heme synthesis occurs primarily in bone marrow and the liver, porphyrias may be classified as erythropoietic or hepatic.

Post-test care — The patient may resume restricted medications.

Interfering factors
- Increased urine urobilinogen levels can interfere with test results by affecting the reagent used in the PBG screening test.
- Oral contraceptives and griseofulvin can elevate levels; rifampin turns urine red-orange, interfering with results.
- Pregnancy and menstruation may increase porphyrin levels.
- Treatment with the following drugs may cause false-positive test results: griseofulvin, tetracycline, barbiturates, chloral hydrate, chlorpropamide, sulfonamides, meprobamate, and chlordiazepoxide. These drugs should be discontinued at least 10 days before the test, if possible.
- Failure to send a random specimen to the laboratory within 1 hour of collection may lead to oxidation of urobilinogen and yield misleading results.
- Failure to send the 24-hour specimen in a light-protected container or to prevent bacterial proliferation may cause misleading test results.

Urine porphyrin levels in porphyria				
Porphyria	Porphyrin precursors		Porphyrins	
	Aminolevulinic acid	Porpho-bilinogen	Uroporphyrins	Copro-porphyrins
Erythropoietic porphyria	Normal	Normal	Highly increased	Increased
Erythropoietic protoporphyria	Normal	Normal	Normal	Normal
Acute inter-mittent por-phyria	Highly increased	Highly increased	Variable	Variable
Variegate porphyria	Highly increased during acute attack	Normal or slightly in-creased; highly increased during acute attack	Normal or slightly in-creased; may be highly in-creased during acute attack	Normal or slightly in-creased; may be highly in-creased during acute attack
Coproporphy-ria	Increased during acute attack	Increased during acute attack	Not applicable	May be highly increased during acute attack
Porphyria cutanea tarda (associated with other he-patic dis-eases; genetic causes pos-sible)	Variable	Variable	Highly increased	Increased

Potassium, serum

This test, a quantitative analysis, measures serum levels of potassium, the major intracellular cation. Small amounts of potassium may also be found in extracellular fluid. Vital to homeostasis, potassium maintains cellular osmotic equilibrium and helps regulate muscle activity (it's essential in maintaining electrical conduction within the cardiac and skeletal muscles). Potassium also helps regulate enzyme activity and acid-base balance and influences kidney function. Potassium levels are affected by variations in the secretion of adrenal steroid hormones, and by fluctuations in pH, serum glucose levels, and serum sodium levels. A reciprocal relationship appears to exist between potassium and sodium; a substantial intake of one element causes a corresponding decrease in the other. Although it readily conserves sodium, the body has no efficient method for conserving potassium. Even in potassium depletion, the kidneys continue to excrete potassium; therefore, potassium deficiency can develop rapidly and is quite common.

Because the kidneys daily excrete nearly all the ingested potassium, a dietary intake of at least 40 mEq/day (mmol/day) is essential. (A normal diet usually includes 60 to 100 mEq [mmol/day] potassium.)

Purpose
• To evaluate clinical signs of potassium excess (hyperkalemia) or potassium depletion (hypokalemia)
• To monitor renal function, acid-base balance, and glucose metabolism
• To evaluate neuromuscular and endocrine disorders
• To detect the cause of arrhythmias

Patient preparation
Explain the purpose of the test. Inform the patient that restriction of food or fluids is not required before the test and that the test requires a blood sample.

Check the patient's medication history for use of diuretics or other drugs that may influence test results. If these medications must be continued, note this on the laboratory slip.

Procedure
Perform a venipuncture, and collect the sample in a 10- to 15-ml *red-top* tube. Draw the sample immediately after applying the tourniquet, because a delay may elevate the potassium level by allowing leakage of intracellular potassium into the serum. Handle the sample gently to avoid hemolysis.

Values
Normally, serum potassium levels range from 3.8 to 5.5 mEq/liter (mmol/L).

Implications of results
Abnormally high serum potassium levels are common in patients with burns, crushing injuries, diabetic ketoacidosis, and myocardial infarction — conditions in which excessive cellular potassium enters the blood. Hyperkalemia may also indicate reduced sodium excretion, possibly because of re-

Causes of altered serum potassium levels

Hypokalemia	Hyperkalemia
Inadequate intake	**Excessive intake**
Anorexia nervosa	Antibiotics (potassium salts)
Dietary deficiency of meat and vegetables	Sodium substitutes
Pica (eating clay, which prevents absorption of potassium)	Potassium supplements
I.V. therapy deficient in potassium supplementation	Blood transfusion (old blood)
Increased excretion	**Decreased excretion**
Cushing's syndrome	Acute renal failure
Diuresis	Hypoaldosteronism
Diaphoresis	Nephritis
GI losses (vomiting, diarrhea)	
Hyperaldosteronism	
Hypomagnesemia	
Laxative abuse	
Renal tubular acidosis	
Thyrotoxicosis	
Disorders of cellular metabolism	**Disorders of cellular metabolism**
Alkalosis	Acidosis
Excessive licorice ingestion	Addison's disease
Familial periodic paralysis	Cell necrosis (resulting from burns, chemotherapy, hemolysis, trauma)
Insulin excess	Hypoaldosteronism
Leukemia	Insulin deficiency
Megaloblastic anemia	
Drug therapy	**Drug therapy**
Aldosterone	Aldosterone antagonists
Ammonium chloride	Amphotericin B
Cortisone	Antibiotics (potassium salts)
Ethacrynic acid	Cyclosporine
Furosemide	Epinephrine
Gentamicin	Heparin
Insulin	Lithium
Laxatives	Potassium chloride
Prednisone	Potassium-sparing diuretics
Thiazide diuretics	Tetracycline

nal failure (preventing normal sodium-potassium exchange) or Addison's disease (caused by the absence of aldosterone, with consequent potassium buildup and sodium depletion). (See *Causes of altered serum potassium levels*.)

► *Clinical alert:* Observe a patient with hyperkalemia for weakness, malaise, nausea, diarrhea, colicky pain, muscle irritability progressing to flaccid paralysis, oliguria, and bradycardia. Electrocardiography (ECG) reveals a prolonged PR interval; wide QRS complex; tall, tented T wave; and ST-segment elevation.

Below-normal potassium values often result from aldosteronism or Cushing's syndrome (marked by hypersecretion of adrenal steroid hormones), loss of body fluids (as in long-term diuretic therapy), or excessive licorice ingestion (because of the aldosterone-like effect of glycyrrhizic acid).

➤ *Clinical alert:* Observe a patient with hypokalemia for decreased reflexes; rapid, weak, irregular pulse; mental confusion; hypotension; anorexia; muscle weakness; and paresthesia. ECG shows a flattened T wave, ST-segment depression, and U-wave elevation. In severe cases, ventricular fibrillation, respiratory paralysis, and cardiac arrest can develop.

Post-test care If a hematoma develops at the venipuncture site, applying warm soaks eases discomfort.

Interfering factors
- Excessive or rapid potassium infusion, spironolactone or penicillin G potassium therapy, or renal toxicity from administration of amphotericin B, methicillin, or tetracycline increases serum potassium levels.
- Insulin and glucose administration, diuretic therapy (especially with thiazides, but not with triamterine, amiloride, or spironolactone), or I.V. infusions without potassium decrease serum potassium levels.
- Excessive hemolysis of the sample or a delay in drawing blood after applying a tourniquet increases potassium levels.

Potassium, urine

This quantitative test measures urine levels of potassium, a major intracellular cation that helps regulate acid-base balance and neuromuscular function. Potassium imbalance may cause such signs and symptoms as muscle weakness, nausea, diarrhea, confusion, hypotension, electrocardiogram (ECG) changes, and even cardiac arrest.

Most commonly, a serum potassium test is performed to detect hyperkalemia (abnormally high levels) or hypokalemia (abnormally low levels). A urine potassium test may be done to evaluate hypokalemia when a history and physical examination fails to uncover the cause. Potassium is filtered through the renal glomeruli and absorbed through the tubules, and adequate excretion of potassium requires that the distal tubules and collecting ducts secrete potassium into the urine. Thus, measuring urine potassium levels can determine if hypokalemia results from a renal disorder, such as renal tubular acidosis, or an extrarenal disorder, such as malabsorption syndrome.

Purpose
- To determine whether hypokalemia is caused by renal or extrarenal disorders
- To aid evaluation of renal disease
- To aid evaluation of electrolyte and acid-base balances
- To aid in assessment of hypokalemia

Patient preparation
Explain the purpose of the test. Inform the patient that the test requires either a random or timed (8-, 12-, or 24-hour) urine specimen. If it's to be collected at home, teach the correct technique. Tell the patient not to contaminate the specimen with toilet tissue or stool. Check the patient's history for medications that may alter test results. If they must be continued, note this on the laboratory slip.

Procedure
Collect the urine specimen. If appropriate, refrigerate the specimen, or place it on ice during the collection period. Send the specimen to the laboratory immediately or refrigerate it.

Values
Normal potassium excretion is 26 to 123 mmol/day. In a patient with hypokalemia and normal kidney function, potassium concentration will be less than 20 mmol/day, indicating that potassium loss is most likely the result of a GI disorder, such as malabsorption syndrome.

Implications of results
In a patient with hypokalemia, urine potassium levels of less than 3 mmol/L indicate renal losses that may result from such disorders as aldosteronism, renal tubular acidosis, or chronic renal failure. Increased urine potassium levels may result from extrarenal disorders, such as dehydration, starvation, Cushing's disease, or salicylate intoxication.

Post-test care
- Patient may resume restricted medications.
- Administer potassium supplements, monitor serum levels as needed, provide dietary supplements and nutritional counseling, and replace volume loss with I.V. or oral fluids.

> *Clinical alert:* Monitor the hypokalemic patient for diminished reflexes; rapid, weak, irregular pulse; mental confusion; hypotension; anorexia; muscle weakness; and paresthesias. Watch for ECG changes and signs of ventricular fibrillation, respiratory paralysis, and cardiac arrest.

Interfering factors

- Excess dietary potassium increases urine potassium levels.
- When potassium losses result from excessive vomiting or stomach suctioning, urine potassium levels will not reflect actual potassium depletion.
- Potassium-wasting medications, such as ammonium chloride and thiazide diuretics, increase potassium levels.
- Failure to collect all urine and incorrect storage of the specimen alters results.
- Urine potassium levels are decreased in Addison's disease and kidney disease.

Progesterone, plasma

Progesterone, an ovarian steroid hormone secreted by the corpus luteum, causes thickening and secretory development of the endometrium in preparation for implantation of the fertilized ovum. Progesterone levels, therefore, peak during the midluteal phase of the menstrual cycle. Progesterone may prolong the surge of luteinizing hormone after ovulation. If implantation doesn't occur, progesterone (and estrogen) levels drop sharply and menstruation begins about 2 days later.

During pregnancy, the placenta releases about 10 times the normal monthly amount of progesterone to maintain the pregnancy. Increased secretion begins toward the end of the first trimester and continues until delivery. Progesterone prepares the endometrium for implantation of the fertilized ovum, decreases myometrial excitability, stimulates vaginal epithelial proliferation, and stimulates growth of the breasts during pregnancy.

This radioimmunoassay is a quantitative analysis of plasma progesterone levels and provides reliable information about corpus luteum function in fertility studies or placental function in pregnancy. Serial determinations are recommended. Although plasma levels provide accurate information, progesterone can also be monitored by measuring urine pregnanediol, a metabolite of progesterone.

Purpose	• To assess corpus luteum function as part of infertility studies
	• To evaluate placental function during pregnancy
	• To aid in confirming ovulation (test results support basal body temperature readings)

Patient preparation	Explain the purpose of the test. Inform the patient that she needn't restrict food or fluids before the test and that the test requires a blood sample. Inform her that the test may be repeated at specific times coinciding with phases of her menstrual cycle or with each prenatal visit.

Procedure	Perform a venipuncture, and collect the sample in a 7-ml *green-top* (heparinized) tube.
	Completely fill the collection tube; then invert it gently at least 10 times to mix the sample and anticoagulant adequately. Send the sample to the laboratory immediately.
	Indicate the date of the patient's last menstrual period on the laboratory slip. If the patient is pregnant, also indicate the month of gestation.

Values	Normal values during menstruation —
	Follicular phase: less than 150 ng/dl (4.8 nmol/L)
	Luteal phase: about 300 ng/dl (9.5 nmol/L; rises daily during periovulation)
	Midluteal phase: 2,000 ng/dl (63.6 nmol/L)
	Normal values during pregnancy —
	First trimester: 1,500 to 5,000 ng/dl (47.7 to 159 nmol/L)
	Second and third trimesters: 8,000 to 20,000 ng/dl (254 to 636 nmol/L)

Implications of results	Elevated progesterone levels may indicate ovulation, luteinizing tumors, ovarian cysts that produce progesterone, or adrenocortical hyperplasias and tumors that produce progesterone along with other steroidal hormones.
	Low progesterone levels are associated with panhypopituitarism, Turner's syndrome, ovarian failure, adrenogenital syndrome, placental insufficiency, toxemia of pregnancy, threatened spontaneous abortion, and fetal death.

Post-test care	If a hematoma develops at the venipuncture site, applying warm soaks eases discomfort.

Interfering factors

- Hemolysis caused by excessive agitation of the sample may affect test results.
- Progesterone, estrogen, or adrenocorticoid therapy may interfere with accurate test results.

Prolactin

Lactogenic hormone, lactogen

Similar in molecular structure and biological activity to human growth hormone, prolactin is a polypeptide hormone secreted by the anterior pituitary gland under control of a hypothalamic inhibiting factor, purportedly the neurotransmitter dopamine. Prolactin induces lactation. It is secreted in males and nonpregnant females, but its function is unknown. Elevated prolactin levels occur in patients with reduced dopamine levels, with hypothalamic or pituitary injury, and with pituitary microadenomas. Prolactin levels rise in response to sleep, physical or emotional stress, and hypoglycemia.

This radioimmunoassay is a quantitative analysis of serum prolactin levels, which normally rise 10- to 20-fold during pregnancy, corresponding to concomitant elevations in human placental lactogen levels. After delivery, prolactin secretion falls to basal levels in mothers who don't breast-feed. However, prolactin secretion increases during breast-feeding, apparently as a result of a stimulus triggered by suckling that curtails the release of prolactin-inhibiting factor by the hypothalamus. This, in turn, allows transient elevations of prolactin secretion by the pituitary. This test is considered useful in patients suspected of having pituitary tumors, which can secrete prolactin in excessive amounts.

Purpose

- To facilitate diagnosis of pituitary dysfunction, possibly caused by pituitary adenoma
- To aid diagnosis of hypothalamic dysfunction
- To evaluate secondary amenorrhea and galactorrhea

Patient preparation

Explain that this test helps evaluate hormonal secretion. Inform the patient that she need not restrict food or fluids, or limit physical activity before the test, and that the test will require a blood sample. Encourage the patient to relax for about one-half hour before the test. Withhold drugs, such as chlorpromazine, methyldopa, and metoclopramide, that may influence serum prolactin levels. If they must be continued, note this on the laboratory slip.

Procedure Perform a venipuncture at least 2 hours after the patient wakes; samples drawn earlier are likely to show sleep-induced peak levels. Collect the sample in a 7-ml *red-top* tube. Handle the sample gently to prevent hemolysis.

Values Normal values range from undetectable to 20 ng/ml (0 to 23 µmg/L) in nonlactating females.

Implications of results Abnormally high prolactin levels (greater than 100 ng/ml [100 µg/L]) suggest autonomous prolactin production by a pituitary adenoma, especially when amenorrhea or galactorrhea is present (Forbes–Albright syndrome). Rarely, hyperprolactinemia also may result from other endocrine disorders, such as hypothyroidism, acromegaly, and hypothalamic or pituitary disorders that depress prolactin-inhibiting factor. Idiopathic hyperprolactinemia may be associated with anovulatory infertility.

Decreased prolactin levels in a lactating mother cause failure of lactation and may be associated with postpartum pituitary infarction (Sheehan's syndrome).

Post-test care
- If a hematoma develops at the venipuncture site, applying warm soaks eases discomfort.
- The patient may resume discontinued medications.

Interfering factors
- Failure to take into account physiologic variations related to sleep or stress may invalidate test results.
- Pretest use of ethanol, haloperidol, morphine, metoclopramide, methyldopa, estrogens, phenothiazines, amphetamines, tricyclic antidepressants, procainamide derivatives, and reserpine raises prolactin levels.
- Pretest use of apomorphine, ergot alkaloids, and levodopa lowers prolactin levels.
- Radioactive scan performed within 1 week before the test or recent surgery may interfere with test results.
- Hemolysis caused by excessive agitation of the sample may interfere with accurate determination of test results.

Propranolol, plasma

Propranolol is a beta-adrenergic receptor blocking agent (beta blocker) used in the treatment of hypertension, angina pectoris, myocardial infarction, and mitral valve prolapse. Propranolol competes with norepinephrine and epinephrine at their beta receptor sites and thereby attenuates some effects of sympathetic nervous system activity. Many of propranolol's effects are mediated by blockade of cardiac beta$_1$ receptors, which induces a slowing of heart rate and reduction in myocardial oxygen demand.

Plasma levels greater than 30 ng/mL (114 nmol/L) are generally required for clinical response; beta blockade is complete at 100 ng/mL (380 nmol/L); higher levels cause no additional improvement in most patients with angina pectoris. Propranolol is metabolized by the liver and undergoes significant first-pass hepatic metabolism, which results in low oral bioavailability (less than 50%) and probably contributes to the variability in plasma levels commonly observed in patients who receive comparable dosages. Because propranolol has a wide margin of safety, and because definite clinical end points exist for monitoring therapeutic response (such as blood pressure measurements in hypertensive patients or heart rate measurements during exercise in angina patients), measuring plasma propranolol levels is not routine. However, such monitoring may be useful in the management of patients who do not show the expected clinical response.

Propranolol is assayed by high performance liquid chromatography or gas chromatography.

Purpose
- To verify that propranolol dosage is adequate to maintain a therapeutic level
- To assess patient compliance

Patient preparation
Explain the purpose of the test and inform the patient that a blood sample is required.

Procedure
Obtain a venous blood sample. The blood should be collected just before administration of the next dose (trough level). This test requires 2 ml of plasma in a *green-top* tube (heparinized) or *lavender-top* tube (EDTA).

Note: Rubber stoppers in some commercially available collection tubes contain plasticizers which displace propranolol from serum-binding proteins; the free propranolol subsequently binds to red blood cells yielding spuriously low results. To avoid this problem, blood should be collected and processed in tubes without stoppers.

Values

The therapeutic range of propranolol is 50 to 100 ng/ml (190 to 3,800 nmol/L).

Toxicity may occur at serum levels greater than 1,000 ng/ml (3,800 nmol/L).

Implications of results

Plasma levels within therapeutic range confirm appropriate dosage and compliance.

Post-test care

If a hematoma develops at the venipuncture site, applying warm soaks eases discomfort.

Interfering factors

• Incorrect timing of sample collection may yield misleading results.
• Use of collection tubes with plasticized stoppers causes spuriously low plasma levels.

Prostate gland biopsy

Prostate gland biopsy is the needle excision of a prostate tissue specimen for histologic examination. A perineal, transrectal, or transurethral approach may be used; the transrectal approach is usually used for high prostatic lesions. Indications include potentially malignant prostatic hyperplasia and prostatic nodules.

Purpose

• To confirm prostate cancer
• To determine the cause of prostatic hyperplasia

Patient preparation

Describe the procedure, answer the patient's questions, and tell him the test provides a tissue specimen for microscopic study.

Make sure that the patient or an appropriate family member has signed a consent form. Check the patient's history for hypersensitivity to the anesthetic or to other medications. For a transrectal approach, the bowel is prepared by administration of enemas until the return is clear. An antibacterial agent may be administered P.O. or I.V. to minimize the risk of infection. Just before the biopsy, check vital signs and administer a sedative, as ordered.

Tell the patient to remain still during the procedure and to follow instructions.

Procedure   *Perineal approach:* The patient is placed in left lateral, knee-chest, or lithotomy position, and the perineal skin is cleaned. After the local anesthetic is administered, a 2-mm incision may be made into the perineum. The examiner immobilizes the prostate gland by inserting a finger into the rectum and introduces the biopsy needle into a prostate lobe. The needle is rotated gently, pulled out about 5 mm, and reinserted at another angle. The procedure is repeated at several areas. Specimens are placed immediately in a labeled specimen bottle containing 10% formaldehyde solution. Pressure is exerted on the puncture site, which is then bandaged.

Transrectal approach: This approach may be performed on outpatients without administering an anesthetic. The patient is placed in a left lateral position. A curved needle guide is attached to the finger palpating the rectum. The biopsy needle is pushed along the guide, into the prostate gland. As the needle enters the prostate, the patient may experience pain. The needle is rotated to cut off the tissue and is then withdrawn. The specimen is placed immediately in a labeled specimen bottle containing 10% formaldehyde solution.

Transurethral approach: An endoscopic instrument is passed through the urethra, permitting direct viewing of the prostate gland and passage of a cutting loop. The loop is rotated to chip away pieces of tissue and is then withdrawn. The specimen is placed immediately in a labeled specimen bottle containing 10% formaldehyde solution.

➤ *Clinical alert:* Complications may include transient, painless hematuria and bleeding into the urethra and bladder.

Findings   Normally, the prostate gland consists of a thin, fibrous capsule surrounding the stroma, which is made up of elastic and connective tissues and smooth-muscle fibers. The epithelial glands, found in these tissues and muscle fibers, drain into the chief excreting ducts.

Implications of results   Histologic examination can confirm cancer, but further tests are required to check for possible extension of the tumor. Bone scans, bone marrow biopsy, and serum acid phosphatase determinations help identify the stage of prostate cancer. Acid phosphatase and prostate-specific antigen levels usually rise in metastatic prostate cancer; they tend to be lower in cancer that's confined to the prostatic capsule. In the latter case, radical surgery and irradiation, although controversial, can provide a high cure rate. If discovery of cancer is delayed (this is common because symptoms are generally absent in early stages and most men don't have regular rectal examinations), treatment necessitates estrogen therapy because continued growth of the tumor depends on testosterone secretion.

Histologic examination can also detect benign prostatic hyperplasia, prostatitis, tuberculosis, lymphomas, and rectal or bladder cancers.

Post-test care
- Check vital signs immediately after the procedure, every 2 hours for 4 hours, and then every 4 hours.
- Observe the biopsy site for a hematoma and for signs of infection, such as redness, swelling, and pain. Watch for urine retention or frequency and for hematuria.

Interfering factor
Failure to obtain an adequate tissue specimen or to place the specimen in formaldehyde solution may interfere with accurate test results.

Prostate-specific antigen

Until 1994, digital rectal examination and measurement of prostatic acid phosphatase (PAP) were the primary methods of monitoring the progression of prostate cancer. In 1994, the Food and Drug Administration approved the prostate-specific antigen (PSA) test to screen for prostate cancer in men over age 50. However, PSA should be combined with digital examination for optimal results.

PSA is also used to monitor prostate cancer and evaluate the patient's response to treatment. Biochemically and immunologically distinct from PAP, PSA is present in varying concentrations in normal, benign hyperplastic, and malignant prostatic tissue, as well as in metastatic prostate cancer.

Purpose
- To detect prostate cancer
- To monitor the course of prostate cancer and aid evaluation of cancer treatment

Patient preparation	Explain the purpose of the test. Tell the patient to fast before the test and that the test requires a blood sample.
Procedure	Perform a venipuncture, and collect the sample in a 7-ml *red-top* tube. Handle the sample gently to prevent hemolysis, and send it to the laboratory immediately. If prolonged storage is necessary, freeze the sample at $-4\,°F$ $(-20°\,C)$.
Precautions	Collect the blood sample either before digital prostate examination or at least 48 hours after examination to avoid false-high PSA levels.
Values	Normal serum values for PSA are less than or equal to 2.7 ng/ml in males under age 40 and less than or equal to 4 ng/ml (μg/L) in males age 40 or older.
Implications of results	Approximately 80% of patients with prostate cancer have pretreatment PSA values greater than 4 ng/ml (μg/L). This percentage varies (higher in advanced stages, lower in early stages).
	PSA levels equal to or higher than 2.7 ng/ml in males under age 40, and PSA levels equal to or higher than 4 ng/ml in males age 40 or older indicate prostate cancer.
Post-test care	If a hematoma develops at the venipuncture site, applying warm soaks eases discomfort.
Interfering factors	• Hemolysis caused by excessive agitation of the sample can interfere with accurate determination of test results.
	• Recent prostatic manipulation will alter test results if performed previous to the test.

Protein C, plasma

Protein C, a vitamin-K dependent protein, is produced in the liver and circulates in the plasma. After activation by thrombin in the presence of the capillary endothelial cofactor thrombomodulin, it is a potent anticoagulant, which acts by deactivating coagulation factors Va and VIIIa.

Congenital deficiencies of protein C are associated with a predisposition to thromboembolic disease. Most affected individuals are heterozygous. Rare, homozygous deficiency of protein C is characterized by rapidly fatal thrombosis in the perinatal period, a syndrome known as purpura fulminans.

Protein C is measured functionally and by immunoassay. The assay is standardized by plasma pooled from a large group of normal donors.

This test is used to investigate the cause of otherwise unexplained thrombosis and to establish patterns of inheritance. A positive finding for heterozygous deficiency is used for informational purposes only, because the clinical significance of the deficiency isn't fully understood and corrective interventions are largely experimental.

Purpose	To investigate the cause of idiopathic venous thrombosis
Patient preparation	Explain the purpose of the test and that the test requires a blood sample. Testing is best performed after resolution of acute thrombi. Check the patient's history for warfarin-type anticoagulants, which will affect test results.
Procedure	Perform a venipuncture, and collect the sample using a 3-ml *blue-top* vacuum tube or a special syringe and anticoagulant provided by the coagulation laboratory. (Sample collection for this test is usually done by laboratory personnel.) Send the sample to the laboratory immediately.
Findings	Normal range is 50% to 150% of the population mean, which is standardized by each laboratory.
Implications of results	Identification of protein C deficiency in idiopathic venous thrombosis is vital in determining whether patients require continued antithrombotic therapy. Family testing is also important in identifying other individuals potentially at risk. Low protein C levels are found in neonates and are associated with liver disease, warfarin therapy, vitamin K deficiency, acute thrombosis, and disseminated intravascular coagulation.
Post-test care	If a hematoma develops at the venipuncture site, applying warm soaks eases discomfort.
Interfering factor	Anticoagulant therapy and acute thrombosis may alter test results.

Protein electrophoresis, serum

This test measures serum albumin and globulins, the major blood proteins, in an electric field by separating the proteins according to their size, shape, and electric charge at pH 8.6. Because each protein fraction moves at a different rate, this movement separates the fractions into recognizable and measurable bands.

Albumin, which comprises more than 50% of total serum protein, maintains oncotic pressure (preventing leakage of capillary plasma) and transports substances that are insoluble in water alone, such as bilirubin, fatty acids, hormones, and drugs. Four types of globulins exist — $alpha_1$, $alpha_2$, beta, and gamma. The first three types act primarily as carrier proteins that transport lipids, hormones, and metals through the blood. The fourth type, gamma globulin, is an important component in the body's immune system.

The usual clinical indication for this test is suspected hepatic disease, protein deficiency, or multiple myelomatosis.

Purpose
: To aid diagnosis of hepatic disease, protein deficiency, blood dyscrasias, renal disorders, and GI and neoplastic diseases, especially multiple myeloma or monoclonal gammopathies

Patient preparation
: Explain the purpose of the test. Inform the patient that restriction of food or fluids is not required before the test and that the test requires a blood sample.

Check the patient's medication history for drugs that may influence serum protein levels. If they must be continued, note this on the laboratory slip.

Procedure
: Perform a venipuncture, and collect the sample in a 7-ml *red-top* tube.

Note: This test must be performed on a serum sample to avoid measuring the fibrinogen fraction.

Values
: Normally, total serum protein levels range from 6.6 to 7.9 g/dl (66 to 79 g/L). The albumin fraction ranges from 3.3 to 4.5 g/dl (33 to 45 g/L). The alpha$_1$-globulin fraction ranges from 0.1 to 0.4 g/dl (1 to 40 g/L); alpha$_2$-globulin ranges from 0.5 to 1 g/dl (5 to 10 g/L). Beta globulin ranges from 0.7 to 1.2

Clinical implications of abnormal protein levels

The chart below lists the disorders that result from abnormal protein levels. The total protein level is indicative of a general disorder, whereas the serum albumin and globulin levels are indicative of specific diseases or disorders.

Total proteins	Albumin	Globulins
Increased levels		
Chronic inflammatory disease (such as rheumatoid arthritis or early-stage Laënnec's cirrhosis) Dehydration Diabetic acidosis Fulminating and chronic infections Monocytic leukemia Multiple myeloma Vomiting, diarrhea	Dehydration	*Alpha$_1$* (α_1) Acute infections Malignancies Pregnancy Tissue necrosis *Alpha$_2$* (α_2) Acute infections Acute myocardial infarction Advanced malignancies Nephrotic syndrome Rheumatic fever Rheumatoid arthritis Trauma, burns *Beta* (β) Biliary cirrhosis Cushing's disease Diabetes mellitus Hypothyroidism Malignant hypertension Nephrotic syndrome *Gamma* (γ) Chronic active liver disease Drugs (tolazamide, tubocurarine, anticonvulsants) Hodgkin's disease Myeloma (compact band) Rheumatoid arthritis Systemic lupus erythematosus (SLE)

(continued)

g/dl (7 to 12 g/L); gamma globulin ranges from 0.5 to 1.6 g/dl (5 to 16 g/L).

Implications of results

For common findings, see *Clinical implications of abnormal protein levels.*

Decreased albumin and elevated globulins suggest chronic liver disease. Normal albumin with increased gamma globulin suggests myeloprolifera-

Clinical implications of abnormal protein levels *(continued)*		
Total proteins	**Albumin**	**Globulins**
Decreased levels		
Benzene and carbon tetra-chloride poisoning Blood dyscrasias Congestive heart failure Hemorrhage Hepatic dysfunction Hodgkin's disease Hyperthyroidism Malabsorption Malnutrition Nephroses Severe burns Surgical and traumatic shock Toxemia of pregnancy Uncontrolled diabetes mellitus	Acute cholecystitis Collagen diseases Diarrhea Drugs (acetaminophen, azathioprine, cyclophospha-mide, niacin, estrogen, dextran) Hepatic disease Hodgkin's disease Hyperthyroidism Malnutrition Metastatic carcinoma Nephritis or nephrosis Peptic ulcer Plasma loss from burns Rheumatoid arthritis Sarcoidosis SLE	*Alpha₁ (α₁)* Genetic deficiency of alpha$_1$-antitrypsin *Alpha₂ (α₂)* Hemolytic anemia Severe hepatic disease *Beta (β)* Hypocholesterolemia *Gamma (γ)* Drugs (BCG vaccine, metho-trexate) Inherited immunoglobulin deficiencies Lymphocytic leukemia Lymphosarcoma Nephrotic syndrome

tive disease (leukemia, Hodgkin's disease) or certain chronic infectious diseases (tuberculosis, chronic hepatitis). A monoclonal band suggests myelomatosis and requires testing by immunofixation electrophoresis.

Post-test care If a hematoma develops at the venipuncture site, applying warm soaks eases discomfort.

Interfering factors
- Pretest administration of a contrast dye (such as sulfobromophthalein) causes false-high total protein levels. Pregnancy and cytotoxic agents may lower serum albumin.
- Use of plasma instead of serum introduces a fibrinogen band which may alter test results.

Protein S, plasma

Protein S is a vitamin K-dependent cofactor produced in the liver, which serves as a cofactor for protein C. Protein S circulates in two forms, one that is free in plasma and another that forms a complex with C4b-binding protein. It is the free form that functions as a cofactor for protein C.

Most laboratories measure free and total plasma protein S levels by immunoassay.

Inherited deficiencies of protein S are associated with a predisposition to thromboembolic disease, and most affected individuals are heterozygous.

Purpose   To investigate the cause of idiopathic venous thrombosis

Patient preparation   Explain the purpose of the test, and tell the patient that the test requires a blood sample. Testing is best performed after resolution of acute thrombi. Check the patient's history for warfarin-type anticoagulants, which will affect test results.

Procedure   Perform a venipuncture, and collect the sample using a 3-ml *blue-top* vacuum specimen tube or a special syringe and anticoagulant provided by the coagulation laboratory. (Sample collection for this test is usually done by laboratory personnel.) Send the sample to the laboratory immediately.

Values   Normal total plasma protein S levels are 0.6 to 1.24 units/ml with free protein S levels of 0.28 to 0.61 units/ml.

Implications of results   Identification of protein S deficiency in idiopathic venous thrombosis is important in determining whether patients require continued antithrombotic therapy. Family testing is also important to identify other individuals potentially at risk. Low protein S levels may be seen in liver disease, warfarin therapy, vitamin K deficiency, acute thrombosis, disseminated intravascular coagulation, pregnancy, systemic lupus erythematosus, and in neonates.

Post-test care   If a hematoma develops at the venipuncture site, applying warm soaks eases discomfort.

Interfering factor   Anticoagulant therapy and acute thrombosis may alter test results.

Protein, urine

This is a quantitative test for proteinuria. Normally, the glomerular membrane allows only proteins of low molecular weight to enter the filtrate. The renal tubules then reabsorb most of these proteins, typically excreting a small amount that's undetectable by a screening test. A damaged glomerular capillary membrane and impaired tubular reabsorption allow excretion of proteins in the urine.

A qualitative screening often precedes this test. A positive result requires quantitative analysis of a 24-hour urine specimen by acid precipitation tests. Electrophoresis can detect Bence-Jones proteins, hemoglobins, myoglobins, or albumin.

Purpose
To aid diagnosis of pathologic states characterized by proteinuria, primarily renal disease

Patient preparation
Explain the purpose of the test. Inform the patient that the test usually requires a 24-hour urine collection, and teach the correct collection method. Tell the patient not to contaminate the urine with toilet tissue or stool.

Check the patient's medication history for drugs that may affect test results. Review your findings with the laboratory, and restrict medications before the test as appropriate.

Procedure
Collect a 24-hour urine specimen. A special specimen container can be obtained from the laboratory. Refrigerate the specimen or place it on ice during the collection period.

Values
Normal values show up to 150 mg of protein excreted in 24 hours.

Implications of results
Proteinuria strongly suggests renal disease. When proteinuria is present in a single specimen, 24-hour urine collection is subsequently required to identify specific renal abnormalities.

Proteinuria can result from glomerular leakage of plasma proteins (a major cause of protein excretion), from overflow of filtered proteins of low molecular weight (when these are present in excessive concentrations), from impaired tubular reabsorption of filtered proteins, and from the presence of renal proteins derived from the breakdown of kidney tissue.

Persistent proteinuria indicates renal disease resulting from increased glomerular permeability. *Minimal* proteinuria, however, is most often associated with renal diseases in which glomerular involvement is not a major factor, such as chronic pyelonephritis.

Moderate proteinuria (0.5 to 4 g/day) occurs in several types of renal disease — acute or chronic glomerulonephritis, amyloidosis, toxic nephropathies — or in diseases in which renal failure often develops as a late complication (diabetes or heart failure, for example). *Heavy* proteinuria (more than 4 g/day) is commonly associated with nephrotic syndrome.

When accompanied by an elevated white blood cell count, proteinuria indicates urinary tract infection; proteinuria with hematuria indicates local or diffuse urinary tract disorders. Other pathologic states (infections and lesions of the central nervous system, for example) also can result in detectable amounts of proteins in the urine.

Many drugs (such as amphotericin B, gold preparations, aminoglycosides, polymyxins, and trimethadione) inflict renal damage, causing true proteinuria. This makes the routine evaluation of urine proteins essential during such treatment.

In all forms of proteinuria, fractionation test results obtained by electrophoresis provide more precise information than the screening test. For example, excessive hemoglobin in the urine indicates intravascular hemolysis; elevated myoglobin suggests muscle damage; albumin, increased glomerular permeability; and Bence-Jones proteins, multiple myeloma.

Not all forms of proteinuria have pathologic significance. *Benign* proteinuria can result from changes in body position. *Functional* proteinuria is associated with emotional or physiologic stress and is usually transient.

Post-test care The patient may resume withheld medications.

Interfering factors
- Administration of tolbutamide, para-aminosalicylic acid, acetazolamide, sodium bicarbonate, penicillin, sulfonamides, iodine contrast media, and cephalosporins may cause false-positive results in acid precipitation tests.
- Contamination of the urine specimen with heavy mucus, vaginal or prostatic secretions, or the presence of numerous white blood cells can alter test results, regardless of laboratory method.
- Extremely dilute urine (which may result from forcing fluids) may depress protein values and cause false-negative results.

Prothrombin time (PT)

Pro time

This test measures the time required for a fibrin clot to form in a citrated plasma sample after addition of calcium ions and tissue thromboplastin (source of tissue factor and phospholipid), and compares this time with a control sample of plasma. Because this test reaction bypasses the intrinsic coagulation pathway and doesn't involve platelets, the prothrombin time (PT) is used to evaluate the extrinsic coagulation sequence, including factors V, VII, X, prothrombin (II), and fibrinogen (I). PT is the test of choice for monitoring oral anticoagulant therapy.

Results are reported in seconds for both the patient and the plasma control. Because test results are affected by the reagent used, a standardized system of reporting results has been developed to allow comparisons between laboratories. The World Health Organization's international normalized ratio (INR) converts PT to the ratio of the patient's PT or the control PT using the World Health Organization's reference reagent.

Purpose
- To evaluate the extrinsic coagulation system
- To monitor response to oral anticoagulant therapy
- To aid diagnosis of conditions associated with abnormal bleeding
- To identify patients at risk for excessive bleeding during surgical or other invasive procedures
- To differentiate deficiencies of specific clotting factors
- To monitor the effects on hemostasis of certain diseases (for example, hepatic disease or protein deficiency)

Patient preparation
Explain the purpose of the test. Inform the patient that restriction of food or fluids is not necessary and that the test requires a blood sample.

Check the patient's history for use of medications that may interfere with the test.

When appropriate, explain to the patient that this test monitors the effects of anticoagulant medications. If so, the test will be performed daily when therapy begins and will be repeated at longer intervals when medication levels stabilize.

Procedure | Perform a venipuncture, avoiding excessive probing of the site. Collect the sample in a 7-ml *blue-top* tube. Completely fill the collection tube, and invert it gently several times to mix the sample and the anticoagulant adequately. If the tube isn't filled to the correct volume, an excess of citrate appears in the sample.

Send the sample to the laboratory promptly. If transport is delayed more than 4 hours, and the sample is kept at room temperature, factor V may deteriorate, prolonging the PT; if the sample is refrigerated, factor VII may be activated, shortening the PT.

Values | Normally, PT values range from 9.6 to 11.8 seconds in males, and from 9.5 to 11.3 seconds in females. However, values vary, depending on the source of tissue thromboplastin and the type of sensing devices used to measure clot formation. In a patient receiving oral anticoagulants, PT is usually maintained between one and a half and two times the normal control.

For laboratories reporting results as INRs, normal values are 1.0 to 1.2 seconds. Recommended therapeutic INR for most patients on oral anticoagulants is 2.0 to 3.0 seconds.

Implications of results | Prolonged PT may indicate deficiencies in fibrinogen, prothrombin, or factor V, VII, or X (specific assays can pinpoint such deficiencies); vitamin K deficiency; or hepatic disease. Or it may result from oral anticoagulant therapy. Prolonged PT that exceeds two and a half times the control value is commonly associated with abnormal bleeding.

Post-test care | If a hematoma develops at the venipuncture site, applying warm soaks eases discomfort.

Interfering factors |
- Hemolysis caused by excessive probing during venipuncture or agitation of the sample may interfere with accurate test results.
- Failure to mix the sample and anticoagulant adequately or to send the sample to the laboratory promptly may alter test results.
- Fibrin or fibrin split products in the sample, or plasma fibrinogen levels less than 100 mg/dl (1.0 g/L) can prolong PT.
- Falsely prolonged results may occur if the sample is drawn from a heparinized line or if the col-

lection tube is not filled to capacity with blood; then the amount of anticoagulant is excessive for the blood sample.

Pyruvate kinase (PK)

The erythrocyte or red blood cell (RBC) enzyme pyruvate kinase (PK) takes part in the anaerobic metabolism of glucose (Embden-Meyerhof pathway). Abnormally low PK levels, revealed by RBC enzyme assay, are inherited as an autosomal recessive trait and may result in a nonspherocytic RBC membrane defect associated with congenital hemolytic anemia. Acquired PK deficiency is usually caused by drug ingestion or metabolic hepatic disease.

Although PK deficiency is uncommon, it is the most prevalent congenital nonspherocytic hemolytic anemia after glucose-6-phosphate dehydrogenase (G6PD) deficiency. PK assay confirms PK deficiency when RBC enzyme deficiency is the suspected cause of anemia.

Purpose
- To differentiate PK-deficient hemolytic anemia from other congenital hemolytic anemias (for example, G6PD deficiency), or from acquired hemolytic anemia
- To detect PK deficiency in asymptomatic, heterozygous inheritance

Patient preparation
Explain the purpose of the test. Inform the patient that restriction of food or fluids is not required before the test and that this test requires a blood sample.

Check patient history for recent blood transfusion, and note such information on the laboratory slip.

Procedure
Perform a venipuncture, and collect the sample in a 7-ml *lavender-top* tube. Completely fill the collection tube, and invert it gently several times to mix the sample and the anticoagulant.

Values
In a routine assay (ultraviolet), red cell PK levels range from 2 to 8.8 U/g of hemoglobin; in the low substrate assay, 0.9 to 3.9 U/g of hemoglobin.

Implications of results	Low red cell PK levels confirm PK deficiency, and allow differentiation between the PK-deficient hemolytic anemia and other inherited disorders.
Post-test care	If a hematoma develops at the venipuncture site, applying warm soaks eases discomfort.
Interfering factors	• Failure to use a collection tube with the proper anticoagulant or to adequately mix the sample and anticoagulant may interfere with accurate determination of test results.
	• Hemolysis caused by excessive agitation of the sample may affect test results.
	• Because PK levels in white blood cells (WBCs) remain normal in hemolytic anemia, the laboratory must remove WBCs from the sample to prevent inaccurate results.
	• Failure to notify the laboratory of recent blood transfusions may interfere with accurate determination of PK levels.

Q-R

Quinidine, serum

Quinidine is a broad spectrum cardiac antiarrhythmic drug used to treat atrial fibrillation or flutter, atrial or ventricular premature contractions, and ventricular tachycardias. Quinidine exerts its effects, at least in part, by decreasing myocardial excitability, automaticity, and conductivity that, in turn, prolongs the refractory period and the duration of the action potential. Quinidine tends to cause an overall decrease in myocardial contractility. Common adverse reactions include GI toxicity (nausea, vomiting, anorexia, diarrhea), cinchonism (blurred vision, tinnitus, tremor), and paradoxical increase in the frequency of cardiac arrhythmias.

Hepatic metabolism accounts for clearance of 60% to 80% of the drug, while 10% to 30% is excreted unchanged in the urine. The drug's average half-life is 5 to 8 hours, but may be prolonged, resulting in increased serum quinidine levels in patients with advanced hepatic or renal disease or congestive heart failure (CHF). Drugs that induce the hepatic microsomal P-450 enzyme (such as phenobarbital or phenytoin) can significantly shorten the half-life and thus decrease serum quinidine levels; hepatic microsomal enzyme inhibitors (cimetidine) can have the opposite effect. The therapeutic response and the frequency of adverse reactions are related to the serum quinidine level.

Quinidine is assayed by enzyme immunoassay, fluorescence polarization immunoassay, and, less frequently, by high-performance liquid chromatography.

Purpose
- To monitor quinidine dosage for optimal therapeutic effect and to minimize adverse effects, which occur more often at supratherapeutic serum levels
- To evaluate compliance
- To detect toxic drug levels, which can produce arrhythmia

Patient preparation
Explain the purpose of this test and that the test requires a blood sample.

Procedure | A venous blood sample is collected when the drug has reached a steady-state serum level. Attainment of steady-state serum quinidine levels occurs 3 to 4 days after initial therapy or adjustment of the total daily dosage. Unless toxicity is suspected, serum levels should not be measured before steady state because such testing yields results that are uninterpretable. The 1-ml serum sample should be collected just before the administration of the next dose (trough level).

Values | *Therapeutic range:* 2 to 7 mg/ml (6.2 to 21.7 µmol/L)
Toxic range: greater than 8 mg/ml (24.8 µmol/L).
The interpretation of test results depends on the assay method used. Newer methods are more specific and are generally associated with lower values for therapeutic range and toxicity. Using older methods, the following values are valid—
Therapeutic range: 2 to 6 mg/ml (6.2 to 18.5 µmol/L)
Toxic range: greater than 8 mg/ml (24.8 µmol/L).

Implications of results | Newer assay methods are more specific for quinidine and generally yield lower plasma level values. Using these new methods, a reduction of premature ventricular contractions has been reported with plasma quinidine levels less than 1 µg/ml.
Serum quinidine levels should be interpreted in light of the patient's current and past clinical status. High levels of quinidine are associated with cardiac conduction defects (up to a 50% widening of the QRS complex), ventricular tachycardia, ventricular flutter, frequent premature ventricular contractions, or complete atrioventricular block. Hearing disturbances such as tinnitus, visual problems, headache, vertigo, or confusion may also accompany high levels of quinidine.

Post-test care | If a hematoma develops at the venipuncture site, applying warm soaks eases discomfort.

Interfering factors |
- Incorrect timing of sample collection may cause misleading test results.
- Factors that may reduce quinidine levels include hypoalbuminemia and medications that activate hepatic enzyme activity or compete for albumin binding.

- Factors that may elevate quinidine levels include CHF and impaired renal or liver function. For example, decreased renal function in elderly patients commonly reduces renal excretion of quinidine.

Radioactive iodine uptake test

The radioactive iodine uptake (RAIU) test evaluates thyroid function by measuring the amount of orally ingested iodine 123 (^{123}I) or iodine 131 (^{131}I) that accumulates in the thyroid gland after 6 and 24 hours. An external single counting probe measures the radioactivity in the thyroid as a percentage of the original dose, thus indicating the ability of the gland to trap and retain iodine. When performed concurrently with radionuclide thyroid imaging, the RAIU test helps differentiate Graves' disease from hyperfunctioning toxic adenoma. Blood tests indicative of thyrotoxicosis combined with a low iodine uptake as determined by the RAIU test suggest thyroiditis. Indications for this test include abnormal results of chemical tests used to evaluate thyroid function.

Purpose
- To evaluate thyroid function
- To aid diagnosis of hyperthyroidism or hypothyroidism
- In combination with other tests, to help distinguish between primary and secondary thyroid disorders

Patient preparation
Explain to the patient that this test assesses thyroid function, and instruct the patient to fast from midnight before the test. Also explain that after receiving the radioactive iodine capsule or liquid, the patient will be scanned 6 and 24 hours later to determine the amount of radioactive substance present in the thyroid gland — an indicator of thyroid function. Assure the patient that the test is painless and that the small amount of radioactivity used for the procedure is harmless.

Check the patient's history for past or present iodine exposure, which may interfere with test results. If the patient has previously undergone radiologic tests using contrast media or nuclear medicine procedures, or is currently receiving iodine preparations or thyroid medications, note this on the request slip.

Because the amount of iodine used in this test is similar to the amount obtained through dietary intake, a history of iodine hypersensitivity is not considered a contraindication to the test.

Procedure

At 6 and 24 hours after administration of an oral dose of radioactive iodine, the patient's thyroid is scanned by placing the anterior portion of his neck in front of an external single counting probe. The amount of radioactivity that the probe detects is compared with the amount in the original dose to determine the percentage of radioactive iodine retained by the thyroid.

Precautions

Radioactive iodine uptake testing is contraindicated during pregnancy and lactation because of iodine uptake by the fetus or nursing child.

Findings

After 6 hours, 3% to 16% of the radioactive iodine should have accumulated in the thyroid; after 24 hours, 8% to 29%. The remaining radioactive iodine is excreted in the urine.

Local variations in the normal range of iodine uptake may occur because of regional differences in dietary iodine intake and procedural differences among individual laboratories.

Implications of results

Below-normal percentages of iodine uptake may indicate hypothyroidism, subacute thyroiditis, or iodine overload. Above-normal percentages may indicate hyperthyroidism, early Hashimoto's thyroiditis, hypoalbuminemia, lithium ingestion, or iodine-deficient goiter. In hyperthyroidism, the rate of turnover may be so rapid that the 24-hour measurement yields false-normal results.

Post-test care

The patient may resume a light diet 2 hours after taking the oral dose of ^{123}I or ^{131}I and a normal diet after the study is complete.

Interfering factors

• Renal failure, diuresis, severe diarrhea, X-ray contrast media studies, ingestion of iodine preparations (including iodized salt, cough syrups, and some multivitamins) or of other drugs (thyroid hormones, thyroid hormone antagonists, salicylates, penicillin, antihistamines, anticoagulants, corticosteroids, and phenylbutazone) can decrease iodine uptake, thereby interfering with accurate determination of iodine uptake test results.

- Iodine-deficient diet or ingestion of phenothiazines can increase iodine uptake, interfering with accurate determination of test results.

Radioallergosorbent test (RAST)

The radioallergosorbent test (RAST) measures IgE antibodies in serum by radioimmunoassay and helps determine specific allergens to which an individual might be generating an immune response. Careful selection of specific allergens, based on the patient's clinical history, is thus crucial for effective testing. Results of assays for specific immunoglobulin E (IgE) antibodies correlate with in vivo tests for allergy, including skin tests.

Although intradermal skin testing is the preferred means for diagnosing IgE-mediated hypersensitivity, RAST may be more useful when a skin disorder makes accurate reading of skin tests difficult, when a patient requires continual antihistamine therapy, or when skin tests are negative but the patient's clinical history supports IgE-mediated hypersensitivity.

In RAST, a sample of the patient's serum is exposed to a panel of specific antigens selected according to the patient's history. The IgE in the patient's serum forms a complex with those antigens to which it is sensitive. Radiolabeled anti-IgE antibody is then added, and this binds to the IgE-antigen complexes. After centrifugation, the amount of radioactivity in the particulate material is directly proportional to the amount of IgE antibodies present. Test results are compared with control values and represent the patient's reactivity to a specific allergen.

Purpose
- To identify allergens to which the patient has an immediate (IgE-mediated) hypersensitivity, for example, in patients with asthma, dermatitis, or allergic rhinitis; or in patients with systemic reactions to chemicals, drugs, or insect venom
- To monitor response to desensitization therapy

Patient preparation
Explain to the patient that this test may detect the cause of allergy or that it monitors the effectiveness of treatment. Inform the patient that the test re-

quires a blood sample. If the patient is scheduled for a radioactive scan, be sure the sample is collected before the scan.

Procedure

Perform a venipuncture, and collect the sample in a 7-ml *red-top* tube. Generally, 1 ml of serum is sufficient for five allergen assays. Be sure to note on the laboratory slip the specific allergens to be tested.

Findings

RAST results are interpreted in relationship to a control or reference serum that differs among laboratories.

Implications of results

Elevated serum IgE levels suggest hypersensitivity to the specific allergen or allergens used.

Post-test care

If a hematoma develops at the venipuncture site, applying warm soaks eases discomfort.

Interfering factor

Radioactive scan within 1 week before sample collection may alter test results.

Raji cell assay

This assay is performed to detect the presence of circulating immune complexes that contain immunoglobulin and complement and to study the Raji lymphoblastoid cell line. Identifying these cells, which have complement receptors, is helpful in evaluating autoimmune disease.

Purpose

• To detect circulating immune complexes
• To aid the study of autoimmune disease

Patient preparation

Explain the purpose of this test, and inform the patient that the test requires a blood sample.

Procedure

Obtain a venous blood sample and send it to the laboratory promptly for assay.

Values

Normal values range from 0 to 12 µg antihemophilic globulin (AHG) Eq/ml. 12 to 25 µg AHG Eq/ml is considered borderline.

Implications of results

A positive Raji cell assay can detect immune complexes including those found in viral, microbial, and parasitic infections, metastasis, autoimmune disorders, and drug reactions. This test may also detect immune complexes associated with celiac disease, cirrhosis, Crohn's disease, cryoglobulinemia, dermatitis herpetiformis, sickle cell anemia, and ulcerative colitis.

Post-test care
If a hematoma develops at the venipuncture site, applying warm soaks eases discomfort.

Interfering factor
Hemolysis of the sample can impair correct interpretation of results.

Renal biopsy, percutaneous

Percutaneous renal biopsy is needle excision of a core of kidney tissue to obtain a specimen for histologic examination using light, electron, and immunofluorescent microscopy. Such examination provides valuable information about glomerular and tubular function. Acute and chronic glomerulonephritis, pyelonephritis, renal vein thrombosis, amyloid infiltration, and systemic lupus erythematosus produce characteristic histologic changes in the kidneys. Complications of percutaneous biopsy may include bleeding, hematoma, arteriovenous fistula, and infection. Noninvasive procedures, especially renal ultrasonography and computed tomography scan, have largely replaced percutaneous renal biopsy in many hospitals.

Purpose
• To aid diagnosis of renal parenchymal disease
• To monitor progression of renal disease and to assess the effectiveness of treatment

Patient preparation
Explain that this test helps diagnose kidney disorders, and instruct the patient to restrict food and fluids for 8 hours before the test.

Tell the patient that blood and urine specimens are collected and tested before the biopsy, and that other tests, such as intravenous pyelography, ultrasonography, or an erect film of the abdomen, may also be performed to help determine the biopsy site.

Make sure the patient or an appropriate family member has signed a consent form. Check the patient's history for hemorrhagic tendencies and hypersensitivity to the local anesthetic. Approximately 30 minutes to 1 hour before the biopsy the patient may receive a mild sedative to promote relaxation and ease. Inform the patient that a local anesthetic will be given but may cause a pinching pain when the needle is inserted through the back into the kidney. Check vital signs, and tell the patient to void just before the test.

Procedure　The patient is placed in a prone position on a firm surface, with a sandbag beneath his abdomen. The patient is asked to take a deep breath while his kidney is being palpated. A 7″ (17.8 cm) 20G needle is used to inject the local anesthetic into the skin at the biopsy site. Instruct the patient to hold his breath and remain immobile while the needle is inserted just below the angle formed by the intersection of the lowest palpable rib and the lateral border of the sacrospinal muscle. The needle is directed through the back muscles, the deep lumbar fascia, the perinephric fat, and the kidney capsule. After the needle is inserted, tell the patient to take several deep breaths. If the needle swings smoothly during deep breathing, it has penetrated the kidney capsule. After the penetration depth is marked on the needle shaft, instruct the patient to hold his breath and remain as still as possible while the needle is withdrawn, injecting the local anesthetic into the back tissues.

After a small incision is made in the anesthetized skin, instruct the patient to hold his breath and remain immobile while a Vim-Silverman needle with stylet is inserted through the incision, down the tract of the infiltrating needle, to the measured depth. Tell the patient to breathe deeply. If the characteristic needle swing occurs, instruct the patient to hold his breath and remain still while the tissue specimen is obtained. After the tissue is examined immediately under a hand lens to ensure that the specimen contains tissue from both cortex and medulla, the tissue is placed on a saline-soaked gauze pad and placed in a properly labeled container. If an adequate tissue specimen has not been obtained, the procedure is repeated immediately. After an adequate specimen is secured, apply pressure to the biopsy site for 3 to 5 minutes to stop superficial bleeding. Then, apply a pressure dressing.

Send the tissue specimen to the laboratory immediately.

Precautions　Percutaneous renal biopsy is contraindicated in a patient with renal tumors, severe bleeding disorder, markedly reduced plasma or blood volume, severe hypertension, hydronephrosis, perinephric abscess, advanced renal failure with uremia, or only one kidney.

Findings
Normally, a section of kidney tissue shows Bowman's capsule (the area between two layers of flat epithelial cells), the glomerular tuft, and the capillary lumen. The tubule sections differ depending on the area of tubule involved. The proximal tubule is one layer of columnar epithelial cells with microvilli that form a brush border. The descending Henle's loop has flat epithelial cells, unlike the ascending, distal convoluted and collecting tubules, which are lined with columnar epithelial cells.

Implications of results
Histologic examination of renal tissue can reveal malignant disease or renal disease. Malignant tumors include Wilms' tumor, usually present in early childhood, and renal cell carcinoma, most prevalent in persons over age 40. Diseases indicated by characteristic histologic changes include disseminated lupus erythematosus, amyloid infiltration, acute and chronic glomerulonephritis, renal vein thrombosis, and pyelonephritis.

Post-test care
• The patient should lie flat without moving for at least 12 hours after the test to prevent bleeding. Check vital signs for significant changes every 15 minutes for 4 hours, then every 30 minutes for 4 hours, then every hour for 4 hours, and finally every 4 hours.
• Examine all urine for blood; small amounts may be present after biopsy but should disappear within 8 hours. Occasionally, hematocrit may be monitored after the procedure, to screen for internal bleeding.
• Encourage fluid intake to initiate mild diuresis, which minimizes colic and obstruction from blood clotting within the renal pelvis.
• The patient may resume a normal diet.

Interfering factor
Failure to obtain an adequate tissue specimen, to store the specimen properly, or to send the specimen to the laboratory immediately may interfere with accurate determination of test results.

Renin activity, plasma

Renin secretion is the first stage of the renin-angiotensin-aldosterone cycle that controls the body's sodium-potassium balance, fluid volume, and blood pressure. Renin is an enzyme released by the juxtaglomerular cells of the kidneys in response to decreased fluid volume, serum sodium, and renal perfusion pressure. It catalyzes the conversion of angiotensinogen, an alpha$_2$-globulin plasma protein, to angiotensin I, which in turn is converted into angiotensin II by hydrolysis. Angiotensin II, a vasoconstrictor, stimulates release of aldosterone. When present in excessive amounts, angiotensin II causes renal hypertension.

The plasma renin activity (PRA) test is a screening procedure for patients with essential, renal, or renovascular hypertension. When supplemented by other special tests, the PRA can help establish the cause of hypertension. For instance, sampling blood obtained from both renal veins by renal vein catheterization and analyzing the renal venous renin ratio can identify renovascular disorders. Indexing renin levels against urinary sodium excretion can help identify primary aldosteronism. A sodium-depleted plasma renin test can then confirm this.

Some experts believe that essential hypertension with low, normal, and high renin levels should be treated differently, and the PRA test can categorize the disease for appropriate therapy.

PRA is measured by radioimmunoassay of a peripheral or renal blood sample, and results are expressed as nanograms of angiotensin I formation per milliliter of plasma per hour of incubation. Patient preparation is crucial and may take up to 1 month.

Purpose
- To assess renin activity in patients with hypertension of unknown cause
- To help plan the best treatment for essential hypertension
- To help identify hypertension linked to unilateral (sometimes bilateral) renovascular disease
- To help identify renal artery stenosis as the cause of hypertension
- To help identify primary aldosteronism (Conn's syndrome) resulting from aldosterone-secreting adrenal adenoma
- To confirm primary and secondary aldosteronism (sodium-depleted plasma renin test)

Patient
preparation

Explain to the patient that this test helps determine the cause of hypertension. The patient must maintain a normal-sodium diet (3 g/day) and must discontinue use of diuretics, antihypertensives, vasodilators, oral contraceptives, and licorice for 2 to 4 weeks before the test. For the sodium-depleted renin test, the patient will receive a diuretic and limit sodium intake for 3 days before the test.

Because posture influences renin secretion, the patient must maintain the required position (recumbent or upright) for 2 hours before the test.

Before renal catheterization, make sure that the patient or responsible family member has signed an informed consent form. Describe the procedure and encourage the patient to ask questions and express concerns. Ask about possible allergies to radiographic dyes.

Procedure

The procedure varies according to the method for obtaining the sample and factors to be controlled.

Peripheral vein sample, normal salt or salt-depleted: Perform a venipuncture, and collect the sample in a 7-ml *lavender-top* tube.

Because renin is very unstable, the sample must be drawn into a chilled syringe and collection tube, placed on ice, and sent to the laboratory immediately. Completely fill the collection tube, and invert it gently several times to mix the sample and the anticoagulant.

Renal vein catheterization: After a site is prepared for femoral vein catheterization, a catheter is advanced to the kidneys, through the femoral vein, under fluoroscopic control. Blood samples are obtained from both renal veins and the vena cava. The samples are placed in chilled *lavender-top* tubes labeled to identify the collection sites. The tubes should be inverted gently several times (to allow mixing with the anticoagulant), placed on ice, and sent to the laboratory immediately.

Values

Levels of plasma renin activity and of aldosterone decrease with advancing age.

Peripheral vein, sodium-depleted, upright: For adults ages 20 to 39, the range is from 2.9 to 24 ng/ml/hour (0.8 to 6.5 ng/L/second); mean, 10.8 ng/ml/hour (3.0 ng/L/second). For adults age 40 and over, the range is from 2.9 to 10.8 ng/ml/hour (0.8 to 3.0 ng/L/second); mean, 5.9 ng/ml/hour (1.8 ng/L/second).

Peripheral vein, normal sodium, upright: For adults ages 20 to 39, the range is from 1 to 4.3 ng/ml/hour (0.3 to 1.2 ng/L/second); mean, 1.9 ng/ml/hour (0.5 ng/L/second). For adults age 40 and over, the range is from 1 to 3 ng/ml/hour (0.3 to 0.8 ng/L/second); mean, 1.5 ng/ml/hour (0.4 ng/L/second).

Renal vein assay: The renal venous renin ratio (the renin level in the renal vein compared to the level in the inferior vena cava) is less than 1.5:1.

Implications of results

Elevated renin levels may occur in essential hypertension (uncommon), malignant and renovascular hypertension, cirrhosis, hypokalemia, hypovolemia caused by hemorrhage, renin-producing renal tumors (Bartter's syndrome), and adrenal hypofunction (Addison's disease). High renin levels may also be found in chronic renal failure with parenchymal disease, end-stage renal disease, and transplant rejection.

Decreased renin levels may indicate hypervolemia caused by a high-sodium diet, salt-retaining steroids, primary aldosteronism, Cushing's syndrome, licorice ingestion syndrome, or essential hypertension with low renin levels.

High serum and urine aldosterone levels, with low plasma renin activity, help identify primary aldosteronism; in the sodium-depleted renin test, low plasma renin confirms primary aldosteronism and differentiates it from secondary aldosteronism (characterized by increased renin).

Post-test care

• If a hematoma develops at the peripheral venipuncture site, applying warm soaks eases discomfort.

• The patient may resume diet and medications restricted before the test.

➤ *Clinical alert:* After renal vein catheterization, apply pressure to the catheterization site for 10 to 20 minutes to prevent extravasation. The patient should be restricted to bed rest for 8 hours after this procedure. Monitor vital signs, and check the catheterization site for bleeding or hematoma every half hour for 2 hours, then every hour for 4 hours. Check distal pulses for signs of thrombus formation and arterial occlusion (cyanosis, loss of pulse, coolness of skin).

Interfering factors

- Failure to use the proper anticoagulant in the collection tube, to completely fill it, or to adequately mix the sample and the anticoagulant may influence renin levels. (EDTA helps preserve angiotensin I; heparin does not.)
- Failure to chill the collection tube and syringe, or failure to chill and send the sample to the laboratory immediately promotes breakdown of renin.
- Renin levels may be affected by failure to observe diet restrictions and to maintain required patient positioning for at least 2 hours before the test.
- Levels are increased by salt intake, diuretic therapy, oral contraceptives, severe blood loss, antihypertensive agents, vasodilators, licorice ingestion, and pregnancy.
- Salt-retaining steroid therapy and antidiuretic therapy decrease renin levels.

Respiratory syncytial virus (RSV) antibodies, serum

Respiratory syncytial virus (RSV), a member of the paramyxovirus group, is the major viral cause of severe lower respiratory tract disease in infants but may cause infections in persons of any age. RSV infections are most common and produce the most severe disease during the first 6 months of life, and they particularly afflict patients confined to nursing homes. Initial infection involves viral replication in epithelial cells of the upper respiratory tract but, in younger children especially, the infection spreads to the bronchi, bronchioli, and even to the parenchyma of the lungs.

Immunoglobulin G (IgG) and immunoglobulin M (IgM) class antibodies can be easily quantified using the indirect immunofluorescence test. Specific results for IgM are obtained only after separation of this class antibody from IgG. Prevalence of IgG antibodies to RSV is extremely high (greater than 95%), especially in adults.

Purpose

To diagnose infections caused by RSV

Patient preparation

Explain the purpose of this test, and inform the patient that the test requires a blood sample.

Procedure
: Perform a venipuncture to collect 5 ml of sterile blood in a *red-top* tube. Allow the blood to clot for at least 1 hour at room temperature. Handle the sample gently to prevent hemolysis. Transfer the serum to a sterile tube or vial and send it to the laboratory. If transfer must be delayed, store the serum at 39.2° F (4° C) for 1 to 2 days, or for longer periods, at –4° F (–20° C) to avoid microbial contamination.

Values
: Sera from patients who have never been infected with RSV will have no detectable antibodies to the virus (less than 1:5). In infants, serologic diagnosis of RSV infections is difficult because of the presence of maternal IgG antibodies; thus in infants, the presence of IgM antibodies is most significant.

Implications of results
: The diagnosis of RSV infection can be ruled out in patients whose serum samples have no detectable antibodies to the virus. The qualitative presence of IgM or a four-fold or greater increase in IgG antibodies indicates active RSV infection.

Post-test care
: If a hematoma develops at the venipuncture site, applying warm soaks eases discomfort.

Interfering factor
: Hemolysis of the sample may interfere with accurate determination of test results.

Reticulocyte count

Reticulocytes are nonnucleated, immature red blood cells (RBCs) that remain in the peripheral blood for 24 to 48 hours before becoming mature RBCs. Reticulocytes are generally larger than mature RBCs, and contain ribosomes, a centriole, particles of Golgi vesicles, and mitochondria. Because reticulocytes retain remnants of normoblasts (their precursors), they absorb supravital stains, such as new methylene blue or brilliant cresyl blue. They sometimes can be distinguished from other blood cells in a peripheral blood smear as metachromatic cells.

In this test, reticulocytes in a whole blood sample are counted and expressed as a percentage of the total RBC count. The reticulocyte count is useful in the evaluation of anemia and is an index of effective erythropoiesis and bone marrow response to anemia. Because the manual method for counting reticulocytes is imprecise, values may be reported as being below normal, normal, or above normal.

Purpose
- To aid in distinguishing between hypoproliferative and hyperproliferative anemias
- To help assess blood loss, bone marrow response to anemia, and therapy for anemia

Patient preparation

Tell the patient this test helps detect anemia or monitors its treatment. Inform the patient that the test requires a blood sample. If the patient is an infant or child, explain to the parents (and to the child who is old enough to understand) that a small amount of blood will be drawn from a finger or earlobe.

Withhold antimalarials, antipyretics, azathioprine, chloramphenicol, corticotropin, dactinomycin, furazolidone (from infants), levodopa, methotrexate, phenacetin, and sulfonamides, as appropriate. If such medications must be continued, note this on the laboratory slip.

Procedure

Perform a venipuncture, and collect the sample in a 7-ml *lavender-top* tube. Completely fill the collection tube and invert it gently several times to mix the sample and the anticoagulant. Handle the sample gently to prevent hemolysis.

Values

Reticulocytes comprise 0.5% to 2% of the total RBC count. In infants, the percentage is normally higher, ranging from 3.2% at birth to 0.7% at age 12 weeks.

Implications of results

A low reticulocyte count indicates hypoproliferative bone marrow (hypoplastic anemia) or ineffective erythropoiesis (pernicious anemia). A high reticulocyte count indicates a bone marrow response to anemia caused by hemolysis or blood loss. The reticulocyte count rises after effective therapy for iron deficiency anemia or pernicious anemia.

Post-test care
- If a hematoma develops at the venipuncture site, applying warm soaks eases discomfort.
- The patient may resume withheld medications.
- When monitoring a patient with an abnormal reticulocyte count, look for trends in repeated tests or gross changes in the numerical value.

Interfering
factors

- False-negative test results can be caused by aza-thioprine, chloramphenicol, dactinomycin, and methotrexate. False-positive test results can be caused by antimalarials, antipyretics, furazoli-done (in infants), and levodopa. Sulfonamides can cause false-negative or false-positive results.
- Failure to use the proper anticoagulant in the col-lection tube or to adequately mix the sample and anticoagulant may present accurate determina-tion of the reticulocyte count.
- Prolonged tourniquet constriction may alter test results.
- Hemolysis caused by excessive agitation of the sample may affect test results.

Rheumatoid factor (RF)

The rheumatoid factor (RF) test is the most useful immunologic test for confirming rheumatoid ar-thritis (RA). In this disease, "renegade" immuno-globulin G (IgG) or immunoglobulin M (IgM) anti-bodies react with IgG to produce immune complexes, complement activation, and tissue de-struction. How these molecules become antigenic is still unknown, but they may be altered by aggre-gating with viruses or other antigens. These im-mune complexes can migrate from the synovial flu-id to other areas of the body, causing vasculitis, subcutaneous nodules, or lymphadenopathy. The IgG or IgM molecules that react with altered IgG are called rheumatoid factors. Agglutination and flocculation tests (the sheep cell agglutination test and the latex fixation test) can detect RF. In the sheep cell test, rabbit IgG adsorbed onto sheep red blood cells (RBCs) is mixed with the patient's se-rum in serial dilutions; in the latex fixation test, hu-man IgG adsorbed onto latex particles is mixed with the patient's serum. Visible agglutination indi-cates the presence of RF. The last tube dilution to show visible agglutination is used as the titer. The sheep cell agglutination test is the better diagnostic method for confirming RA; the latex fixation test is the better screening method. RF can also be mea-sured by enzyme-linked immunoabsorbent assay and nephelometry.

Purpose

To confirm RA, especially when clinical diagnosis is doubtful

Patient preparation	Explain that this test helps confirm RA and that the test requires a blood sample.

Procedure	Perform a venipuncture, and collect the sample in a 7-ml *red-top* tube.

Findings	Normal RF titer is less than 1:20; normal rheumatoid screening test is nonreactive.

Implications of results	Positive RF titers are found in 80% of patients with RA. Titers greater than 1:80 tend to be associated with RA (although high titers can be present in other disorders); titers between 1:20 and 1:80 are difficult to interpret, because they occur in many other diseases, such as systemic lupus erythematosus, scleroderma, polymyositis, tuberculosis, infectious mononucleosis, Hansen's disease, syphilis, sarcoidosis, chronic hepatic disease, subacute bacterial endocarditis, and chronic pulmonary interstitial fibrosis. In addition, 5% of the general population, including up to 25% of elderly people, have positive RF titers.

Conversely, a negative RF titer doesn't rule out RA; 20% to 25% of patients with RA lack reactive RF titers, and RF itself isn't reactive until 6 months after onset of active disease. Repeating the test is sometimes useful. However, correlation between RF and RA is inconclusive, and positive diagnosis always requires correlation with clinical status.

Post-test care	• Because a patient with RA may be immunologically compromised from the disease or from corticosteroid therapy, keep the venipuncture site covered with a clean, dry bandage for 24 hours. Check regularly for signs of infection. • If a hematoma develops at the venipuncture site, applying warm soaks eases discomfort.

Interfering factors	• Inadequately activated complement may cause false-positive results. • Serum with high lipid or cryoglobulin levels may cause false-positive test results and requires repetition of the test after restriction of fat intake. • Serum with high IgG levels may cause false-negative results through competition with IgG on the surface of latex particles or sheep RBCs used as substrate.

Rh typing

The Rh system classifies blood by the presence or absence of the $Rh_o(D)$ antigen on the surface of red blood cells (RBCs). In this test, a patient's RBCs are tested with serum containing anti-$Rh_o(D)$ antibodies and are observed for agglutination. If agglutination occurs, the $Rh_o(D)$ antigen is present, and the patient's blood is type Rh-positive; if agglutination does not occur, the antigen is absent, and the patient's blood is type Rh-negative. Occasionally, the D antigen is weakly expressed on RBCs, requiring additional techniques, such as antiglobulin phase testing, to detect agglutination. This is known as the D^u variant.

Rh typing is performed routinely on prospective blood donors and on blood recipients before transfusion. Rh-compatible blood should be transfused whenever possible to prevent Rh sensitization. Persons with D^u variants are considered Rh-positive donors. Even though the D antigen is weakly expressed on these cells, it is still capable of inducing sensitization to the D antigen. D^u variant recipients may receive either Rh-positive or Rh-negative blood.

Purpose
- To establish blood type according to the Rh system
- To help determine the compatibility of donor blood before transfusion
- To determine if the pregnant patient will need a $Rh_o(D)$ immune globulin injection

Patient preparation
Explain that this test determines or verifies blood group — an important step in ensuring safe transfusion. Inform the patient that the test requires a blood sample.

Check the patient's history for recent administration of dextran, I.V. contrast media, or drugs that may alter results.

Procedure
Identify the patient by asking him his name and examining his wristband to assure that both patient name and identifying number are correct. Next, perform a venipuncture, and collect the sample in a 10- to 15-ml *lavender-top* or *red-top* tube.

The sample must be properly labeled, according to your laboratory's policy and Food and Drug Administration regulations. Mislabeled samples cannot be accepted for testing and must be discarded.

Implications of Rh$_o$(D) typing test results

Classified as Rh$_o$(D)-positive, Rh$_o$(D)-negative, or Rh(D^u)-positive, donor blood may be transfused only if it's compatible with the recipient's blood, as follows.

Rh$_o$(D) recipient types	Compatible Rh$_o$(D) donor types	Incompatible Rh$_o$(D) donor types
Rh$_o$(D)-positive	Rh$_o$(D)-positive or Rh$_o$(D)-negative	None
Rho$_o$(D)-negative	Rh$_o$(D)-negative	Rh$_o$(D)-positive
Rh(D^u)-positive	Rh(D^u)-positive, Rh$_o$(D)-negative, or Rh$_o$(D)-positive	None

Findings and implications of results

Blood is classified as Rh-positive, Rh-negative, or Rh$_o$-D^u-positive (see *Implications of Rh$_o$(D) typing test results*).

If an Rh-negative woman delivers an Rh-positive infant or aborts a fetus whose Rh-type is unknown, she should receive a Rh$_o$(D) immune globulin injection within 72 hours. This measure will prevent Rh sensitization and subsequent hemolytic disease of the newborn in future births.

Post-test care

- If a hematoma develops at the venipuncture site, applying warm soaks eases discomfort.
- Encourage the patient to carry a blood-group identification card for protection in an emergency. Most laboratories provide such a card.

Interfering factors

- Recent administration of dextran or I.V. contrast media may result in cellular aggregation resembling antibody-mediated agglutination.
- If the patient has received blood in the past 3 months, circulating donor cells may be present and can cause a mixed field typing reaction if, for example, an Rh-positive patient received an emergency transfusion of Rh-negative blood. To prevent such reactions, provide the Blood Bank with the patient's prior transfusion history.
- Methyldopa, cephalosporins, or levodopa may cause a positive direct antiglobulin test (Coombs' test). This will result in a false-positive reaction

during testing for the D^u variant. Special saline testing reagents that do not require antiglobulin phase testing are commercially available; inquire if your hospital's supply department stocks them.
- RBCs from patients with autoimmune hemolytic anemia or multiple myeloma may spontaneously agglutinate when tested with protein-rich typing reagents.

Rotavirus antigen, feces

Rotaviruses are the most frequent cause of infectious diarrhea in infants and young children; these organisms are associated with approximately 50% of pediatric hospitalizations for gastroenteritis. Clinical features of rotavirus infection include diarrhea, vomiting, fever, and abdominal pain. This infection is most prevalent in children (ages 3 months to 2 years) during the winter months. In contrast to the severe clinical illness it causes in hospitalized infants, this infection may cause only mild symptoms in adults.

Human rotaviruses do not replicate efficiently in the usual laboratory cell cultures. Therefore, detection of the typical virus particles in stool specimens by electron microscopy has been replaced by sensitive, specific enzyme immunoassays that can provide results within minutes or a few hours (depending on the assay) after the specimen is received in the laboratory.

Purpose
To obtain a laboratory diagnosis of rotavirus gastroenteritis

Patient preparation
Explain the purpose of this test and that the test requires a stool specimen. The specimens should be collected during the acute stages of clinical infection to ensure detection of the viral antigens by enzyme immunoassay.

Procedure
A stool specimen (1 g in a screw-capped tube or vial) is preferable for the detection of rotaviruses. If a microbiological transport swab is used, it must be heavily stained with feces to be diagnostically productive for rotavirus.

Precautions
- Do not use collection containers containing preservatives, transport media, metal ions, deter-

gents, and serum. All will interfere with the immunoassay.
- Store stool specimens for up to 24 hour at 35.6° F to 46.4° F (2° C to 8° C). If a longer period of storage or shipment is necessary, freeze specimens at –4° F (–20° C) or colder. Repeated freezing and thawing will cause the specimen to deteriorate and yield misleading results. Do not store the specimen in a self-defrosting freezer.

Findings   The detection of rotavirus by enzyme immunoassay is laboratory evidence of current infection with the organism.

Implications of results   Rotavirus can infect all age groups, and the severity of disease is generally greater in young children than in adults.

Rotavirus infections are easily transmitted in group settings such as nurseries for children, day-care centers, and nursing homes. Transmission is presumed to occur from person-to-person by the fecal-oral route. Nosocomial spread of this viral infection can have significant medical and economic effects in a hospital setting.

Post-test care   Provide fluid and electrolyte replacements to avoid dehydration caused by vomiting and diarrhea.

Interfering factor   Collecting the specimen in containers with preservatives, transport media, metal ions, detergents, or serum will interfere with detection of the virus.

Rubella antibodies
Hemagglutin inhibition (HI) test

Although rubella (German measles) is generally a mild viral infection in children and young adults, it can produce severe infection in the fetus, resulting in spontaneous abortion, stillbirth, or congenital rubella syndrome.

Because rubella infection normally induces immunoglobulin G (IgG) and immunoglobulin M (IgM) antibody production, measuring rubella antibodies can determine present infection and immunity resulting from past infection. The hemagglutination inhibition (HI) test, the most commonly used serologic test for rubella antibodies, is indicated to diagnose rubella in pregnant patients and others possibly exposed to the infection, and to determine susceptibility to it in children and women of childbearing age. (Selective protein index assay, passive hemagglutination, latex agglutination, and complement fixation tests also can diagnose rubella.)

In this test, serial dilutions of the patient's serum are mixed with rubella virus antigen and goose erythrocytes and then incubated. If rubella antibodies are present, they inhibit hemagglutination. The antibody titer is the highest dilution of serum that totally inhibits hemagglutination. The test for rubella requires two serum samples: one 3 days after onset of rash (acute titer); another, 2 to 3 weeks later (convalescent titer). The test for immunity requires one sample.

Purpose

- To diagnose rubella infection, especially congenital infection
- To determine susceptibility to rubella in children and in women of childbearing age

Patient preparation

Explain that this test diagnoses or evaluates susceptibility to German measles. Inform the patient that she needn't restrict food or fluids before the test and the that this test requires a blood sample (if a current infection is suspected, a second blood sample will be needed in 2 to 3 weeks to identify a rise in the titer).

Procedure

Perform a venipuncture, and collect the sample in a 7-ml *red-top* tube. Handle the sample gently to prevent hemolysis.

Values

A titer less than 1:8 or 1:10 (depending on the test) indicates susceptibility to rubella; a titer greater than 1:10, adequate protection against rubella.

Implications of results

The HI antibodies normally appear 2 to 4 days after the onset of the rash, peak in 2 to 3 weeks, then slowly decline but remain detectable for life. In rubella infection, acute serum titers range from 1:8 to 1:16; convalescent serum titers, from 1:64 to 1:1,024 (or possibly higher). A fourfold rise or greater from the acute to the convalescent titer indicates a recent rubella infection.

Because maternal antibodies cross the placenta and persist in the infant's serum for up to 6 months, congenital rubella can be detected only after this period. An antibody titer greater than 1:8 in an infant age 6 months or older who hasn't been exposed to rubella postnatally confirms congenital rubella.

Post-test care
- If a hematoma develops at the venipuncture site, applying warm soaks eases discomfort.
- When appropriate, instruct the patient to return for an additional blood test.
- If a woman of childbearing age is found susceptible to rubella (titer of 1:8 or less), explain that vaccination can prevent rubella, and that she must wait at least 3 months after the vaccination before becoming pregnant, or risk permanent damage or death to the fetus.
- If a pregnant patient is found susceptible to rubella, instruct her to return for follow-up rubella antibody tests to detect possible subsequent infection.
- If the test confirms rubella in a pregnant patient, provide emotional support. As needed, refer her for appropriate counseling.

Interfering factor
Hemolysis caused by excessive agitation of the sample may interfere with accurate determination of test results.

S

Salicylates, serum

This quantitative test uses a ferric chloride color reaction to measure serum salicylate levels. In unconscious or uncooperative patients, such testing may follow detection of salicylates in a qualitative urine screening.

Absorbed rapidly from the upper GI tract, acetylsalicylic acid in therapeutic doses produces peak blood levels in 30 to 45 minutes, and it is quickly hydrolyzed to salicylic acid and bound to albumin. However, with toxic doses, serum salicylate levels may rise for 6 to 10 hours after ingestion; thus, serial sampling is recommended for 24 hours following overdose to accurately determine toxicity.

Purpose
- To confirm toxicity suspected from history or onset of symptoms
- To monitor therapeutic levels of serum salicylate, especially in the treatment of patients with rheumatoid arthritis, juvenile rheumatoid arthritis, or osteoarthritis

Patient preparation

Explain the purpose of this test, and inform the patient that the test requires a blood sample.

If the test is being performed for medicolegal purposes, make sure that the patient or a responsible family member has signed a consent form. Check the patient's medication history for recent use of salicylates (aspirin, salicylic acid, sodium salicylate). *Note:* Many over-the-counter combinations, especially cold remedies, contain salicylates. Record the amount of salicylate ingested.

Procedure

Perform a venipuncture, and collect the sample in a 7-ml *red-top* tube. Handle the sample gently to prevent hemolysis, and send it to the laboratory immediately or refrigerate it.

For a medicolegal test, observe the appropriate precautions.

Values

The usual total serum salicylate concentration associated with analgesia and antipyresis is 30 to 100 µg/ml (0.2 to 0.7 mmol/L). The usual total serum salicylate concentration required for anti-inflammatory effect is 150 to 300 µg/ml (1.1 to 2.2 mmol/L); however for treatment of rheumatic fever, many clinicians believe a total serum salicylate concentration of 250 to 350 µg/ml (1.8 to 2.5 mmol/L) is associated with optimum therapeutic effect. Most patients experience toxicity when the total serum salicylate concentration exceeds 300 µg/ml (2.2 mmol/L).

Implications of
results

Therapeutic dosage is adjusted based on the reported serum level. Treatment of toxicity is adjusted based on the level of toxicity noted, clinical status, and time-dependent nomogram.

Post-test care

If a hematoma develops at the venipuncture site, applying warm soaks eases discomfort.

Interfering
factors

• Hemolysis caused by excessive agitation of the sample can cause false-high serum salicylate levels.
• Antacids and food lower serum salicylate levels; ammonium chloride and other urine acidifiers elevate levels.

Sedatives and hypnotics

Depending on the drug being measured, this test determines the serum, plasma, or whole blood level of a sedative or hypnotic by colorimetry, photometry, or spectrophotometry. These central nervous system (CNS) depressants (including benzodiazepines, chloral derivatives, and glutethimide) are used to treat anxiety, alcohol withdrawal symptoms, and sleep disorders, and to prepare patients for anesthesia.

Sedatives and hypnotics, alone or in combination with other drugs or alcohol, are commonly used in suicide attempts. As drugs of abuse, they may cause psychological dependence; after prolonged or high-dose usage, they produce physical dependence. Generally absorbed rapidly after oral administration, sedatives and hypnotics are metabolized in the liver and excreted in urine and feces.

Purpose

To check for toxicity suspected from history or after onset of such symptoms of CNS depression as confusion, depression, diminished reflexes, hypotension, somnolence, or coma

Patient
preparation

Explain that this test determines the level of seda-tives or hypnotics in the blood and that the test re-quires a blood sample.

If the test is being performed for medicolegal purposes, make sure that the patient or a responsi-ble family member has signed a consent form. Check the patient's recent medication history for names and dosage schedules of all drugs ingested.

Procedure

Perform a venipuncture, and collect the sample in a 7-ml *red-top* tube. Send the sample to the laborato-ry immediately, or refrigerate it.

For a medicolegal test, observe appropriate pre-cautions.

Values

Therapeutic and toxic levels depend on the specific drug, as shown:

Drug	Therapeutic (μg/ml)	Toxic (μg/ml)
Chlordiazepoxide	5 to 10	$\geq$ 15
Diazepam	0.2 to 0.8	$\geq$ 5.0
Ethchlorvynol	5 to 10	$\geq$ 20
Glutethimide	0.2 to 7	$\geq$ 10
Methyprylon	< 10	$\geq$ 30

Implications of
results

Identification of a sedative or hypnotic drug and its serum concentration confirms toxicity and guides its treatment.

Post-test care

If a hematoma develops at the venipuncture site, applying warm soaks eases discomfort.

Interfering
factor

Ethanol elevates diazepam levels.

Semen analysis

Inexpensive, technically simple, and reasonably de-finitive, semen analysis is usually the first test per-formed to evaluate male fertility. The procedure for analyzing semen for infertility usually includes measuring the volume of seminal fluid, assessing sperm counts, and microscopic examination. Sperm are counted in much the same way that white blood cells, red blood cells, and platelets are counted on an anticoagulated blood sample. Stain-ing and microscopic examination of a drop of semen permits the evaluation of the motility and morphology of the spermatozoa.

Abnormal semen may require further testing (such as liver, thyroid, pituitary, and adrenal function tests) to identify the underlying cause and screen for metabolic abnormalities (such as diabetes mellitus). Significantly abnormal semen — indicated by such signs as greatly decreased sperm count or motility or marked increase in morphologically abnormal forms — may require testicular biopsy.

Semen analysis can also be used to detect semen on a rape victim, to identify the blood group of an alleged rapist, or to prove sterility in a paternity suit. Some laboratories offer specialized semen tests, such as screening for antibodies to spermatozoa.

Purpose	• To evaluate male fertility in an infertile marriage (most common use)
	• To substantiate the effectiveness of vasectomy

For medicolegal purposes:
- To detect semen on the body or clothing of a suspected rape victim or at the crime scene
- To identify blood group substances to exonerate or incriminate a criminal suspect (rare)
- To rule out paternity on grounds of complete sterility (rare)

Patient preparation

For evaluation of fertility: Provide written instructions, and inform the patient that the most desirable specimen requires masturbation, ideally in the doctor's office or a laboratory. Instruct him to follow the prescribed period of continence before the test because it may increase his sperm count. Some clinicians specify a fixed number of days, usually between 2 and 5; others advise a period of continence equal to the usual interval between episodes of sexual intercourse.

If the patient prefers to collect the specimen at home, emphasize the importance of delivering the specimen to the laboratory within 3 hours after collection. Warn him not to expose the specimen to extreme temperatures or to direct sunlight (which can also increase its temperature). Ideally, the specimen should remain at body temperature until liquefaction is complete (about 20 minutes). To deliver a semen specimen to the laboratory during cold weather, the patient must protect the specimen from exposure to cold, for example, by keeping the specimen container in a coat pocket on the way to the laboratory.

Alternatives to collection by masturbation include coitus interruptus or the use of a condom. For collection by coitus interruptus, instruct the patient to withdraw immediately before ejaculation during intercourse and to deposit the ejaculate in a suitable specimen container. For collection by condom, the patient should first wash the condom with soap and water, rinse it thoroughly, and allow it to dry completely. (Powders or lubricants applied to the condom may be spermicidal.) Following collection, the patient should tie the condom, place it in a glass jar, and promptly deliver it to the laboratory.

Fertility may also be determined by collecting semen postcoitally from the female to assess the ability of the spermatozoa to penetrate the cervical mucus and remain active. For the postcoital cervical mucus test, instruct the patient to report for examination during the ovulatory phase of her menstrual cycle, as determined by basal temperature records, and as soon as possible after sexual intercourse (within 8 hours). Explain to the patient scheduled for this test that she'll be placed in the lithotomy position and that the doctor will insert a speculum in the vagina to collect the specimen. She may feel some pressure, but no pain, during this procedure.

For semen collection from rape victim: Explain to the patient that a semen specimen will be obtained from her vagina. Prepare her for insertion of the speculum as you would the patient scheduled for postcoital examination. *Note:* Don't lubricate the vaginal speculum. Oil or grease hinders examination of spermatozoa by interfering with smear preparation and staining and by inhibiting sperm motility through toxic ingredients. Instead, moisten the speculum with water or physiologic saline solution.

Handle the victim's clothes as little as possible. If her clothes are moist, put them in a paper bag, not a plastic bag (which causes seminal stains and secretions to mold). Label the bag properly, and send it to the laboratory immediately. Provide emotional support by speaking to the patient calmly and reassuringly. Encourage her to express her fears and anxieties.

If the rape victim is scheduled for vaginal lavage, tell her to expect a cold sensation when saline solution is instilled to wash out the specimen. To help her relax during this procedure, instruct her to breathe deeply and slowly through her mouth. Just before the test, instruct the victim to urinate, but warn her not to wipe the vulva afterward because this may remove semen.

Equipment   *For semen collection from masturbation, coitus interruptus, or with a condom:* clean plastic specimen container (for example, disposable urine or sputum container, with lid)

   For collection of a postcoital specimen: clean plastic specimen container, vaginal speculum, rubber gloves, cotton-tipped applicators, glass microscope slides with frosted ends, 1-ml tuberculin syringe (without a cannula or needle)

   For semen collection from a rape victim: clean plastic specimen container; vaginal speculum; rubber gloves; cotton-tipped applicators; glass microscope slides with frosted ends; physiologic (0.85%) saline solution; Pap sticks; Coplin jars containing 95% ethanol; large syringe, rubber bulb, or other device suitable for vaginal lavage

Procedure   To obtain a semen specimen for a fertility study, ask the patient to collect semen in a clean, plastic specimen container.

   Instruct the male patient who wants to collect the specimen during coitus interruptus to prevent any loss of semen during ejaculation.

   Before postcoital examination, the examiner wipes any excess mucus from the external cervix and collects the specimen by direct aspiration of the cervical canal, using a 1-ml tuberculin syringe without a cannula or needle.

   A specimen is obtained from the vagina of a rape victim by direct aspiration, saline lavage, or a direct smear of vaginal contents, using a Pap stick or, less desirably, a cotton-tipped applicator. Dried smears are usually collected from the suspected rape victim's skin by gently washing the skin with a small piece of gauze moistened with physiologic saline solution. Prepare direct smears on glass microscopic slides after labeling the frosted end. Immediately place smeared slides in Coplin jars containing 95% ethanol.

   Note: Use extreme caution in securing, labeling, and delivering all specimens required for medicolegal purposes. You may be asked to testify as to when, where, and from whom the specimen was obtained; the specimen's general appearance and identifying features; steps taken to ensure the specimen's integrity; and when, where, and to whom the specimen was delivered for analysis. If your hospital or clinic uses routing slips for such specimens, fill them out carefully, and submit them to the permanent medicolegal file.

Deliver all specimens, regardless of source or method of collection, to the laboratory promptly. Protect semen specimens for fertility studies from extremes of temperature and direct sunlight during delivery to the laboratory.

Values

Normal semen volume ranges from 0.7 to 6.5 ml. Paradoxically, the semen volume of males in infertile couples is frequently increased. Continence for 1 week or more results in progressively increased semen volume (sperm counts increase with abstinence up to 10 days; sperm motility progressively decreases; and sperm morphology stays the same). Liquefied semen is generally highly viscid, translucent, and gray-white, with a musty or acrid odor. After liquefaction, specimens of normal viscosity can be poured in drops. Normally, semen is slightly alkaline, with a pH of 7.3 to 7.9.

Other normal characteristics of semen: it coagulates immediately and liquefies within 20 minutes; normal spermatozoa count ranges from 20 to 150 million/ml (20 to 150×10^9/L); at least 40% of spermatozoa have normal morphology; at least 20% of spermatozoa show progressive motility within 4 hours of collection.

The normal postcoital cervical mucus test shows at least ten motile spermatozoa per microscopic high-power field; spinnbarkeit (a measurement of the tenacity of the mucus) of at least 4″ (10 cm). These findings indicate adequate spermatozoa and receptivity of the cervical mucus.

Implications of results

Abnormal semen is not synonymous with infertility. Only one viable spermatozoon is needed to fertilize an ovum. Although a normal sperm count is more than 20 million/ml (20×10^9/L), many males with sperm counts below 1 million/ml have fathered normal children. Only males who can't deliver *any* viable spermatozoa in their ejaculates during sexual intercourse are absolutely sterile. Nevertheless, subnormal sperm counts, decreased sperm motility, and abnormal morphology are usually associated with decreased fertility. Other tests may be necessary to evaluate the patient's general health, metabolic status, or function of specific endocrine systems (pituitary, thyroid, adrenal, or gonadal).

Post-test care
- Inform a patient who is undergoing infertility studies that test results should be available in 24 hours.
- Refer the suspected rape victim to an appropriate specialist for counseling — a gynecologist, psychiatrist, clinical psychologist, nurse specialist, member of the clergy, or representative of a community support group, such as Women Organized Against Rape.

Interfering factors
- Delayed delivery of the specimen, exposure of the specimen to extremes of temperature or direct sunlight, or the presence of toxic chemicals in the specimen container or condom can decrease the number of viable sperm.
- An incomplete specimen — from faulty collection by coitus interruptus, for example — diminishes the volume of the specimen.

Siderocyte stain

Siderocytes are red blood cells (RBCs) containing particles of nonhemoglobin iron known as siderotic granules. In newborns, siderotic granules are normally present in normoblasts and reticulocytes during hemoglobin synthesis. However, the spleen removes most of these granules from normal RBCs, and they disappear rapidly with age. In adults, an elevated siderocyte level usually indicates abnormal erythropoiesis, as occurs in congenital spherocytic anemia, chronic hemolytic anemias (such as the thalassemias), pernicious anemia, hemochromatosis, toxicities (such as lead poisoning), infection, or severe burns. An elevated siderocyte level may also follow splenectomy because the spleen normally removes siderotic granules.

Purpose
To aid differential diagnosis of the anemias and hemochromatosis and help detect toxicities

Patient preparation
Explain the purpose of this test, that the test requires a blood sample, and that additional tests may be required.

Procedure
The siderocyte stain test measures the number of circulating siderocytes. Venous blood is drawn into a 7-ml *lavender-top* tube or, for infants and children, collected in a microcollection tube or pipette and smeared directly on a 3″ × 1″ glass slide. When the

blood smear is stained, siderotic granules appear as purple-blue specks clustered around the periphery of mature erythrocytes. Cells containing these granules are counted as a percentage of total RBCs.

Findings | Normally, newborns have a slightly elevated siderocyte level, which reaches the normal adult value of 0.5% of total RBCs in 7 to 10 days.

Implications of results | In patients with pernicious anemia, the siderocyte level is 8% to 14%; with chronic hemolytic anemia, 20% to 100%; with lead poisoning, 10% to 30%; and with hemochromatosis, 3% to 7%. A high siderocyte level mandates additional testing — including bone marrow examination — to determine the cause of abnormal erythropoiesis.

Post-test care | If a hematoma develops at the venipuncture site, applying warm soaks eases discomfort.

Interfering factors | None

Skin tests, delayed hypersensitivity

Skin testing, also referred to as an *anergy panel,* is one of the most important methods for evaluating the cellular immune response of a patient with severe recurrent infection, infection caused by unusual organisms, or suspected disorder associated with delayed hypersensitivity. Because diminished delayed hypersensitivity may be associated with a poor prognosis in patients with certain malignant diseases, this test also may be useful in determining prognosis in such patients. A positive test reaction shows that the afferent, central, and efferent limbs of the immune response are intact, and that the patient can maintain a nonspecific inflammatory response to infection.

Skin tests employ new and recall antigens. New antigens—those not previously encountered by the patient, such as dinitrochlorobenzene (DNCB)—evaluate the secondary immune response; these antigens include candidin, trichophytin, streptokinase-streptodornase, purified protein derivative, staphage lysate, mumps, and mixed respiratory vaccine, among others. The specific antigens chosen for this test are those to which exposure is common and which will usually provoke an immune response.

In skin tests, a small amount of antigen (or group of antigens) is injected intradermally or applied topically, and the test site is later examined for a visible reaction. Skin tests have only limited value in infants because their immune systems are immature and inadequately sensitized.

Purpose

- To evaluate primary and secondary immune responses
- To assess effectiveness of immunotherapy when the patient's immune response is augmented by adjuvants (such as the bacille Calmette-Guérin [BCG] vaccine) or other means (transfer factor, levamisole)
- To diagnose fungal diseases (coccidioidomycosis, histoplasmosis), bacterial diseases (tuberculosis, brucellosis, Hansen's disease), and viral diseases (infectious mononucleosis)
- To monitor the course of certain diseases, such as Hodgkin's disease and coccidioidomycosis

Patient preparation

Explain the purpose of this test and describe the procedure, which involves application or injection of small doses of antigens. Tell the patient that it takes about 10 minutes for each antigen to be administered and that reactions should appear in 48 to 72 hours. Explain that some antigens (such as DNCB) are readministered after 2 weeks or, if the test is negative, that a stronger dose of antigen may be given.

Check the patient's history for hypersensitivity to any of the test antigens; if not listed in his history, ask the patient if he's had a skin test previously and, if so, what his reactions were. Check for previous BCG vaccination or tuberculosis. If the patient's history reveals no sensitivity or hypersensitivity, it's appropriate to test with intermediate-strength antigens.

If skin tests are planned, the standardized hospital procedure must be checked. Since many antigens are approved by the Food and Drug Administration (FDA) for use as vaccines but not for skin testing, check with the pharmacy about FDA approval for this purpose. If the tests require the patient's informed consent, such as for the use of DNCB in research studies, follow appropriate guidelines.

Equipment *DNCB test:* DNCB, sterile gauze pad and tape, gloves, surgical mask, alcohol sponges, acetone, cotton-tipped applicator

Recall antigen test: 1-ml tuberculin syringes, 25G ⅝″ needles, alcohol sponges, antigens, syringe filled with diluted epinephrine (1:1,000), extra needle and syringe containing allergy test diluent, pen

Procedure *DNCB test:* Wear gloves and a mask to avoid sensitizing yourself to DNCB. Dissolve DNCB in acetone. Position the patient's forearm comfortably, ventral side up, with his elbow slightly flexed. Clean a small, hairless area midway between the wrist and elbow with an alcohol sponge, allow it to dry, and apply the prescribed amount of DNCB (sensitizing dose) with a cotton-tipped applicator. Allow this to dry; then cover the area with a sterile gauze pad for 24 to 48 hours.

Instruct the patient to watch for a spontaneous flare reaction 10 to 14 days after application of DNCB. (If a reaction occurs, a lower dose of the test solution can be used for the challenge dose of DNCB.)

After 14 days, apply a challenge dose of DNCB to the same spot and in the same manner. Inspect the site 48 to 96 hours after application of DNCB for reactivity. The challenge dose can be repeated 2 weeks later (1 month after the sensitizing dose) when test results are negative.

Recall antigen test: Inject each antigen being tested intradermally, using a separate tuberculin syringe, on the patient's forearm. Circle each injection site with a pen and label each according to the antigen given. Instruct the patient to avoid washing off the circles until the test is completed. Then, inject the control allergy diluent on the other forearm.

Inspect injection sites for reactivity after 48 and 72 hours. Record induration and erythema in millimeters. A negative test at the first concentration of antigen should be confirmed using a higher concentration.

Stored antigens in lyophilized (freeze-dried) form should be refrigerated and protected from light. Reconstitute them shortly before use, and check their expiration dates.

Precautions • If the patient is suspected of hypersensitivity to the antigens, apply them first in low concentrations.

- Because excess DNCB can burn the patient's skin, apply only the prescribed amount.
- If the forearms are not free from disease (for example, if the patient has atopic dermatitis), use other sites, such as the back.
- Observe the patient carefully for signs of anaphylactic shock—urticaria, respiratory distress, and hypotension. If such signs develop, administer epinephrine, as appropriate.

Findings
In the DNCB test, a positive reaction (erythema, edema, induration) appears 48 to 96 hours after the second (challenge) dose; 95% of the population reacts positively to DNCB. In the recall antigen test, a positive response (5 mm or more of induration at the test site) appears 48 hours after injection.

Implications of results
In the DNCB test, failure to react to the challenge dose indicates diminished delayed hypersensitivity. In the recall antigen test, a positive response to less than two of the six test antigens, a persistent unresponsiveness to intradermal injection of higher-strength antigens, or a generalized diminished reaction (causing a combined induration of less than 10 mm) indicates diminished delayed hypersensitivity.

Diminished delayed hypersensitivity can result from conditions such as Hodgkin's disease (common); sarcoidosis; liver disease; congenital immunodeficiency disease, such as DiGeorge syndrome, ataxia-telangiectasia, and Wiskott-Aldrich syndrome; uremia; acute leukemia; viral diseases, such as influenza, infectious mononucleosis, measles, mumps, and rubella; fungal diseases, such as coccidioidomycosis and cryptococcosis; bacterial diseases, such as Hansen's disease and tuberculosis; and terminal cancer. Diminished delayed hypersensitivity can also result from immunosuppressant or steroid therapy or viral vaccination.

Post-test care
- Monitor the patient closely for severe local reactions that may occur at the test site, such as pain, blistering, swelling, induration, itching, and ulceration. Scarring or hyperpigmentation may result. Also observe for swelling and tenderness in the lymph nodes at the elbow or axillary region. Check for tachycardia and fever, although these rarely occur. Symptoms generally appear in 15 to 30 minutes.

- Tell the patient who experiences hypersensitivity that corticosteroids will control the reaction, but skin lesions may persist for 10 to 14 days. Advise the patient to avoid scratching or otherwise disturbing the affected area.

Interfering factors

- Use of antigens that have expired, or been exposed to heat and light or to bacterial contamination, interferes with accurate testing.
- Incorrect injection technique—subcutaneous instead of intradermal injection—may produce negative results.
- Inaccurate dilution of antigens or an error in reading or timing test results causes inaccurate test results.
- A strong immediate reaction to the antigen at the site of injection may cause a false-negative delayed reaction.

Small-bowel biopsy

Small-bowel biopsy helps evaluate diseases of the intestinal mucosa that may cause malabsorption or diarrhea. Using a capsule, it produces larger specimens than does endoscopic biopsy and allows removal of tissue from those areas beyond an endoscope's reach.

Several types of capsules are available, all similar in design and use. The Carey capsule, for example, is a spring-loaded, two-piece capsule, ⅜″ (8 mm) in diameter and 1″ (2.5 cm) long. A mercury-weighted bag is attached to one end of the capsule; a thin polyethylene tube about 5′ (1.5 m) long is attached to the other end. After the bag, capsule, and tube are in place in the small bowel, suction applied to the tube causes the mucosa to enter the capsule. Continued suction closes the capsule, cutting off the piece of tissue within.

The biopsy sample verifies diagnosis of some diseases, such as Whipple's disease, and may help confirm others, such as tropical sprue. Capsule biopsy is an invasive procedure, but it causes little pain and complications are rare.

Purpose

To help diagnose diseases of the intestinal mucosa

Patient preparation

Describe the procedure, and explain that this test helps identify intestinal disorders. Tell the patient to restrict food and fluids for at least 8 hours before the test. Reassure the patient that the procedure causes little discomfort. Administer a sedative, as ordered.

Make sure that the patient or a responsible family member has signed a consent form. Ensure that coagulation tests have been performed and that the results are recorded on the patient's chart.

Withhold aspirin and anticoagulants, as appropriate. If they must be continued, note this on the laboratory slip.

Procedure   Check the tubing and the mercury bag for leaks. Lightly lubricate the tube and the capsule with a water-soluble lubricant, and moisten the mercury bag with water. Spray the back of the patient's throat with a local anesthetic, as ordered, to decrease gagging during passage of the tube. Ask the patient to sit upright. The capsule is then placed in his pharynx, and he is asked to flex his neck and swallow as the examiner advances the tube about 20″ (50 cm). (If a local anesthetic is used to control the gag reflex, the patient must not receive any fluids to help him swallow the capsule.) The patient is placed on his right side; the examiner then advances the tube another 20″. The tube's position must be checked by fluoroscopy or by instilling air through the tube and listening with a stethoscope for air to enter the stomach.

Next, the tube is advanced 2″ to 4″ (5 to 10 cm) at a time to pass the capsule through the pylorus. Talking to the patient about food may stimulate the pylorus and help advance the capsule. When fluoroscopy confirms that the capsule has passed the pylorus, keep the patient on his right side to allow the capsule to move into the second and third portions of the small bowel. Tell the patient that he may hold the tube loosely to one side of his mouth if this is more comfortable. Capsule position is checked again by fluoroscopy.

When the capsule is at or beyond the ligament of Treitz, the biopsy sample can be taken. The patient is placed supine so that the capsule's position can be verified fluoroscopically. A 100-ml glass syringe is placed on the end of the tube, and steady suction is applied to close the capsule and cut off a tissue specimen. Suction is maintained on the syringe as the tube and capsule are removed; then the suction is released. This opens the capsule and exposes the specimen, mucosal side down. The specimen is gently removed with forceps, placed mucosal side up on a piece of mesh, and placed in a biopsy bottle with the required fixative. The specimen should be sent to the laboratory immediately.

Precautions
- Keep suction equipment nearby to prevent aspiration if the patient vomits.
- Do not allow the patient to bite the tubing.
- Biopsy is contraindicated in patients unable to cooperate, in those taking aspirin or anticoagulants, and in those with uncontrolled coagulation disorders.

Findings
A normal small-bowel biopsy specimen consists of fingerlike villi, crypts, columnar epithelial cells, and round cells.

Implications of results
Small-bowel tissue that reveals histologic changes in cell structure may indicate abetalipoproteinemia, Whipple's disease, eosinophilic enteritis, lymphangiectasia, lymphoma, and such parasitic infections as giardiasis and coccidiosis. Abnormal specimens may also suggest celiac sprue, tropical sprue, infectious gastroenteritis, intraluminal bacterial overgrowth, folate and vitamin B_{12} deficiency, radiation enteritis, and malnutrition, but such disorders require further studies.

Post-test care
The patient may resume a normal diet after confirming return of the gag reflex.

➤ *Clinical alert:* Complications are rare. However, watch for signs of hemorrhage, bacteremia with transient fever and pain, and bowel perforation. Tell the patient to report abdominal pain or bleeding.

Interfering factors
- Mechanical failure of the biopsy capsule or any hole in the tubing can prevent removal of a tissue sample.
- Incorrect specimen handling or positioning may alter test results.
- Failure to fast before the biopsy may yield a poor specimen or cause vomiting and aspiration.
- Failure to place the specimen in fixative or a delay in transport may alter test results.

Sodium, serum

This test measures serum levels of sodium, the major extracellular cation. Sodium affects body water distribution, maintains osmotic pressure of extra-cellular fluid, and helps promote neuromuscular function; it also helps maintain acid-base balance and influences chloride and potassium levels. Sodium is absorbed by the intestines and is excreted primarily by the kidneys; a small amount is lost through the skin.

Because extracellular sodium concentration helps the kidneys to regulate body water (decreased sodium levels promote water excretion and increased levels promote retention), serum levels of sodium are evaluated in relation to the amount of water in the body. For example, a sodium deficit (hyponatremia) refers to a decreased level of sodium in relation to the body's water level. The body normally regulates this sodium-water balance through aldosterone, which inhibits sodium excretion and promotes its reabsorption (with water) by the renal tubules. Low sodium levels stimulate aldosterone secretion; elevated sodium levels depress aldosterone secretion.

Purpose	• To evaluate fluid-electrolyte and acid-base balance, and related neuromuscular, renal, and adrenal functions • To evaluate the effects of drug therapy (such as diuretics) on serum sodium levels
Patient preparation	Explain that this test determines the sodium content of blood. Inform the patient that restriction of food or fluids is not required before the test and that this test requires a blood sample. Check the patient's medication history for use of diuretics and other drugs that influence sodium levels. If these medications must be continued, note this on the laboratory slip.
Procedure	Perform a venipuncture, and collect the sample in a 10- to 15-ml *red-top* tube. Handle the sample gently to prevent hemolysis.
Values	Normally, serum sodium levels range from 135 to 145 mEq/liter (mmol/L).
Implications of results	Sodium imbalance can result from a loss or gain of sodium or from a change in water volume. Serum sodium results must be interpreted in light of the patient's state of hydration.

Elevated serum sodium levels (hypernatremia) may be caused by inadequate water intake, water loss in excess of sodium (as in diabetes insipidus, impaired renal function, prolonged hyperventilation, profuse sweating, and, occasionally, severe vomiting or diarrhea), and sodium retention (as in aldosteronism). Hypernatremia can also result from excessive sodium intake.

➤ *Clinical alert:* In a patient with hypernatremia and associated loss of water, observe for signs of thirst, restlessness, dry and sticky mucous membranes, flushed skin, oliguria, and diminished reflexes. However, if increased total body sodium causes water retention, observe for hypertension, dyspnea, and edema.

Abnormally low serum sodium levels (hyponatremia) may result from inadequate sodium intake or excessive sodium loss caused by profuse sweating, gastric suctioning, diuretic therapy, diarrhea, vomiting, adrenal insufficiency, burns, or chronic renal insufficiency with acidosis. Urine sodium determinations are frequently more sensitive to early changes in sodium balance and should always be evaluated simultaneously with serum sodium findings. Hyponatremia may also be seen with excess water intake or retention, as in congestive heart failure, malnutrition, chronic liver disease, diabetes mellitus, and nephrotic syndrome.

➤ *Clinical alert:* In a patient with hyponatremia, watch for apprehension, lassitude, headache, decreased skin turgor, abdominal cramps, and tremors that may progress to seizures.

Post-test care If a hematoma develops at the venipuncture site, applying warm soaks eases discomfort.

Interfering factors
- Most diuretics suppress serum sodium levels by promoting sodium excretion; lithium, chlorpropamide, and vasopressin suppress levels by inhibiting water excretion.
- Corticosteroids elevate serum sodium levels by promoting sodium retention. Antihypertensives, such as methyldopa, hydralazine, and reserpine, may cause sodium and water retention.
- Hemolysis caused by excessive agitation of the sample may interfere with accurate determination of test results.

Sodium and chloride, urine

This test determines urine levels of sodium, the major extracellular cation, and of chloride, the major extracellular anion. Less significant than serum levels (and, consequently, performed less frequently), measurement of urine sodium and urine chloride concentrations is used to evaluate renal conservation of these two electrolytes and to confirm serum sodium and chloride values.

Sodium and chloride help maintain osmotic pressure, and water and acid-base balance. After these ions are absorbed by the intestinal tract, they are regulated by the kidneys and rise and fall in tandem. The kidneys maintain constant serum levels of sodium and of chloride — even at the risk of dehydration or edema — or they excrete excessive amounts. Normal ranges of sodium and chloride in the urine may vary greatly with dietary salt intake and perspiration.

Purpose
- To help evaluate fluid and electrolyte imbalance
- To monitor the effects of a low-salt diet
- To help evaluate renal and adrenal disorders

Patient preparation
Explain the purpose of this test, that no special restrictions are necessary before the test, and that it requires a 24-hour urine specimen. If the specimen will be collected at home, teach the patient the proper collection technique. Tell the patient not to contaminate the specimen with toilet tissue or stool.

Check the patient's history for medications that may influence test results.

Procedure
Collect a random or timed urine specimen in a plastic urine container without preservatives.

Values
Normal urine sodium excretion ranges from 27 to 280 mmol/day; normal urine chloride excretion, from 110 to 250 mmol/day, depending on intake; and normal urine sodium-chloride excretion, from 5 to 20 g/day (mmol/day).

Implications of results
Usually, urine sodium and urine chloride levels are parallel, rising and falling in tandem. Abnormal sodium and chloride levels may indicate the need for more specific determination. Elevated urine sodium levels may reflect increased salt intake, adrenal failure, salicylate toxicity, diabetic acidosis, salt-

losing nephritis, and water-deficient dehydration. Decreased urine sodium levels suggest decreased salt intake, diuresis, primary aldosteronism, acute renal failure, congestive heart failure (CHF), and syndrome of inappropriate antidiuretic hormone.

Elevated urine chloride levels may result from water-deficient dehydration, salicylate toxicity, diabetic acidosis, adrenocortical insufficiency (Addison's disease), and salt-losing renal disease. Decreased levels may result from excessive diaphoresis, CHF, or hypochloremic metabolic alkalosis after prolonged vomiting or gastric suctioning.

To evaluate fluid-electrolyte imbalance, urine levels must be correlated with results of serum electrolyte studies.

Post-test care   None

Interfering factors
- Failure to collect all urine during the timed test period may interfere with accurate test results.
- Ammonium chloride, potassium chloride, and halogens (such as bromine, fluorine, and iodine) elevate urine chloride levels.
- Sodium bicarbonate and thiazide diuretics raise urine sodium levels; corticosteroids suppress them.

Sperm antibody assay

This direct assay, known as immunobead, is performed to detect immunologic infertility by determining whether or not a male or his partner have antibodies directed against his sperm cells. In direct methods, viable sperm coated with antisperm antibodies (from a test fluid) are incubated with polyacrylamide beads coated with anti-immunoglobulin antibodies. A positive reaction shows motile sperm with attached beads. Current consensus holds that some type of direct method provides the most meaningful results. Several other types of assays can be used to perform this analysis. For example, indirect assays such as enzyme-linked immunosorbent assay (ELISA), which use serum as a test fluid, identify the formation of antigen-antibody complexes during the assay and visualize them by colorimetric changes in the medium.

Purpose   • To detect immunologic infertility

- To detect antisperm antibodies in test fluids
- To determine the isotype of sperm antibodies
- To determine the binding site on the sperm of any antisperm antibody

Patient preparation

Explain the purpose of the test, and inform the patient about specimen collection.

Procedure

For a test using serum, obtain a venous blood sample and allow the blood to clot. After collection, the serum should be heated to 138.2° F (56° C) for 30 minutes before assay. If seminal plasma will be tested, a semen specimen should be obtained and treated as for a semen analysis. If cervical mucus will be tested, a specimen should be collected as near as possible to the time of ovulation. The cervical mucus is then incubated with an agent such as bromelin to liquefy the sample for further processing.

Sperm cells are incubated in the test fluid of interest for approximately 1 hour to expose the sperm cells to any antisperm antibodies that are present in the fluid. The resulting sperm-antibody complex is then incubated with beads coated with either anti-immunoglobulin G, anti-immunoglobulin A, or anti-immunoglobulin M antibodies. A complex will then be formed between any antibody-bound sperm and the appropriate beads. Positive reactions can then be observed under the microscope as motile sperm with attached beads. In addition, it can determine the proportion of bound sperm, the immunoglobulin isotype, and the site of binding. The site of binding may have implications for the potential infertility effect.

Precautions

- Blood sample collection for this assay should be undertaken with the same precautions as for any other blood sample. Cervical mucus collection should be collected with the same care as that of a postcoital test. Semen collection should be as for a semen analysis.
- All test fluids should be treated by laboratory personnel as potentially infectious.

Findings

Under normal conditions, sperm-bead binding should be negative. However, some specimens may show low levels (10%) of sperm binding to immunobeads without clinical significance. Binding to the extreme tip of the sperm tail may occur frequently without clinical significance.

Implications of results

If the sperm antibody assay confirms the presence of antisperm antibodies, several points should be considered. First, no common treatment has yet been identified to counteract the presence of anti-sperm antibodies. A procedure that has not been widely accepted is treatment with steroids. While such treatment can lower the antibody titer, the potential side effects and inconsistent clinical result (pregnancy) argue against this protocol. More recently, some effort has been given to collection of the semen specimen directly into a culture medium containing high protein levels. The specimen is then processed and inseminated artificially. This treatment might be effective in males with antibodies against their own spermatozoa. However, the efficacy of this procedure is still unconfirmed.

Information regarding the binding site can be useful. The presence of these antibodies can interfere with the transport of spermatozoa through the cervix and thus impair their ability to reach the site of fertilization. This is most likely when antibody binding is directed against tail components of the sperm; antibody binding directed against elements of the sperm head can impair attachment of the sperm to the egg and consequently inhibit fertilization. To overcome impaired sperm transport, intra-uterine insemination of appropriately prepared sperm specimens has met with some success. Finally, the antibody isotype can suggest whether the immune response elicited by the sperm is local or systemic.

Post-test care

None

Interfering factors

- High incidence of sperm-reactive antibodies in the sera of fertile men and women can interfere with accurate test results with ELISA.
- Different methods of fixing spermatozoa can cause variation in ability of ELISA to detect sperm-reactive antibodies.
- Improper specimen collection or failure to deliver it to the laboratory promptly many prevent accurate test results.

Sputum culture

Bacteriologic examination of sputum — material raised from the lungs and bronchi during deep coughing — is an important aid to the management of lung disease. During passage through the throat and oropharynx, sputum specimens are commonly contaminated with indigenous bacterial flora, such as alpha-hemolytic streptococci, *Neisseria* species, diphtheroids, and some haemophili, pneumococci, staphylococci, and yeasts, such as *Candida*. Pathogenic organisms most often found in sputum include *Streptococcus pneumoniae, Klebsiella pneumoniae (and other Enterobacteriaceae), Haemophilus influenzae, Staphylococcus aureus, Pseudomonas aeruginosa,* and *Mycobacterium tuberculosis.* (*M. tuberculosis* may also be found using special bacteriology techniques.) Other agents, such as *Pneumocystis carinii,* the Legionellae, *Mycoplasma pneumoniae,* and respiratory viruses may exist in the sputum and can cause lung disease, but usually require other diagnostic techniques.

The usual method of specimen collection is expectoration (which may require ultrasonic nebulization, hydration, physiotherapy, or postural drainage); other methods include tracheal suctioning or bronchoscopy.

A Gram's stain of expectorated sputum must be examined to ensure that it's a representative specimen of secretions from the lower respiratory tract (many white blood cells [WBCs] and few epithelial cells) rather than one contaminated by oral flora (few WBCs and many epithelial cells). Careful examination of an acid-fast smear of sputum may provide presumptive evidence of a mycobacterial infection, such as tuberculosis.

Purpose

To isolate and identify the cause of a pulmonary infection, thus aiding diagnosis of respiratory diseases (most frequently bronchitis, pneumonia, lung abscess, and tuberculosis, in that order)

Patient preparation

Explain that this test helps to identify the organism causing respiratory tract infection. Tell the patient the test requires a sputum specimen. If the suspected organism is *Mycobacterium tuberculosis,* tell the patient that at least three morning specimens may be required.

Results are usually available within 48 to 72 hours. However, because cultures for tuberculosis may take several weeks, diagnosis of this disorder generally depends on clinical symptoms, a smear for acid-fast bacilli, chest X-ray, and response to a purified protein derivative skin test.

If the specimen will be collected by expectoration, the patient should be encouraged to help sputum production by increasing fluid intake the night before collection. Teach the patient how to expectorate by taking three deep breaths and forcing a deep cough. Emphasize that sputum isn't the same as saliva, which will be rejected for culturing. Tell him not to brush his teeth or use mouthwash before the specimen collection, although he may rinse his mouth with water.

If the specimen will be collected by tracheal suctioning, tell the patient he'll experience transient discomfort as the catheter passes into the trachea.

If the specimen will be collected by bronchoscopy, instruct the patient to fast for 6 hours before the procedure. Make sure that the patient or a responsible family member has signed a consent form. Tell the patient that a local anesthetic will be given just before the test, to minimize discomfort during passage of the tube.

Equipment *For expectoration:* sterile, disposable, impermeable container with a tight-fitting cap; 10% sodium chloride solution, acetylcysteine, propylene glycol, or sterile or distilled water aerosols to induce cough, as ordered; leakproof bag

For tracheal suctioning: size 16 or size 18 French suction catheter, water-soluble lubricant, sterile gloves, sterile specimen container or in-line specimen trap, normal saline solution

For bronchoscopy: bronchoscope, local anesthetic, sterile needle and syringe, sterile specimen container, normal saline solution, bronchial brush, sterile gloves

Procedure *Expectoration:* Instruct the patient to cough deeply and expectorate into the container. If the cough is nonproductive, chest physiotherapy, heated aerosol spray (nebulization), or intermittent positive pressure breathing with the prescribed aerosol may be used to induce sputum. Using aseptic technique, close the container securely. Dispose of equipment properly; seal the container in a leakproof bag before sending it to the laboratory.

Tracheal suctioning: Administer oxygen to the patient before and after the procedure, if necessary. Attach the sputum trap to the suction catheter. Using sterile gloves, lubricate the catheter with normal saline solution, and pass the catheter through the patient's nostril, without suction. (The patient will cough when the catheter passes through the larynx.) Advance the catheter into the trachea. Apply suction for no longer than 15 seconds to obtain the specimen. Stop suction, and gently remove the catheter. Discard the catheter and gloves in the proper receptacle. Then, detach the in-line sputum trap from the suction apparatus and cap the opening.

Bronchoscopy: After a local anesthetic is sprayed into the patient's throat or the patient gargles with a local anesthetic, the bronchoscope is inserted through the pharynx and trachea, into the bronchus. Secretions are then collected with a bronchial brush or aspirated through the inner channel of the scope, using an irrigating solution, such as normal saline solution, if necessary. After the specimen is obtained, the bronchoscope is removed.

Label the container with the patient's name. Include on the laboratory slip the nature and origin of the specimen, the date and time of collection, the initial diagnosis, and any current antibiotic therapy. Send the specimen to the laboratory immediately after collection.

Precautions
- Tracheal suctioning is contraindicated in patients with esophageal varices or cardiac disease.
- During tracheal suctioning, suction for only 5 to 10 seconds at a time. Never suction longer than 15 seconds. If the patient becomes hypoxic or cyanotic, remove the catheter immediately, and administer oxygen.
- Because the patient may cough violently during suctioning, wear a mask to avoid exposure to respiratory pathogens.
- Don't use more than 20% propylene glycol with water as an inducer for a specimen scheduled for tuberculosis culturing because higher concentrations inhibit the growth of *M. tuberculosis*. (If propylene glycol isn't available, use 10% to 20% acetylcysteine with water or sodium chloride.)

➤ *Clinical alert:* In a patient with asthma or chronic bronchitis, watch for aggravated bronchospasms with use of more than 10% concentration of sodium chloride or acetylcysteine in an aerosol.

Findings
Flora commonly found in the respiratory tract include alpha-hemolytic streptococci, *Neisseria* spe-

cies, and diphtheroids. However, the presence of normal flora doesn't rule out infection.

Implications of
results

Because sputum is invariably contaminated with normal oropharyngeal flora, interpretation of a culture isolate must relate to the patient's overall clinical condition. Isolation of *M. tuberculosis* is always a significant finding.

Post-test care

• After tracheal suctioning, offer the patient a drink of water.
• Good mouth care should be provided, or the patient should have the opportunity to clean his mouth and rinse with mouthwash.

➤ *Clinical alert:* After bronchoscopy, observe the patient carefully for signs of hypoxemia (cyanosis), laryngospasm (laryngeal stridor), bronchospasm (paroxysms of coughing or wheezing), pneumothorax (dyspnea, cyanosis, pleural pain, tachycardia), perforation of the trachea or bronchus (subcutaneous crepitus), or trauma to respiratory structures (bleeding). Also, check for difficulty in breathing or swallowing. Don't give liquids until the gag reflex returns.

Interfering
factors

• Improper collection or handling of the specimen may interfere with accurate determination of results.
• Failure to report current or recent antibiotic therapy prevents correct interpretation of decreased bacterial growth.
• Sputum collected over an extended period may allow pathogens to deteriorate or become overgrown by commensals and will not be accepted as a valid specimen by most laboratories.

Stool culture

Bacteriologic examination of feces is valuable for identifying pathogens that cause overt GI disease (such as typhoid and dysentery) and carrier states. Normal bacterial flora in feces include many species and several potentially pathogenic organisms. The most common pathogenic organisms of the GI tract are *Shigella, Salmonella,* and *Campylobacter jejuni;* other pathogenic organisms include *Vibrio cholerae, V. parahaemolyticus, Clostridium botulinum, C. difficile, C. perfringens, Staphylococcus aureus,* pathogenic strains of *Escherichia coli, Bacillus cereus, Yersinia enterocolitica,* and *Aeromonas hydrophila.* Identification of these organisms is vital not only for treating and preventing potentially fatal complications (especially in a debilitated patient) but also for confining these severe infectious diseases. A sensitivity test may follow isolation of the pathogen.

Some virus groups, such as rotavirus and parvovirus, which also cause GI symptoms, can only be detected by immunoassay or electron microscopy. Viral stool culture may detect other organisms, such as enterovirus, which can cause aseptic meningitis.

Purpose

- To identify pathogenic organisms causing GI disease
- To identify carrier states

Patient preparation

Explain that this test helps determine the cause of GI symptoms or may establish whether or not the patient is a carrier of infectious organisms. Inform the patient that restrictions of food or fluids is not required before the test, and that the test may require the collection of a stool specimen on 3 consecutive days.

Check the patient's history for dietary patterns and recent antibiotic therapy, and for recent travel that might suggest endemic infections or infestations.

Equipment

Tongue blade; 8-oz waterproof container with tight-fitting lid or sterile cotton-tipped applicator and commercial sterile collection and transport system; bedpan (if needed)

Procedure

Collect a stool specimen directly into the container or, if the patient isn't ambulatory, into a clean, dry bedpan. Then, using a tongue blade, transfer the specimen to the transport container. To collect a specimen from the rectum, insert the applicator past the anal sphincter, rotate it gently, and withdraw it. Then, place the applicator in the appropriate container. If the patient uses a bedpan or a diaper, avoid contaminating the stool specimen with urine.

If the specimen is to be processed for a viral test, check with the laboratory for the proper collection procedure before obtaining a specimen.

Label the specimen with the patient's name and identification number, the name of the doctor, the date and time of collection, the suspected cause of enteritis and current antibiotic therapy on the laboratory slip.

Send the specimen to the laboratory immediately; be sure to include mucoid and bloody portions. The specimen should always be representative of the first, middle, and last portion of the feces passed. Use aseptic technique when handling the specimen. Put the specimen container in a leak-proof bag before transporting it to the laboratory.

Findings
From 96% to 99% of normal fecal flora reportedly consist of anaerobes, including non–spore-forming bacilli, clostridia, and anaerobic streptococci. The remaining 1% to 4% consist of facultative anaerobes, including gram-negative bacilli (predominantly *E. coli* and other Enterobacteriaceae, plus small amounts of *Pseudomonas*), gram-positive cocci (mostly enterococci), and a few yeasts.

Implications of results
Isolation of some pathogens (such as *Salmonella, Shigella, Campylobacter, Yersinia,* and *Vibrio*) indicates bacterial infection in patients with acute diarrhea and may require antibiotic sensitivity tests. Because normal fecal flora may include *Clostridium difficile, E. coli,* and other organisms, isolation of these may require further tests to demonstrate invasiveness or toxin production. Isolation of pathogens such as *C. botulinum* indicates food poisoning; however, the pathogens must also be isolated from the contaminated food. In a patient receiving long-term antibiotic therapy, isolation of large numbers of *Staphylococcus aureus* or yeast, such as *Candida,* may indicate infection. (Asymptomatic carrier states are also indicated by these enteric pathogens.) Isolation of enteroviruses requires special virologic techniques.

If a stool culture shows no unusual growth, detection of viruses by immunoassay or electron microscopy may diagnose nonbacterial gastroenteritis. Increased polymorphonuclear leukocytes in fecal material may indicate an invasive pathogen.

Post-test care
None

Interfering
factors

- Improper collection technique or the presence of urine in the specimen may injure or destroy some enteric pathogens.
- Antibiotic therapy may decrease bacterial growth in the specimen.
- Failure to transport the specimen promptly or, if delivery is delayed, to use a transport medium that stabilizes pH (such as a buffered glycerol medium) may result in loss of some enteric pathogens or overgrowth of nonpathogenic organisms.

Sweat test

The sweat test quantitatively measures electrolyte concentrations (primarily sodium and chloride) in sweat, usually through pilocarpine iontophoresis (pilocarpine is a sweat inducer). This test is used almost exclusively in children to confirm cystic fibrosis, a congenital condition that raises the sodium and chloride electrolyte levels in sweat.

Sweat glands are found over most body surfaces. When stimulated by the sympathetic nerves, these glands secrete a watery solution that contains sodium chloride, most plasma components (except proteins), urea, and lactate ions. Elevated sodium and chloride sweat concentrations may also occur in persons predisposed to cystic fibrosis, such as those with family histories of the disease, or in those suspected of having the disease because of malabsorption syndrome or failure to thrive.

Purpose

To confirm cystic fibrosis

Patient
preparation

Because this test is usually performed on a child, explain the test as simply as possible (if the child is old enough to understand). Inform the patient that restrictions of diet, medication, or activity are not required before the test. Tell the child he may feel a slight tickling sensation during the procedure but won't feel any pain. If he becomes nervous or frightened during the test, offer a book, television, or other appropriate diversion.

Encourage the parents to assist with preparations and to stay with their child during the test. Their presence will minimize the child's anxiety.

Equipment

Analyzer, two skin chloride electrodes (positive and negative), distilled water, two standardizing solutions (chloride concentrations), pilocarpine pads, 2″ × 2″ sterile gauze pads (kept in airtight container), forceps (for handling pads), straps (for securing electrodes), gram scale, normal saline solution

Procedure   With distilled water, wash the test area and dry it. (For iontophoresis, the flexor surface of the right forearm is commonly used; the right thigh, when the patient's arm is too small to secure electrodes, as with an infant.) Place a gauze pad saturated with premeasured pilocarpine solution on the positive electrode; place the pad saturated with normal saline solution on the negative electrode. Apply both electrodes to the test area and secure them with straps.

Lead wires to the analyzer — which are attached in a manner similar to that used for electrocardiogram electrodes — are given a current of 4 milliamperes in 15 to 20 seconds. This process (iontophoresis) is continued at 15- to 20-second intervals for 5 minutes. After iontophoresis, remove both electrodes. Discard the pads, clean the skin with distilled water, then dry it.

Using forceps, place a dry gauze pad or filter paper (previously weighed on a gram scale) on the pilocarpine-treated area. Cover the pad or filter paper with a slightly larger piece of plastic, and seal the edges of the plastic with waterproof adhesive tape. Leave the gauze pad or filter paper in place for about 30 to 40 minutes. (The appearance of droplets on the plastic usually indicates induction of an adequate amount of sweat.)

Remove the pad or filter paper with the forceps, place it immediately in the weighing bottle, and insert the stopper in the bottle. (The difference between the first and second weights indicates the weight of the sweat specimen collected.)

Make sure at least 100 mg of sweat is collected for analysis. Carefully seal the gauze pad or filter paper in the weighing bottle, and send the bottle to the laboratory immediately.

Precautions   Always perform iontophoresis on the right arm (or right thigh) rather than on the left.

➤ *Clinical alert: Never* perform iontophoresis on the chest, especially in a child, because the current can induce cardiac arrest.

To prevent electric shock, use battery-powered equipment, if possible. Stop the test immediately if the patient complains of a burning sensation, which usually indicates that the positive electrode is exposed or positioned improperly. Adjust the electrode, and continue the test.

Values
Normal sodium values in sweat range from 10 to 30 mEq/liter. Normal chloride values range from 10 to 35 mEq/liter (mmol/L).

Implications of results
Abnormal sodium values range from 50 to 130 mEq/liter (mmol/L). Abnormal chloride values range from 50 to 110 mEq/liter (mmol/L). Sodium and chloride concentrations of 50 to 60 mEq/liter (mmol/L) strongly suggest cystic fibrosis. Concentrations greater than 60 mEq/liter (mmol/L), with typical clinical features, confirm the diagnosis. Only a few conditions other than cystic fibrosis cause elevated sweat electrolyte levels — most notably, untreated adrenal insufficiency, as well as type I glycogen storage disease, vasopressin-resistant diabetes insipidus, meconium ileus, and renal failure. However, cystic fibrosis is the only condition that increases sweat electrolyte levels above 80 mEq/liter (mmol/L).

In females, sweat electrolyte levels fluctuate cyclically: chloride concentrations usually peak 5 to 10 days before onset of menses, and most women retain fluid before menses. Males also show fluctuations (up to 70 mEq/liter [mmol/L]).

Post-test care
• Wash the test area with soap and water, and dry it thoroughly.
• If the test area looks red, reassure the patient that this is normal and will disappear within a few hours.
• The patient may resume his usual activities.

Interfering factors
• Failure to obtain an adequate amount of sweat (common in neonates) prevents proper testing.
• Salt depletion (common during hot weather) may cause false-normal test results.
• Failure to clean the skin thoroughly or to use sterile gauze pads may cause false-high results.
• Failure to seal the gauze pad or filter paper carefully may cause false-high electrolyte levels because of evaporation.

Synovial fluid analysis

Synovial fluid is normally a viscid, colorless-to-pale-yellow liquid found in small amounts in the diarthrodial (synovial) joints, bursae, and tendon sheaths. It's thought to be produced by the dialysis of plasma across the synovial membrane and by the secretion of hyaluronic acid, a mucopolysaccharide. Although its functions aren't clearly understood, synovial fluid probably lubricates the joint space, nourishes the articular cartilage, and protects the cartilage from mechanical damage while stabilizing the joint.

In synovial fluid aspiration, or arthrocentesis, a sterile needle is inserted into a joint space — most commonly the knee — under strict aseptic conditions, to obtain a fluid specimen for analysis. This procedure is indicated in patients with undiagnosed articular disease and symptomatic joint effusion — the excessive accumulation of synovial fluid.

Although rare, complications associated with synovial fluid aspiration include joint infection and hemorrhage leading to hemarthrosis (accumulation of blood within the joint).

Purpose
- To aid differential diagnosis of arthritis, particularly septic or crystal-induced arthritis
- To identify the cause and nature of joint effusion
- To relieve the pain and distention resulting from accumulation of fluid within the joint
- To administer local drug therapy, usually corticosteroids

Patient preparation

Describe the procedure and explain that this test helps determine the cause of joint inflammation and swelling and also helps relieve the associated pain. If glucose testing of synovial fluid is to be included, the patient must fast for 6 to 12 hours before the test; otherwise, restriction of food or fluids is not required before the test. Inform the patient that a local anesthetic will be given, but the needle will cause transient pain when it penetrates the joint capsule.

Make sure that the patient or a responsible family member has signed a consent form. Check the patient's history for hypersensitivity to iodine compounds (such as povidone-iodine), procaine, lidocaine, or other local anesthetics. A sedative may be administered as needed.

Equipment   Surgical detergent; skin antiseptic (usually tincture
of povidone-iodine); alcohol sponges; local anesthetic (1% or 2% procaine or lidocaine); sterile, disposable 1½″, 25G needle; sterile, disposable 1½″ to
2″, 20G needle; sterile 5-ml syringe for injecting anesthetic; sterile 20-ml syringe for aspiration; 3-ml
syringe for administering a sedative; 2″ × 2″ sterile
gauze pads; sterile dressings; sterile drapes; elastic
bandage; tubes for culture and cytologic, clot, and
glucose analyses; anticoagulants (heparin, EDTA,
and potassium oxalate); venipuncture equipment
   For corticosteroid administration: corticosteroid
suspension, such as hydrocortisone, 2-ml and 5-ml
syringes (or one 10-ml syringe if procaine and a corticosteroid are to be injected simultaneously)

Procedure   Instruct the patient to assume a supine position
with the knee fully extended and explain that this
position must be maintained throughout the procedure. Warn that insertion of the needle will probably cause some discomfort. (A sedative is sometimes ordered for a young child.) Clean the skin
over the puncture site with surgical detergent and
alcohol. Paint the site with tincture of povidone-iodine, and allow it to air-dry for 2 minutes. After the
local anesthetic is administered, the aspirating needle is quickly inserted through the skin, subcutaneous tissue, and synovial membrane, into the joint
space. As much fluid as possible is aspirated into
the syringe; a minimum of 10 to 15 ml should be
obtained, although a lesser amount is usually adequate for analysis. The joint (except for the area
around the puncture site) may be wrapped with an
elastic bandage to compress the free fluid into this
portion of the sac, ensuring maximal collection of
fluid.
   If a corticosteroid is being injected, the syringe is
detached, leaving the needle in the joint, and the
syringe containing the corticosteroid attached to
the needle instead. After the corticosteroid is injected and the needle withdrawn, wipe the puncture
site with alcohol. Apply pressure to the site for
about 2 minutes to prevent bleeding, then apply a
sterile dressing.
   Add anticoagulants to the specimen, according
to the laboratory tests requested. Gently invert the
tube several times to mix the specimen and anticoagulant adequately. *For cultures,* obtain 2 to 5 ml of
synovial fluid and, if possible, inoculate the medium
immediately. Otherwise, add 1 or 2 drops of heparin

Normal synovial fluid values

	Range	Mean
pH	7.3 to 7.43	7.38
White blood cells (WBCs) per mm^3	13 to 180	63
WBC differential count		
Polymorphonuclear	0 to 25	7
Lymphocytes	0 to 78	24
Monocytes	0 to 71	48
Clasmatocytes	0 to 26	10
Synovial lining cells	0 to 12	4
Total protein (g/dl)	1.2 to 3.0	1.8
Albumin (%)	56 to 63	60
Globulin (%)	37 to 44	40
Hyaluronate (g/dl)		0.3

Adapted with permission from McCarty, D. (ed). *Arthritis & Allied Conditions: A Textbook of Rheumatology,* 12th ed. Baltimore: Williams & Wilkins, 1992.

to the specimen. *For cytologic analysis,* add 5 mg of EDTA or 1 or 2 drops of heparin to 2 to 5 ml of synovial fluid. *For glucose analysis,* add potassium oxalate, as specified by the laboratory, to 3 to 5 ml of synovial fluid. *For crystal examination,* add heparin, if specified by the laboratory. *For other studies,* such as general appearance and clot evaluation, obtain 2 to 5 ml of synovial fluid, but don't add an anticoagulant.

Send the properly labeled specimens to the laboratory immediately — gonococci are particularly labile. If a white blood cell (WBC) count is being performed, clearly label the specimen "Synovial Fluid" and "Caution — Don't use acid diluents." If glucose is being measured, perform a venipuncture to obtain a blood sample for glucose analysis.

Precautions   Adhere to strict aseptic technique throughout aspiration to prevent contamination of joint space or the synovial fluid specimen.

Findings   Examination of synovial fluid in the laboratory can take many forms. Routine examination includes gross analysis for color, clarity, quantity, viscosity, pH, and the presence of a mucin clot, as well as

Examples of diseases producing fluids of different groups

Noninflammatory (Group I)	Inflammatory† (Group II)	Purulent† (Group III)	Hemorrhagic (Group IV)
Osteoarthritis	Rheumatoid arthritis	Bacterial infections	Trauma, especially fracture
Early rheumatoid arthritis	Reiter's syndrome	Tuberculosis	Neuroarthropathy (Charcot's joint)
Trauma	Crystal synovitis, acute (gout, pseudogout, other)		Blood dyscrasia (such as hemophilia)
Osteochondritis dissecans	Psoriatic arthritis		Tumor, especially pigmented villo-nodular synovitis or hemangioma
Osteochondromatosis	Arthritis of inflammatory bowel disease		
Crystal synovitis, chronic or subsiding acute (gout and pseudogout)	Viral arthritis		Chondrocalcinosis
Systemic lupus erythematosus*	Rheumatic fever		Anticoagulant therapy
Polyarteritis nodosa*	Behçet's syndrome		Joint prostheses
Scleroderma	Fat droplet synovitis		Thrombocytosis
Amyloidosis (articular)			Sickle cell trait or disease
Polymyalgia rheumatica			Myeloproliferative disease
High-dose cortico-steroid therapy			

* May occasionally be inflammatory.
† As a disease in these groups remits, the exudate (fluid) passes through a group I phase before returning to normal.

Adapted with permission from McCarty, D. (ed). *Arthritis & Allied Conditions: A Textbook of Rheumatology*, 12th ed. Baltimore: Williams & Wilkins, 1992.

microscopic analysis for WBC count and differential. Special examination includes microbiological analysis for formed elements (including crystals) and bacteria, serologic analysis, and chemical analysis for such components as glucose, protein, and enzymes. (See *Normal synovial fluid values,* page 584.)

Implications of results	Examination of synovial fluid may reveal various diseases (see *Examples of diseases producing fluids of different groups,* above, and *Gross analysis of joint fluid,* page 586) including noninflammatory disease (traumatic arthritis and osteoarthritis), inflammatory disease (systemic lupus erythematosus, rheumatic fever, pseudogout, gout, and rheumatoid arthritis), and septic disease (tuberculous and septic arthritis).

Gross analysis of joint fluid

Criteria	Normal	Noninflammatory (Group I)	Inflammatory (Group II)	Purulent (Group III)
Volume (knee)	< 4 ml	often > 4 ml	often > 4 ml	often > 4 ml
Color	Clear to pale yellow	Xanthochromic	Xanthochromic to white	White
Clarity	Transparent	Transparent	Translucent to opaque	Opaque
Viscosity	Extremely high	High	Low	Extremely low, may be high with coagulase-positive staphylococcus
Mucin clot*	Good	Fair to good	Fair to poor	Poor
Spontaneous clot	None	Often	Often	Often

* Recent effusions do not give firm clot because of serum admixture.

Adapted with permission from McCarty, D. (ed). *Arthritis & Allied Conditions: A Textbook of Rheumatology,* 12th ed. Baltimore: Williams & Wilkins, 1992.

Post-test care
- Apply ice or cold packs to the affected joint for 24 to 36 hours after aspiration, to decrease pain and swelling. Use pillows to support painful joints. If a large quantity of fluid was aspirated, apply an elastic bandage to stabilize the joint.
- If the patient's condition permits, he may resume normal activity immediately after the procedure. However, warn against excessive use of the joint for a few days after the test, even though pain and swelling may have subsided. Excessive use may cause transient pain, swelling, and stiffness.
- Carefully handle the dressings and linens of patients who have drainage from the joint space, especially if septic arthritis is confirmed or suspected.
- The patient may resume his usual diet.

➤ *Clinical alert:* Monitor the patient for increased pain or fever, which may indicate joint infection.

Interfering
factors

- Acid diluents added to the specimen for WBC count precipitate the mucin and alter the cell count.
- Failure to mix the specimen and the anticoagulant adequately or to send the specimens to the laboratory immediately may cause inaccurate test results.
- Failure to follow pretest dietary restrictions can affect glucose levels.
- Contamination of the specimen can invalidate test results.

T

Testosterone

The principal androgen secreted by the interstitial cells of the testes (Leydig's cells), testosterone induces puberty in the male and maintains male secondary sex characteristics.

Testosterone production begins to increase at onset of puberty, under the influence of luteinizing hormone (LH) from the anterior pituitary, and continues to rise during adulthood. Testosterone inhibits gonadotropin secretion by a negative feedback mechanism similar to that of ovarian hormones in females. Production begins to taper off at about age 40, eventually dropping to approximately one-fifth the peak level by age 80. In females, the adrenal glands and the ovaries secrete small amounts of testosterone.

This radioimmunoassay measures plasma or serum testosterone levels and, when combined with plasma gonadotropin levels (follicle-stimulating hormone and LH), reliably aids evaluation of gonadal dysfunction in males and females.

Purpose
- To facilitate differential diagnosis of male sexual precocity before age 10 (true precocious puberty must be distinguished from pseudoprecocious puberty)
- To aid differential diagnosis of hypogonadism (primary hypogonadism must be distinguished from secondary hypogonadism)
- To evaluate male infertility or other sexual dysfunction
- To evaluate hirsutism and virilization in females

Patient preparation
Explain that this test helps evaluate secretion of male sex hormone. Inform the patient that restriction of food or fluids is not required and that the test requires a blood sample.

Procedure
Perform a venipuncture, and collect the sample in a 7-ml *red-top* tube. Use a *green-top* (heparinized) tube if plasma is to be collected. Indicate the patient's age, sex, and history of hormone therapy on the laboratory slip. Handle the sample gently to prevent hemolysis, and send it to the laboratory.

The sample is stable at room temperature and requires no refrigeration or preservative for up to 1 week. Frozen samples are stable for at least 6 months.

Values

Normal levels of testosterone are as follows —
Males: 300 to 1,200 ng/dl (10.5 to 42 nmol/L)
Females: 30 to 95 ng/dl (1.0 to 3.0 nmol/L)
Prepubertal children: in males, less than 100 ng/dl (3.5 nmol/L); in females, less than 40 ng/dl (1.5 nmol/L).

Testosterone values vary slightly among laboratories.

Implications of results

Elevated testosterone levels in prepubertal males may indicate true sexual precocity, caused by excessive gonadotropin secretion, or pseudoprecocious puberty, caused by secretions of male hormone by a testicular tumor. They can also indicate congenital adrenal hyperplasia, which results in virilization and precocious puberty in males (between ages 2 and 3) and pseudohermaphroditism and milder virilization in females (during and after puberty). Increased testosterone levels can also occur with a benign adrenal tumor or cancer, hyperthyroidism, or incipient puberty. In females with ovarian tumors or polycystic ovary syndrome, testosterone levels may rise slightly, leading to hirsutism.

Depressed testosterone levels can indicate primary hypogonadism (testicular failure, as in Klinefelter's syndrome) or secondary hypogonadism (hypogonadotropic eunuchoidism) resulting from hypothalamic-pituitary dysfunction. Depressed testosterone levels can also follow orchiectomy, testicular or prostatic cancer, delayed male puberty, estrogen therapy, or cirrhosis of the liver.

Post-test care

If a hematoma develops at the venipuncture site, applying warm soaks eases discomfort.

Interfering factors

• Exogenous sources of estrogens or androgens can interfere with test results. Estrogens decrease free testosterone levels by increasing sex hormone-binding globulin (SHBG), which binds testosterone; androgens can elevate these levels. Both thyroid and growth hormones decrease SHBG and increase levels of free testosterone. Other pituitary-based hormones may also influence test results.

- Hemolysis caused by excessive agitation of the sample may affect test results.

Tetrahydrocannabinol (THC), urine

Delta-9 tetrahydrocannabinol, commonly referred to as THC, is the major psychologically active constituent of the marijuana plant (*Cannabis sativa*). Ingestion of THC results in intoxication, of varying severity, depending on the dose and frequency of use. Of the several THC metabolites identified in human urine, the major one is 11-nor-Δ-tetrahydrocannabinol-9-carboxylic acid (THC-COOH), which exists in urine in the free or conjugated state as a glucuronide.

To determine marijuana use, most analytic techniques for THC metabolites in urine are directed toward THC-COOH. The length of time THC metabolites remain in the body varies, depending on the individual's metabolic rate, frequency and amount of drug use, and time of last ingestion. Generally, analysis can detect drug ingestion up to 6 weeks after the last ingestion in a chronic user and up to 3 days after the last ingestion in an occasional user.

The analysis is usually carried out in two stages, screening and confirmation testing. Immunoassays (radioimmunoassays or enzyme immunoassays) are the most commonly used methods for screening urine specimens for THC metabolites. Confirmation of immunoassay results requires any of several chromatographic techniques. However, gas chromatography-mass spectrometry (GCMS) is the most reliable method known and the one most recommended for confirmation, particularly when the test results are needed for forensic purposes.

Purpose To determine the presence and level of THC metabolites in the body

Patient preparation Explain that this test determines recent use of marijuana or hashish and that the test requires a urine specimen. Inform the patient that restriction of food or fluids is not required. Teach the proper collection techniques. Make sure that the patient or a responsible family member has signed an appropriate consent form. Thoroughly check the patient's recent medication history, noting time and route of administration of all drugs.

Procedure   Collect a random urine specimen. The first morning void usually contains higher levels than later voids.

Send the specimen to the laboratory immediately. If the specimen will be sent to an outside laboratory for analysis or, if testing will be delayed for more than 72 hours, freeze the specimen to minimize decomposition.

Findings   Normally, no THC metabolites are found in urine.

Implications of results   A positive test for THC metabolites confirmed by GCMS indicates ingestion of marijuana or hashish or passive exposure through inhalation. (However, a THC-COOH level higher than 20 ng/dl [200 µg/L] usually indicates drug ingestion rather than passive exposure.)

Post-test care   None

Interfering factor   Delayed analysis of an unfrozen specimen may result in misleading test results.

Throat culture

A throat culture is used primarily to isolate and identify group A beta-hemolytic streptococci (*Streptococcus pyogenes*) — thereby allowing early treatment of streptococcal pharyngitis — and to prevent sequelae, such as rheumatic heart disease or glomerulonephritis. This test is also used to screen for carriers of *Neisseria meningitidis*. Rarely, a throat culture may be used to identify *Corynebacterium diphtheriae, Bordetella pertussis*, or *N. gonorrhoeae*.

This test requires swabbing the throat, streaking a culture plate, and allowing the organisms to grow, for isolation and identification of pathogens. Culture results necessitate correlation with the patient's clinical status and recent antibiotic therapy and the amount of normal flora.

Purpose   • To isolate and identify pathogens, such as group A beta-hemolytic streptococci, *C. diphtheriae, B. pertussis*, and *N. gonorrhoeae*
• To screen asymptomatic carriers of pathogens, especially carriers of *N. meningitidis*

Patient
preparation

Explain the purpose of this test and that restriction of food or fluids is not required. Describe the procedure, and warn the patient that he may gag when the throat is swabbed.

Check the patient's medication history for recent antibiotic therapy. Determine his immunization history if it's relevant to the preliminary diagnosis. Procure the throat specimen before antibiotic therapy begins.

Equipment

Tongue blade, sterile cotton-tipped applicator and culture tube with a transport medium (or commercial collection and transport system)

Procedure

Tell the patient to tilt his head back and close his eyes. With the throat well illuminated, check for inflamed areas, using a tongue blade. Swab the tonsillar areas from side to side; include any inflamed or purulent sites. Don't touch the tongue, cheeks, or teeth with the cotton-tipped applicator. Immediately place the applicator in the culture tube. If using a commercial sterile collection and transport system, crush the ampule and force the applicator into the medium to keep the applicator moist. To protect the specimen and prevent its exposure to pathogens, use aseptic technique during the procedure, and observe proper precautions when sending the specimen to the laboratory.

Note recent antibiotic therapy on the laboratory slip. Label the specimen, including the date and time of collection, and the origin of the specimen. Also indicate the suspected organism, especially *C. diphtheriae,* which requires a culture using two applicators and a special growth medium; *B. pertussis,* which requires a nasopharyngeal culture and a special growth medium; and *Neisseria* organisms, which require cultures using enriched selective media.

Send the specimen to the laboratory immediately to prevent bacterial growth or deterioration. If a commercial sterile collection and transport system is not being used, keep the container upright during transport.

Findings

Normal throat flora include nonhemolytic and alpha-hemolytic streptococci, *Neisseria* organisms, staphylococci, diphtheroids, some haemophilii, pneumococci, yeasts, and enteric gram-negative rods.

Implications of
results

Possible pathogens identified in a culture include group A beta-hemolytic streptococci (*S. pyogenes*), which can cause scarlet fever or pharyngitis; *Candida albicans*, which can cause thrush; *Corynebacterium diphtheriae*, which can cause diphtheria; and *B. pertussis* and *N. gonorrhoeae*, which can cause whooping cough. The laboratory report should indicate the prevalent organisms and the quantity of pathogens found.

Post-test care None

Interfering
factors

- Failure to report recent or current antibiotic therapy on the laboratory slip may cause erroneous evaluation of bacterial growth.
- Failure to send the specimen to the laboratory promptly may permit bacterial growth or deterioration.
- Failure to use the proper transport media may cause the specimen to dry out and the bacteria to die.

Thyroid biopsy

Thyroid biopsy is the excision of a thyroid gland tissue specimen for histologic examination. This procedure is indicated in patients with thyroid enlargement or nodules (even if serum triiodothyronine [T_3] and serum thyroxine [T_4] levels are normal), breathing and swallowing difficulties, vocal cord paralysis, weight loss, hemoptysis, and a sensation of fullness in the neck. Thyroid biopsy commonly is performed when noninvasive tests, such as thyroid ultrasonography and scan, are abnormal or inconclusive.

Thyroid tissue may be obtained with a hollow needle after a local anesthetic is administered or during open (surgical) biopsy under general anesthesia. Open biopsy, performed in the operating room, is obviously more complex and provides more accurate information than needle biopsy. In open biopsy, the surgeon obtains a tissue specimen from the exposed thyroid gland, and sends it to the histology laboratory for rapid analysis. This method also permits direct examination and immediate excision of suspicious thyroid tissue.

Coagulation studies should always precede thyroid biopsy.

Purpose
- To differentiate between benign and malignant thyroid disease
- To help diagnose Hashimoto's thyroiditis, subacute granulomatous thyroiditis, hyperthyroidism, and nontoxic nodular goiter

Patient preparation

Describe the procedure and answer the patient's questions. Explain that this test permits microscopic examination of a thyroid tissue specimen. Inform the patient that restriction of food or fluids is not required (unless the patient will receive general anesthesia). Make sure that the patient or a responsible family member has signed a consent form. Check for hypersensitivity to anesthetics or analgesics.

Tell the patient that a local anesthetic will be given to minimize pain during the procedure, but warn that some pressure may be felt when the tissue specimen is procured. Advise the patient that he may have a sore throat the day after the test. The patient may benefit from administration of a sedative 15 minutes before biopsy.

Procedure

For needle biopsy, the patient is placed in a supine position, with a pillow under the shoulder blades. (This position pushes the trachea and thyroid forward and allows the neck veins to fall backward.) The skin over the biopsy site is then prepared. As the examiner prepares to inject the local anesthetic, warn the patient not to swallow. After the anesthetic is injected, the carotid artery is palpated, and the biopsy needle is inserted parallel to and about 3″ (7.5 cm) from the thyroid cartilage, to prevent damage to the deep structures and larynx. When the specimen is obtained, the needle is removed, and the specimen placed immediately in formaldehyde because cell breakdown in the tissue specimen begins after excision.

Apply pressure to the biopsy site to stop bleeding. If bleeding continues for more than a few minutes, press on the site for up to an additional 15 minutes. Apply an adhesive bandage. Bleeding may persist in a patient with abnormal prothrombin time (PT) or abnormal activated partial thromboplastin time (APTT), or in a patient with a large vascular thyroid, with distended veins.

Precautions Thyroid biopsy should be performed cautiously in patients with coagulation defects indicated by abnormal PT or APTT.

Findings Histologic examination of normal tissue shows fibrous networks dividing the gland into pseudolobules that comprise follicles and capillaries. Cuboidal epithelium lines the follicle walls and contains the protein thyroglobulin, which stores T_4 and T_3.

Implications of results Malignant tumors appear as well encapsulated, solitary nodules of uniform but abnormal structure. Papillary carcinoma is the most common thyroid malignancy. Follicular carcinoma, a less common form, strongly resembles normal cells.

Benign tumors — such as nontoxic nodular goiter — demonstrate hypertrophy, hyperplasia, and hypervascularity. Distinct histologic patterns characterize subacute granulomatous thyroiditis, Hashimoto's thyroiditis, and hyperthyroidism.

Because malignant tumors of the thyroid gland are frequently multicentric and small, a negative histologic report doesn't rule out malignant disease.

Post-test care
- For comfort, place the patient in semi-Fowler's position. Suggest that putting both hands behind his neck when attempting to sit up avoids undue strain on the biopsy site.
- Keep the biopsy site clean and dry.

➤ *Clinical alert:* Watch for signs of bleeding, tenderness, or redness at the biopsy site. Observe for difficult breathing caused by edema or hematoma, with resultant tracheal collapse. Check the back of the neck and the patient's pillow for bleeding every hour for 8 hours. Report bleeding immediately.

Interfering factor Failure to obtain a representative tissue specimen or to place the specimen in formaldehyde solution may prevent accurate determination of test results.

Thyroid-stimulating hormone (TSH), neonatal

Neonatal thyrotropin

This radioimmunoassay confirms congenital hypothyroidism after an initial screening test detects low serum thyroxine (T_4) levels. Normally, thyroid-stimulating hormone (TSH) levels surge soon after birth, triggering a rise in thyroid hormone, which is essential for neurologic development. However, in primary congenital hypothyroidism, the thyroid gland doesn't respond to TSH stimulation, resulting in diminished thyroid hormone levels and elevated TSH levels. Early detection and treatment of congenital hypothyroidism is critical in preventing mental retardation and cretinism. Increasingly, neonatal TSH testing is being used as the first-line screening test for congenital hypothyroidism, replacing T_4.

Purpose To confirm diagnosis of congenital hypothyroidism

Patient preparation Explain to the parents the purpose of the test. Emphasize the test's importance in detecting the disorder early so that prompt therapy can prevent irreversible brain damage.

Equipment *For a filter paper sample:* alcohol or povidone-iodine sponges, sterile lancet, specially marked filter paper, $2'' \times 2''$ sterile gauze pads, adhesive bandage, labels
For a serum sample: venipuncture equipment

Procedure *For a filter paper sample:* Assemble the necessary equipment and wash your hands thoroughly. Wipe the infant's heel with an alcohol or povidone-iodine sponge, then dry it thoroughly with a gauze pad. Perform a heelstick. Squeezing the infant's heel gently, fill the circles on the filter paper with blood. Make sure the blood saturates the paper. Gently apply pressure with a gauze pad to ensure hemostasis at the puncture site. Allow the filter paper to dry, label it appropriately, and send it to the laboratory.
For a serum sample: Perform a venipuncture and collect the sample in a 5-ml *red-top* tube. Label the sample and send it to the laboratory immediately.

Values At age 1 to 2 days, TSH levels are normally 25 to 30 µIU/ml (U/L). Thereafter, levels for infants and children are normally similar to adult levels.

Implications of results Neonatal TSH levels must be interpreted in light of T_4 concentrations. Elevated TSH accompanied by decreased T_4 indicates primary congenital hypothyroidism (thyroid gland dysfunction). Depressed

TSH and T_4 may be present in secondary congenital hypothyroidism (pituitary or hypothalamic dysfunction). Normal TSH accompanied by depressed T_4 may be caused by a congenital defect in thyroxine-binding globulin (in this case, free thyroxine would be normal) or may indicate transient congenital hypothyroidism caused by prematurity or prenatal hypoxia. A complete thyroid workup must be performed to confirm the cause of hypothyroidism before treatment can begin.

Post-test care
If a hematoma develops at the venipuncture site, apply warm soaks. Heelsticks require no special care.

Interfering factors
- Corticosteroids, T_3, and T_4 lower TSH levels; lithium carbonate, potassium iodide, excessive topical resorcinol, and TSH injection elevate TSH levels.
- Failure to let a filter paper sample dry completely may alter test results.
- Excessive agitation of a serum sample may cause hemolysis and may interfere with accurate testing.

Thyroid-stimulating hormone (TSH), serum, high sensitivity
Thyrotropin

Thyroid-stimulating hormone (TSH) is a glycoprotein secreted by the anterior pituitary gland after stimulation by thyrotropin-releasing hormone (TRH) from the hypothalamus. TSH stimulates an increase in the size, number, and secretory activity of thyroid cells and stimulates the release of triiodothyronine (T_3) and thyroxine (T_4). These hormones exert a generalized effect on total body metabolism and are essential for normal growth and development.

This test measures serum TSH levels by radioimmunoassay. It's a reliable test for primary hypothyroidism and helps determine whether hypothyroidism results from thyroid gland failure, or from pituitary or hypothalamic dysfunction. Normal serum TSH levels rule out primary hypothyroidism because the absence of thyroid hormone in the serum stimulates pituitary hypersecretion of TSH through negative feedback.

Purpose
- To distinguish between primary and secondary hypothyroidism
- To confirm or rule out primary hypothyroidism
- To monitor drug therapy in patients with primary hypothyroidism
- To diagnose hyperthyroidism

Patient preparation
Explain that this test helps assess thyroid gland function, and tell the patient that the test requires a blood sample. As appropriate, withhold corticosteroids, thyroid hormones, and other drugs that may influence test results. If these medications must be continued, note this on the laboratory slip. Keep the patient relaxed and recumbent for 30 minutes before the test.

Procedure
Perform a venipuncture between 6 a.m. and 8 a.m.; collect the sample in a 5-ml *red-top* tube. Handle the sample gently to prevent hemolysis.

Values
Normal values for adults and children largely depend on the assay used; but values range from 0.25 to 3.5 mIU/ml (U/L).

Implications of results
TSH levels that exceed 10 µIU/ml (U/L) suggest primary hypothyroidism. TSH levels may be slightly elevated in euthyroid patients with certain disorders.

TSH levels less than 0.1 mIU/ml indicate secondary hypothyroidism (with inadequate secretion of TSH or TRH), hyperthyroidism (Graves' disease) or thyroiditis; both are marked by hypersecretion of thyroid hormones, which suppresses TSH release.

Post-test care
If a hematoma develops at the venipuncture site, applying warm soaks eases discomfort.

Interfering factors
- Failure to observe restrictions of medications may cause spurious test results. Aspirin, corticosteroids, T_3, and heparin lower TSH levels; lithium carbonate and potassium iodide raise them.
- Radioactive scan performed within 1 week before the test may influence test results.
- Falsely elevated TSH levels may occur in patients with choriocarcinoma, hydatidiform mole, embryonal carcinoma of the testes; and in pregnant or postmenopausal patients.

- Hemolysis caused by excessive agitation of the sample may affect test results.

Thyroid-stimulating hormone, sensitive (s-TSH), serum

s-TSH assay

The thyroid-stimulating hormone (TSH, or thyrotropin) modulates metabolism by regulating production of thyroid hormones thyroxine (T_4) and triiodothyronine (T_3). Usually, TSH production is inversely related to the levels of these hormones. Low T_4 or T_3 levels, associated with primary hypothyroidism, cause TSH elevation. High T_4 or T_3 levels, associated with primary hyperthyroidism, cause TSH suppression.

Purpose
- To differentiate diagnosis of primary hypothyroidism from pituitary hyperthyroidism
- To monitor therapy in hypothyroidism or hyperthyroidism (radioiodine or surgery)

Patient preparation
Explain that this test helps evaluate thyroid function and that the test requires a blood sample.

Procedure
Perform a venipuncture, and collect the sample in a *red-top* tube.

Handle the sample gently, and send it to the laboratory immediately. Note on the laboratory slip if the patient received radioactive iodine 48 hours before the test.

Values
Normal serum values vary among assay methods but usually range between 0.4 to 10 mIU/liter (U/L).

Implications of results
TSH levels are high in primary hypothyroidism, and are low in hyperthyroidism. Low levels of TSH occur with excessive thyroid replacement. Hypothyroid patients who have a head injury may have a normal TSH level.

Post-test care
If a hematoma develops at the venipuncture site, applying warm soaks eases discomfort.

Interfering factors
- Hemolysis caused by excessive agitation of the sample affects test results.
- TSH levels may be affected by dopamine, glucocorticoids, and severe illness.

Thyroid-stimulating immunoglobulin, serum
TSI, TSIg, thyroid-stimulating antibody, thyroid-stimulating autoantibody

Thyroid stimulating immunoglobulin (TSI) is an immunoglobulin present in the blood of most patients with Graves' disease. This autoantibody reacts with cell-surface receptors that usually combine with thyroid-stimulating hormone (TSH). TSI reacts with these receptors, activates intracellular enzymes, and promotes epithelial cell activity outside the normal feedback regulation mechanism for TSH.

TSI stimulates the thyroid gland to produce and excrete excessive amounts of thyroid hormones.

Purpose
To diagnose Graves' disease and hyperthyroidism

Patient preparation
Explain that this test helps evaluate thyroid function and that the test requires a blood sample.

Procedure
Perform a venipuncture, and collect a 5-ml sample of blood in a *red-top* tube. Handle the sample gently to prevent hemolysis. Note on the laboratory slip if the patient received radioactive iodine 48 hours before the test.

Findings
TSI is not normally present in the serum. However, 4% of normal patients show false-positive levels.

Implications of results
Increased levels of TSI are associated with Graves' disease and hyperthyroidism.

Post-test care
If a hematoma develops at the venipuncture site, applying warm soaks eases discomfort.

Interfering factors
- Administration of radioactive iodine within 48 hours of the test may alter test results.
- Hemolysis caused by excessive agitation of the sample may interfere with accurate test results.

Thyroxine, free, and triiodothyronine, free, serum

These tests, often done simultaneously, measure serum levels of free thyroxine (FT_4) and free triiodothyronine (FT_3), the minute portions of T_4 and T_3 not bound to thyroxine-binding globulin (TBG) and other serum proteins. As the active components of T_4 and T_3, these unbound hormones enter target cells and are responsible for the thyroid gland's effects on cellular metabolism. Because levels of circulating FT_4 and FT_3 are regulated by a feedback mechanism that adusts total hormone levels to compensate for changes in binding protein concentrations, measurement of free hormone levels is the best indicator of thyroid function. Disagreement exists as to whether FT_4 or FT_3 is the better indicator; therefore, laboratories commonly measure both. The disadvantages of these tests include a cumbersome and difficult laboratory method, inaccessibility, and cost. This test may be useful in the 5% of patients in whom sensitive TSH and total T_4 tests fail to produce diagnostic results.

Purpose
- To measure the metabolically active form of the thyroid hormones
- To aid diagnosis of hyperthyroidism or hypothyroidism

Patient preparation
Inform the patient that this special test helps evaluate thyroid function and that the test requires a blood sample.

Procedure
Draw venous blood into a 7-ml *red-top* tube. Handle the sample gently to prevent hemolysis.

Values
Normal range for FT_4 is from 1 to 3 ng/dl (13 to 39 pmol/L); for FT_3, from 0.2 to 0.6 ng/dl (3 to 9 pmol/L). Values vary, depending on the laboratory.

Implications of results
Elevated FT_4 and FT_3 levels indicate hyperthyroidism, unless peripheral resistance to thyroid hormone is present. T_3 toxicosis, a rare form of hyperthyroidism, yields high FT_3 levels, with normal or low FT_4 values. Low FT_4 levels usually indicate hypothyroidism, except in patients receiving replacement therapy with T_3. Patients receiving thyroid agents may have varying levels of FT_4 and FT_3, de-

pending on the thyroid preparation used and the time of sample collection.

Post-test care   If a hematoma develops at the venipuncture site, applying warm soaks eases discomfort.

Interfering   Except for hemolysis that can result from exces-
factors   sive agitation of the sample, this test is virtually free of interfering factors. Agents that compete with T_4 and T_3 binding to TBG increase FT_4 fraction; this does not affect in vitro TBG studies because of serum dilution. Depending on the dosage, thyroid therapy may increase FT_4 or FT_3 levels. However, these medications should not be withheld; serial tests may be performed to evaluate thyroid function.

Thyroxine (T_4), serum

Thyroxine (T_4) is secreted by the thyroid gland in response to thyroid-stimulating hormone (TSH) from the pituitary gland and, indirectly, to thyrotropin-releasing hormone (TRH) from the hypothalamus. The rate of T_4 secretion is normally regulated by a complex system of negative and positive feedback involving the thyroid, anterior pituitary, and hypothalamus. Through the iodination of the amino acid tyrosine, monoiodotyrosine (T_1) and diiodotyrosine (T_2) are formed. Two T_2 molecules join to form a single T_4 molecule. (T_3 is formed by the joining of a T_1 molecule and a T_2 molecule.)

Only a fraction of T_4 (about 0.3%) circulates freely in the blood; the rest binds strongly to plasma proteins, primarily thyroxine-binding globulin (TBG). This minute fraction is responsible for the clinical effects of thyroid hormone on body cells and tissues. Because of the tenacity of TBG's binding power, T_4 survives in the plasma for a relatively long time, with a half-life of about 6 days. This radioimmunoassay, one of the most common diagnostic indicators of thyroid function, measures the total circulating T_4 level when TBG is normal. Free thyroxine, the active hormone, can also be measured directly, thereby avoiding erroneous results due to abnormalities and fluctuations of TBG.

Purpose   • To evaluate thyroid function
• To aid diagnosis of hyperthyroidism and hypothyroidism

- To monitor response to treatment with antithyroid medication in hyperthyroidism, and to monitor response to thyroid replacement therapy in hypothyroidism

Patient preparation

Explain that this test helps evaluate thyroid gland function. Inform the patient that fasting or restriction of physical activity is not required, and that the test requires a blood sample.

As appropriate, withhold medications that may interfere with test results. If such medications must be continued, note this on the laboratory slip. (If this test is being performed to monitor thyroid therapy, the patient continues to receive daily thyroid replacement.)

Procedure

Perform a venipuncture, and collect the sample in a 7-ml *red-top* tube. Send the sample to the laboratory immediately so that the serum may be separated. Handle the sample gently to prevent hemolysis.

Values

Normally, total T_4 levels range from 5 to 13.5 mcg/dl (64 to 174 nmol/L) and free T_4 levels range from 1 to 3 ng/dl (13 to 39 pmol/L).

Implications of results

Abnormally elevated levels of T_4 are consistent with primary and secondary hyperthyroidism, including excessive T_4 (L-thyroxine sodium) replacement therapy (factitious or iatrogenic hyperthyroidism). Conversely, subnormal levels suggest primary or secondary hypothyroidism, or may be caused by T_4 suppression by normal, elevated, or replacement levels of T_3. In doubtful cases of hypothyroidism, TSH levels or TRH test may be indicated.

A normal T_4 level, however, is no guarantee of euthyroidism; for example, normal levels occur in T_3 thyrotoxicosis and in some cases of mild hypothyroidism. In the presence of overt signs of hyperthyroidism, therefore, further testing is necessary.

Post-test care

- If a hematoma develops at the venipuncture site, applying warm soaks eases discomfort.
- The patient may resume discontinued medications.

Interfering factors

- Hemolysis caused by excessive agitation or stasis of the sample may interfere with accurate test results.

- Hereditary factors and some hepatic diseases can decrease or increase TBG concentration; protein-wasting diseases (nephrotic syndrome) and androgens may also reduce TBG. Thus, TBG levels can interfere with accurate determination of total T_4 levels.

Thyroxine-binding globulin (TBG), serum

This test measures the serum level of thyroxine-binding globulin (TBG), the predominant protein carrier for circulating thyroxine (T_4) and triiodothyronine (T_3). Values for TBG levels may be identified by radioimmunoassay.

Any condition that affects TBG levels and subsequent binding capacity also affects the amount of free T_4 (FT_4) and free T_3 (FT_3) in circulation. This can be clinically significant because only FT_4 and FT_3 are metabolically active.

Purpose
- To determine T_4 binding capacity for differentiation of patients with high T_4 levels caused by hyperthyroidism and individuals with normally high T_4 levels
- To identify TBG abnormalities

Patient preparation
Inform the patient that this test helps evaluate thyroid function and that the test requires a blood sample.

Withhold estrogens, perphenazine, and tamoxifen because these medications can increase TBG levels. If these medications must be continued, note this on the laboratory slip. (For example, they may be continued to determine if prescribed drugs are affecting TBG levels.) Also note on the laboratory slip if the patient received radioactive isotopes during the past week.

Procedure
Draw venous blood into a *red-top* tube. Handle the sample gently to prevent hemolysis.

Values
Normal values range from 25 to 52 µg/dl (270 to 669 nmol/L).

Implications of results
TBG levels rise during pregnancy and may be high in infants. Hepatitis and other liver diseases may also increase TBG levels. Low TBG levels may be

present in chronic liver disease, nephrosis, acromegaly, and large amounts of glucosteroids, androgens, and anabolic steroids.

Patients with TBG abnormalities require additional testing, such as the serum FT_3 and the serum FT_4 tests, to evaluate thyroid function more precisely.

Post-test care
- If a hematoma develops at the venipuncture site, applying warm soaks eases discomfort.
- The patient may resume discontinued medications.

Interfering factors
- Estrogens (including oral contraceptives), tamoxifen, and perphenazine elevate TBG levels.
- Androgens, prednisone, phenytoin, and high doses of salicylates depress TBG levels.
- Hemolysis caused by excessive agitation of the sample may interfere with accurate determination of test results.

Tocainide, serum

This quantitative analysis, done by high-performance liquid chromatography, measures serum levels of tocainide hydrochloride to identify subtherapeutic, therapeutic, and potentially toxic doses during initial dose titration and maintenance therapy. An oral antiarrhythmic agent, tocainide has Class 1B antiarrhythmic properties similar to those of lidocaine and, like lidocaine, is indicated for the treatment of ventricular arrhythmias.

Purpose
- To monitor therapeutic levels of tocainide
- To detect drug toxicity and monitor its treatment

Patient preparation
Explain that this test helps determine the safest and most effective dosage of tocainide. Inform the patient that restriction of foods or fluids is not required before the test and that the test requires a blood sample. Before sample collection, review the patient's history for use of other drugs.

Procedure
Perform a venipuncture, and collect a trough-level or peak-level sample, as ordered, in a *red-, green-,* or *lavender-top* tube, as directed by the testing laboratory. Record the date and time of the last drug dose

and the time of sample collection on the laboratory slip.

Handle the sample gently to prevent hemolysis, and send it to the laboratory immediately.

Values
The therapeutic range for serum tocainide is 4 to 10 µg/ml.

Implications of results
Trough levels guide the adjustment of therapeutic dosage; peak levels can detect toxicity and monitor its treatment. Because adverse effects of tocainide (commonly GI disturbances, vertigo, dizziness, blurred vision, paresthesias, tremor) increase with greater drug concentration, even within the therapeutic range, the lowest effective dose should be prescribed for long-term therapy. At therapeutic serum concentrations, 24-hour continuous electrocardiogram tracings help determine the optimum dose.

Therapeutic effects of tocainide are more likely when serum concentrations are within the therapeutic range. If a patient doesn't receive therapeutic benefit, although serum concentrations are at the upper end of the therapeutic range, administration of another antiarrhythmic drug should be considered.

Patients with tocainide concentrations in the toxic range require immediate assessment for severe central nervous system and cardiovascular effects. Serious toxic effects can be minimized by reducing the dose immediately when serum concentrations fall within the toxic range.

Post-test care
If a hematoma develops at the venipuncture site, applying warm soaks eases discomfort.

Interfering factor
Hemolysis caused by excessive agitation of the sample can interfere with accurate determination of test results.

TORCH test

This test is performed to detect exposure to pathogens involved in congenital and neonatal infections. TORCH is an acronym for *t*oxoplasmosis, *o*ther (viruses), *r*ubella, *c*ytomegalovirus, *h*erpes (viruses), and syphilis. These pathogens are commonly associated with congenital or neonatal infections that are not clinically apparent and may cause severe central nervous system impairment. This test confirms such infection serologically by detecting specific immunoglobulin M (IgM)-associated antibodies in an infant's blood.

Purpose
To aid diagnosis of acute, congenital, and intrapartum infections

Patient preparation
Explain the purpose of this test, and mention that the test requires a blood sample.

Procedure
Obtain a 3-ml sample of venous or cord blood. Send it to the laboratory promptly for serologic testing.

Findings
Normal test result is negative for TORCH agents.

Implications of results
Toxoplasmosis is diagnosed by sequential examination that shows rising antibody titers, changing titers and serologic conversion from negative to positive; a titer of 1:256 suggests recent *Toxoplasma* infection. Approximately two-thirds of infected infants are asymptomatic at birth; one-third show signs of cerebral calcifications and choroidoretinitis.

In infants less than 6 months old, rubella infection is associated with a marked and persistent rise in complement-fixing antibody titer over time. Persistence of rubella antibody in an infant after age 6 months strongly suggests congenital infection. Congenital rubella is associated with cardiac anomalies, neurosensory deafness, growth retardation and encephalitic symptoms.

Detection of herpes antibodies in cerebrospinal fluid, with signs of herpetic encephalitis, and persistent herpes virus type 2 antibody levels confirms herpes simplex infection in a neonate without obvious herpetic lesions.

Post-test care
If a hematoma develops at the venipuncture site, applying warm soaks eases discomfort.

Interfering factors
None

Transferrin, serum

Siderophilin

A quantitative analysis of serum transferrin levels, this test evaluates iron metabolism. Transferrin, a glycoprotein that is formed in the liver, transports circulating iron obtained from dietary sources and from the breakdown of red blood cells by reticulo-endothelial cells. Most of this iron is transported to bone marrow for use in hemoglobin synthesis; some is converted to hemosiderin and ferritin and is stored in these forms in the liver, the spleen, and bone marrow. Inadequate transferrin levels may therefore lead to impaired hemoglobin synthesis and, possibly, anemia. Transferrin, normally about 30% saturated with iron, is measured directly by immunoassay; a serum iron level is usually obtained simultaneously.

Purpose
- To determine the iron-transporting capacity of the blood
- To evaluate iron metabolism in iron deficiency anemia

Patient preparation
Explain that this test helps determine the cause of anemia. Inform the patient that restriction of food or fluids is not required and that the test requires a blood sample. Check the patient's medication history for drugs that may influence transferrin levels.

Procedure
Perform a venipuncture, and collect the sample in a 10- to 15-ml *red-top* tube. Handle the sample gently, and send it to the laboratory immediately.

Values
Normal serum transferrin values range from 250 to 390 µg/dl (45 to 65 µmol/L), of which 65 to 170 µg/dl (12 to 30 µmol/L) are usually bound to iron.

Implications of results
Depressed serum levels may indicate inadequate production of transferrin because of hepatic damage or excessive protein loss from renal disease. Decreased transferrin levels may also result from acute or chronic infection, malignant disease, malnutrition, and nephrotic syndrome.

Elevated serum transferrin levels with decreased serum iron occur in iron deficiency anemia.

Post-test care
If a hematoma develops at the venipuncture site, applying warm soaks eases discomfort.

Interfering
factors
- Late pregnancy or the use of oral contraceptives may raise transferrin levels.
- Hemolysis caused by excessive agitation of the sample may affect test results.

Triglycerides, serum

This test provides quantitative analysis of triglycerides, the main storage form of lipids, which constitute about 95% of fatty tissue. Although not in itself diagnostic, serum triglyceride analysis permits early identification of hyperlipemia (characteristic in nephrotic syndrome and other conditions). Hypertriglyceridemia is an independent risk factor in coronary artery disease (CAD).

Triglycerides consist of one molecule of glycerol bonded to three molecules of fatty acids (usually some combination of stearic, oleic, and palmitic). Thus, degradation of triglycerides leads directly to production of fatty acids. Together with carbohydrates, these compounds furnish energy for metabolism. Serum triglycerides are associated with several lipoproteins, primarily chylomicrons and very-low-density lipoproteins. When present in serum, chylomicrons produce a cloudiness that interferes with many laboratory tests.

Purpose
- To determine the risk of CAD
- To screen for hyperlipemia
- To identify disorders associated with altered triglyceride levels

Patient
preparation

Explain that this test helps detect disorders of fat metabolism, and tell the patient the test requires a blood sample. Advise him to abstain from food for 12 to 14 hours before the test and from alcohol for 24 hours before the test.

As appropriate, withhold medications that may alter test results (antilipemics, corticosteroids, estrogen, and some diuretics).

Procedure

Perform a venipuncture, and collect a serum sample in a 7-ml *red-top* tube. A plasma sample is acceptable if a serum sample can't be collected but usually yields slightly lower values that do not correlate reliably with normal serum range.

Send the sample to the laboratory immediately. Some redistribution may occur among lipids.

Values

Triglyceride values are age-related. Some controversy exists over the most appropriate normal ranges, but the following are fairly widely accepted:

Age	Triglycerides	
	mg/dl	**nmol/L**
0 to 29	10 to 140	0.1 to 1.55
30 to 39	10 to 150	0.1 to 1.65
40 to 49	10 to 160	0.1 to 1.75
50 to 59	10 to 190	0.1 to 2.10

Implications of results

Increased or decreased serum triglyceride levels merely suggest a clinical abnormality, and additional tests are required for a definitive diagnosis. For example, measurement of cholesterol may also be necessary because cholesterol and triglycerides vary independently. High levels of triglyceride and cholesterol reflect an exaggerated risk of atherosclerosis or CAD.

Mild-to-moderate increase in serum triglyceride levels indicates biliary obstruction, diabetes, nephrotic syndrome, endocrinopathies, or excessive consumption of alcohol. Markedly increased levels without an identifiable cause reflect congenital hyperlipoproteinemia and necessitate lipoprotein phenotyping to confirm diagnosis.

Decreased serum triglyceride levels are rare, occurring primarily in malnutrition or abetalipoproteinemia. In the latter, the serum is virtually devoid of beta-lipoproteins and triglycerides because the body lacks the capacity to transport preformed triglycerides from the epithelial cells of the intestinal mucosa or from the liver.

Post-test care

• If a hematoma develops at the venipuncture site, applying warm soaks eases discomfort.
• The patient may resume restricted medications and diet.

Interfering factors

• A plasma sample may produce slightly lower values than a serum sample.
• Failure to comply with dietary restrictions may interfere with accurate determination of test results.
• Ingestion of alcohol within 24 hours of the test may cause elevated triglyceride levels. In fact, excessive alcohol consumption is a common cause of excessive levels of triglycerides. A fatty liver is

an early manifestation of this metabolic phenomenon.

- Cholestyramine lowers cholesterol but may have no effect on triglycerides. Colestipol lowers cholesterol but may raise or have no effect on triglycerides.
- Long-term use of corticosteroids raises triglyceride levels, as does use of oral contraceptives, estrogen, furosemide, and miconazole.
- Clofibrate, dextrothyroxine, heparin, sulfonylureas, norethindrone, androgens, ascorbic acid, gemfibrozil, and niacin lower cholesterol and triglyceride levels.
- Certain drugs have a variable effect: Probucol inhibits transport of cholesterol from the intestine and may also affect cholesterol synthesis. It lowers cholesterol but has a variable effect on triglycerides.

Triiodothyronine (T_3), serum

This highly specific radioimmunoassay measures total (bound and free) serum content of triiodothyronine (T_3) to investigate clinical indications of thyroid dysfunction. T_3, the more potent thyroid hormone, is an amine derived from the joining of monoiodotyrosine (T_1) and diiodotyrosine (T_2). Like T_4 secretion, T_3 secretion occurs in response to thyroid-stimulating hormone (TSH) released by the pituitary gland and, secondarily, to thyrotropin-releasing hormone from the hypothalamus through a complex negative feedback mechanism.

Although T_3 is present in the bloodstream in minute quantities and is metabolically active for only a short time, its impact on body metabolism dominates that of T_4. Another significant difference between the two major thyroid hormones is that T_3 binds less firmly to thyroxine-binding globulin (TBG). Consequently, T_3 persists in the bloodstream for a short time; half disappears in about 1 day, while half of T_4 disappears in 6 days.

Purpose
- To aid diagnosis of T_3 toxicosis
- To aid diagnosis of hypothyroidism and hyperthyroidism
- To monitor clinical response to thyroid replacement therapy in hypothyroidism (in the rare circumstances when T_3 replacement is given)

Patient preparation	Explain that this test helps to evaluate thyroid gland function. Inform the patient that this test requires a blood sample. As appropriate, withhold medications, such as corticosteroids, propranolol, and cholestyramine, that may influence thyroid function. If such medications must be continued, record this information on the laboratory slip.

Procedure	Draw venous blood into a 7-ml *red-top* tube. Send the sample to the laboratory as soon as possible to avoid stasis and to allow early separation of serum from the clotted blood. Handle the sample gently to prevent hemolysis. If a patient must receive thyroid preparations such as T_3 (liothyronine sodium), note the time of administration on the laboratory slip. Otherwise, T_3 levels are not reliable.

Values	Serum T_3 levels normally range from 90 to 230 ng/dl (1.5 to 3.5 nmol/L). These values may vary with the laboratory performing this test.

Implications of results	Serum T_3 and T_4 levels usually rise and fall in tandem. However, in T_3 toxicosis, only T_3 levels rise, whereas total and free T_4 levels remain normal. T_3 toxicosis occurs in patients with Graves' disease (rare), toxic adenoma, or toxic nodular goiter. T_3 levels also surpass T_4 levels in patients receiving thyroid replacement containing more T_3 than T_4. In a person living in an iodine-deficient geographic area, the thyroid gland may produce larger amounts of the more cellularly active T_3 than of T_4 in an effort to maintain the euthyroid state. Generally, T_3 levels appear to be a more accurate diagnostic indicator of hyperthyroidism, but it is only needed as an adjunct to a suppressed high sensitivity TSH level. In some patients with hypothyroidism, T_3 levels may fall within the normal range and may not be diagnostically significant. A rise in serum T_3 levels normally occurs during pregnancy as a result of a physiologic increase in TBG. Low T_3 levels may appear in euthyroid patients with systemic illness (especially hepatic or renal disease), during severe acute illness, or following trauma or major surgery; in such patients, however, TSH levels are within normal limits. Low serum T_3 levels are sometimes found in euthyroid patients with malnutrition.

Post-test care
- If a hematoma develops at the venipuncture site, applying warm soaks eases discomfort.
- The patient may resume discontinued medications.

Interfering factors
- Markedly increased or decreased TBG levels influence test results regardless of cause.
- Failure to take into account medications that affect T_3 levels, such as corticosteroids, clofibrate, and propranolol, influences test result.
- Hemolysis caused by excessive agitation of the sample can influence test results.

Triiodothyronine resin uptake (T₃RU)

T_3 uptake ratio

This test indirectly measures free thyroxine (FT_4) levels by demonstrating the availability of serum protein-binding sites for T_4. A known amount of radioactive triiodothyronine (T_3), which exceeds the capacity of thyroxine-binding globulin (TBG) to bind to it, and a resin are added to a serum sample. The radioactive hormone combines with unoccupied sites on the TBG; any leftover hormone remains free and available for binding to the resin particles. After the resin is separated from the serum, the amount of radioactivity remaining on the TBG or bound to resin is measured by radioimmunoassay; it is expressed as a percentage of the total amount of the T_3 added initially. T_3 resin uptake does not measure serum T_3 and should not be used alone, but in combination with T_4 measurement.

The results of T_3 resin uptake (T_3RU) are frequently combined with a T_4 radioimmunoassay or competitive protein-binding test ($T_4[D]$) to determine the free thyroxine index, a mathematical calculation that is thought to reflect FT_4 by correcting for TBG abnormalities. The T_3RU is considered a valuable ancillary test for thyroid gland dysfunction.

Purpose
- To aid diagnosis of hypothyroidism and hyperthyroidism when TBG is abnormal
- To assist diagnosis of primary disorders of TBG levels, such as nephrotic syndrome

Patient preparation	Explain that this test helps evaluate thyroid status and that the test requires a blood sample. As appropriate, withhold medications, such as estrogens, androgens, phenytoin, salicylates, or thyroid preparations, that may interfere with test results. If these medications must be continued, note this on the laboratory slip.
Procedure	Draw venous blood into a 7-ml *red-*, *lavender-* or *green-top* tube. Handle the collection tube gently to prevent hemolysis.
Values	Normally, 25% to 34% of T_3 binds to the resin. The concentration of T_3RU ranges from 0.1 to 1.35; the value may vary, depending on the laboratory method used.
Implications of results	T_3RU concentration increases in hyperthyroidism; in such disorders as malnutrition and nephrotic syndrome, when TBG concentration decreases; and when high doses of aspirin, phenylbutazone, and phenytoin displace T_4 from TBG. T_3 concentration decreases in hypothyroidism; during pregnancy when TBG concentration increases; during menopause or treatment of osteoporosis when estrogen is given as a contraceptive; and with perphenazine administration.
Post-test care	• If a hematoma develops at the venipuncture site, applying warm soaks eases discomfort. • The patient may resume discontinued medications.
Interfering factors	• Diagnostic or therapeutic administration of radioactive material interferes with accurate test results. • Hemolysis caused by excessive agitation of the sample may interfere with accurate test results.

Triiodothyronine (T_3) thyroid suppression test

The triiodothyronine (T_3) thyroid suppression test measures the thyroid gland's metabolic response to administration of oral T_3. The test also helps determine if areas of excessive iodine uptake in the thyroid (hot spots) are autonomous (as in some cases of Graves' disease) or if they reflect pituitary overcompensation (as in iodine-deficient goiter). Autonomous hot spots function independently of pituitary control. However, hot spots caused by iodine deficiency stem from reduced thyroxine (T_4) production, which decreases T_3 production and increases thyroid-stimulating hormone (TSH) production. In turn, increased TSH production overstimulates the thyroid and causes excessive iodine uptake.

Normally, T_3 administration will decrease the uptake of iodine by the thyroid gland.

Purpose

To help determine the cause of excessive iodine uptake by the thyroid gland

Patient preparation

Explain that this test helps evaluate thyroid function and describe the procedure for T_3 and schedule of administration for T_3 and radioactive iodine. Advise the patient to avoid foods that contain iodine (such as shellfish and iodized salt) before the test.

Procedure

After a baseline reading of thyroid function is obtained by a radioactive iodine uptake (RAIU) test, a 75- to 100-mcg dose of T_3 is administered for 5 to 10 days (for example, 25 mcg every 8 hours for 5 days). During the last 2 days of T_3 administration, RAIU tests are repeated to assess thyroid response. (Normally, T_3 acts through a negative feedback mechanism to suppress pituitary release of TSH; TSH suppression then suppresses thyroid function and iodine uptake.)

Findings

In euthyroid patients with normal thyroid uptake, administration of T_3 suppresses uptake to at least 50% of baseline.

Implications of results

Suppression of RAIU to at least 50% of baseline shows that the hot spot is under pituitary control and suggests iodine deficiency as the cause of increased iodine uptake. Failure to suppress RAIU by 50% suggests autonomous thyroid hyperfunction, possibly caused by Graves' disease or a toxic thyroid nodule. RAIU may or may not be suppressed in patients with thyroid cancer.

Post-test care

Patient may resume a normal diet and restricted medications.

Interfering factor Failure to restrict ingestion of iodine may interfere with accuracy of test results.

Tuberculin skin tests
Mantoux test

This skin test is used to screen for previous *Mycobacterium tuberculosis* infection and is performed in patients with findings that suggest this infection. In both the old tuberculin (OT) and purified protein derivative (PPD) tests, intradermal injection of the tuberculin antigen causes a delayed hypersensitivity reaction in patients with active or dormant tuberculosis; sensitized lymphocytes gather at the injection site and cause erythema, vesiculation, or induration that peaks within 24 to 48 hours and persists for at least 72 hours.

The most accurate tuberculin test method, the Mantoux test, employs a single-needle intradermal injection of PPD, permitting precise measurement of dosage and accurate interpretation of results.

Purpose
• To determine exposure to *M. tuberculosis*
• To identify persons who need diagnostic investigation for tuberculosis

Patient preparation
Explain that this test helps detect tuberculosis. Tell the patient the test requires an intradermal injection, which may cause transient discomfort.

➤ *Clinical alert:* Check the patient's history for active tuberculosis, the results of previous skin tests, or hypersensitivities. Don't perform a skin test if the patient has had tuberculosis or a positive reaction to previous skin tests. If the patient has had an allergic reaction to acacia, don't perform an OT test because this product contains acacia.

If performing a tuberculin test on an outpatient, instruct the patient to return at the specified time so that test results can be read. Inform the patient that a positive reaction to a skin test appears as a red, hard, raised area at the injection site. Warn that the area may itch, and advise against scratching it. Reassure the patient that a positive reaction doesn't always indicate active tuberculosis.

Equipment
Alcohol sponges; vial of intermediate-strength PPD with 5 tuberculin units per 0.1 ml and 1-ml tuberculin syringe with ½″ or ⅝″ 25G or 26G needle for the

Mantoux test; epinephrine (1:1,000) and a 3-ml syringe (for emergency use)

Procedure

The patient is seated, with arm extended and supported on a flat surface. Clean the volar surface of the upper forearm with alcohol; allow the area to dry completely.

Mantoux test: Perform an intradermal injection.

Tuberculin skin tests are read 48 to 72 hours after injection.

Precautions

• Tuberculin skin tests are contraindicated in patients with active tuberculosis.
• Don't perform a skin test on body areas with excessive hair, acne, or insufficient subcutaneous tissue (such as over a tendon or bone).
• Have epinephrine available to treat a possible anaphylactoid or acute hypersensitivity reaction.

Findings

In tuberculin skin tests, normal findings show negative or minimal reactions.

Mantoux test: In patients with human immunodeficiency virus (HIV) and other immunocompromised disorders, positive test results are indicated by indurations of more than 5 mm in diameter; in patients at risk for HIV or other immunocompromised disorders, more than 10 mm; and in otherwise normal patients, more than 15 mm.

Implications of results

A positive tuberculin reaction indicates previous infection by tubercle bacilli. It does not distinguish between an active and dormant infection, nor does it provide a definitive diagnosis. If a positive reaction occurs, sputum smear and culture, chest radiography, or other tests may be indicated.

In the Mantoux test, induration of 5 to 9 mm in diameter indicates a borderline reaction; larger induration, a positive reaction. Because patients infected with atypical mycobacteria other than tubercle bacilli may have borderline reactions, repeat testing is necessary.

If the first PPD is negative, a second, two-step test is needed to detect the booster phenomenon.

Post-test care

If ulceration or necrosis develops at the injection site, applying cold soaks or a topical corticosteroid eases discomfort.

Interfering factors	• Subcutaneous injection, usually indicated by erythema more than 10 mm in diameter without induration, invalidates the test.
	• Corticosteroids and other immunosuppressants, and live-vaccine viruses (measles, mumps, rubella, or polio) given within the past 4 to 6 weeks may suppress skin reactions.
	• Elderly persons and patients with viral infection, malnutrition, febrile illness, uremia, immunosuppressive disorders, or miliary tuberculosis may have suppressed skin reactions.
	• If less than 10 weeks has passed since infection with tuberculosis, the skin test may be negative.
	• Improper dilution, dose, or storage of the tuberculin interferes with accurate testing.

Tubular reabsorbed phosphate, plasma and urine

Because tubular reabsorbed phosphate (TRP) is closely regulated by the parathyroid hormone (PTH), measuring urine and plasma phosphate, accompanied by creatinine clearance measurement, provides an indirect method of evaluating parathyroid function. PTH (also called parathormone) helps maintain optimum blood levels of ionized calcium and controls renal excretion of calcium and phosphate. Specifically, PTH stimulates reabsorption of calcium and inhibits reabsorption of phosphate from the glomerular filtrate. A regulatory feedback mechanism causes PTH secretion to diminish as ionized calcium levels return to normal. In primary hyper-parathyroidism, excessive secretion of PTH disrupts this calcium-phosphate balance.

This test is indicated to detect hyperparathyroidism in persons with clinical signs of this disorder and borderline or normal values for serum calcium, phosphate, and alkaline phosphatase.

Purpose	• To evaluate parathyroid function
	• To aid diagnosis of primary hyperparathyroidism
	• To aid differential diagnosis of hypercalcemia

Patient preparation	Explain to the patient that this test evaluates the function of the parathyroid glands and requires a blood sample and a 24-hour urine collection.
	Teach the patient how to maintain a normal phosphate diet for 3 days before the test, because low

phosphate intake (less than 500 mg/day) may elevate tubular reabsorption values, and a high-phosphate diet (3,000 mg/day) may lower them. Common nutritional sources of phosphorus include legumes, nuts, milk, egg yolks, meat, poultry, fish, cereals, and cheese. These foods should be eaten in moderate amounts. Instruct the patient to fast from midnight the night before the test.

As appropriate, withhold drugs, such as amphotericin B, chlorothiazide diuretics, furosemide, and gentamicin, that are known to influence test results. If these medications must be continued throughout the test period, note this on the laboratory slip.

Procedure First, perform a venipuncture, and collect the sample in a 10-ml *red-top* tube. Handle the collection tube gently to prevent hemolysis. Then, instruct the patient to void and discard the urine; record this as time zero. Collect a 24-hour urine specimen. Tell the patient to avoid contaminating specimens with toilet paper or stool. (Occasionally, a 4-hour collection may be used instead.)

After the venipuncture, allow the patient to eat and encourage fluid intake to maintain adequate urine flow.

Keep the urine specimen container refrigerated or on ice during the collection period. At the end of the collection period, label the specimen and send it to the laboratory immediately.

Findings Renal tubules normally reabsorb 80% or more of phosphate. Normal TRP ranges from 84% to 95%. TRP is reported as the percentage of phosphate reabsorbed.

Implications of results Reabsorption of less than 74% of phosphate strongly suggests primary hyperparathyroidism, but requires additional studies to confirm primary hyperparathyroidism as the cause of hypercalcemia. Direct assay of PTH is indicated. Chest and bone X-rays and bone scans should be performed because bony metastasis is the most common cause of hypercalcemia. Depressed reabsorption occurs in a small number of patients who have renal calculi but no parathyroid tumor. However, normal reabsorption occurs in roughly one-fifth of patients with parathyroid tumor. Increased reabsorption of phosphate may result from uremia, renal tubular disease, osteomalacia, sarcoidosis, and myeloma.

Post-test care
- If a hematoma develops at the venipuncture site, applying warm soaks eases discomfort.
- The patient may resume restricted medications and diet.

Interfering factors
- Hemolysis caused by excessive agitation of the blood sample may alter test results.
- Failure to collect all urine during the test period may interfere with accurate determination of test results.
- Failure to follow guidelines for pretest diet restrictions and phosphate intake may alter test results.
- Amphotericin B and chlorothiazide diuretics may diminish reabsorption; furosemide and gentamicin may enhance it.

U

Uric acid, serum

Used primarily to detect gout, this test measures serum levels of uric acid, the major end metabolite of purine. Large amounts of purines are present in nucleic acids and are derived from dietary and endogenous sources. Uric acid clears the body by glomerular filtration and tubular secretion. However, uric acid is not soluble at a pH of 7.4 or lower. Disorders of purine metabolism, rapid destruction of nucleic acids (as occurs in gout), excessive cellular turnover (as in leukemia), and conditions marked by impaired renal excretion (as in renal failure) characteristically raise serum uric acid levels.

Purpose
- To confirm diagnosis of gout
- To help detect kidney dysfunction

Patient preparation
Explain the purpose of this test, that restriction of food or fluids is not required before the test, and that the test requires a blood sample.

Check the patient's medication history for any drugs that may influence uric acid levels.

Procedure
Perform a venipuncture, and collect the sample in a 10- to 15-ml *red-top* tube. Handle the sample gently to prevent hemolysis.

Values
Uric acid concentrations in men normally range from 4.3 to 8 mg/dl (260 to 480 µmol/L); in women, from 2.3 to 6 mg/dl (140 to 360 µmol/L).

Implications of results
Increased serum uric acid levels may indicate gout, although levels don't correlate with the severity of disease or impaired renal function. Uric acid levels may also rise in congestive heart failure, glycogen storage disease (type I, von Gierke's disease), acute infectious diseases (such as infectious mononucleosis), hemolytic or sickle cell anemia, hemoglobinopathies, polycythemia, leukemia, lymphoma, metastatic malignant disease, and psoriasis.

Depressed uric acid levels may indicate defective tubular absorption (as in Fanconi's syndrome and Wilson's disease) or acute hepatic atrophy.

Post-test care   If a hematoma develops at the venipuncture site, applying warm soaks eases discomfort.

Interfering
factors

- Loop diuretics, ethambutol, vincristine, pyrazinamide, thiazides, and low doses of salicylates may raise uric acid levels. When uric acid is measured by the colorimetric method, false elevations may be caused by acetaminophen, ascorbic acid, levodopa, and phenacetin.
- Starvation, a high-purine diet, stress, and alcohol abuse may raise uric acid levels.
- Aspirin in high doses, coumarin, clofibrate, allopurinol, corticotropin, and phenothiazines may decrease uric acid levels.

Uric acid, urine

A quantitative analysis of urine uric acid levels, this test supplements serum uric acid testing in identifying disorders that alter production or excretion of uric acid (such as leukemia, gout, and renal dysfunction). Derived from dietary purines in organ meats (liver, kidney, and sweetbread [thymus or pancreas]) and from endogenous nucleoproteins, uric acid (as urate) is found normally in the blood and other tissues in amounts totaling about 1 g. Urate is formed primarily in the liver, although the intestinal mucosa is also involved in its production. As the chief end product of purine catabolism, urate passes from the liver through the bloodstream into the kidneys, where roughly 50% is excreted daily in the urine. Renal urate metabolism is complex, involving glomerular filtration, tubular secretion, and a second reabsorption by the renal tubules.

The most specific laboratory method for detecting uric acid is spectrophotometric absorption, after treatment of the specimen with the enzyme uricase.

Purpose   To detect enzyme deficiencies and metabolic disturbances that affect uric acid production

Patient
preparation

Explain the purpose of this test, that restriction of food or fluids is not required before the test, and that the test requires a 24-hour urine specimen. Teach the patient the proper collection technique.

Check the patient's medication history for recent use of drugs that may influence uric acid levels. If these medications must be continued, note this on the laboratory slip.

Procedure

Collect a 24-hour urine specimen. Send the specimen to the laboratory immediately at the end of the collection period.

Values

Normal urine uric acid values vary with diet but generally range from 250 to 750 mg/day (1.5 to 4.5 mmol/day).

Implications of results

Elevated urine uric acid levels may result from chronic myeloid leukemia, polycythemia vera, multiple myeloma, and early remission in pernicious anemia, and may occur in lymphosarcoma and lymphatic leukemia during radiotherapy. High levels also result from tubular reabsorption defects, such as Fanconi's syndrome and hepatolenticular degeneration (Wilson's disease).

Low urine uric acid levels occur in gout (when associated with normal uric acid production but inadequate excretion), and in severe renal damage, such as that resulting from chronic glomerulonephritis, diabetic glomerulosclerosis, and collagen disorders.

Post-test care

The patient may resume medications withheld before the test.

Interfering factors

- Drugs that decrease urine uric acid excretion include diuretics, including benzthiazide, furosemide, ethacrynic acid, and pyrazinamide. Low doses of salicylates, phenylbutazone, and probenecid also lower uric acid levels; high doses of these drugs cause levels to rise above normal. Allopurinol, a drug used to treat gout, increases uric acid excretion.
- Urine uric acid concentrations rise with a high-purine diet and fall with a low-purine diet.
- Failure to observe drug restrictions or to collect all urine during the test period may alter test results.

Urinalysis (UA), routine

Routine urinalysis is an important, commonly used screening test for urinary and systemic pathologic conditions. Abnormal findings suggest disease and mandate further urine or blood tests to identify it.

The elements of routine urinalysis include the evaluation of physical characteristics (color, odor, and opacity); the determination of specific gravity and pH; the detection and rough measurement of protein, glucose, and ketone bodies; and the examination of sediment for blood cells, casts, and crystals.

Urinalysis methods include visual examination for appearance; reagent strip screening for pH, protein, glucose, and ketone bodies; refractometry for specific gravity; and microscopic inspection of centrifuged sediment for cells, casts, and crystals.

Purpose
- To screen for renal or urinary tract disease
- To help detect metabolic or systemic disease

Patient preparation
Explain that this test aids diagnosis of renal or urinary tract disease. Also inform the patient that restriction of food or fluids is not required and that the test requires a urine specimen. Check the patient's history for recent use of medications that may affect test results.

Procedure
Collect a random urine specimen of at least 15 ml. A first-voided morning specimen contains the greatest concentration of solutes. *Note:* If the patient is being evaluated for renal colic, strain the specimen to catch stones or stone fragments. Place an unfolded 4″ × 4″ gauze pad or a fine-mesh sieve over the specimen container, and carefully pour the urine through the gauze or sieve. Send the specimen to the laboratory immediately, or refrigerate it if analysis will be delayed longer than 1 hour.

Findings
See *Normal findings in routine urinalysis* for a listing of normal test results.

Implications of results
Variations in urinalysis findings may result from diet, nonpathologic conditions, specimen collection time, and other factors. The following benign variations are commonly nonpathologic:

Specific gravity: Urine becomes darker and its odor becomes stronger as the specific gravity increases. Specific gravity is highest in the first-voided morning specimen.

Urine pH: Greatly affected by diet and medications, urine pH influences the appearance of urine and the composition of crystals. An alkaline pH (above 7.0) — characteristic of a diet high in vegetables, citrus fruits, and dairy products, but low in

Normal findings in routine urinalysis

Element	Finding
Macroscopic	
Color	Straw
Odor	Slightly aromatic
Appearance	Clear
Specific gravity	1.005 to 1.020
pH	4.5 to 8.0
Protein	None
Glucose	None
Ketones	None
Other sugars	None
Microscopic	
Red blood cells	0 to 3/high-power field
White blood cells	0 to 4/high-power field
Epithelial cells	Few
Casts	None, except occasional hyaline casts
Crystals	Present
Yeast cells	None
Parasites	None

meat — causes turbidity and the formation of phosphate, carbonate, and amorphous crystals. An acid pH (below 7.0) — typical of a high-protein diet — produces turbidity and formation of oxalate, cystine, amorphous urate, and uric acid crystals. Urine that remains at room temperature before being tested will often become alkaline caused by bacterial degradation of urea to ammonia. An alkaline urine sample may yield false-positive test results for protein on urine test strips.

Protein: Normally absent from urine, protein can appear in urine in a benign condition known as orthostatic (postural) proteinuria. This condition is most common during the second decade of life, is intermittent, appears after prolonged standing, and disappears after recumbency. Transient benign proteinuria can also occur with fever, exposure to cold, emotional stress, or strenuous exercise.

Sugars: Also usually absent from urine, sugars may appear under normal conditions. The most common sugar in urine is glucose. Transient, nonpathologic glycosuria may result from emotional stress or pregnancy and may follow ingestion of a high-carbohydrate meal. Other sugars — fructose, lactose, and pentose — rarely appear in urine under nonpathologic conditions. (Lactosuria, however, may occur during pregnancy and lactation.)

Red blood cells (RBCs): Hematuria may occasionally follow strenuous exercise.

The following abnormal findings generally suggest pathologic conditions.

Color: Changes in color can result from diet, drugs, and some metabolic, inflammatory, or infectious diseases.

Odor: In diabetes mellitus, starvation, and dehydration, a fruity odor accompanies formation of ketone bodies. In urinary tract infection, a fetid odor is common. Maple syrup urine disease and phenylketonuria also cause distinctive odors.

Turbidity: Turbid urine may contain blood cells, bacteria, fat, or chyle, suggesting renal infection.

Specific gravity: Low specific gravity (less than 1.005) occurs with a high fluid intake and is characteristic of diabetes insipidus, nephrogenic diabetes insipidus, acute tubular necrosis, and pyelonephritis. Fixed specific gravity, in which values remain 1.010 regardless of fluid intake, occurs in chronic glomerulonephritis with severe renal damage. High specific gravity (greater than 1.020) occurs in nephrotic syndrome, dehydration, acute glomerulonephritis, congestive heart failure, liver failure, and shock.

pH: Alkaline urine pH may result from Fanconi's syndrome, urinary tract infection, and metabolic or respiratory alkalosis. Acid urine pH is associated with pyrexia and all forms of acidosis.

Protein: Proteinuria suggests renal diseases, such as nephrosis, glomerulosclerosis, glomerulonephritis, nephrolithiasis, polycystic kidney disease, and renal failure. Proteinuria can also result from multiple myeloma.

Sugars: Glycosuria usually indicates diabetes mellitus but may also result from pheochromocytoma, Cushing's syndrome, acromegaly, and increased intracranial pressure. Galactosuria, fructosuria, and pentosuria generally suggest rare hereditary metabolic disorders. However, an alimentary form of pentosuria and fructosuria may follow excessive pentose or fructose ingestion, resulting in failure to metabolize the sugar. Because the renal tubules fail to reabsorb pentose or fructose, these sugars spill over into the urine.

Ketones: Ketonuria occurs in diabetes mellitus when cellular energy needs exceed available cellular glucose. In the absence of glucose, cells metabolize triglyceride, an alternate energy supply. Ketone bodies — the end products of incomplete fat metabolism — accumulate in plasma and are excreted in urine. Ketonuria may also occur in conditions of acutely increased metabolic demand associated with decreased food intake, such as diarrhea, vomiting, or malnutrition.

Cells: Hematuria (the presence of intact RBCs) indicates bleeding within the genitourinary tract and may result from infection, obstruction, inflammation, trauma, tumors, glomerulonephritis, renal hypertension, lupus nephritis, renal tuberculosis, renal vein thrombosis, hydronephrosis, pyelonephritis, scurvy, malaria, parasitic infection of the bladder, subacute bacterial endocarditis, polyarteritis nodosa, and hemorrhagic disorders. Numerous white blood cells (WBCs) in urine usually suggest urinary tract inflammation, especially cystitis or pyelonephritis. WBCs and WBC casts in urine suggest renal infection. An excessive number of epithelial cells suggests renal tubular degeneration.

Casts (plugs of gelled proteinaceous material [high molecular weight mucoprotein]): Casts form in the renal tubules and collecting ducts by agglutination of protein cells or cellular debris and are flushed loose by urine flow. Excessive numbers of casts indicate renal disease. Hyaline casts are associated with renal parenchymal disease, inflammation, and trauma to the glomerular capillary membrane; epithelial casts, with renal tubular damage, nephrosis, eclampsia, amyloidosis, and heavy metal poisoning; coarse and fine granular casts, with acute or chronic renal failure, pyelonephritis, and

(Text continues on page 630.)

Drugs that influence routine results of urinalysis

Color change

Alcohol (light, because of diuresis)
Chlorpromazine hydrochloride (dark)
Chlorzoxazone (orange to purple-red)
Deferoxamine mesylate (red)
Dyes in many foods, especially candies
Fluorescein sodium I.V. (yellow-orange)
Furazolidone (brown)
Iron salts (black)
Levodopa (dark)
Methylene blue (blue-green)
Metronidazole (dark)
Nitrofurantoin (brown)
Oral anticoagulants, indanedione
    derivatives (orange)
Phenazopyridine (orange-red,
    orange-brown, or red)
Phenolphthalein (red to purple-red)
Quinacrine (deep yellow)
Rifampin (red-orange)
Sulfasalazine (orange-yellow)
Sulfobromophthalein (red)

Odor

Antibiotics
Paraldehyde
Vitamins

Increased specific gravity

Albumin
Dextran
Glucose
Radiopaque contrast media

Decreased pH

Ammonium chloride
Ascorbic acid
Diazoxide
Methenamine
Metolazone

Increased pH

Acetazolamide
Amphotericin B
Mafenide
Sodium bicarbonate
Potassium citrate

False-positive result for proteinuria

Acetazolamide (Combistix or Labstix)
Aminosalicylic acid (sulfosalicylic acid
    or Exton's method)
Cephalothin in large doses
    (sulfosalicylic acid method)
Nafcillin (sulfosalicylic acid method)
Sodium bicarbonate (all methods)
Tolbutamide (sulfosalicylic acid method)
Tolmetin (sulfosalicylic acid method)

True proteinuria

Amikacin
Amphotericin B
Bacitracin
Gentamicin
Gold preparations
Kanamycin
Neomycin
Netilmicin
Phenylbutazone
Polymyxin B
Streptomycin
Tobramycin
Trimethadione

True proteinuria or false-positive result

Penicillin in large doses
    (except with Ames reagent strips);
    however, some penicillins cause true
    proteinuria.
Sulfonamides (sulfosalicylic acid method)

False-positive result for glycosuria

Aminosalicylic acid (Benedict's test)
Ascorbic acid (Clinistix, Diastix, or
    Tes-Tape); in large doses (Clinitest
    tablets)
Cephalosporins (Clinitest tablets)
Chloral hydrate (Benedict's test)
Chloramphenicol (Benedict's test
    or Clinitest tablets)
Isoniazid (Benedict's test)
Levodopa (Clinistix, Diastix, or Tes-
    Tape); in large doses (Clinitest tablets)
Methyldopa (Tes-Tape)

Drugs that influence routine results of urinalysis *(continued)*

False-positive result for glycosuria
(continued)

Nalidixic acid (Benedict's test or Clinitest tablets)
Nitrofurantoin (Benedict's test)
Penicillin G in large doses (Benedict's test)
Phenazopyridine (Clinistix, Diastix, or Tes-Tape)
Probenecid (Benedict's test or Clinitest tablets)
Salicylates in large doses (Clinitest tablets, Clinistix, Diastix, or Tes-Tape)
Streptomycin (Benedict's test)
Tetracycline (Clinistix, Diastix, Tes-Tape)
Tetracyclines, because of ascorbic acid buffer (Benedict's test or Clinitest tablets)

True glycosuria

Ammonium chloride
Asparaginase
Carbamazepine
Corticosteroids
Dextrothyroxine
Lithium carbonate
Nicotinic acid (large doses)
Phenothiazines (long-term)
Thiazide diuretics

Increased white blood cells

Allopurinol
Ampicillin
Aspirin toxicity
Kanamycin
Methicillin

Hematuria

Amphotericin B
Coumarin derivatives
Methenamine in large doses
Methicillin
Para-aminosalicylic acid
Phenylbutazone
Sulfonamides

False-positive result for ketonuria

Levodopa (Ketostix or Labstix)
Phenazopyridine (Ketostix or Gerhardt's reagent strip shows atypical color)
Phenolsulfonphthalein (Rothera's test)
Phenothiazines (Gerhardt's reagent strip shows atypical color)
Salicylates (testing with Gerhardt's reagent strip shows reddish color)
Sulfobromophthalein (Bili-Labstix)

True ketonuria

Ether (anesthesia)
Insulin (excessive doses)
Isoniazid (intoxication)
Isopropyl alcohol (intoxication)

Casts

Amphotericin B
Aspirin toxicity
Bacitracin
Ethacrynic acid
Furosemide
Gentamicin
Griseofulvin
Isoniazid
Kanamycin
Neomycin
Penicillin
Radiographic agents
Streptomycin
Sulfonamides

Crystals (if urine is acidic)

Acetazolamide
Aminosalicylic acid
Ascorbic acid
Nitrofurantoin
Theophylline
Thiazide diuretics

chronic lead intoxication; fatty and waxy casts, with nephrotic syndrome, chronic renal disease, and diabetes mellitus; RBC casts, with acute glomerular nephritis, renal infarction, subacute bacterial endocarditis, vascular disorders, sickle cell anemia, scurvy, blood dyscrasias, malignant hypertension, collagen disease, and acute inflammation; and WBC casts, with acute pyelonephritis and glomerulonephritis, nephrotic syndrome, pyogenic infection, and lupus nephritis.

Crystals: Some crystals normally appear in urine, especially when it's left standing. Oxalate crystals can be profuse in children, and cystine crystals (cystinuria) reflect an inborn error of metabolism.

Other components: Yeast cells and parasites in urinary sediment reflect genitourinary tract infection, as well as contamination of external genitalia. Yeast cells, which may be mistaken for RBCs, can be identified by their ovoid shape, lack of color, variable size, and, frequently, signs of budding. The most common parasite in sediment is *Trichomonas vaginalis,* a flagellated protozoan that commonly causes vaginitis, urethritis, and prostatovesiculitis.

Post-test care None

Interfering factors
- Failure to follow proper collection procedure, to send the specimen to the laboratory immediately, or to refrigerate the specimen may interfere with accurate determination of test results.
- Strenuous exercise before routine urinalysis may cause transient myoglobinuria, producing misleading results and inaccurate diagnosis.
- Many drugs can influence the results of this test. (See *Drugs that influence routine results of urinalysis,* pages 628 and 629.)

Urinary calculi

Urinary calculi are insoluble substances most commonly formed of the mineral salts calcium oxalate, calcium phosphate, magnesium ammonium phosphate, urate, or cystine that may appear anywhere in the urinary tract. These calculi (or stones) range in size from microscopic to several centimeters. Calculi usually possess well-defined nuclei composed of bacteria, fibrin, blood clots, or epithelial cells, enclosed in a protein matrix. Mineral salts accumulate around this matrix in layers, causing progressive enlargement.

Formation of calculi can result from dehydration, increased excretion of mineral salts, urinary stasis, pH changes, and decreased protective substances. Calculi commonly form in the kidney, pass into the ureter, and are excreted in the urine. Because not all calculi pass spontaneously, they may require surgical extraction. Calculi don't always cause symptoms; but when they do, hematuria and renal colic are common. When calculi obstruct the ureter, they may cause severe flank pain, dysuria, urine retention, and urinary frequency and urgency.

To test for urinary calculi, the patient's urine must be carefully strained. Qualitative chemical analysis then reveals their composition to help identify their causes.

Purpose   To detect and identify calculi in the urine

Patient preparation   Explain that this test detects urinary stones, and that, if such stones are found, laboratory analysis will reveal their composition. Inform the patient that the test requires collection of a urine sample and that restriction of food or fluids is not required. The patient's symptoms may or may not subside immediately after excretion of any stones. The patient may require medication to control pain.

Equipment   Strainer (such as an unfolded 4″ × 4″ dressing or a fine-mesh sieve), specimen container

Procedure   After the patient voids into the strainer, inspect the strainer carefully. Such calculi may be very small and may look like gravel or sand. Document the appearance of the calculi and the number, if possible. Then, place the calculi in a properly labeled container, and send the container to the laboratory immediately for prompt analysis.

Precautions   The patient who has received analgesics before collection of the urine specimen should have the strainer and urinal or bedpan within his reach (he may be drowsy and unable to get out of bed to void).

Findings   Normally, calculi are not present in the urine.

Causes and incidence of urinary calculi

Calcium oxalate calculi (incidence, 72%) usually result from idiopathic hypercalciuria, a condition that reflects excessive absorption of calcium from the bowel.

Calcium phosphate calculi (incidence, 2%) usually result from primary hyperparathyroidism, which causes excessive resorption of calcium from bone.

Cystine calculi (incidence, 3%) result from primary cystinuria, an inborn error of metabolism that prevents renal tubular reabsorption of cystine.

Magnesium ammonium phosphate calculi (incidence, 15%) result from the presence of urea-splitting organisms, such as *Proteus*, which raises ammonia concentration and makes urine alkaline.

Urate calculi (incidence, 8%) result from gout, dehydration (causing elevated uric acid levels), acidic urine (pH 5.0), or hepatic dysfunction.

Implications of results

More than half of all calculi in urine are of mixed composition, containing two or more mineral salts; calcium oxalate is the most common component. Determining the composition of calculi helps identify various metabolic disorders (see *Causes and incidence of urinary calculi*).

Post-test care

- Observe for severe flank pain, dysuria, urine retention, and urinary frequency or urgency. Hematuria should subside.
- Inform the patient of dietary limits to prevent formation of calculi.

Interfering factors

None

Urinary tract brush biopsy

Retrograde brush biopsy of the urinary tract may be performed to obtain a renal tissue specimen when X-rays show a lesion in the renal pelvis or calyx. It can also be used to obtain specimens from other areas of the urinary tract. However, retrograde brush biopsy is contraindicated in patients with acute urinary tract infection or an obstruction at or below the biopsy site.

Purpose   To obtain a specimen of renal tissue

Patient
preparation

Explain the purpose of this test, describe the procedure, and warn the patient that the test will cause some discomfort. Make sure the patient or a responsible family member has signed an appropriate consent form. Because this procedure requires the use of a contrast agent and a general, local, or spinal anesthetic, check the patient's history for hypersensitivity to anesthetics, contrast media, or iodine-containing foods, such as shellfish. Just before the biopsy procedure, the patient may receive a sedative.

After a sedative and an anesthetic have been administered, the patient is placed in the lithotomy position. Using a cystoscope, the doctor passes a guide wire up the ureter and then advances a urethral catheter over the guide wire. Contrast medium is instilled through the catheter, which is positioned next to the lesion under fluoroscopic guidance. The contrast medium is washed out with normal saline solution to prevent cell distortions caused by the dye. A nylon or steel brush is passed through the catheter and the lesion is brushed. This procedure is repeated at least six times, using a new brush each time.

As each brush is removed from the catheter, a smear is made for Papanicolaou staining and the brush tip is cut off and placed in formalin for 1 hour. The biopsy specimen is then removed from the brush tip for histologic examination. When the last brush is withdrawn, the catheter is irrigated with normal saline solution to remove additional cells. These cells are also sent for histologic examination.

Findings   Biopsy results are reported as malignant or benign.

Implications of
results

Results of the urinary tract brush biopsy differentiate malignant from benign lesions, which may have appeared similar on X-rays.

Post-test care

• Because brush biopsy may cause such complications as perforation, sepsis, hemorrhage, or contrast medium extravasation, careful observation of the patient is required after this test. The time, color, and amount of voiding must be recorded, and the patient must be watched for signs of hematuria and abdominal or flank pain.

- The patient may require administration of analgesics and antibiotics.

Interfering factors

None

Urine concentration

The kidneys normally concentrate or dilute urine according to fluid intake. When intake is excessive, the kidneys excrete more water in the urine; when intake is limited, they excrete less. To make such variation possible, the distal segment of the renal tubules adjusts its permeability to water in response to the antidiuretic hormone (ADH), which, with renal blood flow, determines urine concentration or dilution.

This test measures specific gravity or osmolality; it evaluates renal capacity to concentrate urine in response to fluid deprivation or to dilute urine in response to fluid overload (see *Dehydration test for diabetes insipidus* for a related test). Specific gravity, the ratio of urine mass to an equal volume of water, is high in small volumes of output (concentrated urine) and low in large volumes (dilute urine). Osmolality, a more sensitive index of renal function, measures the number of osmotically active ions or particles present per kilogram of water. Osmolality is high in concentrated urine and low in dilute urine. Specific gravity is measured by a urinometer or urine refractometer; osmolality, by the effect of solute particles on the freezing point of a fluid.

Dilution tests, measuring the ability of the kidney to handle a large (1.0 or 1.5 L) waterload, contribute little to diagnosis and are potentially hazardous. They are no longer performed.

Purpose

- To evaluate renal tubular function
- To detect renal impairment

Patient preparation

Explain the purpose of this test, that the test requires several urine specimens, and how many specimens will be collected and when. Instruct the patient to discard any urine voided during the night.

Withhold diuretics, as appropriate.

The patient should eat a high-protein meal and drink only 200 ml of fluid the night before the test. Then, instruct the patient to restrict food and fluids for at least 14 hours. (Some concentration tests re-

Dehydration test for diabetes insipidus

The dehydration test measures urine osmolality, which reflects renal concentrating capacity after a period of dehydration and after subcutaneous injection of the pituitary hormone vasopressin. Comparison of the two osmolality values permits reliable diagnosis of diabetes insipidus, a metabolic disorder characterized by vasopressin (antidiuretic hormone) deficiency. Simply measuring urine osmolality after a period of water deprivation doesn't itself confirm vasopressin deficiency; however, subsequent injection of vasopressin raises urine osmolality beyond normal limits only in patients with diabetes insipidus.

To achieve dehydration, withhold fluids the evening before and the morning of the test. Collect a urine specimen at hourly intervals in the morning for osmolality measurement. At noon, or after osmolality increases less than 30 mOsm/kg each hour for 3 consecutive hours, draw a blood sample for osmolality measurement. If serum osmolality exceeds 288 mOsm/kg, the level of adequate dehydration, inject 5 units of vasopressin subcutaneously. Within an hour, collect a urine specimen for osmolality measurement.

➤ *Clinical alert*: During dehydration, weigh the patient and monitor vital signs every 2 hours; a 2-lb (1-kg) weight loss normally accompanies adequate dehydration. In a patient with polyuria exceeding 10 liters/day, withhold fluids only during the morning of the test; if his weight loss exceeds 4 lb (2 kg), discontinue the test.

In a patient with normal neurohypophyseal function, urine osmolality after vasopressin injection doesn't rise more than 9% of the maximum dehydration osmolality. A larger increase indicates diabetes insipidus. In a patient with polyuria caused by renal disease, potassium depletion, or nephrogenic diabetes insipidus, urine osmolality increases slightly during dehydration but not at all after vasopressin injection.

quire that water be withheld for 24 hours but permit relatively normal food intake.) The patient must limit salt intake at the evening meal to prevent excessive thirst. Emphasize to the patient that adherence to these restrictions is necessary to obtain accurate results.

Procedure   Collect urine specimens at 6 a.m., 8 a.m., and 10 a.m.

The patient who is unable to urinate into the specimen containers should have a clean bedpan, urinal, or toilet specimen pan. The collection device must be rinsed after each use. If the patient is catheterized, the drainage bag should be emptied before the test. The specimens are then collected from the catheter, and the catheter is clamped between collections.

Precautions Concentration tests should be used cautiously in patients with polyuria because hypovolemic circulatory collapse can occur.

Values Specific gravity ranges from 1.025 to 1.032 and osmolality rises above 800 mOsm/kg of water in patients with normal renal function.

Implications of results Decreased renal capacity to concentrate urine in response to fluid deprivation may indicate tubular epithelial damage, decreased renal blood flow, loss of functional nephrons, or pituitary or cardiac dysfunction.

Post-test care
• After the final specimen is collected, the patient should have a balanced meal or a snack.
• Be sure the patient voids within 8 to 10 hours after the catheter is removed.

Interfering factors
• Failure to adhere to dietary and fluid restrictions may interfere with accurate determination of test results.
• Diuretics increase urine volume and dilution, thereby lowering specific gravity; nephrotoxic drugs cause tubular epithelial damage, thereby decreasing renal concentrating ability.
• Patients who have been markedly overhydrated for several days before the test may have depressed concentration values; those who are dehydrated or have electrolyte imbalances may retain fluids, leading to inaccurate results.

Urine culture

Laboratory examination and culture of urine are necessary for evaluation of urinary tract infections (UTIs), most commonly bladder infections. Although urine in the kidneys and bladder is normally sterile, some bacteria are usually present in the urethra. Consequently, urine may contain a variety of organisms. Nevertheless, bacteriuria generally results from prevalence of a single type of bacteria; the presence of more than two distinct bacterial species in a urine specimen strongly suggests contamination during collection. However, a single negative culture doesn't always rule out UTI, as occurs in chronic, low-grade pyelonephritis.

Thus, isolation of known pathogenic bacteria doesn't necessarily confirm UTI because specimens are commonly contaminated by organisms from the urethra and external genitalia. To distinguish between true bacteriuria and contamination, it is necessary to know the number of organisms in a milliliter of urine, estimated by a culture technique called a colony count. Additionally, the presence of pyuria may signal renal disease. Clean-voided midstream collection is considered the method of choice.

Purpose To diagnose UTI

Patient preparation Explain that this test helps detect UTI, that the test requires a urine specimen and that no restriction of food or fluids is necessary. Provide instruction on how to collect a clean-catch midstream specimen; emphasize that external genitalia must be cleaned thoroughly. Or, if appropriate, explain catheterization or suprapubic aspiration and inform the patient that he may experience discomfort during specimen collection. Tell the patient with suspected tuberculosis that specimen collection may be necessary on three consecutive mornings.

Check the patient's medication history for current antibiotic therapy.

Equipment Sterile specimen cup, towelettes, or sterile water, cleaning solution (such as aqueous green soap), and cotton balls or sterile gauze sponges (commercial clean-catch urine kits are available; many include instructions in several languages)

Procedure Collect a urine specimen. Collect at least 3 ml of urine, but don't fill the specimen cup more than halfway. Seal the cup with a sterile lid, and send the specimen to the laboratory immediately. If transport is delayed longer than 30 minutes, store the specimen at $39.2°F$ ($4°C$) or place it on ice.

Record the suspected diagnosis, the collection time and method, current antibiotic therapy, and fluid- or drug-induced diuresis on the laboratory slip.

Findings   Culture results of sterile urine are normally reported as "no growth." Usually, this finding indicates the absence of UTI.

Implications of results

Bacterial counts of 100,000 or more organisms/ml (1×10^8/L) of a single microbial species indicate probable UTI. Counts under 100,000/ml (1×10^8/L) may be significant, depending on the patient's age, sex, history, and other individual factors. However, counts under 10,000/ml (1×10^7/L) usually suggest that the organisms are contaminants, except in symptomatic patients, those with urologic disorders, or those whose urine specimens were collected by suprapubic aspiration. A special test for acid-fast bacteria isolates *Mycobacterium tuberculosis,* which indicates tuberculosis of the urinary tract.

Isolation of more than two species of organisms, or of vaginal or skin organisms, usually suggests contamination and requires a repeat culture. However, polymicrobial infection may occur after prolonged catheterization or urinary diversion, such as an ileal conduit.

Post-test care   None

Interfering factors

- Improper collection technique may contaminate the specimen.
- Fluid- or drug-induced diuresis and antibiotic therapy may lower bacterial counts.
- Failure to refrigerate the specimen or to send it to the laboratory immediately may lead to inaccurate colony counts.

Urine cytology

Epithelial cells line the urinary tract and exfoliate easily into the urine. Consequently, a simple cytologic examination of these cells can aid diagnosis of urinary tract disease. Although urine cytology is not done routinely, it's particularly useful for detecting cancer and inflammatory diseases of the renal pelvis, ureters, bladder, and urethra. In fact, it's especially useful for detecting bladder cancer in high-risk groups, such as smokers, people who work with aniline dyes, and patients who have received treatment for bladder cancer. Urine cytology can also detect cytomegalovirus (CMV) infection and other viral diseases, and it can determine whether bladder lesions that appear on X-rays are benign or malignant.

Purpose
- To aid diagnosis of cancer and inflammatory diseases of the ureters, urethra, bladder, and renal pelvis
- To detect bladder cancer in high-risk groups
- To detect cytomegalic inclusion disease and other viral diseases

Patient preparation

Explain the purpose of this test, that the test requires a urine specimen, and teach the patient the correct method for collecting the specimen.

Procedure

To perform the test, the patient must collect a 100- to 300-ml clean-catch urine specimen 3 hours after the last voiding (not the first-voided specimen of the morning). The urine specimen is sent to the cytology laboratory immediately so that it can be examined before the cells begin to degenerate.

The specimen is prepared in one of three ways and stained with Papanicolaou's stain—

Centrifuge: After the urine is spun down, the sediment is smeared on a glass slide and stained for examination.

Filter: Urine is poured through a filter that traps the cells so that they can be stained and examined directly.

Cytocentrifuge: After the urine is centrifuged, the sediment is resuspended and placed on slides, which are spun in a cytocentrifuge and stained for examination.

Findings and implications of results

Normal urine is relatively free of cellular debris but should have some epithelial and squamous cells that appear normal under a microscope. Identification of malignant cells or any other signs of malignant disease may indicate cancer of the kidney, renal pelvis, ureters, bladder, or urethra. It could also indicate a metastatic tumor. An overgrowth of epithelial cells, an excessive number of red blood cells, or the presence of white blood cells or atypical cells may indicate a lower urinary tract inflammation, which can result from prostatic hyperplasia, urinary calculi, bladder diverticula, strictures, or malformations. Large intranuclear inclusions may indicate a CMV infection, which usually affects the renal tubular epithelium. This viral infection typically occurs in cancer patients undergoing chemotherapy and transplant recipients receiving immuno-suppressant drugs. Cytoplasmic inclusion bodies may also indicate measles and may precede its characteristic Koplik's spots.

Post-test care   None

Interfering factor   Delayed transfer to the laboratory may cause deterioration of the cellular elements in the specimen.

Urobilinogen, fecal

Urobilinogen, the end product of bilirubin metabolism, is a brown pigment formed by bacterial enzymes in the small intestine. It's excreted in feces or reabsorbed into portal blood, where it is returned to the liver and reexcreted in bile; a small amount of urobilinogen is also excreted in urine. Because bilirubin metabolism depends on a properly functioning hepatobiliary system and a normal erythrocyte life span, measurement of fecal urobilinogen is a useful indicator of hepatobiliary and hemolytic disorders. However, this test is rarely performed because serum bilirubin and urine urobilinogen can be measured more easily, and because handling potentially hepatitis-contaminated material poses grave risks to nursing and laboratory personnel.

Purpose   To aid diagnosis of hepatobiliary and hemolytic disorders

Patient preparation   Explain the purpose of this test, that restriction of food or fluids is not required, and that the test requires collection of a random stool specimen.

Withhold broad-spectrum antibiotics, sulfonamides, and salicylates for 2 weeks before the test. If these medications must be continued, note this on the laboratory slip.

Procedure   Collect a 48-hour stool specimen into a light-resistant collection container. (Urobilinogen breaks down to urobilin on exposure to light.) Tell the patient not to contaminate the stool specimen with toilet tissue or urine.

Send the specimen to the laboratory immediately. If transport or testing is delayed more than 30 minutes, refrigerate the specimen; if testing is being performed by an outside laboratory, freeze the specimen.

Values Normally, fecal urobilinogen values range from 50 to 300 mg/day (85 to 510 μmol/d).

Implications of results Low levels or absence of urobilinogen in feces indicates obstructed bile flow (the result of intrahepatic disorders such as hepatocellular jaundice caused by cirrhosis or hepatitis); extrahepatic disorders (such as tumor of the head of the pancreas, the ampulla of Vater, or the bile duct); and choledocholithiasis. Low fecal urobilinogen levels are also associated with depressed erythropoiesis, as occurs in aplastic anemia.

Elevated fecal urobilinogen levels are typical in hemolytic jaundice; thalassemia; and hemolytic, sickle cell, and pernicious anemias.

Post-test care The patient may resume medications withheld before the test.

Interfering factors
- Broad-spectrum antibiotics can depress fecal urobilinogen levels by inhibiting bacterial growth in the colon. Sulfonamides, which react with the reagent used in this test, and large doses of salicylates can raise fecal urobilinogen levels.
- Contamination of the specimen or failure to collect it in a light-resistant container prevents accurate testing.

Urobilinogen, urine

This test detects impaired liver function by measuring urine levels of urobilinogen, the colorless, water-soluble compound that results from the reduction of bilirubin by intestinal bacteria. Up to 50% of intestinal urobilinogen returns to the liver, where some of it is resecreted into bile and back into the intestine through the enterohepatic circulation. Small amounts of circulating urobilinogen enter the circulation and are excreted in the urine (urobilinogenuria).

Eliminated in large amounts in the feces (50 to 250 mg/day) and in small amounts in the urine (1 to 4 mg/day), urobilinogen reflects bile pigment metabolism. Consequently, absent or altered urobilinogen levels can indicate hepatic damage or dysfunction. Complete bile duct obstruction results in a complete lack of urobilinogen in the urine and feces. Urine urobilinogen can also indicate hemolysis of red blood cells, which increases bilirubin production and causes increased production and excretion of urobilinogen. Quantitative analysis of urine urobilinogen involves the addition of Ehrlich's reagent to a 2-hour urine specimen. The resulting color reaction is read promptly by spectrophotometry. (See also *Random specimen for urobilinogen*.)

Purpose
- To aid diagnosis of extrahepatic obstruction, such as blockage of the common bile duct
- To aid differential diagnosis of hepatic and hematologic disorders

Patient preparation
Explain the purpose of this test and that the test does not require restriction of fluids or food. Tell the patient that the test requires a 2-hour urine specimen, and teach the proper collection method.

Check the patient's medication history for drugs that may affect urine urobilinogen levels. Review your findings with the laboratory and restrict such drugs before the test, as appropriate.

Procedure
Most laboratories request a random urine specimen; others prefer a 2-hour specimen, usually collected in the afternoon, preferably between 1 p.m. and 3 p.m. when urobilinogen levels peak.

Send the specimen to the laboratory immediately. This test must be performed within 30 minutes of collection because urobilinogen quickly oxidizes to an orange compound called urobilin.

Values
Normally, urine urobilinogen values in females range from 0.1 to 1.1 Ehrlich units/2 hours; in males, from 0.3 to 2.1 Ehrlich units/2 hours.

Implications of results
Absence of urine urobilinogen may result from complete obstructive jaundice or treatment with broad-spectrum antibiotics, which destroy the intestinal bacterial flora. Low urine urobilinogen levels may result from congenital enzymatic jaundice (hyperbilirubinemia syndromes) or from treatment with drugs that acidify urine, such as ammonium chloride or ascorbic acid.

Elevated levels may indicate cirrhosis, hemolytic jaundice, or hepatitis.

| **Random specimen for urobilinogen** |

Quantitative tests for urinary urobilinogen excretion can also be done with reagent strips, such as Bili-Labstix or N-Multistix (dip-and-read test).

To perform such tests, collect a clean-catch urine specimen in a clean, dry container — preferably during the afternoon when urine urobilinogen levels peak — and test the specimen immediately. A fresh urine specimen is essential for reliable results because urobilinogen is very unstable when exposed to room temperature and light. Dip the strip into the urine and, while removing it, start timing the reaction. Carefully remove excessive urine by tapping the edge of the strip against the container or a clean, dry surface, to prevent color changes along the edge of the test area. When using N-Multistix or a similar product for multiple testing), hold the strip in a horizontal position to prevent mixing of chemicals from adjacent reagent areas. Place the strip near the color block on the bottle, and carefully compare the colors. Read the results at 45 seconds. The results correspond to Ehrlich units per deciliter (units/dl) of urine.

Normal: yellow-green to yellow = 0.1 to 1 Ehrlich unit/dl

Positive: yellow-orange = 2 Ehrlich units/dl

medium yellow-orange = 4 Ehrlich units/dl

light brown-orange = 8 Ehrlich units/dl

brown-orange = 12 Ehrlich units/dl

Normally, a random specimen contains small amounts of urobilinogen. This test cannot determine the *absence* of urobilinogen in the specimen being tested.

Para-aminosalicylic acid may cause unreliable results with this reagent strip test. Drugs containing azo dyes (phenazopyridine) mask test results by causing a golden color.

Post-test care The patient may resume diet and drugs restricted before the test.

Interfering factors
- The following drugs affect the test reagent and may interfere with determination of urobilinogen levels: para-aminosalicylic acid, phenazopyridine, procaine, methenamine mandelate, phenothiazines, and sulfonamides.
- Highly alkaline urine, which may be caused by acetazolamide or sodium bicarbonate, may elevate urobilinogen levels.

Urogenital secretions, examination for trichomonads

Microscopic examination of urine or vaginal, ure-thral, or prostatic secretions can detect urogenital infection by *Trichomonas vaginalis* — a parasitic, sexually transmitted flagellate protozoan. This test is performed more often on females than on males. Males with trichomoniasis may have symptoms of urethritis or prostatitis.

Purpose To confirm trichomoniasis

Patient preparation Explain to the patient that this test helps to deter-mine the cause of urogenital infection. Tell the fe-male patient that the test requires a specimen of vaginal secretions or urethral discharge. Instruct her not to douche before the test. Tell the male pa-tient the test requires a specimen of urethral or prostatic secretions.

Equipment Cotton-tipped applicator, test tube containing small amount of normal saline solution (or transport me-dia), vaginal speculum, specimen cup (if a urine specimen is required)

Procedure *Vaginal secretions:* With the patient in lithotomy po-sition, an unlubricated vaginal speculum is inserted and discharge is collected with a cotton-tipped ap-plicator. The applicator is then placed in the tube containing normal saline solution or transport me-dia, and the speculum is removed.

Prostatic material: After prostatic massage, ure-thral secretions are collected with a cotton-tipped applicator, and the applicator is placed in normal saline solution.

Urethral discharge: Collect the discharge with a cotton-tipped applicator, and place the applicator in normal saline solution.

Urine: Include the first portion of a voided ran-dom specimen (not the midstream portion).

If possible, obtain the urogenital specimen be-fore treatment with a trichomonacide begins. Label the specimen appropriately, including the date and time of collection. Send the specimen to the labora-tory immediately because trichomonads are not easily identified while still motile.

Findings	Trichomonads are normally absent from the urogenital tract. In approximately 25% of infected females and most infected males, trichomonads may be present without associated pathology.
Implications of results	Presence of trichomonads confirms trichomoniasis.
Post-test care	Provide perineal care, as appropriate.
Interfering factors	• Failure to send the specimen to the laboratory immediately will result in the trichomonads' losing their motility. • Improper collection technique may interfere with detection of trichomonads. • Collection of the specimen after trichomonacide therapy begins decreases the number of parasites in the specimen.

Uroporphyrinogen I synthase

Uroporphyrinogen I synthetase, porphobilinogen deaminase

This test measures blood levels of uroporphyrinogen I synthase, an enzyme that converts porphobilogen to uroporphyrinogen during heme biosynthesis. Uroporphyrinogen I synthase is normally present in erythrocytes, fibroblasts, lymphocytes, liver cells, and amniotic fluid cells. However, a hereditary deficiency can reduce uroporphyrinogen I synthase levels by 50% or more, resulting in acute intermittent porphyria (AIP). An autosomal-dominant disorder of heme biosynthesis, AIP remains latent until certain factors (some sex hormones and drugs, a low-carbohydrate diet, or an infection) can activate it.

Traditional urine tests can also detect AIP during an acute episode. But the test for uroporphyrinogen I synthase can detect AIP even during its latent phase. Thus, it can identify affected individuals before their first acute episode. Moreover, its specificity for AIP can differentiate AIP from other porphyrias.

Enzyme activity is determined by measuring the conversion rate of porphobilinogen to uroporphyrinogen by fluorometry. If levels are indeterminate, urine and stool tests for aminolevulinic acid (ALA) and porphobilinogen may be ordered because excretion of those porphyrin precursors increases substantially during an acute episode of AIP and may increase slightly during the latent phase.

Purpose
: To aid diagnosis of AIP

Patient preparation
: Explain the purpose of this test, that the test requires fasting for 12 to 14 hours before the test but does not limit water, and that the test requires a blood sample.

  If the patient's hematocrit values are available, record them on the laboratory slip. As appropriate, withhold any medications that may decrease enzyme levels. If they must be continued, note this on the laboratory slip.

Procedure
: Perform a venipuncture and collect the sample in a 10-ml *green-top* tube. Handle the sample gently to prevent hemolysis, and send it to the laboratory promptly. Do not freeze the sample.

Values
: Normal values for uroporphyrinogen I synthase are 8.1 to 16.8 nmol/second/liter for females and 7.9 to 14.7 nmol/second/liter for males.

Implications of results
: Decreased levels generally indicate latent or active AIP; symptoms differentiate these phases. Levels below 6.0 and 8.0 nmol/second/liter are indeterminate. Indeterminate results may require urine and stool tests for porphyrin precursors ALA and porphobilinogen to support the diagnosis.

Post-test care
:
- If a hematoma develops at the venipuncture site, applying warm soaks eases discomfort.
- The patient may resume diet and medications restricted before the test.
- If the patient has AIP, nutritional and genetic counseling are recommended. Teach the patient to avoid a low-carbohydrate diet, alcohol, and such drugs as estrogens, steroid hormones, barbiturates, sulfonamides, phenytoin, griseofulvin, and others that may precipitate an acute episode. Emphasize the need to seek care for all infections promptly because they may also precipitate an acute episode.

Interfering
factors

- Hemolytic and hepatic diseases may elevate levels of uroporphyrinogen I synthase.
- Hemolysis caused by excessive agitation of the sample may cause inaccurate results.
- Freezing the sample will invalidate the test.
- The patient's failure to fast before the test may increase enzyme levels.
- A low-carbohydrate diet, alcohol, infection, and certain drugs may increase enzyme levels.

V

Valproic acid, serum

Valproic acid is an antiseizure drug used to treat absence (petit mal) seizures and, secondarily, generalized tonic-clonic and myoclonic seizures, partial epilepsies, and febrile seizures. Valproic acid appears to exert its pharmacologic activity by potentiating gamma-aminobutyric acid pathways in the central nervous system. Valproic acid is measured by the enzyme-multiplied immunoassay technique.

Purpose
- To determine if drug dosage is appropriate for optimizing therapeutic efficacy while minimizing adverse effects.
- To assess patient compliance, particularly in patients who show a poor therapeutic response
- To assess suspected toxicity

Patient preparation
Explain the purpose of this test, that the test requires a blood sample, and that the patient need not restrict food or fluids. Peak serum concentrations occur within 1 to 4 hours; for consistency, monitor trough concentrations and collect the sample within one hour prior to the next dose, if possible.

Procedure
Perform a venipuncture, and collect a 0.5-ml (or more) sample in a *red-top* tube.

Values
The therapeutic range for valproic acid ranges from 50 to 100 µg/ml. Concentrations of 120 µg/ml or greater are usually considered toxic.

Implication of results
Approximately 2 to 4 days are required to achieve a steady-state serum concentration. Likewise, any change in the total daily dose will require 2 to 4 days to establish a new steady state. Most patients show a favorable response when serum concentrations are maintained in the therapeutic range. Doses that elevate serum concentrations above 100 µg/ml usually do not provide additional therapeutic benefits and may increase the frequency of adverse effects.

Post-test care   If a hematoma develops at the venipuncture site, applying warm soaks eases discomfort.

Interfering factor   Coadministered anticonvulsants that induce hepatic microsomal enzymes (for example, carbamazepine, phenytoin, phenobarbital, primidone) will increase the clearance of valproic acid and reduce its serum concentration; a compensatory increase in dosage may be required to maintain a therapeutic serum concentration.

Vanillylmandelic acid (VMA), urine

Using spectrophotofluorometry, this test determines urine levels of vanillylmandelic acid (VMA), the catecholamine metabolite that is normally most prevalent in the urine. VMA is the product of hepatic conversion of epinephrine and norepinephrine, and its levels in urine reflect endogenous production of these major catecholamines. This test helps detect catecholamine-secreting tumors — primarily pheochromocytoma — and helps evaluate the function of the adrenal medulla, the primary site of catecholamine production. This test is performed preferably on a 24-hour urine specimen (not a random specimen) to overcome the effects of diurnal variations in catecholamine secretion. Other catecholamine metabolites — metanephrine, normetanephrine, and homovanillic acid (HVA) — may be measured at the same time.

Purpose   • To help detect pheochromocytoma, neuroblastoma, and ganglioneuroma
   • To evaluate adrenal medullary function

Patient preparation   Explain the purpose of this test. Tell the patient to restrict foods and beverages containing phenolic acid, such as coffee, tea, bananas, citrus fruits, chocolate, and vanilla, for 3 days before the test and to avoid stressful situations and excessive physical activity during the urine collection period. Tell the patient that the test requires collection of a 24-hour urine specimen, and teach the proper collection technique.

   Check the patient's medication history for drugs that may affect test results. Review your findings with the laboratory and withhold these drugs before the test, as appropriate.

Procedure
Collect a 24-hour urine specimen in a bottle containing a preservative, to keep the specimen at a pH of 3.0.

Refrigerate the specimen or keep it on ice during the collection period. When the collection is completed, send the specimen to the laboratory immediately.

Values
Normally, urine VMA values range from 0.7 to 6.8 mg/day (3 to 35 μmol/day).

Implications of results
Elevated urine VMA levels occur in pheochromocytoma. Slight-to-moderate elevations occur in neuroblastomas and ganglioneuromas. Elevated catecholamine levels occur in pheochromocytoma, progressive muscular dystrophy, myasthenia gravis, neuroblastomas, and ganglioneuromas.

Further testing, such as measurement of urine HVA levels to rule out pheochromocytoma, is necessary for precise diagnosis (see *Urine determinations in diagnosis of catecholamine-secreting tumors*). When pheochromocytoma is confirmed, the patient may be tested for multiple endocrine neoplasia, an inherited condition commonly associated with pheochromocytoma. (Family members of a patient with confirmed pheochromocytoma should be carefully evaluated for multiple endocrine neoplasia as well.)

Post-test care
The patient may resume medications, normal diet, and activity restricted before the test.

Interfering factors
• Epinephrine, norepinephrine, lithium carbonate, and methocarbamol may raise urine VMA levels. Chlorpromazine, guanethidine, reserpine, monoamine oxidase inhibitors, and clonidine may lower VMA levels. Levodopa and salicylates may raise or lower VMA levels.

• Failure to observe drug and dietary restrictions, to collect all urine during the test period, or to store the specimen properly may interfere with test results.

• Excessive physical exercise or emotional stress may raise VMA levels.

<hr>

Urine determinations in diagnosis of catecholamine-secreting tumors

Although a pheochromocytoma is a catecholamine-producing tumor, causing hypersecretion of epinephrine and norepinephrine by the adrenal medulla, it does not cause hypertension or elevate levels of urine catecholamines in every patient. Thus, an analysis of one or more catecholamine metabolites offers diagnostic support to an analysis of total catecholamines.

When urine levels of catecholamines remain normal in the presence of hypertension, an elevated vanillylmandelic acid (VMA) level may signal a tumor. Or the metanephrine level may be high, while VMA and catecholamines levels remain essentially unchanged. A VMA assay is also an alternative method when catecholamine analysis has been compromised by interfering food or drugs. Elevated excretion of homovanillic acid (HVA) typically indicates a malignant pheochromocytoma, although the incidence of malignancy is extremely low.

Measurement of urine VMA levels is useful in diagnosing two neurogenic tumors: neuroblastoma, a common soft-tissue tumor that's a leading cause of death in infants and young children; and ganglioneuroma, a well-defined tumor of the sympathetic nervous system that occurs in older children and young adults. Both tumors primarily produce dopamine and cause the expected high readings of the dopamine metabolite HVA, especially when they are malignant tumors. However, both types of tumors also cause abnormal increases in urine VMA levels.

<hr>

Venereal Disease Research Laboratory (VDRL) test

The Venereal Disease Research Laboratory (VDRL) test is widely used to screen for primary and secondary syphilis (see *Rapid plasma reagin [RPR] card test,* page 652, an alternative screening test). This flocculation test demonstrates the presence of reagin — an antibody relatively specific for *Treponema pallidum,* the spirochete that causes syphilis — in a serum sample, after addition of an antigen consisting of cardiolipin and lecithin (two specific and reactive substances) and cholesterol. After the antigen complex is mixed with the serum on a slide, the sample is rotated and examined microscopically. If flocculation occurs, the sample is diluted until it no longer appears. The last dilution to show visible flocculation is reported as the titer of the antibody.

Rapid plasma reagin (RPR) card test

This rapid, macroscopic serologic test is an acceptable substitute for the Venereal Disease Research Laboratory (VDRL) test in diagnosis of syphilis. The rapid plasmin reagin (RPR) card test, available as a kit, uses a cardiolipin antigen to detect reagin, the antibody relatively specific to the causative agent of syphilis. In the RPR test, the patient's serum is mixed with cardiolipin on a plastic-coated card that is rotated mechanically and examined with the unaided eye. If flocculation occurs, the test sample is diluted until no visible reaction occurs. The last dilution to show visible flocculation is the titer of the reagin antibody.

In the RPR test, as in the VDRL test, normal serum shows no flocculation.

Although the test has diagnostic significance during the first two stages of syphilis, transient or permanent biological false-positive reactions can make accurate interpretation difficult. A biological false-positive reaction can result from viral or bacterial infection, an immune complex disease such as systemic lupus erythematosus (SLE), chronic systemic illness, or nonsyphilitic treponemal disease. In advanced syphilis, the VDRL test may be negative in more than a third of infected persons.

A serum sample is used in the VDRL test, but this test may also be performed on a specimen of cerebrospinal fluid (CSF), obtained by lumbar puncture, to test for tertiary syphilis. However, the VDRL test of CSF is less sensitive than the fluorescent treponemal antibody absorption test.

Purpose	• To screen for primary and secondary syphilis • To confirm primary or secondary syphilis in the presence of syphilitic lesions • To monitor response to treatment
Patient preparation	Explain the purpose of this test. Inform the patient that the test requires a blood sample and that restriction of food, fluids, or medication is not required. The patient should, however, abstain from alcohol for 24 hours before the test.
Procedure	Perform a venipuncture, and collect the sample in a 7-ml *red-top* tube. Handle the sample carefully to prevent hemolysis.

Findings	Normal serum shows no flocculation and is reported as a nonreactive test.
Implications of results	Definite flocculation is reported as a reactive test; slight flocculation is reported as a weakly reactive test. A reactive VDRL test occurs in about 50% of patients with primary syphilis and in nearly all patients with secondary syphilis. In a patient with syphilitic lesions, a reactive VDRL test is diagnostic. In a patient without evident lesions, a reactive VDRL test necessitates repeated testing. However, biological false-positive reactions can result from conditions unrelated to syphilis, for example, infectious mononucleosis, malaria, Hansen's disease, hepatitis, SLE, rheumatoid arthritis, and nonsyphilitic treponomal diseases, such as pinta or yaws. (See *Sensitivity of syphilis tests,* page 654.)

A nonreactive VDRL test doesn't rule out syphilis because *T. pallidum* causes no detectable immunologic changes in the serum for 14 to 21 days after infection. However, dark-field microscopic examination of exudate from suspicious lesions can aid early diagnosis by identifying the causative spirochetes.

A reactive VDRL test result on a CSF specimen indicates neurosyphilis, which can follow the primary and secondary stages in untreated persons.

Post-test care	• If a hematoma develops at the venipuncture site, applying warm soaks eases discomfort. • If the test is nonreactive or borderline but syphilis hasn't been ruled out, instruct the patient to return for follow-up testing. Explain that borderline test results don't necessarily mean the patient is free from the disease. • If the test is reactive, explain the importance of proper treatment. Provide further information about venereal disease and how it is spread, and emphasize the need for antibiotic therapy. Patients with syphilis may also be infected with other sexually transmitted diseases; be prepared to test the patient. Prepare the patient to expect mandatory inquiries from public health authorities. If the test is reactive but the patient shows no clinical signs of syphilis, explain that many uninfected persons show false-positive reactions. However, emphasize the need for further specific tests to rule out syphilis.

Sensitivity of syphilis tests

The fluorescent treponemal antibody absorption (FTA-ABS) test — which uses a strain of the *Treponema pallidum* antigen itself as a reagent — is more sensitive than the Venereal Disease Research Laboratory (VDRL) test or the rapid plasma reagin (RPR) card test in detecting all stages of untreated syphilis, but its complex testing method and incidence of false-positive results make it an impractical screening tool. The VDRL and RPR tests are preferred for wide-scale screening and also when primary and secondary syphilis are suspected. In advanced syphilis, when the VDRL test may be negative for more than one-third of infected persons, the FTA-ABS test is preferred for sensitivity and is also the most reliable confirmation of a positive VDRL.

The VDRL test can be used to monitor response to treatment for syphilis. Untreated syphilis produces antibody titers that are low in the primary stage (less than 1:32), elevated in the secondary stage (greater than 1:32), and variable in the tertiary stage. Successful therapy markedly reduces titers, with two-thirds of patients reverting to a nonreactive VDRL result, especially during the first two stages of disease. Third-stage therapy seldom produces a nonreactive VDRL, but maintenance of low-reactive values during the 6- to 12-month period after therapy indicates success. A subsequent rise in antibody titers signals reinfection. By comparison, the FTA-ABS test results usually remain positive after treatment.

A significant number of patients with infectious diseases show temporary false-positive VDRL test results. Chronic false-positive VDRL and FTA-ABS test readings are associated with immune complex diseases, such as systemic lupus erythematosus.

Interfering factors

- Ingestion of alcohol within 24 hours of the test can produce transient, nonreactive results.
- Abnormalities of immune function can cause nonreactive results.
- The presence of SLE can cause a false-positive VDRL test result.
- Presence of anticardiolipin antibodies can interfere with accurate test results.
- Hemolysis of the sample can interfere with accurate test results.

Virus culture

Many viruses replicate in cell cultures and can be identified according to their characteristic cytopathic effect (CPE). Usually, each of three tubes or microtiter plates containing monolayers of diploid fibroblast, primary monkey kidney, and epithelial cells are inoculated. Collectively, the function of these cells is analogous to the differential media: each cell type has an optimal susceptibility and produces a distinct CPE for each individual or group of viruses. For example, members of the herpesvirus group (cytomegalovirus [CMV], varicella-zoster virus [VZV], and herpes simplex virus [HSV]) replicate most rapidly and exclusively in diploid fibroblast cells; orthomyxoviruses and paramyxoviruses replicate only in primary monkey kidney cells; replication of enteroviruses (echovirus, coxsackievirus, poliovirus) requires all three cell types. Cell cultures are examined by light microscopy, usually on a daily basis for evidence of CPEs. Laboratory diagnosis of a viral infection by this method requires 1 to 2 days for some HSV or enterovirus strains; CMV produces CPEs after an average of 9 days.

Purpose   To aid diagnosis of viral infections

Patient preparation   Explain the purpose of this test, and describe the procedure for collecting the specimen for culture.

Procedure   Specimens should be collected during the prodromal and acute stages of clinical infection to ensure the best chance of recovering a virus in cell cultures.

Collect a specimen for culture into the appropriate collection device as listed below —

Throat, skin, rectum, eye, or genital area: viral transport swab or media

Feces, urine, or cerebrospinal fluid (CSF): sterile screw-capped tube or vial

Sputum, bronchoalveolar lavage tissue, or bronchial washings: sterile screw-capped jar

Blood: sterile tube with anticoagulant (preferably with EDTA).

Precautions   Specimens should be transported to the laboratory as soon as possible after collection. If the anticipated time between collection and inoculation into cell cultures is more than 1 to 2 hours, the specimen should be transported at 39.2° F (4° C). Do not freeze the specimen or allow it to become dry.

Findings
: Normally, viruses are not detected by routine cell cultures used for diagnostic virology. Recovery of a virus by culture frequently indicates the etiology of infection, especially if the virus was recovered from a specimen of blood or CSF.

Implications of results
: Because viruses can infect many target organs, interpretation of results regarding etiology requires consideration of clinical presentation and other laboratory results.

Post-test care
: None

Interfering factor
: Administration of antiviral drugs before collection of the specimen may prevent recovery of virus.

Vitamin A, serum

Retinol

Blood levels of vitamin A reflect the amount of this vitamin and carotene ingested and absorbed by the intestine. Carotene is converted to vitamin A (retinol) in the intestinal absorptive cells and by hepatocytes. Because the absorption of fat-soluble vitamins is impaired when fat absorption is poor, low carotene and vitamin A levels indicate malabsorption syndrome. The blood level of vitamin A is influenced by recent ingestion of carotene, which exists in yellow or orange vegetables and fruits and in leafy green vegetables.

Vitamin A supports normal vision and prevents night blindness, maintains epithelial cells as barriers to infection, and is necessary for normal growth of bone, teeth, and soft tissues. Vitamin E and thyroxine strengthen vitamin A utilization.

In children, vitamin A deficiency causes skeletal growth impairment, blindness, dysfunction of the intestinal mucosa, xerophthalmos, renal medullary cornification, and increased respiratory tract infections. In adults, the most common effect of vitamin A deficiency is night blindness; more serious effects are rare.

Decreased blood levels of vitamin A are associated with lipid malabsorption, biliary obstruction, low-fat diets, biliary cirrhosis, liver disease, and excessive ingestion of mineral oil.

Purpose
: • To detect hypervitaminosis

- To evaluate xerophthalmia, blindness, keratomalacia, and impaired skeletal growth related to vitamin A deficiency

Patient preparation Explain the purpose of this test and that the test requires a blood sample. Advise the patient to fast for 8 hours before the test and to omit vitamin supplements containing vitamin A for 24 hours before the test. Check the patient's history for use of drugs that may interfere with accurate test results.

Procedure Perform a venipuncture and collect a blood sample into a chilled 15-ml *red-top* tube. Protect the sample from exposure to light, which may influence test results, and handle it gently to prevent hemolysis. Keep the sample on ice, and send it to the laboratory promptly.

Values *Normal concentration of vitamin A:* 30 to 95 mg/dl (1.05 to 3.32 mmol/L)
Normal concentration of carotene: in infants, 0 to 40 mg/dl (0 to 0.8 mmol/L); in children, 40 to 130 mg/dl (0.8 to 2.4 mmol/L); and in adults, 50 to 200 mg/dl (0.93 to 3.72 mmol/L)

Implications of results Elevated levels of vitamin A are commonly associated with excessive vitamin intake and with pregnancy, use of oral contraceptives, myxedema, nephritis, hyperlipidemia, and hypercholesterolemia. Decreased levels may result from inadequate nutritional intake — because absorption of vitamin A requires the presence of fats and bile — or from conditions that cause lipid malabsorption or biliary obstruction.

Vitamin A intoxication in children can cause tender swelling over the long bones, and hyperostoses; in adults, it can cause calcification of pericapsular, ligamentous, and subperiosteal structures. Large daily doses can induce headache, nausea, anorexia, epistaxis, weakness, and dermatitis.

Post-test care If a hematoma develops at the venipuncture site, applying warm soaks eases discomfort.

Interfering factors
- Failure to observe dietary and drug restrictions before the test may alter test results.
- Incorrect handling of the sample — for example, exposing it to light — causes deterioration.

- Hemolysis caused by excessive agitation of the sample alters test results.
- Decreased levels may result from excessive ingestion of mineral oil, which interferes with the absorption of all fat-soluble vitamins.
- Serum levels of vitamin A do not correspond well to liver stores because of homeostatic control exercised by the liver.
- False-high levels may be associated with pregnancy or use of oral contraceptives and with hyperlipidemia, hypercholesterolemia, diabetes, nephritis, and myxedema.

Vitamin B$_{12}$ absorption
Schilling test

The test for vitamin B$_{12}$ absorption, the Schilling test, measures urinary excretion of vitamin B$_{12}$ (cyanocobalamin) after administration of standard doses of radioactive and nonradioactive vitamin B$_{12}$. The test also differentiates intrinsic factor deficiency from malabsorption syndromes. The first stage of the test detects deficient urinary excretion of vitamin B$_{12}$; the second stage, performed 3 days later with the intrinsic factor added to the vitamin B$_{12}$ doses, confirms the cause.

Hematopoiesis requires the extrinsic factor (vitamin B$_{12}$), which is acquired through diet and is absorbed with the aid of the intrinsic factor, produced by the gastric mucosa. Absence or deficiency of the intrinsic factor disrupts red blood cell formation and leads to pernicious anemia. Dietary deficiency of vitamin B$_{12}$ is rare.

Purpose
- To diagnose Crohn's disease of the terminal ileum
- To diagnose other small-intestine adsorption defects
- To assess vitamin B$_{12}$ absorption to diagnose malabsorption resulting from lack of the intrinsic factor

Patient preparation
Explain that this test evaluates the body's ability to absorb vitamin B$_{12}$. Advise the patient to stop taking B vitamins 3 days before the test. Instruct the patient to fast from midnight before the test. Inform the patient that the test may be performed in two stages; during each stage, an oral dose of medication and an injection are followed by a 24-hour urine

specimen collection. Check the patient's history for exposure to radioactive materials within the preceding 10 days.

Procedure   *First stage (without intrinsic factor):* The patient is instructed to void and then discard the urine. After the patient receives 0.5 mcg of vitamin B$_{12}$ tagged with radioactive cobalt orally, a 24-hour urine collection begins. After 2 hours, 1,000 mcg of nonradioactive vitamin B$_{12}$ is administered I.M. to saturate tissue-binding sites and to permit some excretion of radioactive vitamin B$_{12}$ in the urine.

Second stage (with intrinsic factor): Five days later, the patient voids and discards the urine. The patient receives 0.5 mcg of radioactive vitamin B$_{12}$ orally, followed by 60 mg of the intrinsic factor; then a 24-hour urine collection begins. After 2 hours, 1,000 mcg of nonradioactive vitamin B$_{12}$ is administered I.M. Abnormal results after vitamin B$_{12}$ administration indicates that the problem is not pernicious anemia, but a malfunction of the lower GI tract.

In a patient with elevated blood urea nitrogen levels, collect the urine for 48 hours because impaired renal function may slow excretion of vitamin B$_{12}$. Tell the patient not to contaminate the urine specimen with toilet tissue or stool.

Note: Obtain vitamin B$_{12}$, folate levels, and bone marrow examinations before this test. Refrigerate the specimens or place them on ice during the collection period.

Findings   Normally, 8% to 40% of the original oral dose of radioactive vitamin B$_{12}$ appears in the 24-hour urine specimen, but values vary with the laboratory and procedure used.

Implications of results   Patients who excrete normal amounts of radioactive vitamin B$_{12}$ in the first stage of this test require no further testing. Those who excrete less than 8% of the dose need the second stage of this test to confirm pernicious anemia. After administration of the intrinsic factor with vitamin B$_{12}$, most patients with pernicious anemia excrete normal amounts of radioactive vitamin B$_{12}$; the others excrete normal amounts after I.V. infusion of vitamin B$_{12}$. Poor adsorption of vitamin B$_{12}$ (less than 6%), with or without the intrinsic factor, implies intestinal malabsorption.

Post-test care
- After receiving radioactive vitamin B$_{12}$ I.M., the patient should eat a balanced meal.
- Inform the patient with depressed vitamin B$_{12}$ excretion in the first stage of this test that additional testing is needed and will probably be performed in 3 to 5 days.
- Ensure that the vitamin B$_{12}$ absorption test is completed before other isotope tests are performed.

Interfering factors
- Failure to collect all urine during the test period, to store the specimen properly, or to observe the required fast interferes with accuracy of test results.
- Radioisotope scans before the test will affect test results.
- Fecal contamination of the specimens (feces contains some unabsorbed B$_{12}$) will affect test results.

Vitamin B$_{12}$, serum

Cyanocobalamin, antipernicious anemia factor, extrinsic factor

This radioisotopic assay of competitive binding is a quantitative analysis of serum vitamin B$_{12}$ levels. This test is usually performed concurrently with measurement of serum folic acid levels because deficiencies of vitamin B$_{12}$ and folic acid are the two most common causes of megaloblastic (pernicious) anemia. A water-soluble vitamin containing cobalt, vitamin B$_{12}$ is essential to hematopoiesis, deoxyribonucleic acid synthesis and growth, and myelin synthesis and central nervous system (CNS) integrity. Ingested almost exclusively in animal products, such as meat, shellfish, butter, cheese, milk, and eggs, vitamin B$_{12}$ is absorbed from the ileum, after forming a complex with the intrinsic factor, and is stored in the liver. A clinical vitamin B$_{12}$ deficiency takes years to develop because almost total conservation is provided by a cyclic pathway (enterohepatic circulation) that allows reabsorption of the vitamin B$_{12}$ normally excreted in the bile. Deficiency of the intrinsic factor, however, causes malabsorption of vitamin B$_{12}$ and may result in pernicious anemia.

Purpose	• To aid differential diagnosis of megaloblastic anemia, which may be caused by a deficiency of vitamin B$_{12}$ or folic acid • To aid differential diagnosis of CNS disorders that affect peripheral and spinal myelinated nerves
Patient preparation	Explain that this test, which requires a blood sample, determines the amount of vitamin B$_{12}$ in the blood. Also instruct the patient to observe an overnight fast before the test. Check the patient's history for use of drugs — such as methotrexate, pyrimethamine, triamterene, pentamide, isethionate, trimethoprim, phenytoin, barbiturates, cycloserine, aminosalicylic acid, and oral contraceptives — which interfere with B$_{12}$ absorption.
Procedure	Perform a venipuncture, and collect the sample in a 7-ml *red-top* tube. Handle the sample gently to prevent hemolysis, and send it to the laboratory immediately. Draw the sample before B$_{12}$ therapy or transfusions begin.
Values	Normally, serum vitamin B$_{12}$ values range from 250 to 1,100 pg/ml (150 to 810 pmol/L).
Implications of results	Decreased serum levels of vitamin B$_{12}$ may indicate inadequate dietary intake of the vitamin, especially if the patient is a strict vegetarian. Low levels are also associated with hypochlorhydria, inflammatory bowel disease, bacterial overgrowth in the small intestine, malabsorption syndromes (such as celiac disease), isolated malabsorption of vitamin B$_{12}$, hypermetabolic states (such as hyperthyroidism), pregnancy, and CNS damage (posterolateral sclerosis or funicular degeneration, for example). Elevated levels of serum vitamin B$_{12}$ are associated with chronic granulocytic leukemia, chronic obstructive pulmonary disease, chronic renal failure, severe congestive heart failure, diabetes mellitus, obesity, and liver disease.
Post-test care	If a hematoma develops at the venipuncture site, applying warm soaks eases discomfort.
Interfering factors	• The patient's failure to observe the overnight fast or the administration of substances that decrease absorption of vitamin B$_{12}$ will alter test results.

- Hemolysis caused by excessive agitation of the sample alters test results.
- Resection of the terminal ileum to treat Crohn's disease prevents B_{12} absorption.

Vitamin C, plasma
Ascorbic acid

This chemical assay measures plasma levels of vitamin C, a water-soluble vitamin required for collagen synthesis and cartilage and bone maintenance. Vitamin C also promotes iron absorption, influences folic acid metabolism, and may be necessary for withstanding the stresses of injury and infection.

After vitamin C is absorbed from the small intestine, it's transported by the blood to the kidneys, oxidized to dehydroascorbic acid, and then stored in the adrenal and salivary glands, pancreas, spleen, testes, and brain. The adrenal glands contain high concentrations of vitamin C that may be depleted by corticotropic stimulation of these glands. Severe vitamin C deficiency, or scurvy, causes capillary fragility, joint abnormalities, and multiple systemic symptoms.

Purpose To assess vitamin C deficiency

Patient preparation Explain that this test, which requires a blood sample, detects the amount of vitamin C in the blood. Instruct the patient to observe an overnight fast before the test.

Procedure Perform a venipuncture, and collect the sample in a 15-ml *green-top* (heparinized) tube (*red-, lavender-,* or *gray-top* tubes may also be used). Handle the sample gently to prevent hemolysis, and send it to the laboratory immediately. If transport is delayed, place the sample on ice.

Values Normally, plasma vitamin C values range from 0.6 to 2 mg/dl (34 to 114 µmol/L).

Implications of results Vitamin C levels diminish during pregnancy, reaching their lowest point immediately postpartum. Depressed levels occur in alcoholism, hyperthyroidism, malabsorption, and renal failure. Levels are also lower in smokers than in nonsmokers. A severe deficiency of vitamin C results in scurvy.

High plasma levels of vitamin C can indicate increased ingestion of the vitamin in amounts far exceeding the recommended daily allowances. Excessive vitamin C is converted to oxalate, which is excreted in the urine. Excessive concentration of oxalate can produce urinary calculi.

Post-test care If a hematoma develops at the venipuncture site, applying warm soaks eases discomfort.

Interfering factors
- Failure to follow dietary restrictions or to transport the sample to the laboratory promptly will alter test results.
- Hemolysis caused by excessive agitation of the sample will alter test results.

Vitamin D$_3$, serum
Calcitriol, cholecalciferol

Vitamin D$_3$, the major form of vitamin D, is endogenously produced in the skin by the sun's ultraviolet rays and occurs naturally in fish liver oils, egg yolks, liver, and butter. Like all other fat-soluble vitamins, vitamin D$_3$ is absorbed from the intestine in the presence of bile salts and is stored in the liver. To become active, this vitamin must be converted to 25-hydroxycholecalciferol, its circulating metabolite; and then to 1,25-dihydroxycholecalciferol, a potent compound — often called a hormone — which controls bone mineralization.

The hormonal function of vitamin D$_3$ closely parallels that of the parathyroid hormone (PTH) in maintaining calcium and phosphorus homeostasis. Low serum calcium and phosphorus levels stimulate production of PTH, which then stimulates renal secretion of 1,25-dihydroxycholecalciferol to promote intestinal absorption of calcium and phosphate. Together, the two hormones stimulate renal absorption of calcium and mobilization of calcium from bone.

This test, a competitive protein-binding assay, determines serum levels of 25-hydroxycholecalciferol after chromatography has separated it from other vitamin D metabolites and contaminants. Clinically useful in evaluating nutritional status and biological activity of vitamin D$_3$, this test is commonly combined with measurement of serum calcium and alkaline phosphatase levels.

Purpose
- To assess vitamin D deficiency
- To evaluate skeletal disease, such as rickets and osteomalacia
- To aid diagnosis of hypercalcemia, hypocalcemia, and hypophosphatemia
- To detect vitamin D toxicity
- To monitor therapy with vitamin D₃

Patient preparation
Explain that this test measures vitamin D in the body, that the patient must fast before the test, and that the test requires a blood sample. Check for drugs that alter test results (for example, corticosteroids or anticonvulsants). If they must be continued, note this on the laboratory slip.

Procedure
Perform a venipuncture, and collect the sample in a 7-ml *red-* or *green-top* tube. Handle the sample carefully to prevent hemolysis, and avoid shaking the tube.

Values
The normal range for serum 25-hydroxycholecalciferol is 10 to 60 ng/ml (25 to 150 nmol/L), depending on the diagnostic method used; the patient's diet and clothing (less clothing exposes a patient to greater amounts of ultraviolet light); and the season.

Implications of results
Low or undetectable levels of vitamin D₃ may result from vitamin D deficiency, which can cause rickets or osteomalacia. Such deficiency may stem from a poor diet, decreased exposure to the sun, or impaired absorption of vitamin D (secondary to hepatobiliary disease, pancreatitis, celiac disease, cystic fibrosis, or gastric or small bowel resection). Low levels may also be related to various hepatic diseases that directly affect vitamin D metabolism.

Elevated levels (over 100 ng/ml) may indicate toxicity caused by excessive self-medication or prolonged therapy. Elevated levels associated with hypercalcemia may be caused by hypersensitivity to vitamin D, as occurs in sarcoidosis.

Post-test care
If a hematoma develops at the venipuncture site, applying warm soaks eases discomfort.

Interfering factors
- Hemolysis of the sample interferes with test results.

- Vitamin D values will vary with the amount of sunlight and during a female patient's menstrual cycle, especially at ovulation.

Von Willebrand's factor (VWF), antigen, plasma

Von Willebrand's factor (VWF) is a mixture of small and large VWF polymers. The VWF antigen test measures the immunologic levels of VWF in plasma. Because VWF is composed of different sized multimers, enzyme-linked immunoabsorbent assay or radioimmunoassay testing is preferred over other methods of antigen quantitation.

VWF is important for platelet adhesion and also serves as the carrier molecule for factor VIII. Severe deficiencies of VWF are associated with abnormal platelet adhesion and deficiencies of circulating factor VIII levels. VWF testing is used to investigate abnormalities in factor VIII levels and to diagnose von Willebrand's disease. Measurement of VWF antigen and factor VIII levels can also determine carrier status for hemophilia A (factor VIII deficiency) because carriers often have lower-than-normal factor VIII-VWF antigen levels. Testing for von Willebrand's disease involves measuring the bleeding time, VWF antigen levels, VWF ristocetin cofactor activity, multimer analysis of plasma VWF, and ristocetin-induced platelet aggregation.

Ristocetin cofactor activity is a functional test of VWF, measuring the latter's ability to interact with platelets in the presence of ristocetin. Multimer testing evaluates whether the most potent, high molecular weight forms of VWF are present. No one test is sensitive and specific for von Willebrand's disease: a profile of test results is required to classify the particular type of von Willebrand's disease.

Purpose
- To aid diagnosis and management of platelet function disorders
- To identify patients with von Willebrand's disease

Patient preparation
Explain the purpose of this test and that the test requires a blood sample. Tell the patient that restriction of food or fluids is not required before the test.

Procedure — Perform a venipuncture, and collect a blood sample in an appropriate container as required by the testing laboratory. Submit the patient's coagulation history with the sample.

Findings — Normal plasma content of VWF antigen is 45% to 185%.

Implications of results — Low or abnormal levels of VWF antigen indicate von Willebrand's disease. Ristocetin cofactor activity and VWF multimer levels are needed to classify which form of von Willebrand's disease the patient has.

Post-test care — If a hematoma develops at the site of venipuncture, applying warm soaks eases discomfort.

Interfering factors —
- Hormonal changes associated with stress or pregnancy and an acute phase response to inflammation or infection can elevate the VWF antigen levels.
- In persons with mild von Willebrand's disease, plasma levels may vary, causing results that make diagnosis difficult.
- Individuals with blood group O have lower levels of VWF antigen.

Von Willebrand's factor (VWF), multimers, plasma

The test for von Willebrand's factor (VWF) measures the composition of plasma VWF using electrophoresis. VWF is a mixture of small and large VWF polymers; the largest polymers (multimers) are the most biologically active. (The large multimers move the slowest.) Plasma is separated on agarose gels and transferred to a membrane; then immunoblotting is performed with a VWF antibody. The patient's multimers are compared with those of a normal plasma pool.

Patients lacking high molecular weight multimers of VWF are missing the most potent forms. This test is used to distinguish type 1 von Willebrand's disease (low antigen levels, but normal multimers) from type 2 in which high molecular multimers of VWF are absent. VWF multimer changes are also observed in thrombotic thrombocytopenic purpura and hemolytic-uremic syndrome.

Purpose
- To aid in the diagnosis of von Willebrand's disease

Patient preparation
Explain the purpose of this test, that the test requires a blood sample, and that the patient need not fast before the test.

Procedure
Perform a venipuncture, and collect a blood sample in an appropriate container as required by the testing laboratory. Submit the patient's coagulation history with the sample.

Findings
The patient's VWF multimers are compared with those of a normal plasma pool.

Implications of results
High molecular weight multimers are deficient in types 2A and 2B von Willebrand's disease, but normal in type 1.

Post-test care
If a hematoma develops at the site of venipuncture, applying warm soaks eases discomfort.

Interfering factors
Severe VWF deficiencies can hinder multimer analysis.

Von Willebrand's factor (VWF), ristocetin cofactor activity, plasma

The test for the ristocetin cofactor activity of von Willebrand's factor (VWF) measures the functional levels of VWF in plasma. Ristocetin, an antibiotic, causes VWF to bind to its receptor on platelets, thereby inducing platelet agglutination. Testing is performed using an aggregometer and standard, fixed platelets. A curve is generated using normal plasma to measure ristocetin cofactor activity in the patient's plasma.

Purpose
- To aid diagnosis of platelet function disorders
- To identify patients with von Willebrand's disease

Patient preparation	Explain the purpose of this test, that the test requires a blood sample, and that the patient need not restrict food or fluids before the test.
Procedure	Perform a venipuncture, and collect a blood sample in an appropriate container as required by the testing laboratory. Submit the patient's coagulation history with the sample.
Findings	Normal plasma levels of VWF ristocetin cofactor activity range from 50 to 200%.
Implications of results	Low levels of ristocetin cofactor activity aid in the diagnosis of von Willebrand's disease. However, antigen levels and multimer analysis are required to classify the type of von Willebrand's disease.
Post-test care	If a hematoma develops at the site of venipuncture, applying warm soaks eases discomfort.
Interfering factors	Platelet aggregation is inhibited by such drugs as aspirin, aspirin compounds, antihistamines, and anti-inflammatory agents.

White blood cell (WBC) count
Leukocyte count

Part of the complete blood count, the white blood cell (WBC) count reports the number of white cells found in a microliter (cubic millimeter) of whole blood by using a hemacytometer or an electronic device, such as a Coulter counter.

On any given day, the WBC count may vary by as much as 2,000/µliter. Such variation can be the result of strenuous exercise, stress, or digestion. The WBC count may rise or fall significantly in certain diseases, but is diagnostically useful only when interpreted in light of the WBC differential and of the patient's current clinical status.

Purpose
- To detect infection or inflammation
- To determine the need for further tests, such as the WBC differential, or bone marrow biopsy
- To monitor response to chemotherapy or radiation therapy

Patient preparation
Explain the purpose of the test, that restriction of food or fluids is not required before the test, that the test requires a blood sample, and that strenuous exercise should be avoided for 24 hours before the test. The patient should also avoid eating a heavy meal before the test.

Inform the patient who is being treated for an infection that this test will be repeated to monitor progress. Review the patient's history for medications that may interfere with accurate determination of test results. Note use of such medications on the laboratory slip.

Procedure
Perform a venipuncture, and collect the sample in a 7-ml *lavender-top* tube. Completely fill the sample collection tube, and invert it gently several times to adequately mix the sample and the anticoagulant.

Values
The WBC count ranges from 4,100 to 10,900/µliter (4.1 to 10.9×10^9/L).

Implications of
results

An elevated WBC count (leukocytosis) usually signals infection, such as an abscess, meningitis, appendicitis, or tonsillitis. A high WBC count may also result from leukemia and tissue necrosis caused by burns, myocardial infarction, or gangrene.

A low WBC count (leukopenia) indicates bone marrow depression that may result from viral infections or from toxic reactions, such as those following treatment with antineoplastics, ingestion of mercury or other heavy metals, or exposure to benzene or arsenicals. Leukopenia characteristically accompanies influenza, typhoid fever, measles, infectious hepatitis, mononucleosis, and rubella. Any unexplained abnormality of the total WBC count requires a WBC differential count to reveal any underlying abnormality.

Post-test care

• If a hematoma develops at the venipuncture site, applying warm soaks eases discomfort.
• The patient may resume normal activity that was restricted before the test.
• Patients with severe leukopenia may have little or no resistance to infection and therefore may require reverse isolation.

Interfering
factors

• Hemolysis caused by excessive agitation of the sample may interfere with accurate determination of test results.
• Exercise, stress, or digestion raises the WBC count, yielding inaccurate results.
• Some drugs, including most antineoplastic agents; anti-infectives, such as metronidazole and flucytosine; anticonvulsants, such as phenytoin derivatives; thyroid hormone antagonists; and nonsteroidal anti-inflammatory drugs, such as indomethacin, lower the WBC count, thereby altering results.

White blood cell (WBC) differential count

Because the white blood cell (WBC) differential count evaluates the distribution and morphology of white cells, it provides more specific information about a patient's immune function than the WBC count. In this test, the laboratory classifies 100 or more white cells in a stained film of peripheral blood according to two major types of leukocytes — granulocytes (neutrophils, eosinophils, and ba-

Reference values: White blood cell differential count

FOR ADULTS

Cells	Relative value	Absolute value
Neutrophils	47.6% to 76.8%	1,950 to 8,400/μliter
Lymphocytes	16.2% to 43%	660 to 4,600/μliter
Monocytes	0.6% to 9.6%	24 to 960/μliter
Eosinophils	0.3% to 7%	12 to 760/μliter
Basophils	0.3% to 2%	12 to 200/μliter

FOR CHILDREN (AGES 6 TO 17)

Cells	Relative value Boys	Girls
Neutrophils	38.5% to 71.5%	41.9% to 76.5%
Lymphocytes	19.4% to 51.4%	16.3% to 46.7%
Monocytes	1.1% to 11.6%	0.9% to 9.9%
Eosinophils	1% to 8.1%	0.8% to 8.3%
Basophils	0.25% to 1.3%	0.3% to 1.4%

sophils) and nongranulocytes (lymphocytes and monocytes) — and determines the percentage of each type. The differential count is the relative number of each type of white cell in the blood. Multiplying the percentage value of each type by the total WBC count provides the absolute number of each type of white cell. Although little is known about the function of eosinophils in the blood, abnormally high levels of these cells are associated with various allergic diseases and reactions to parasites. In such cases, an eosinophil count is sometimes ordered as a follow-up test to the WBC differential count. This test is also appropriate if the differential WBC count shows a depressed eosinophil level.

Purpose
- To evaluate the body's capacity to resist and overcome infection
- To detect and identify various types of leukemia

Interpreting the differential count

To make an accurate diagnosis, the examiner must consider both relative and absolute values of the differential count. Considered alone, relative results may point to one disease, while masking the true pathology that would be revealed by considering the results of the white blood cell (WBC) count. For example, consider a patient whose WBC count is 6,000/µliter, and whose differential count shows 70% lymphocytes and 30% neutrophils. His relative lymphocyte count would seem to be quite high (lymphocytosis); but when this figure is multiplied by the WBC count (6,000 × 70% = 4,200 lymphocytes/µliter), it is well within the normal range.

This patient's neutrophil count, however, is low (30%). When this figure is multiplied by the WBC count (6,000 × 30% = 1,800 neutrophils/µliter), the result is a low absolute number. This low result indicates decreased neutrophil production, which may suggest bone marrow depression.

- To determine the stage and severity of an infection
- To detect allergic reactions
- To assess the severity of allergic reactions (eosinophil count)
- To detect parasitic infections

Patient preparation Explain that this test, which requires a blood sample, helps evaluate immunity and resistance to infection. Inform the patient that restriction of food or fluids is not required but that strenuous exercise should be avoided for 24 hours before the test.

Review the patient's history for use of medications that may interfere with test results.

Procedure Perform a venipuncture, and collect the sample in a 7-ml *lavender-top* tube. Completely fill the collection tube, and invert it gently several times to mix the sample and the anticoagulant adequately. Handle the tube gently to prevent hemolysis.

Values Normal values for the five types of WBCs that are classified in the differential — neutrophils, eosinophils, basophils, lymphocytes, and monocytes — are given for adults and children in *Reference values: White blood cell differential count,* page 671. For an accurate diagnosis, differential test results must always be interpreted in relation to the total WBC count.

Implications of results

Evidence for a wide range of disease states and other conditions is revealed by abnormal differential patterns. (See *Interpreting the differential count.*)

Post-test care

If a hematoma develops at the venipuncture site, applying warm soaks eases discomfort.

Interfering factors

- Hemolysis caused by excessive agitation of the sample may affect test results.
- Failure to use the proper anticoagulant, to completely fill the collection tube, or to mix the sample and anticoagulant adequately may interfere with accurate determination of test results.

Wound culture

A wound culture consists of microscopic analysis of a specimen from a lesion to confirm an infection. Wound cultures may be aerobic (for detection of organisms that usually require oxygen to grow and usually appear in a superficial wound) or anaerobic (for organisms that need little or no oxygen and appear in areas of poor tissue perfusion, such as postoperative wounds, ulcers, or compound fractures). Indications for wound culture include fever and inflammation and drainage in damaged tissue.

Purpose

To identify infectious etiology of wound infection

Patient preparation

Explain that this test identifies infectious microbes and describe the procedure. Tell the patient that a drainage specimen from the wound is withdrawn by a syringe or removed with cotton-tipped applicators.

Equipment

Sterile cotton-tipped applicators and sterile culture tube, or commercial sterile collection and transport system (for aerobic culture); sterile cotton-tipped applicators or sterile 10-ml syringe with 21G needle; special culture tube containing carbon dioxide or nitrogen (for anaerobic culture); sterile gloves; alcohol sponges; sterile gauze and povidone-iodine solution

Procedure   Prepare a sterile field and clean the area around the wound with antiseptic solution.

For aerobic culture, express the wound and remove as much exudate as possible, or insert a cotton-tipped applicator deeply into the wound and gently rotate. Immediately place the applicator in the aerobic culture tube.

For anaerobic culture, insert a cotton-tipped applicator deeply into the wound, gently rotate, and immediately place the applicator in the anaerobic culture tube; or insert the needle into the wound, aspirate 1 to 5 ml of exudate into the syringe, and immediately inject the exudate into the anaerobic culture tube. If the needle is covered with a rubber stopper, the aspirate may be sent to the laboratory in the syringe.

Record on the laboratory slip recent antibiotic therapy, the source of the specimen, and the suspected organism. Label the specimen container appropriately including the wound site and the time of collection.

Precautions
- Clean the area around the wound thoroughly to limit contamination of the culture by normal skin flora, such as diphtheroids, *Staphylococcus epidermidis,* and alpha-hemolytic streptococcus.
- Make sure no antiseptic enters the wound.
- Obtain exudate from the entire wound, using more than one cotton-tipped applicator, as necessary.
- Because some anaerobes die in the presence of even a small amount of oxygen, place the specimen in the culture tube quickly, taking care that no air enters into the tube, and check that double stoppers are secure.
- Keep the specimen container upright, and send it to the laboratory within 15 minutes to prevent growth or deterioration of microbes; or use a transport system with special media.
- Use aseptic technique during the procedure and necessary isolation precautions when sending the specimen to the laboratory.

Findings   Normally, no pathogenic organisms are present in a clean wound.

Implications of results   The most common aerobic pathogens for wound infection include *S. aureus,* Group A beta-hemolytic streptococci, *Escherichia coli* and other Enterobacteriaceae, Group D streptococci including enterococci and *Streptococcus bovis,* and some *Pseudomonas* species; the most common anaerobic pathogens include some *Clostridium* and *Bacteroides* species.

Post-test care Dress the wound, as appropriate.

Interfering factors
- Failure to report recent or current antibiotic therapy may cause erroneous evaluation of bacterial growth.
- Poor collection technique may contaminate or invalidate the specimen; failure to use the proper transport media may cause the specimen to dry up and the bacteria to die.

X-Y-Z

X- and Y-chromatin test
Buccal smears

This test examines stained cells from the buccal mucosa. After exposure to a nuclear stain, many buccal cells from normal females show a 1- to 2-micron chromatin mass at the edge of the nucleus called an X-chromatin or Barr body. Cells of patients with more than two X chromosomes show multiple X-chromatin bodies; cells of patients with only one X chromosome show no X-chromatin bodies. Normal males lack X-chromatin, but usually show Y-chromatin. In most males, part of the Y chromosome fluoresces intensely when stained with quinacrine mustard. This is readily observed as a bright spot in many buccal cells. Both X- and Y-chromatin should be scored with this test regardless of the patient's apparent sex.

Because the results obtained from buccal smears have often been ambiguous and misleading, this test should not be used as a substitute for complete chromosome analysis. The subjective interpretation of X- and Y-chromatin is often erroneous. This test is recommended only in the diagnostic workup for Klinefelter's syndrome. It is sometimes useful in patients with ambiguous genitalia and some sex chromosome syndromes. The test is not recommended for diagnosing Turner's syndrome because nearly 50% of these patients have mosaicism or chromosome structural abnormalities that are not readily identified. Because of these difficulties, some cytogenetic laboratories have discontinued this test and recommend complete chromosome analysis in its place.

Purpose
- To help establish the sex chromosome complement
- To supplement routine chromosome analysis to determine if tissues other than hematopoietic cells might have sex chromosome abnormalities

Patient preparation
Explain that this test requires a painless scraping of surface cells from within the mouth. Because the clinical circumstances for which this test is used

can be particularly sensitive (for example, ambiguous genitalia, intersex syndromes, and mental retardation), and because the results can be complex and ambiguous, the patient usually requires special counseling before and after the test.

Procedure   Because the procedure varies among laboratories, it is important to obtain specific instructions before starting the test and to provide the laboratory with clinical information. This will help the laboratory interpret the results and provide guidance to further cytogenetic testing. Just before collection of the specimen, the patient should rinse his mouth with water to reduce interference from bacteria. Using a sterile metal spatula, scrape any area of the buccal mucosa firmly — but without causing pain or bleeding — to remove surface material and then spread buccal material on the spatula across the surface of a clean microscope slide. The slide is then placed immediately in a Coplin jar containing a fixative solution (methanol and glacial acetic acid, 3:1). Using the same technique, prepare five additional slides, scraping a different area of the mouth each time (for a total of three slides from the left side and three from the right). The slides should be set in a fixative for approximately 1 hour and then allowed to dry at room temperature. Place the microscope slides in an appropriate transport box, and send them at ambient temperature to the laboratory.

Findings   X-chromatin bodies represent the late replicating inactive X chromosome. Thus, patients have one less X-chromatin body than they have X chromosomes. In patients with structurally abnormal X chromosomes, the size of the X-chromatin body may be abnormal, but this is not always apparent. Most laboratories score 200 cells for X-chromatin and 200 cells for Y-chromatin; they process cells from normal controls simultaneously along with the patient's cell specimen for quality control. In normal females, X-chromatin occurs in about $15\% \pm 4\%$ of cells. To avoid overinterpretation from artifacts, accept up to 2% "X-chromatin" values as normal in males, and up to 2% apparent "Y-chromatin" in females. Y-chromatin occurs in about $52\% \pm 14\%$ of cells in most normal males. If any doubt exists about the accuracy of the results, a complete chromosome analysis should be performed.

Implications of results
This test will produce one less X-chromatin body than the number of X chromosomes present in the patient's karyotype. Thus, a person with three X chromosomes would have two X-chromatin bodies in many cells; a person with one X chromosome would have no X-chromatin bodies. In most males, the number of Y-chromatin bodies should reflect the number of Y chromosomes in the karyotype.

Post-test care
The specimen collection for buccal smears is unlikely to have any adverse effects. Problems of post-test care relate mainly to issues surrounding genetic counseling.

Interfering factors
- If the patient's mouth is not properly rinsed before collection of the specimen, bacteria that may stain similar to X- and Y-chromatin could interfere with accurate scoring.
- Outdated reagents, which may contain bacteria, can interfere with the test.
- The strict rules of scoring X-chromatin prevent identifying X-chromatin in all cells in normal females. Similar restrictions for scoring Y-chromatin prevent this test from producing Y-chromatin in all cells of normal males. Thus, the scoring of X-chromatin and Y-chromatin is not perfect. These restrictions, which are necessary for overall test accuracy, prevent the identification of sex chromosome abnormalities in many patients who exhibit mosaicism in the sex chromosomes.
- In about 2% of males, the Y-chromosome band is extremely small. Although this band does not contain clinically significant genes, its apparent absence produces a negative Y-chromatin test.
- In some patients, chromosome bands on one or more of the autosomes can be confused with Y-chromatin in buccal cells. This would produce a false-positive result for Y-chromatin.
- Failure to immerse the microscope slide in fresh fixative can interfere with cell morphology and make identification of X- and Y-chromatin difficult.
- Uneven distribution of the buccal cells over the microscope slide may cause cell clumps or rolling of cells, which can interfere with the test.

Zinc, serum

This test, an analysis by atomic absorption spectroscopy, measures serum levels of zinc, an important trace element. Zinc is found throughout the body but is concentrated primarily in the blood cells, especially in leukocytes. This element is an integral component of more than 80 enzymes and proteins and plays a critical role in enzyme catalytic reactions. For example, zinc is closely linked to the activity of carbonic anhydrase, the enzyme that catalyzes the elimination of carbon dioxide.

Zinc occurs naturally in water and in most foods; high concentrations are found in meat, seafood, dairy products, whole grains, and nuts. Zinc deficiency (hypozincemia) can seriously impair body metabolism, growth, and development. This defect is most apt to develop in patients with certain diseases, such as chronic alcoholism or renal disease, which tend to deplete its body stores. Zinc toxicity is rare but can occur after inhalation of zinc oxide during industrial exposure.

Purpose

To detect zinc deficiency or toxicity

Patient preparation

Inform the patient that this test determines the concentration of zinc in the blood. Inform him he needn't restrict food or fluids before the test and that the test requires a blood sample.

Check the patient's medication history for zinc-chelating agents and other medications that may interfere with the test results.

Procedure

Perform a venipuncture, and collect the sample in a metal-free collection tube. Laboratories provide special kits for this test on request.

Handle the sample gently to prevent hemolysis, and send it to the laboratory immediately. Reliable analysis must begin before platelet disintegration can alter test results.

Values

Normally, serum zinc values range from 66 to 110 µg/dL (10 to 16.8 µmol/L).

Implications of results

Decreased serum zinc levels may indicate an acquired deficiency (caused by insufficient dietary intake or to an underlying disease) or a hereditary deficiency. Markedly depressed serum levels are common in leukemia and may be related to impaired zinc-dependent enzyme systems. Low serum zinc levels are commonly associated with alcoholic cirrhosis of the liver, myocardial infarction, ileitis, chronic renal failure, rheumatoid arthritis, and anemia (such as hemolytic or sickle cell anemia).

Elevated and potentially toxic serum zinc levels may result from accidental ingestion or industrial exposure.

Post-test care   If a hematoma develops at the venipuncture site, applying warm soaks eases discomfort.

Interfering   • Zinc-chelating agents (such as penicillinase) and
factors   corticosteroids decrease serum zinc levels and may interfere with accuracy of test results.
• Hemolysis caused by excessive agitation of the sample, or failure to use a metal-free collection tube or to send the sample to the laboratory immediately will alter test results.

Critical laboratory values

Critical (panic) laboratory values represent severe pathophysiologic states that are life-threatening unless immediate corrective action is taken. The chart below lists critical limits as determined by a national survey of trauma and medical centers in the United States. The chart lists low and high critical limits for tests for clinical chemistry, blood gases and pH, and hematology; it also lists important qualitative results.

Critical values in clinical chemistry

Test	Units	Low	Range	High	Range
Bilirubin	μmol/L	N/A	N/A	257	86 to 513
	mg/dl	N/A	N/A	15	5 to 30
Calcium	mmol/L	1.65	1.25 to 2.15	3.22	2.62 to 3.49
	mg/dl	6.6	5.0 to 8.6	12.9	10.5 to 14.0
Calcium, free	mmol/L	0.78	0.75 to 0.88	1.58	1.50 to 1.63
	mg/dl	3.13	3.01 to 3.53	6.33	6.01 to 6.53
Chloride	mmol/L	75	60 to 90	126	115 to 156
CO_2 content	mmol/L	11	5 to 20	40	35 to 50
Creatinine	μmol/L	N/A	N/A	654	177 to 1,326
	mg/dl	N/A	N/A	7.4	2.0 to 15.0
Glucose	mmol/L	2.6	1.7 to 3.9	26.9	6.1 to 55.5
	mg/dl	46	30 to 70	484	110 to 1,000
Glucose, CSF	mmol/L	2.1	1.1 to 2.8	24.3	13.9 to 38.9
	mg/dl	37	20 to 50	438	250 to 700
Lactate	mmol/L	N/A	N/A	3.4	2.3 to 5.0
	mg/dl	N/A	N/A	30.6	20.7 to 45.0
Magnesium	mmol/L	0.41	0.21 to 0.74	2.02	1.03 to 5.02
	mg/dl	1.0	0.5 to 1.8	4.9	2.5 to 12.2
Osmolality	mmol/kg	250	230 to 280	326	295 to 375
Phosphorus	mmol/L	0.39	0.26 to 0.65	2.87	2.26 to 3.23
	mg/dl	1.2	0.8 to 2.0	8.9	7.0 to 10.0
Potassium	mmol/L	2.8	2.5 to 3.6	6.2 8.0 (Hemo- lyzed)	5.0 to 8.0
Sodium	mmol/L	120	110 to 137	158	145 to 170
Urea nitrogen	mmol/L	N/A	N/A	37.1	14.3 to 107.1
	mg/dl	N/A	N/A	104	40 to 300
Uric acid	μmol/L	N/A	N/A	773	595 to 892
	mg/dl	N/A	N/A	13	10 to 15

(continued)

Critical laboratory values *(continued)*

Critical values in blood gases and pH

Test	Units	Low	Range	High	Range
PCO_2	mm Hg	19	9 to 25	67	50 to 80
	kPa	2.5	1.2 to 3.3	8.9	6.7 to 10.7
pH		7.21	7.00 to 7.35	7.59	7.50 to 7.65
PO_2	mm Hg	43	30 to 55	N/A	N/A
	kPa	5.7	4.0 to 7.3	N/A	N/A
PO_2, newborn	mm Hg	37	30 to 50	92	70 to 100
	kPa	4.9	4.0 to 6.7	12.3	9.3 to 13.3

Critical values in hematology

Fibrinogen	g/liter	0.88	0.5 to 1	7.75	5 to 10
Hematocrit		0.18	0.12 to 0.30	0.61	0.54 to 0.80
Hemoglobin	g/liter	66	40 to 120	199	170 to 300
Partial thromboplastin time	s	N/A	N/A	68	32 to 150
Platelets	$\times 10^9$/L	37	10 to 100	910	555 to 1,000
Prothrombin time	s	N/A	N/A	27	14 to 40
White blood cell count	$\times 10^9$/L	2.0	1.0 to 4.0	37	10.0 to 100.0

Critical qualitative findings

Hematology	• blasts on blood smear • new diagnosis or findings of leukemia • sickle cells (or aplastic crisis)
Microbiology and parasitology	• positive culture or Gram's stain from blood, CSF, or body cavity fluid • positive antigen detection for *Cryptoccocus*, group b streptocci, *Haemophilus influenzae* b, or *Neisseria meningitidis* • positive acid-fast bacillus or culture • *Salmonella*, *Shigella*, or *Campylobacter* on stool culture • malarial parasites
Microscopy and urinalysis	• elevated white blood cell count in CSF • malignant cells, blasts, or microorganisms in CSF or body fluids • positive results for glucose or ketones in urine • pathologic crystals on urinalysis
Blood bank and immunology	• incompatible crossmatch • positive test for syphilis

Source: Kost, Gerald J. "Critical Limits for Urgent Clinician Notification at U. S. Medical Centers," *JAMA* 263(5):704-07, February 2, 1990.

Guide to abbreviations

Abbreviations	Text
<	less than
>	greater than
ABGs	arterial blood gases
ACTH	adrenocorticotropic hormone
ADH	antidiuretic hormone
AFP	alpha-fetoprotein
AHB	alpha hydroxybutyric dehydrogenase
ALT	alanine aminotransferase
ANA	antinuclear antibodies
ASO	antistreptolysin-O
AST	aspartate aminotransferase
BUN	blood urea nitrogen
Ca	calcium
CD	cell dissociation
CEA	carcinoembryonic antigen
Cl	chloride
cm^3	cubic centimeter
CPK	creatine phosphokinase
CRP	C-reactive protein
cu mm (mm^3)	cubic millimeter
dl	deciliter (100 ml)
EBV	Epstein-Barr virus
ELISA	enzyme-linked immunosorbent assay
ESR	erythrocyte sedimentation rate
FSH	follicle-stimulating hormone
FSP	fibrin split products
FTA-ABS	fluorescent treponemal antibody absorption
g	gram
GFR	glomerular filtration rate
GGT	gamma glutamyl transpeptidase
GH	growth hormone
HCG, hCG	human chorionic gonadotropin
HCT, Hct	hematocrit
Hg	hemoglobin
HIV	human immunodeficiency virus
HLA	human leukocyte antigen
IU	international unit
kg	kilogram
L	liter
LAP	leucine aminopeptidase; leukocyte alkaline phosphatase
LD	lactate dehydrogenase
LH	luteinizing hormone

(continued)

Guide to abbreviations *(continued)*

Abbreviations	Text
m^2	square meter
mcg, μg	microgram
mEq	milliequivalent
Mg	magnesium
mg	milligram
MHC	major histocompatibility complex
mIU	milli-international unit
ml, mL	milliliter
mm	millimeter
mM	mmillimole
mm Hg	millimeter of mercury
mmol	millimole
mOsm	milliosmole
mμ	millimicron
mU	milliunit
ng	nanogram
nmol	nanomole
pg	picogram
Pt, Pro time	prothrombin time
PTH	parathyroid hormone
PTT	partial thromboplastin time
RAST	radioallergosorbent test
RF	rheumatoid factor
RPR	rapid plasma reagin test
sec	second
SI	Système Internationale units
SSA	Sjögren's syndrome antigen A
T3	triiodothyronine
T_3RU	triiodothyronine resin uptake
TBG	thyroxine binding globulin
TSH	thyroid-stimulating hormone
TSI	thyroid-stimulating immunoglobulins
μ	micron
U	unit
μg	microgram
μIU	micro-international unit
μliter	microliter
μmol	micromole
μU	microunit
VDRL	Venereal Disease Research Laboratory
WBC	white blood cell

Selected references

Brown, E.A., et al. "Hepatitis C & E: How Much of a Threat?," *Patient Care* 28(9): 105-7, 112, 114-17, May 15, 1994.

Cerda, J.J., et al. "A Revolution in Peptic Ulcer Disease," *Patient Care* 28(9): 18-22, 24-28, 31-32, May 15, 1994.

Chambers, H.F. "Detection of Methicillin-resistant Staphylococci," *Infectious Disease Clinics of North America* 7(2): 425-433, June 1993.

Elias, D. "Understanding Laboratory and Diagnostic Tests," *Nursing RSA Verpleging* 8(9): 41-43, September 1993.

Fischbach, F. *A Manual of Laboratory & Diagnostic Tests*, 4th ed. Philadelphia: J.B. Lippincott Co., 1992.

Gilikison, C.R. "Differential Diagnosis: A Case of Swollen Thyroid...Subacute Thyroiditis," *American Journal of Nursing* 93(12): 16F, 16H-16J, December 1993.

Grady, C., et al. "Laboratory Methods for Diagnosing and Monitoring HIV Infection...ELISA, Western blot, Immunofluorescence," *Journal of Association of Nurses in AIDS Care* 4(2): 11-23, April-June 1993.

Gump, R.S. "How to Detect Diabetic Complications Early," *American Journal of Nursing* 93(11): 16A-B, November 1993.

Higgins, C. "Diabetes Mellitus Test Measures...Biochemistry...Glucose Testing," *Nursing Times* 90(2): 64-66, January 12-18, 1994.

Jacobs, D.S., et al. *Laboratory Test Handbook*, 3rd ed. Baltimore: Williams & Wilkins, 1994.

Martinez, M., et al. "Making Sense of Hypothyroidism: An Approach to Testing and Treatment," *Postgraduate Medicine* 93(6): 135-138, 141-145, 195-197, May 1, 1993.

Mayo Medical Laboratories Test Catalog. Rochester, Minn.: Minservco, Inc., 1994.

Mellico, K.D. "Interpretation of Abnormal Laboratory Values in Older Adults," part 1, *Journal of Gerontological Nursing* 19(1): 39-45, January 1993.

Norris, M.K.G. "Evaluating Serum Triglyceride Levels," *Nursing* 23(5): 31, May 1993.

Peterson, K.J., and Solie, C.J. "Interpreting Lab Values in Chronic Renal Insufficiency," *American Journal of Nursing* 94(5): 56B, 56E, 56H+, May 1994.

Potanovich, L.M. "Lung Cancer Prevention and Detection Update," *Seminars in Oncology* 9(3): 174-179, August 1993.

Proffitt, M.R., and Yen-Lieberman, B. "Laboratory Diagnosis of Human Immunodeficiency Virus Infection," *Infectious Disease Clinics of North America* 7(2): 203-219, June 1993.

Simsir, A., and Burke, D. "Elevation of Cancer Antigen 125 in a Patient with Ascites," *Laboratory Medicine* 25(3): 146-147, March 1994.

Washington, J.A. "Laboratory Diagnosis of Infectious Diseases," *Infectious Disease Clinics of North America* 7(2): xiii-459, June 1993.

Index

t refers to a table

t refers to a table

t refers to a table

t refers to a table